HANDBOOK OF FUNGAL INFECTIONS

Dr. Greeshma Sharma

ALLIED HEALTH PRESS

Handbook of Fungal Infections

Author: **Dr. Greeshma Sharma**

Allied Health Press
4164 Lakeshore Road
Burlington ON L7L 1A4
Canada
www.alliedhealthpress.com
Email: orders@arclereducation.com

ISBN: 978-1-77956-849-6

General Disclaimer:

This book is a summation of information from different sources and encompasses a wide range of medical conditions, the latest therapy methods, principals and techniques that are used in current practice, at the time of publication. This book offers general information with educational purposes, it is not to be applied or relied on for any diagnostic or treatment purposes. Please do not use the data/matter as a substitute for professional diagnosis and treatment. Please consult your healthcare provider or a licensed physician before making any healthcare queries or treatment choices. The medical information and research findings presented in this book are for educational purposes only and should not be used for the treatment of specific individual patients, as individual cases may vary. The author(s), editors(s) and publisher cannot be held accountable and make no guarantees that the information provided in this book will apply to each and individual patient. This book is meant to serve as a basic guideline and other relevant literature sources should be used for more specific information. This text can be a vital resource for students, trainees, and practitioners, covering essential topics. This book encompasses a wide range of medical conditions and the latest therapy options used in current practice. Through the utilization of many different medical studies this book provides the basics of different medical conditions, which can be used as a basic guide from where medical students, trainees and practitioners can extract necessary information. Further, some of the books have graphic images to explain anatomy for medical/educational purposes only. Hence, the book is intended for students or teachers/staff or individuals with a mature outlook looking to learn or enhance their knowledge.

Allied Health Press publishes wide variety of books and eBooks. For more information about Allied Health Press and its products, visit our website at www.alliedhealthpress.com

ABOUT THE AUTHOR

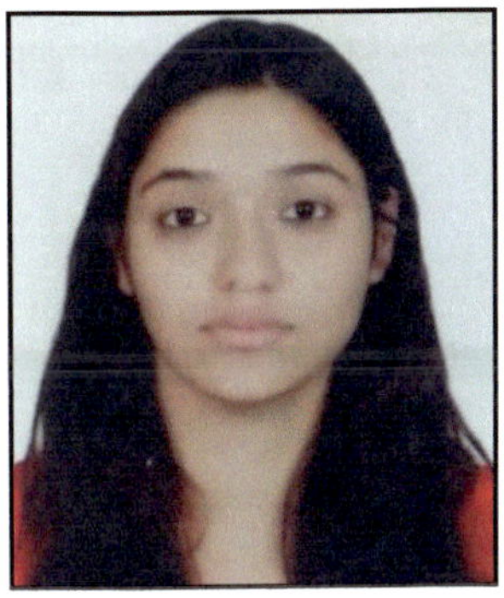

Dr. Greeshma Sharma, holds Ph.D. in Transfusion Medicine from PGIMER, Chandigarh, with a research focus on Neonatal Thrombocytopenia and Neonatal Alloimmune Thrombocytopenia (NAIT). She has completed her M.Sc. in Forensic Biotechnology from NFSU and a B.Sc. in Biological Sciences from Delhi University. She is currently working as a Project Research Scientist I under an ICMR-funded project on NAIT diagnosis and have previous experience as a Junior Research Fellow in DST-funded research. Some of her Publications include articles in Newborn Journal and Vox Sanguinis. She has qualified the UGC-NET (Forensic Science) and have received awards including the Harold Gunson Fellowship (ISBT 2020).

Brief Table of Contents

Detailed Table of Contents

CHAPTER 3

Dermatophytosis 61

CHAPTER 4

Superficial Candidiasis 91

LIST OF FIGURES

PREFACE

Fungi are ubiquitous organisms with diverse functions in the environment ranging from being decomposers in their natural habitats to causing disease in human beings. While many of them coexist harmoniously with human beings, others are known to cause significant illnesses when the body's immune system is compromised. The increasing use of immunosuppressive therapy, the pandemic of chronic diseases, and the HIV/AIDS pandemic have all contributed to a considerable rise in the incidence of fungal diseases detected in routine practice. They manifest themselves from minor skin, nail, or mucous membrane involvement to life-threatening systemic disease. With advances in treatment and diagnostic methods comes the necessity for such knowledge and involvement of these pathogens in clinic practice.

The clinical dilemma presented by fungal infections has driven a growing need for effective diagnostic modalities, successful treatment, and health care provider recognition. Presentation is indolent in some infections and acutely progressive with high morbidity in others. Early accurate recognition and identification are critical. Lack of prior exposure to fungal pathogens, however, predisposes to misdiagnosis or delayed diagnosis. In addition, increasing antifungal resistance adds to the management dilemma. Therefore, there is a pressing need for learning materials that summarize key information in a concise, clinically relevant format for students, clinicians, and laboratory personnel alike.

Handbook of Fungal Infections meets this need by offering a comprehensive and concise overview of mycotic infections within various organ systems. The book, written for students, clinicians, and microbiologists, aims to be both a primer and a clinical handbook. The book integrates required theory with practical diagnostic and management methods, striving to connect theory and practice.

Chapter 1 presents an overview of the basic biology of fungi, including their taxonomy, reproduction, and anatomy. It also explains the mechanisms by which fungi become pathogenic, including host-pathogen interactions and virulence factors. Chapter 2 is fully devoted to laboratory diagnosis, focusing on sampling, microscopy, culture, and emerging molecular technology. The chapter offers the technical skills necessary for the laboratory detection of fungal pathogens.

Chapter 3 covers dermatophytosis, including *Trichophyton, Epidermophyton*, and *Microsporum* infections. Epidemiology, clinical features, and treatment are covered in depth. Chapter 4 covers superficial candidiasis, noting its oral, genital, and intertriginous manifestations. It takes host-associated predispositions into account and resistance problems. Chapter 5 shifts attention to other cutaneous fungal infections like tinea versicolor and cutaneous sporotrichosis and centers on their diagnosis and differentiating them from allied dermatoses.

Chapter 6 describes mould infections of the nails with particular focus on onychomycosis. The chapter gives causative organisms, methods of diagnosis, and treatment considerations like systemic and topical treatment regimens. Chapter 7 covers keratomycosis, the most prevalent cause of corneal blindness, with its presentation, risk factors such as trauma and contact lens wear, and antifungal treatment. Chapter 8 deals with otomycosis, a commonly seen external ear canal infection. It discusses its symptomatology, mycological agents, and treatment modalities.

Chapter 9 is left for aspergillosis, which is a condition with an expansive clinical spectrum from allergic bronchopulmonary presentations to invasive pulmonary infection. Diagnostic algorithms and antifungal stewardship are highlighted. Chapter 10 discusses mucormycosis, a fulminant condition with high morbidity in diabetic and immunocompromised hosts. Early clinical presentations, radiological patterns, and surgical interventions are included alongside pharmacologic therapy.

Chapter 11 presents an overview of cryptococcosis, especially its manifestations in the central nervous system and lungs. The chapter outlines diagnostic techniques, i.e., antigen detection and interpretation of lumbar punctures, and treatment regimen. Chapter 12 presents coccidioidomycosis, encompassing endemicity, primary pulmonary infection, and potential dissemination. Chapter 13 presents blastomycosis, with cutaneous and pulmonary manifestations, and recent advances in diagnosis.

Chapter 14 covers histoplasmosis, often seen with bird or bat feces, and discusses acute and chronic presentations, diagnosis by antigen detection and culture, and treatment. Chapter 15 concludes with paracoccidioidomycosis, a Latin America-endemic systemic mycosis. Clinical presentation, differential diagnosis, and reaction to treatment are also covered.

This book is written for a broad-based readership of medical students, residents, clinical microbiologists, general practitioners, infectious disease specialists, dermatologists, and respiratory physicians. It is an academic study guide as well as a guide to clinical decision-making, providing readers with authoritative evidence-based information and structured advice. Whether as a tutorial tool or bedside pocket reference in practice, this handbook is intended to support evidence-based knowledge and management of fungal infections across various healthcare settings.

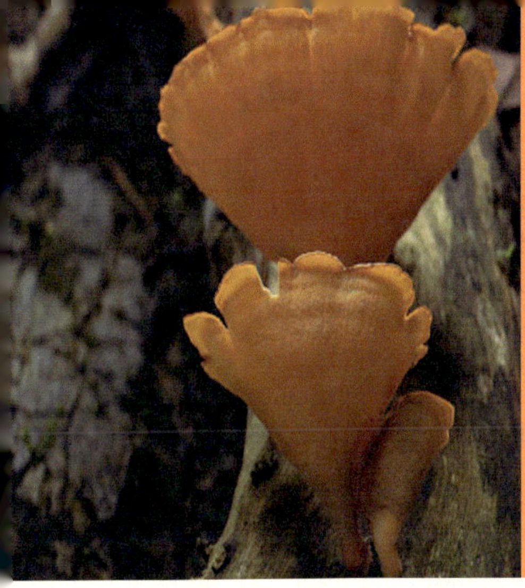

Chapter 1
BASIC MYCOLOGY

Contents

Introduction

Mycology, the scientific study of fungi, is an extremely broad and extensive field that has relevance to biology, ecology, and even medicine. As an independent academic field, mycology studies the strange biological characteristics of fungi, including their taxonomy, physiology, and environmental roles. From a branch of botany, the field has evolved a lot, particularly with advances in molecular biology and DNA sequencing. These developments have bred a revolution in the taxonomy of fungi, allowing scientists to articulate relationships between species of fungi and reveal their ecological significance. Mycology now focuses on emphasizing key roles fungi have in nutrient cycling, symbiotic relations, and the health of ecosystems, and thus places them in greater context as ecosystem contributors and factors in human health. The use of molecular techniques in mycology has transformed traditional approaches to fungal classification and identification. (Abarenkov et al., 2013) points out that molecular data have become essential tools in fungal systematics, enabling scientists to construct more accurate phylogenetic trees and shed light on the evolutionary ties among various fungal groups. The examination of molecular data not only involves high laboratory techniques but also demands consideration of taxon sampling and analytical procedures for the data, which all influence interpretations and implications of research outcomes. With mycology continuously developing in terms of incorporating new technologies, there is a greater focus on the need for interdisciplinarity where mycologists are in close association with geneticists and ecologists to know the complexities of fungal biology and thus lay the groundwork for future developments.

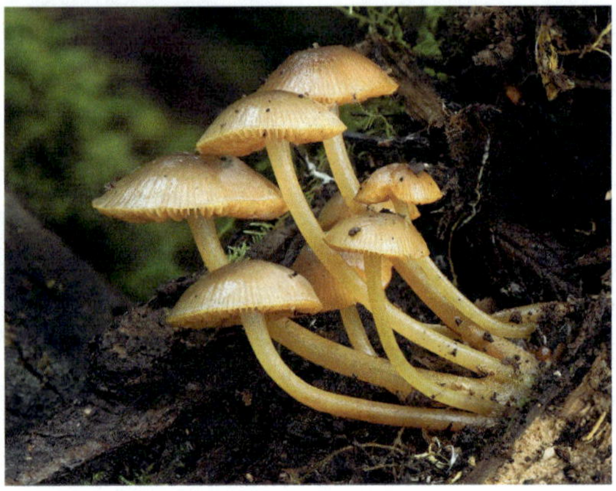

Figure 1.1. Mycology.

Source: https://upload.wikimedia.org/wikipedia/commons/7/70/Mycena_leaiana_var._australis.jpg.

Moreover, significant advancements have been made towards the standardization and registration of fungal taxonomy, making it easier for scientists to navigate this heterogenous domain. MycoBank, established to index and host a central repository of fungal nomenclature, is an indispensable resource for mycologists worldwide. (Amor et al., 2013) discusses the various innovations of MycoBank, including facilitating typing events and including DNA sequence data in its database. This has enabled coherent and standardized reporting of fungal species and their classifications. While challenges continue to plague linking taxonomic names with genetic data, the ongoing refinement of such databases will ultimately result in a better system for the study of fungi whereby mycological research continues to be relevant and accurate in the face of an increasingly dynamic scientific landscape. Through rigorous standardization and adoption of novel approaches, mycology continues to develop as a fundamental area of research with far-reaching consequences for biodiversity and ecological integrity (Figure 1.1).

1.1. Classification of Fungi

Fungal taxonomy is a process that utilizes various morphological, ecological, and molecular processes to properly classify the heterogenous taxon in the fungal kingdom. In the past, fungi were divided into groups based on their reproductive structures as well as their method of spore production, hence the formation of expansive phyla such as Ascomycota and Basidiomycota. However, advances in molecular biology, particularly DNA sequencing, have revealed detailed that many morphological placements of fungi underrepresent true fungal diversity. Such discrepancy demands the application of molecular information to provide improved understanding of the evolutionary relationships and limits of species among fungi, pinpointing the importance of making use of sound DNA sequence data along with good morphological descriptions in systematic mycology (Abarenkov et al., 2014). Fungi are extremely diverse with estimates ranging from 0.8 million to over 5 million species globally (Aaronson et al., 2016). This vast diversity of fungi is critical because they serve critical ecological roles such as serving as decomposers, mutualists, and pathogens. Their ecological significance is realized by virtue of their contribution to nutrient cycling and their interaction with higher plants. For instance, many fungi form mycorrhizal relationships that enhance water and nutrient acquisition by plants, thus maintaining forest health and diversity. Fungi also contribute to human sustenance by providing food and medicinal products; thousands of species are harvested annually for food purposes, and several others for their medicinal properties. A correct classification system that acknowledges these ecological functions is crucial in conservation as well as economic exploitation of fungal materials. Fungal classification remains an active area, and research continues to expand our knowledge of fungal phylogeny and systematics. With the presence of high-throughput sequencing facilities, there is a need for effective and standardized systems of species identification. The process of compiled public databases, such as the NCBI RefSeq Targeted Loci (RTL) database, has enabled the use of re-annotated sequences covering the large orders of fungi (Abarenkov et al., 2014) at ease. These databases enable scientists to conduct in-depth species assignment and improve data quality in fungal research. As our understanding of fungal diversity expands, it becomes increasingly vital to integrate both molecular and morphological classification approaches to capture the full spectrum of fungal biodiversity, thereby contributing to a more accurate and comprehensive framework for Basic Mycology (Figure 1.2).

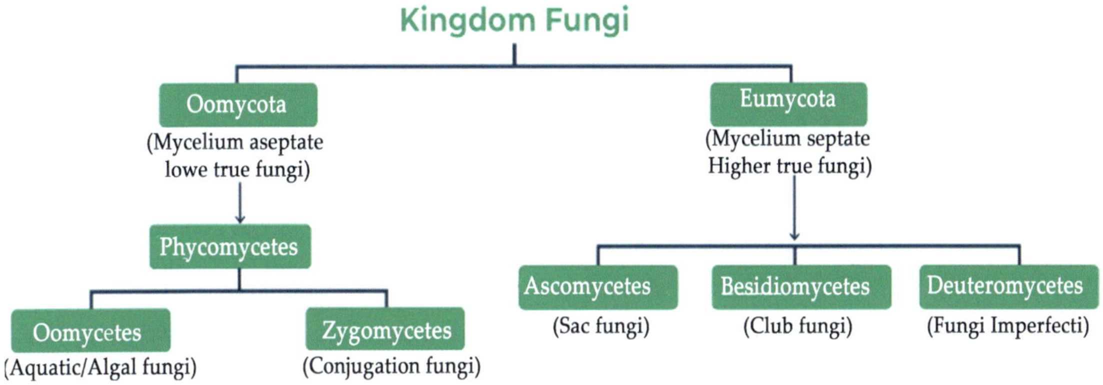

Figure 1.2. The classification of fungi is a complex endeavor that incorporates various morphological, ecological, and molecular approaches to accurately categorize the diverse taxa within this kingdom.

Source: https://media.geeksforgeeks.org/wp-content/uploads/20231003171041/Classification-of-Fungi.png.

1.1.1. Major Groups of Fungi

Fungi, one of the very diverse kingdoms in the domain Eukarya, comprise a number of large groups, each with different life cycles, modes of reproduction, and ecological niches. Ascomycetes, being the largest and most commonly known group, are also commonly called sac fungi and hold important positions in numerous ecological systems. Ascomycetes include yeasts and molds, which play significant roles in fermentation and decomposition processes. Ascomycetes are sexually propagated by the formation of ascospores within a sac-like structure known as an ascus, but asexually they are propagated through spores that are externally formed. Their ecological role is emphasized not just due to their nutrient cycling ability but also due to their relationship with plant and animal life, thus making them central in various food webs and ecosystems (Abarenkov et al., 2013). Another significant division, Basidiomycetes, or club fungi, are most familiar in their fruiting stage, such as mushrooms. This division also plays a major role in cycling nutrients, particularly for the decomposition of lignin and cellulose, which make up primarily wood and plant material. Basidiomycetes both reproduce sexually and asexually, giving rise to diversity in fungal morphology, such as gills, pores, and spines, where the spores are produced. Ecological associations of the fungi with their environments can be observed in symbiotic relationships, such as with plants in mycorrhizal association, which enhance nutrient uptake and plant well-being (Alastruey-Izquierdo et al., 2015).

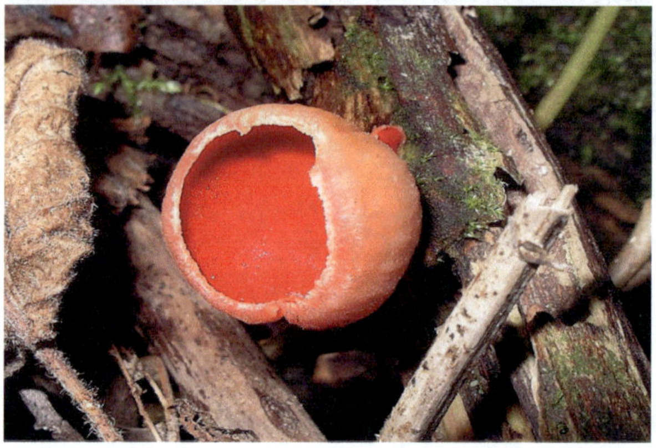

Figure 1.3. Ascomycetes reproduce sexually by forming ascospores within a sac-like structure called an ascus, as well as asexually through spores produced externally.

Source: https://upload.wikimedia.org/wikipedia/commons/6/67/Scarlet_elf_cap_cadnant_dingle.jpg.

Thus, Basidiomycetes are not only major decomposers but also significant producers of ecosystem productivity accelerations. The third significant group, Zygomycetes, consists of copiously growing molds that are normally found in soil and decaying organic matter. They are unique in having a zygospore formed during sexual reproduction that allows them to withstand unfavorable environmental conditions. While most Zygomycetes are saprophytic and assist in decomposing organic material, others develop plant pathogens. Their role in food spoilage cannot be ignored, causing damage to farm crops and food supply chains on a regular basis (Abarenkov et al., 2013). Moreover, Zygomycetes have a complex life cycle with dichotomous asexual reproduction by sporangiospores. Overall, awareness of the major fungal orders provides an insight into their ecological significance, evolutionary trends, and relationships with other organisms, indicating the vital role fungi play in natural and anthropogenic ecosystems (Alastruey-Izquierdo et al., 2015) (Figure 1.3).

1.1.2. Taxonomy and Nomenclature

The mycological discipline is heavily reliant on nomenclature and taxonomy for the identification and classification of the vast diversity of fungal species. Taxonomy is the science that is used to classify living things based on shared characteristics, thus allowing mycologists to place fungi into hierarchical ranks that consist of kingdoms, genera, and species. Nomenclature, on the other hand, is the science of giving names to these organisms so that a given species can be universally recognized by it. This dual approach is not only essential for scholarly discourse but also for practical applications in ecology, agriculture, and medicine. In establishing an open taxonomy, mycologists can share correct information about fungi, aiding research and refining our understanding of their ecological roles. In the past several years, initiatives like MycoBank have transformed the science of fungal nomenclature by providing a central registry of taxonomic information. Established in response to the need for firm taxonomic information, MycoBank is an integrating center linking many collections and databases of fungi, such as Index Fungorum. The International Code of Nomenclature for algae, fungi, and plants (ICN) mandates obligatory registration of fungal names as a condition for valid publication, thus standardizing nomenclatural processes. The improvements introduced by MycoBank, i.e., advanced queries and multilingual interfaces, make access easier for mycologists everywhere.

The ongoing challenge, however, remains to enhance integration of taxonomic names with DNA sequence information, in accordance with the evolving concept of fungal diversity and classification (Amor et al., 2013). The integration of molecular tools in taxonomy has also brought to the fore the importance of accurate DNA sequence information in determining fungal species. Morphological characters are not sufficient to reflect the actual diversity of fungal taxa and, as such, lead to an underestimation of species diversity. The advent of phylogenetics and DNA barcoding has revolutionized the approaches of mycologists in fungal classification, as witnessed in the re-annotation of reference sequences in curated databases like the National Center for Biotechnology Information (NCBI). The databases facilitate the rapid assignment of species in ecological and microbiome research, where high-throughput sequencing is now the norm. The proposal of standards and protocols for improving data quality is meant to enhance the accuracy of identification of fungi and actually bridge the gap between traditional taxonomy and modern molecular techniques and make the science of mycology robust and cohesive (Abarenkov et al., 2014) (Figure 1.4).

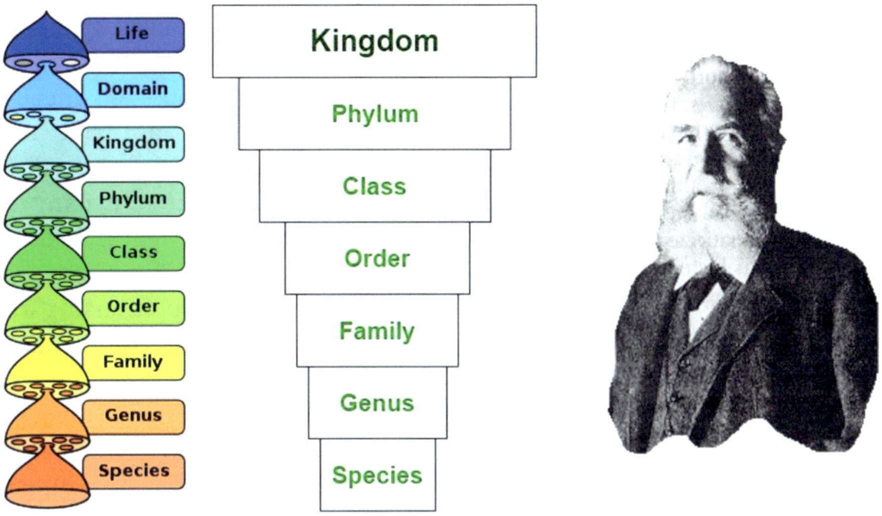

Figure 1.4. Taxonomy serves as the scientific framework that organizes living organisms based on shared characteristics, allowing mycologists to categorize fungi into hierarchical groups, such as kingdoms, genera, and species.

Source: https://biologynotesonline.com/wp-content/uploads/2024/03/Phylum-Definition-Importance-Examples.jpg.

1.1.3. Differences Between Fungi and Other Organisms

It is necessary to understand the differences between fungi and other organisms to understand their function within ecological processes and physiological mechanisms. Fungi lack chlorophyll and therefore do not perform photosynthesis; they are heterotrophs and are able to acquire nutrients by the degradation of organic matter. This specialized nutrition strategy allows fungi to be an integral part of the nutrient cycling in ecosystems. Moreover, the structural components of fungi, such as chitin, separate them from the plant kingdom, where the principal component is cellulose. Chitin provides toughness and defense and is responsible for the capacity of fungi to thrive in various environments. Such fundamental differences demonstrate that fungi occupy a unique place in the bio hierarchy, functioning both as decomposers and symbionts in most of the biological relationships. Compared to animals, which are more or less motile and possess a complex nervous system, fungi are not motile and possess a more primitive way of life. Fungal growth patterns, particularly by hyphal extension, possess a peculiar form of development that marks them as distinct from other organisms. Fungal filamentous structures known as hyphae allow for very high surface area to volume ratios for the uptake and transport of nutrients. These structures also facilitate the ability of fungi to effectively colonize substrates, being capable of adapting to different habitats, as indicated in research where bacterial isolates from fungi had antagonistic characteristics against pathogens, reflecting their ecological adaptability (Felitti et al., 2017). Fungi life cycle can include both asexual and sexual reproductive stages, which is very distinct from the more reliable forms of reproduction among animals and serves to emphasize their resilience and flexibility in a changing environment. Moreover, fungal biochemical pathways are extremely different from those in other kingdoms. For instance, research on biological control methods has demonstrated how fungal metabolites can efficiently combat disease-causing microorganisms without the application of harmful chemicals, offering a promising avenue for sustainable activities (O'Callahan et al., 2012). This ability to produce secondary metabolites that contain antibiotics or antifungal compounds emphasizes the significance of fungi as significant players in health, agriculture, and ecological management. This metabolic variation contributes not only to their survival but also to their ecological significance. By studying these unique features, scientists are able to exploit fungi's potential in a bid to address challenges such as sustainable agriculture and disease management, underscoring their centerpiece role in ecological as well as utilitarian contexts in the discipline of basic mycology.

1.2. Fungal Structure and Function

Fungal morphology is very varied, reflecting adaptations to facilitate their existence in a broad range of ecological niches. Fungi are typically multicellular or unicellular organisms composed of hyphae, branching filaments which collectively constitute a mycelium. The mycelium invades substrates, and uptake of nutrients and growth are facilitated. The cell wall, constructed primarily of chitin, provides structural rigidity and protection against environmental stresses. Also, some fungi exhibit specialized structures, such as fruiting bodies, required for reproduction to ensure spore dispersal. These specializations enable the fungi to thrive in wide-ranging habitats, from soil to rot, thereby showing their vital role in nutrient cycling in ecosystems. Overall, structural features of the fungi form the bases of their functions and illustrate a highly developed relationship among form and ecological function. Functional characteristics of fungi are equally crucial as they define how the organisms interact with their environment. Fungi are heterotrophic, deriving most of their nutrients from decomposition, aided by the breakdown of extracellular enzymes that catabolize intricate organic material. It not only contributes to the growth of fungi but also facilitates recycling of nutrients in environments. Moreover, others symbiotically associate, such as mycorrhizal association with plants that facilitate the absorption of phosphorus, among others. Other strains are pathogenic, for example, those that form biofilms that are treatment-resistant and complicate infection, particularly in the case of human health. For instance, the presence of fungal biofilms such as those of *Candida albicans* illustrates complex patterns of resistance characterized by extracellular matrix formation and operation of efflux pumps, which compromise conventional antifungal therapies (Rajendran et al., 2012). Thus, the functional nature of fungi indicates their ecological significance as well as human importance. The interface of fungal function and structure is an important consideration in understanding their ecological functions as well as possibilities of exploitation. For instance, white-rot fungi show this interaction in ligninolytic enzymes, which are important for bioremediation processes like the degradation of stable pollutants like polychlorinated biphenyls (PCBs). Ligninolytic enzyme secretion, especially laccases, is closely associated with growth potential of various fungal strains, revealing that structural properties affect enzymatic performance (Fonseca et al., 2018). With the help of such potentials, researchers are exploring biotechnological applications with fungi in environmental cleanup and bioconversion processes. This intricate synergy between structural specializations and functional consequences not only emphasizes the ecological relevance of fungi but also presents new opportunities in green practice, highlighting the ongoing necessity of basic mycology to current scientific discourse (Figure 1.5).

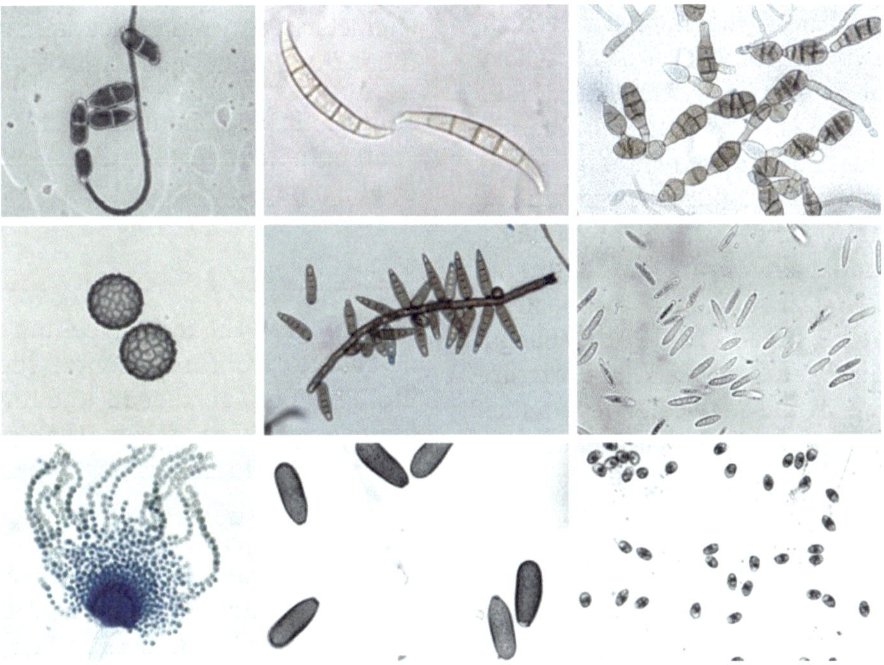

Figure 1.5. Fungal structure exhibits remarkable diversity, reflecting adaptations that enhance their survival across a myriad of ecological niches.

Source: https://media.springernature.com/lw685/springer-static/image/chp%3A10.1007%2F978-3-031-68663-4_3/MediaObjects/502042_1_En_3_Fig17_HTML.jpg.

1.2.1. Cellular Structure of Fungi

The structural arrangement of the fungal cell is characterized by unique features that differentiate them from other kingdoms of life. The cells possess walls that are predominantly composed of chitin, a hard polysaccharide conferring structural strength and protection. Chitin content in fungal cell walls differentiates them from plant cellulose-based walls, which makes fungi resistant to enzymatic hydrolysis and provides them with a support system, necessary for their filamentous nature. Fungi also exhibit a filamentous type of growth known as hyphae, which are elongated thread-like cells that form clumps to form mycelium. Mycelial network is responsible for nutrient uptake because the extensive surface area maximizes contact with substrates and facilitates the acquisition of resources in diverse environments. Fungal cell structure also features compartmentalization, which may be of septate or coenocytic forms. Septate fungi have cross-walls or septa inside them that allow compartalization, which helps to regulate the distribution of resources and cellular processes. The coenocytic fungi lack septa, and this makes them multinucleate where the cytoplasm is free to flow around the hyphal network. This difference in structure is of evolutionary significance and reflects adaptations in various ecological niches. Besides, cellular processes such as reproduction, metabolism, and stress reactions are integrated in the cell organization to facilitate fungi, such as *Aspergillus nidulans*, to endure fluctuating environmental conditions and expand ecological roles in decomposition and nutrient cycling (Chen et al., 2018). Fungal cells possess equally stunning cellular structure and organization at the molecular level, such as essential organelles like mitochondria, endoplasmic reticulum, and Golgi apparatus that play very important roles in metabolic processes. Mitochondria, where aerobic respiration occurs, are required for generating energy, and endoplasmic reticulum and Golgi apparatus are involved in the synthesis and secretion of protein, required for the production of enzymes responsible for the degradation of nutrients. It is important to understand the cell structure of fungi, especially when considering their pathogenicity and biofilm formation that greatly complicates therapeutic regimens in clinical practice. The drug resistance mechanisms demonstrated by fungal biofilms, especially by such species as *Candida albicans*, reflect the highly complex nature of their cell structure and function (Rajendran et al., 2012). This information is central to understanding the intricacies of fungal biology and their relevance in disease and health (Figure 1.6).

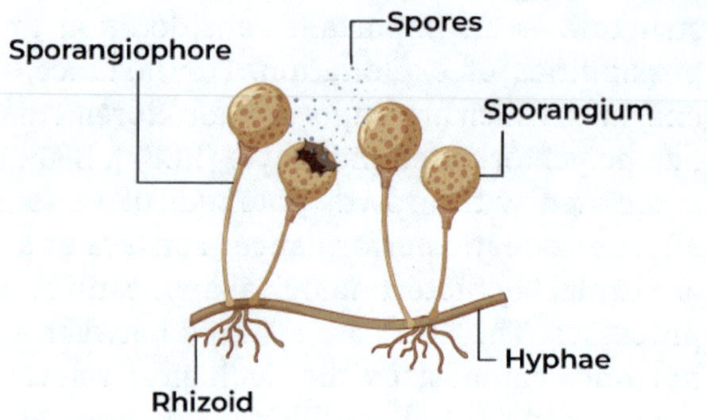

Figure 1.6. The cellular structure of fungi is characterized by unique features that distinguish them from other kingdoms of life.

Source: https://media.geeksforgeeks.org/wp-content/uploads/20240307150934/Structure-of-Fungi.png.

1.2.2. Hyphal Growth and Mycelium

Hyphal growth and mycelium formation in mycology are fundamental ideas in fungal biology. Fungal thread-like organisms, the hyphae, possess a remarkable capacity for elongation and branching to produce a highly networked organ, the mycelium. The mycelium is essential for the absorption of nutrients because the hyphae can penetrate other substrates to transport nutrients back to the fungal body. The process of growth is driven by the uptake and assimilation of these nutrients, which are assimilated into the cellular substance to bring about biomass increase and ensuing reproductive organs. Vegetative reproduction and its physiological process have been explored through model organisms such as *Saccharomyces cerevisiae* and *Schizosaccharomyces pombe*, through which one can elucidate how hyphal growth might be influenced by both external and internal metabolic processes (Boswell et al., 2017).

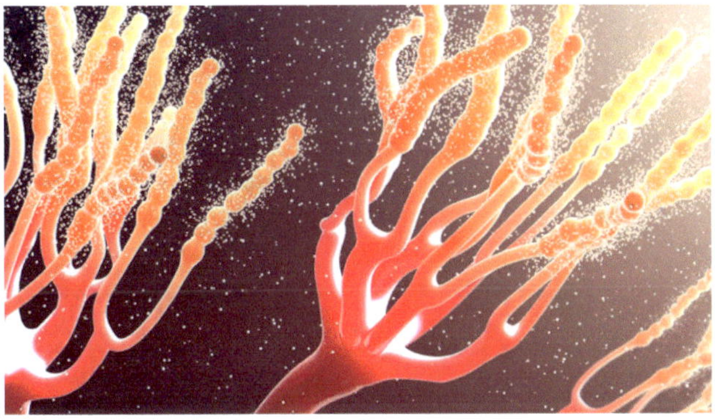

Figure 1.7. Hyphae, the thread-like structures of fungi, exhibit a remarkable ability to elongate and branch, forming a complex network known as mycelium.

Source: https://researchoutreach.org/wp-content/uploads/2022/02/Fungal-minds-Main-Image-1200x675.jpg.

Mycelial networks are not merely nutrient procurement but exhibit sophisticated movement dynamics within their local surroundings. This is highly relevant when dealing with the ecological roles of fungi, as mycelium is able to interact with other organisms and substrates in a multitude of complex manners. Certain recent studies have looked at concepts like informed growth and mycelial translocations, which demonstrate how these organisms respond to environmental cues. Above all, the notion of fungal highways is about highlighting the capacity of mycelium to extend between disconnected sources of nutrients and enable efficient sharing of resources between fungal communities. This framework unlocks the possibilities of interdisciplinarity since integrating fungal biology in the broader framework of movement ecology promises novel methods for deciphering ecosystem behavior and ultimately assembly of communities and species interactions (Aguilar-Trigueros et al., 2019). The effects of mycelium and hyphal growth reach beyond individual organisms into ecological stability and sustainability. As mycelial networks are responsible for decomposing organic matter, they play a key role in nutrient cycling and soil aggregation. Recycling and reuse of cellular material during hyphal development also enable such fungi to adapt and thrive in a variety of environments. The complex interrelationship between structure and function in mycelia highlights the dynamic character of fungal existence. An understanding of these phenomena not only supports the cultivation of useful fungal species for agriculture and bioremediation but also has implications for more general issues of biodiversity and resilience in ecosystems. Thus, hyphal growth and mycelium studies have continued to be a core part in the quest for understanding fungal ecology complexities and diversity of interactions in ecosystems (Boswell et al., 2017) (Figure 1.7).

1.2.3. Reproductive Structures of Fungi

Fungal sex organs are major tools for sexual and asexual reproduction and show the unimaginable diversity of the kingdom. Asexual reproduction is mostly conidium formation as spores on specialized structures such as conidiophores. Gene expression studies in filamentous fungi, such as *Aspergillus nidulans*, have identified regulatory pathways governing conidial development and conserved proteins critical for this process.

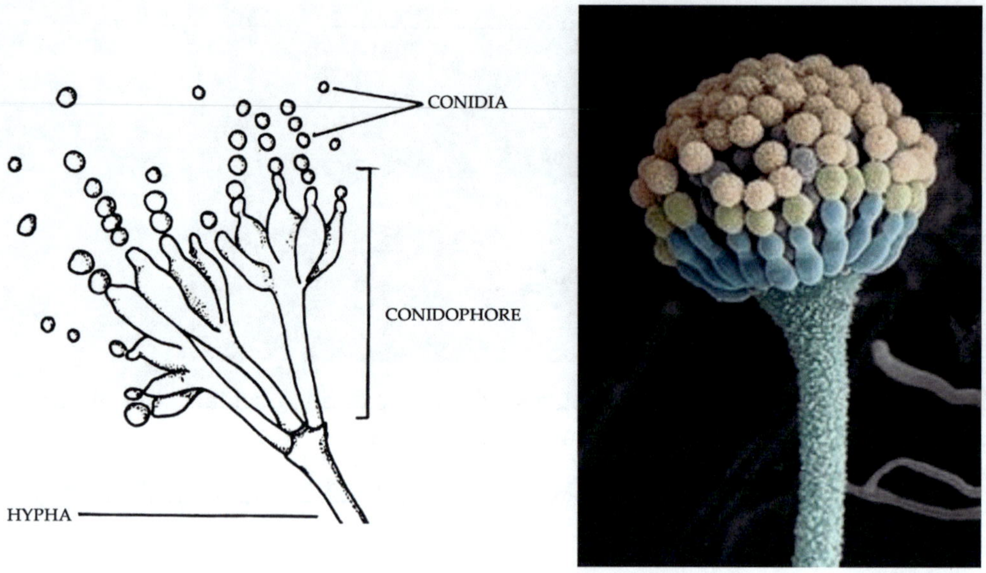

Figure 1.8. Asexual reproduction often occurs through the production of spores, such as conidia, which are formed on specialized structures like conidiophores.

Source: https://biologynotesonline.com/wp-content/uploads/2024/01/Deuteromycetes-Reproduction-Characteristics-Classification-and-Examples.jpeg.

For example, the proteins FlbA and AbaA are significant in various taxa, demonstrating evolutionary significance and intricacy of asexual reproduction in fungi. This establishes how some regulatory pathways are maintained, albeit with variations across different groups, illustrating convergences and divergences in reproductive strategy across the fungal kingdom (Chen et al., 2018). In contrast to asexual reproduction, fungal sexual reproduction typically involves fusion of special hyphae and formation of complex structures like fruiting bodies that bear sexual spores. In addition to genetic recombination, these structures are also important for survival under unfavorable environmental conditions. Sexuality control mechanisms are similarly complex, with mating type (MAT) loci showing wide variation among species. For instance, research on *Aspergillus* species has uncovered varying MAT loci designs in heterothallic and homothallic species, suggesting evolutionary divergence that impacts reproductive modes. Such research assists in the comprehension of how sexual reproduction may transcend what appears to be asexual species, investigating concealed genetic architectures that support an amazing diversity of reproductive behaviors in fungi (Chen et al., 2018). Besides, the importance of fungal reproductive organs in ecology cannot be undermined, particularly when estimating their role in environmental processes. One such example is that of biological soil crusts (BSCs), which are communities usually consisting of various fungi, contributing to stabilization of the soil and cycling of nutrients via reproduction. Asexual reproduction among some fungi included in BSCs demonstrates their capacity for tolerance to extreme environments, for instance, desiccation and temperature variation. Dispersal mechanisms of these fungi enable them to cover extensive areas of land, further solidifying their ecological niche. Once the role played by fungal reproductive structures in soil crust community dynamics is known, scientists are able to better facilitate land management practices in order to ensure the sustainability of such vital ecosystems (Figure 1.8).

1.3. Fungal Ecology

Fungal ecology is an advanced field that explores the wide range of roles played by fungi within various ecosystems. Fungi are not merely decomposers of fallen organic matter; they have intricate relationships with plants, animals, and other microbes. These relationships play a critical role in nutrient cycling and energy transfer within ecosystems. For instance, the relationship between fungi and plant roots, or mycorrhiza, enables plants to uptake more nutrients in return for supplying fungi with essential carbohydrates.

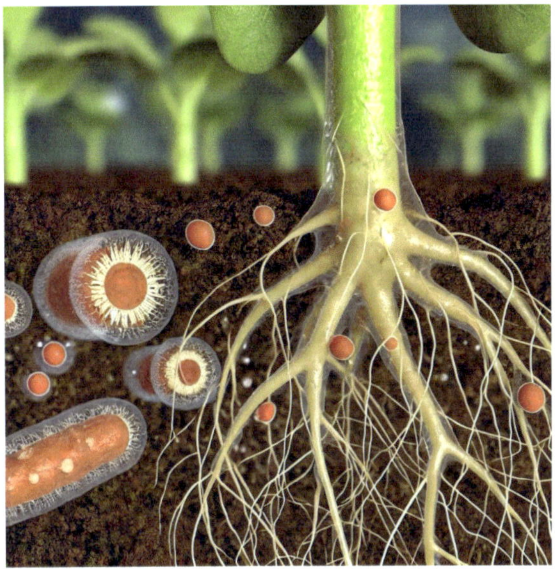

Figure 1.9. The relationship between fungi and plant roots, known as mycorrhiza, facilitates enhanced nutrient absorption for plants while providing fungi with essential carbohydrates.

Source: https://cdn.shopify.com/s/files/1/0723/9450/6454/files/The-Role-of-Mycorrhizal-Fungi-in-Enhancing-Nutrient-Absorption-in-Medicinal-Plants-2b_1.png?v=1738870011.

This symbiotic association demonstrates how fungi contribute to enhancing farming yields and natural ecosystems alike in the same manner. Such relationships are crucial in determining the ecological balance and stability of environments, which are constantly under assault from human-induced elements such as climate change and habitat destruction. In discovering fungal interactions, there occur antagonistic relationships as fundamental elements of ecological processes. Some fungal strains possess antagonistic characteristics against pathogenic organisms, and these can offer valuable biological control mechanisms in agriculture. Various researches have uncovered various genera, including *Acremonium* and *Penicillium*, which show efficacy against fungal pathogens, indicating their nature as biocontrol agents. The studies on these fungi illustrate their ecological functions, whereby they not only suppress harmful organisms but also enhance ecosystem stability and plant health. Such data promote further studies into how such processes are carried out and suggest that taking advantage of such natural links can offer sustainable agricultural options and enhanced ecosystem resilience. The understanding of antagonistic fungi can therefore play a powerful influence on ecological research and actual agricultural application (Felitti et al., 2017). Furthermore, entomopathogenic fungi illustrate another aspect of fungal ecology because they deal with insect populations within their ecosystems. In the past, they were famous for their potential application in pest control, whereas modern studies have unveiled their other ecological role as endophytes and rhizosphere colonizers. These findings highlight that entomopathogenic fungi are not only pathogens but also have the ability to induce plant growth and health under certain conditions. This double duty creates opportunities for using these fungi in integrated pest management, thereby enhancing crop resilience and sustainability. Future research must tackle the complexities of these interactions because it is important to know how such fungi play an ecological role in order to maximize their use and maximize control of pests while providing healthy plant growth. This holistic understanding shall enhance wider application of fungal ecology in agroecology and environmental management (Andrews et al., 2009) (Figure 1.9).

1.3.1. Role of Fungi in Ecosystems

The contribution of fungi to ecosystems is quintessential, as they contribute through their diverse activities in nutrient cycling, soil formation, and ecological sustainability. Fungi, being vital decomposers, decompose organic matter of high complexity, including dead vegetation and animals, and recycle essential nutrients into the soil. Decomposition increases the fertility of soils by making nutrients accessible to the plants for easier uptake. Besides, fungi enter symbiotic relationships with a variety of plants through mycorrhizal relationships, which significantly increase the area for the uptake of water and nutrients. These mechanisms emphasize the role of fungi not only in nutrient cycling but also in maintaining biodiversity in ecosystems through the preservation of mixed communities of plants that rely on such relationships for productive growth and protection against environmental stresses. Moreover, fungi play a fundamentally important role in biological phosphorus mobilization, a key macronutrient often in deficient supply in soils. Various saprotrophic fungi have recently been shown to mobilize phosphorus from insoluble minerals in a wide range of ways, with the result that it is brought into availability for plant assimilation. Some examples are species of *Rhizopus stolonifer* var. stolonifer and *Aspergillus niger* have been found to be rich in phosphorus solubilization activity, which makes them prime candidates as biofertilizers that could enhance agricultural productivity in an environmentally friendly way (Ceci et al., 2017). This phosphorus-enhancing ability not only is beneficial for the growth of plants but also aids in improving the overall efficiency of nutrient utilization in farming systems. By introducing these fungi into agriculture, potential exists for minimizing reliance on nonrenewable phosphate rock and thus for a more sustainable strategy for crop management. Additionally, the continuous development of fungal taxonomy and nomenclature, as represented by improvements in databases such as MycoBank, has far-reaching significance for our comprehension of fungi in ecosystems. They enable the identification and classification of fungi species, paving the way for studies on the ecological role and relationship of fungi. This integration enables scientists to link DNA sequence data with taxonomic information so as to comprehend the vast fungal diversity and individual roles (Amor et al., 2013). As our knowledge advances, it increasingly becomes evident that fungi are not only passive participants in ecosystems but actual agents that determine community patterns by affecting nutrient cycling, plant interactions, and overall ecosystem well-being. Increased insight into these roles, facilitated by enhanced research technologies, will be essential in meeting environmental challenges and promoting sustainability (Figure 1.10).

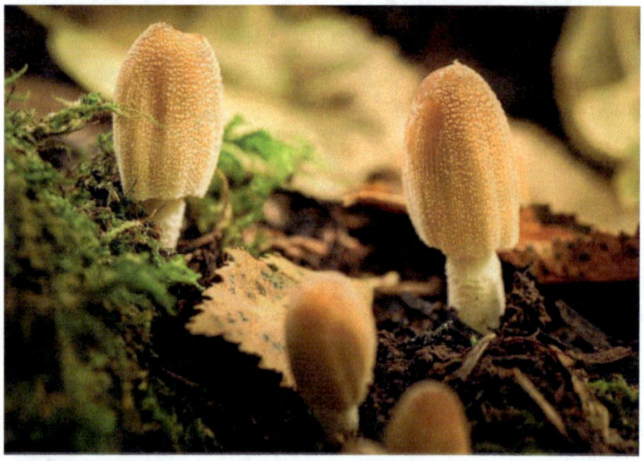

Figure 1.10. As essential decomposers, fungi break down complex organic matter, such as dead plants and animals, returning vital nutrients to the soil.

Source: https://earth.org/wp-content/uploads/2023/07/Untitled-683-%C3%97-1024px-1024-%C3%97-683px-85-1200x675.jpg.

1.3.2. Symbiotic Relationships (e.g., Mycorrhizae)

Symbiotic associations such as mycorrhizae are a significant feature of acquisition of nutrients by plants and ecosystem balance in some ecosystems. Mycorrhizae, the root-fungi plant symbiotic relationship, enhances nutrient uptake by host plants, particularly in the uptake of essential elements such as phosphorus and nitrogen.

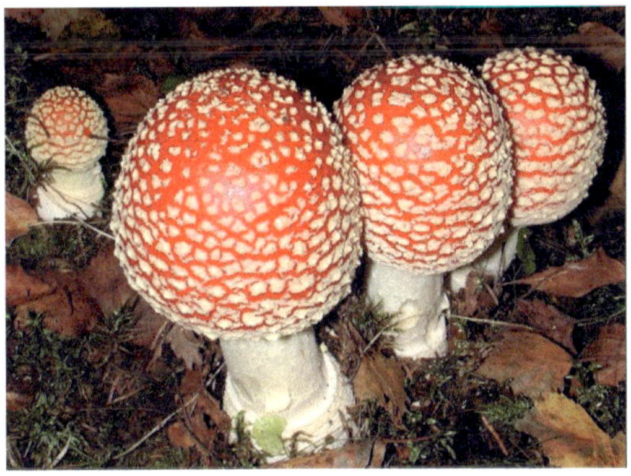

Figure 1.11. Ectomycorrhizal fungi, in particular, form mutualistic associations with many tree species, contributing significantly to their nutrient acquisition capabilities.

Source: https://upload.wikimedia.org/wikipedia/commons/a/a5/Amanita_muscaria_fruit_bodies.jpg.

These fungi extend the root networks reach, allowing increased access to soil resources unavailable to the plants themselves. The intricate relationship between mycorrhizal fungi and plants not only facilitate nutrient exchange but also enhance plant growth and resistance to stress, highlighting the importance of these relationships in terrestrial systems. Mycorrhizal relationships with woody and herbaceous vegetation are complex but vital in maintaining forest productivity. Ectomycorrhizal fungi are particularly symbiotic with many tree species, critically contributing to the trees' ability to take up nutrients. Recent research indicates that the fungi can be affected by changing soil nutrient levels, including phosphorus and nitrogen. As (Victoroff et al., 2020) have explained, the response of ectomycorrhizal fungi to forest nutrient manipulation is insightful into how such symbiotic associations react to environmental changes. Such understanding is thus important for forest management and conservation against the context of a climate where temperatures are rising and nutrient regimes have changed. Besides traditional plant-fungus interactions, symbiotic relationships also entail intricate community dynamics of biological soil crusts (BSCs). BSCs are a combination of organisms like mycorrhizal fungi, lichens, and cyanobacteria that collectively stabilize soil surfaces and allow nutrient cycling. These communities are very tolerant to extreme environmental conditions and are fundamental to enhancing soil quality and fertility. As highlighted in Aanderud et al., (2019), the relationships among these organisms illustrate the intricate network of relationships underlying ecosystem functionality and stability. Furthermore, information regarding how such crust communities form and respond to human-induced impacts is increasing in significance for land management plans aimed at preserving biodiversity and ecosystem health in an evolving environment (Figure 1.11).

1.3.3. Fungi as Decomposers

The contribution of fungi to ecosystems on land is extremely important, especially as decomposers. In contacting organic matter, fungi begin the process of decomposition, decomposing complex biomolecules into simple ones. This process recycles nutrients back to the soil, thereby making them accessible to other living things, even plants. Fungi use enzymes to carry out this process, thus being capable of decomposing lignin, cellulose, and other resistant organic compounds. Their unique biochemical processes differentiate them from bacteria and enable fungi to survive in various environments, ranging from soil on the forest floor to pastures.

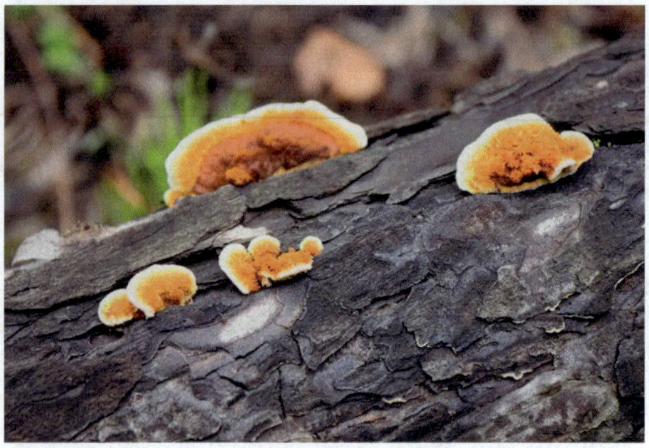

Figure 1.12. The role of fungi in terrestrial ecosystems is profoundly significant, particularly as decomposers.

Source: https://www.tigersafariindia.com/blog/wp-content/uploads/2024/07/tree-mushroom-on-a-tree-trunk-covered-with-green-moss-in-a-forest.jpg.

Thus, the function of fungi in the cycling of nutrients not only promotes plant growth but also enhances overall ecosystem health and endurance. With progressing research, it becomes all the more clear that the identification of the diverse functions of fungi can make ecological conservation more effective (Barron et al., 2014). The role of fungi in ecology is not only limited to simple decomposition; they also have an impact on soil structure and health. Through the degradation of organic matter, fungi help build humus, which boosts soil fertility as well as water retention. Moreover, their mycelium forms symbiotic relationships with plant roots, enabling the sharing of nutrients and enhancing the growth of the plant. This mutualism represents the intricate processes of ecosystems where the decomposer organisms play a crucial role in recycling nutrients and fostering biodiversity. Such appreciation goes against the conventional wisdom of conservation biology that has sought to overlook the function of fungi. While scientists begin using fungi alongside conservation efforts, their worthiness as surrogates to ecosystem integrity and as providers of the most important ecosystem functions increases (Barron et al., 2014). Besides acting as decomposers in terrestrial ecosystems, fungi show a lot of potential in agricultural ecosystems too, that is, in enhancing the provision of nutrients in the soil. A fascinating use is the employment of saprotrophic fungi as biofertilizers, which is increasingly significant as natural nutrient sources, e.g., phosphate rock, become rarer. Fungi of certain species can solubilize phosphorus from insoluble compounds and thus make it accessible for use by plants. These include *Aspergillus niger* and *Rhizopus stolonifer* var. stolonifer have been found to be able to do this, and this is a sign of the biphasic function of fungi in relation to agricultural output and ecosystem well-being. With the development of mycology, there is a requirement for constant research into the relationship between fungi, crop management, and ecosystem health with emphasis on the significance of including these organisms in sustainable agriculture (Figure 1.12).

1.4. Fungi in Human Life

Fungi perform a multifaceted role in human life, much more significant than their historical connotations with decay and illness. Beneficial fungi are crucial for agriculture by way of symbiosis with plant roots to enhance the plants' nutrition uptake. Mycorrhizal symbiosis not only aids plant health and growth but also results in fertile ground. Besides, fungi are also used in biotechnology, for instance in the production of biofuels whereby enzymes in fungi decompose organic matter to forms that can be consumed as energy. Beyond agricultural use, fungi also have a pivotal role in medicine as a source of antibiotics and other pharmaceuticals. The discovery of penicillin from the Penicillium fungus transformed the prevention and treatment of bacterial infections and demonstrated the way in which fungi are not only deliverers of nutrients but also vital players in human health and well-being. The relationship between humans and fungi can be detrimental, though, particularly if pathogenic fungi are involved. Fungal infectious diseases pose severe health threats, particularly to immunocompromised patients.

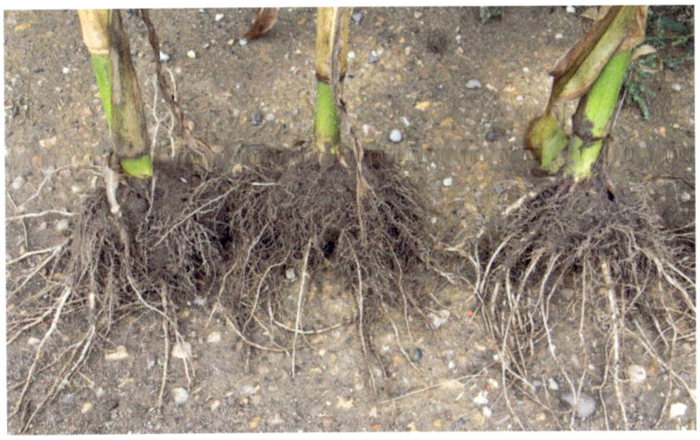

Figure 1.13. Beneficial fungi contribute significantly to agriculture by forming symbiotic relationships with plant roots, enhancing nutrient uptake.

Source: https://cdn.wikifarmer.com/images/detailed/2023/04/The-Importance-of-Mycorrhizae-in-Agriculture-and-Ecosystems.jpg.

For example, *Candida albicans* is a pathogenic fungus that may lead to severe infections in individuals with weakened immune systems. Fungal biofilms, which develop on medical devices and tissues, are difficult to treat due to their mechanisms of resistance. These biofilms are often resistant to antifungal medications and necessitate highly expensive surgical interventions for medical institutions (Rajendran et al., 2012). This fungi dualism of being good and bad calls for great knowledge in fungal biology and ecology to comprehend their complexities in environments that humans inhabit. With advancing science in mycology, there have been resources made available for additional research and application of knowledge regarding fungi, predominantly through open platforms like MycoBank. MycoBank was established in 2004 and serves as an integrated registration system to document fungal taxa for identification and classification purposes. Its features, from complex queries to a multilingual interface, enhance use convenience among researchers worldwide, enhancing global collaboration (Amor et al., 2013). With formal systems of naming needing to grow, the database is set to satisfy demands such as linking taxonomic names to DNA sequence data as well as improving data quality in general. Therefore, MycoBank is not just a repository but a valuable tool in modern mycology, facilitating the identification and understanding of the vast number of fungi impacting us today to become more efficient (Figure 1.13).

1.4.1. Fungi in Food Production

The contribution of fungi towards food production cannot be exaggerated as they also have a significant role to play in fermentation and enhancing the quality of the food. Fungi, or rather yeasts, have an undeniable contribution to the fermentation of foods and beverages like bread, beer, and wine. The capability of yeast to ferment sugars into alcohol and carbon dioxide provides a way to produce leavened bread, which has a light, airy texture because of the carbon dioxide produced. In addition to preserving food, the fermentation process also creates distinctive flavors and aromas that characterize different foods. This critical experience highlights the importance of fungi in food industry and gastronomy, clarifying their various roles in contributing to nutritional value and sensory appeal of the final products. Fungi are also very important in the production of mold-ripened cheeses, where other types of fungi are utilized in developing characteristic flavor and texture. An example is the use of *Penicillium roqueforti* in blue cheese production, which provides it with the characteristic blue veins and odorous flavor.

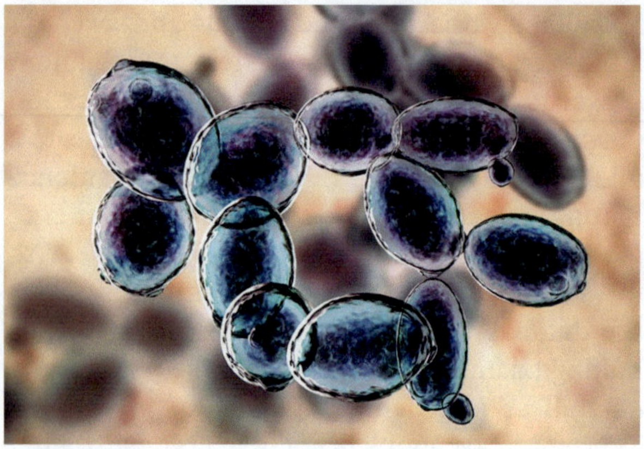

Figure 1.14. Yeasts, a group of fungi, are paramount in the fermentation of various foods and beverages, including bread, beer, and wine.

Source: https://exploreyeast.com/wp-content/uploads/2022/03/Microorganism.jpg.

The enzymatic action of such fungi during aging degrades protein and fat to produce complex flavor profiles highly valued in gourmet cheese. This symbiotic relationship of fungi with food products is one such instance of the sophisticated nature of fungal utilization in food production, highlighting how controlled growth of fungi can lead to culinary innovation. Also, the use of fungi in cheese production not only leads to enhanced flavor but also helps in preservation, highlighting the double-edged benefit of fungi in terms of quality and safety in food production. Apart from fermentation and dairy, fungi are increasingly being viewed to enrich farm process in their role as biofertilizers and nutrient cycling. Certain fungal species, through their establishment of mycorrhizal associations with crops, facilitate increased availability of essential nutrients, i.e., phosphorus. This activity plays a significant role in modern agriculture, given the limited source of phosphate rock, which is a dominant source of phosphorus fertilizers. Research has indicated that saprotrophic fungi can mobilize phosphorus from insoluble sources, thereby contributing to soil fertility and supporting sustainable agricultural practices. Fungi's ability to facilitate nutrient uptake and improve soil health amplifies their significance in food production, illustrating their indispensable role not only in the direct production of food but also in ensuring the growth of food sources through enhanced soil management and resource efficiency. Here, fungi are found to be significant stakeholders in the quest for sustainable food production systems as can be seen from studies confirming the efficacy of various strains of fungi in mobilizing nutrients (Ceci et al., 2017) (Figure 1.14).

1.4.2. Medicinal Uses of Fungi

The history of fungi as a medicinal agent is far-reaching, crossing cultures in which mushrooms and other fungi species have been employed due to their medicinal properties. Most regions have indigenous peoples who have been aware of the medicinal properties of macrofungi since centuries ago. Extensive fieldwork for ethnomycology shows that at least 448 edible mushrooms have been documented, an estimate of how common they are consumed for sustenance, spiritual needs, and medicinal purposes. For instance, fungi like *Ganoderma lucidum* are prized for their immunoenhancing and stress-reducing capacities, a testament to an ancient admiration of fungic value in traditional medicine (Mjaika et al., 2022). Moreover, the diversity of fungal species utilized for medicinal applications reflects a staggering alignment of local knowledge and biodiversity that remains relatively unexploited, emphasizing the necessity of carrying out research on their ecological and pharmacological potentials. In contemporary science, studies of fungi have diversified into pharmacological aspects, leading to numerous fungal derivatives with medical uses. Compounds from fungi such as penicillin in the Penicillium species have revolutionized medicine today. Investigations also indicate that certain fungi possess anti-inflammatory, antioxidant, and anticancer activities, which can be developed for use in drugs. For example, polysaccharides from mushrooms like *Agaricus blazei* have exhibited immunomodulatory activities and have emerged as therapeutic agents of potential interest for complementary cancer therapy (Ndoro et al., 2023). This new school of thinking about fungi not only turns out to be a validation of their customary uses but also opens up possibilities for innovative clinical applications by means of bioprospecting lesser-explored species of fungi, toward reconciling folk remedies with modern medical science. Moreover, the issue of mycotoxin pollution of medicinal fungi is both an opportunity and a challenge to increase safety standards in traditional herbal medicine.

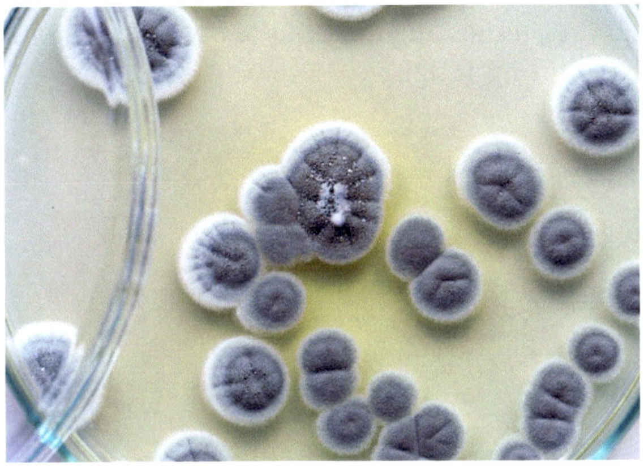

Figure 1.15. Compounds derived from fungi, such as penicillin from Penicillium species, have revolutionized modern medicine.

Source: https://cdn.the-scientist.com/assets/articleNo/72304/aImg/54703/penicillium-jira-2-l.jpg.

Experiments have shown that a large percentage of medicinal plants sold in markets are affected by some fungal species, leading to the production of mycotoxins, which represent gigantic health risks to consumers. For instance, a South African study showed that over 74% of the medicinal plant samples examined had fungi, some that contained toxic mycotoxins in concentrations higher than regulatory levels (Ndoro et al., 2023). This observation necessitates rigorous control of medicinal fungi and fosters the implementation of best practices for their cultivation, production, and trade. Lastly, determination of the safety and efficacy of medicinal fungi through suitable evaluation and adherence to up-to-date health standards is necessary for them to be further applied in health practice (Figure 1.15).

1.4.3. Fungal Pathogens and Diseases

Fungal diseases are a serious issue in agricultural and medical sciences since they result in a broad spectrum of plant and human diseases. Fungal disease can destroy crops in agriculture, leading to heavy economic losses as well as food shortages. Species of genera *Fusarium* and *Alternaria* are well known for their pathogenicity against various plant hosts.

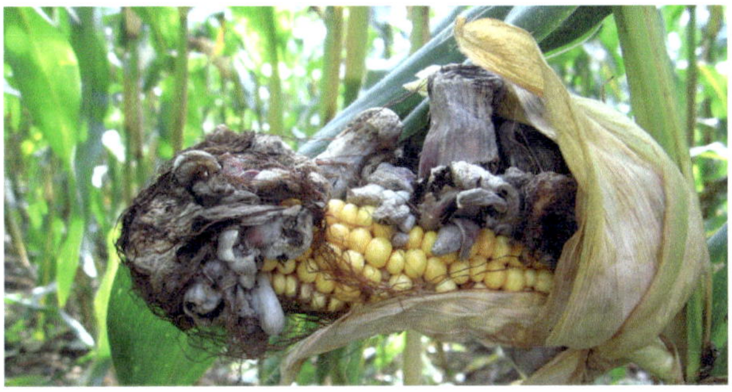

Figure 1.16. Fungal pathogens present a significant challenge in both agricultural and medical fields, as they are responsible for a myriad of diseases affecting plants and humans.

Source: https://www.mpg.de/23579406/header_image-1728982185.jpg?t=eyJ3aWR0aCI6ODQ4LCJmaWxlX2V4dGVuc2lvbiI6ImpwZyIsIm9ial9pZCI6MjM1Nzk0MDZ9--fbf78bb5d9c963c28dc4114fc15f5a43abd7d1df.

These fungi can potentially lead to blight, rot, or wilt, drastically reducing production and affecting the health of the ecosystem. Additionally, studies on antagonistic fungi, such as those in the *Acremonium* genus, have been promising toward biological control methods that can counter these negative effects. Fungal isolation from hosts like *Paspalum dilatatum* indicates potential for the improvement of more environmentally friendly farming methods for fungal pathogen control, reducing the application of chemical methods with harmful environmental implications (Felitti et al., 2017). Within the clinic, fungal pathogens increasingly become an important public health risk, particularly among immunocompromised individuals. Some of the most virulent human pathogens include *Candida* species such as *Candida albicans*, which can form biofilms on medical devices and tissue surfaces. Biofilms make treatment procedures challenging since they are resistant to antifungal medications and need surgery, greatly hindering healthcare systems in terms of finances (Rajendran et al., 2012). The ability of the fungi to avoid immune responses and develop resistance mechanisms underscores the need for new therapeutic modalities. The epidemiology of fungal infections, particularly in high-risk populations, can inform better clinical management and enhanced preventive strategies against fungal infections. Furthermore, the mechanism of interaction between pathogenic fungi and their host is complex and multifaceted. Fungi have a tendency to use various mechanisms for evading host defense, including the formation of biofilms and drug-resistant efflux pumps. For instance, biofilms form a protective matrix that not only shelters fungal cells but also provides difficulty in treatment. The extracellular matrices of fungal infections have been found to be linked with increased virulence and persistence, which makes infections difficult to get rid of. Exploration of such mechanisms is important for developing efficient antifungal drugs and has the potential to revolutionize the management of fungal disease in healthcare settings. As our understanding of these pathogens advances, there is a need to extend investigations into novel solutions that will fight their growing significance as agents of human disease and agricultural production (Rajendran et al., 2012) (Figure 1.16).

1.5. Fungal Diversity

The concept of fungal diversity encompasses a sophisticated matrix of species that contribute not just to biodiversity but also to ecological resilience. There are fungi in every type of ecosystem, from the alpine to the tropical rainforest, with an incredibly diverse set of adaptations that allow them to subsist under a variety of environmental conditions. As an example, recent research has added new species such as *Hebeloma grandisporum* and *H oreophilum*, which now only exist in alpine habitats, indicating the unique ecological niches occupied by fungi.

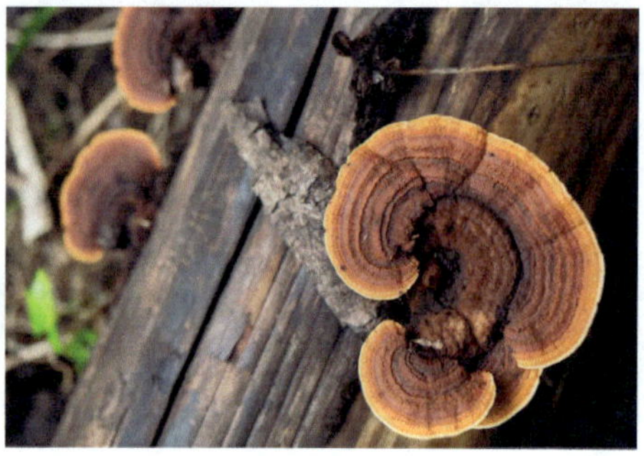

Figure 1.17. Fungi inhabit a variety of ecosystems, from alpine regions to tropical forests, exhibiting a remarkable range of adaptations that allow them to thrive in diverse environmental conditions.

Source: https://www.tigersafariindia.com/blog/wp-content/uploads/2024/07/Fungi-and-its-role-in-environment.jpg.

Moreover, there are several species within the same genus that exist in lowlands or boreal ecosystems, indicating the adaptability and diversity of fungal life forms. This diversity plays critical ecological functions, including nutrient cycling, plant symbiotic relations, and interactions with other microorganisms, thus signifying the importance of conserving fungal biodiversity as ecosystems are under numerous anthropogenic threats. Fungal species taxonomy has proven a challenging feat, driven by longstanding debate and innovation in taxonomic approaches. The Global Consortium for the Classification of Fungi represents a collective endeavor on the part of mycologists worldwide toward a unified framework of perception of the diversity of fungi. It requests input from more than 550 scientists in many fields, and thus creates an electronic database that sets out to revise classifications every two years. By their resolution of contentious issues like the delimitation of species within the genus *Fusarium* and the positioning of 'dark fungal taxa,' this consortium is working towards minimizing variability among scientists and providing stability in the taxonomization of fungi. The dynamism of this endeavor illustrates how various perspectives become aggregations of more encompassing knowledge about the diversity of fungi. Ultimately, the resolution of issues with fungal diversity and classification needs a multidisciplinary approach that takes ecological, genetic, and evolutionary needs into account. With research ongoing to reveal the sheer number of as-yet-unknown species, standardized taxonomy becomes increasingly imperative. Papers published in support of initiatives like the Global Consortium not only enable better classification but also enable better communication between scientists, facilitating collaborations that can accelerate research efforts. Emphasizing strict and ethically appropriate critique in society encourages responsible advancements in classification and creates a better picture of the intricacies of fungal biodiversity. Increasing our understanding of fungi, in this case, means it is critical to advocate for their conservation and research in a manner that their position in ecosystems is realized and preserved for future generations (Figure 1.17).

1.5.1. Overview of Fungal Species

The domain of fungal species is vast and complex, consisting of an humbling amount of diversity that is vital to numerous ecological and biological processes. Fungi are classified into several main groups, including the Ascomycetes, Basidiomycetes, Chytridiomycetes, and Zygomycetes, each characterized by reproductive structures and life cycles that are distinct from the class as a whole. This classification not only reflects their evolutionary past but also accounts for how they interact in ecosystems. For instance, Ascomycetes, or sac fungi, possess a specialized ascus for spore development, making them valuable nutrient cyclers as decomposers in a variety of habitats. Moreover, with advances in molecular techniques, new information has emerged regarding these groupings, revealing the phylogenetic nuances that clean morphological assessments overlook. As a result, contemporary mycology emphasizes the multi-faceted description of fungal diversity by combined employment of scientific techniques (Abarenkov et al., 2013). The incorporation of molecular data into mycology revolutionized fungal species classification and understanding. Application of DNA sequencing technology not only revealed taxonomic relationships but also stressed the sophisticated evolution history of fungal taxa. This molecular method gives a better view of biodiversity since the genetic dissimilarities and similarities in most instances explain relationships that were previously obscure. Using the capability to compare a number of genes, researchers can construct reliable phylogenetic trees that give comprehensive information on how fungi evolved. Adherence to rigorous taxonomic criteria, including ensuring that genera stay monophyletic and adequately supported by enough phylogenetic data, is necessary for the construction of accurate classifications (Ammirati et al., 2015). Thus, the integration of molecular data into mycology is not only a procedural improvement but a paradigm shift that fosters improved understanding of fungal ecology and evolution. When analyzing the ecological importance of fungal species, their diverse roles within symbiotic associations, both pathogenic and beneficial, must be considered.

Mycorrhizal fungi, for example, have symbiotic associations with plant roots, facilitating nutrient uptake and improving plant health. The association is particularly important in soils with limited nutrients, where mycorrhizal webs can greatly augment the productivity of plants. Conversely, there are opportunistic fungi within the fungal group that are pathogenic to plant and animal welfare, for instance, fungi that bring about differing forms of blight in plants or infections in humans. Such duality underscores the importance of acknowledging fungal diversity and extent in ecological studies. Furthermore, studies on the fungal genera are consistently revealing their as yet unrealized potential, for instance, in biotechnology and medicine. By exploiting the unique properties of specific fungi, researchers seek to discover innovative solutions to nature and health challenges, highlighting the indispensable role of fungi in natural and human-dominated ecosystems (Figure 1.18).

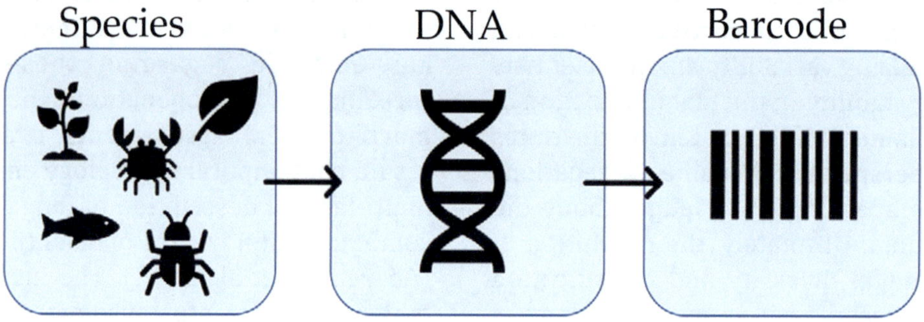

Figure 1.18. Employing DNA sequencing technologies has not only clarified taxonomic relationships but also highlighted the intricate evolutionary lineage of various fungal taxa.

Source: https://upload.wikimedia.org/wikipedia/commons/b/bd/DNA_Barcoding.png.

1.5.2. Unique Adaptations of Fungi

Fungi possess an incredible array of strange adaptations that allow them to live in diverse ecological niches. One of the most intriguing of these adaptations is how they reproduce and can be either sexual or asexual reproduction. For instance, certain species of the genus *Aspergillus*, that is *Aspergillus nidulans*, have been extensively studied due to their complex system of regulation that governs sporulation. It has been studied that while some of the genes that are linked with asexual reproduction are maintained in most fungi, others like BrlA are more restricted, suggesting they have had an intricate evolutionary history influencing their reproductive manner. Such adaptation does not only allow fungi to live under varied environmental conditions but also allows for genetic variation, which is vital for their capacity to endure and adapt in changing environments (Chen et al., 2018). One of the fascinating adaptations exists among the yeast species, that is, in their survival with plants and animals. Yeasts belonging to the Ascomycota and Basidiomycota phyla have evolved to thrive in different environments, like soil and water, which proves their evolutionary acumen. Their unicellular or hyphal form of growth provides flexibility in adaptation to nutrient availability and environmental pressures, which is a prerequisite in competitive environments. Yeast species such as *Saccharomyces cerevisiae* are significant in human business, showing the potential to exploit resources for fermentation.

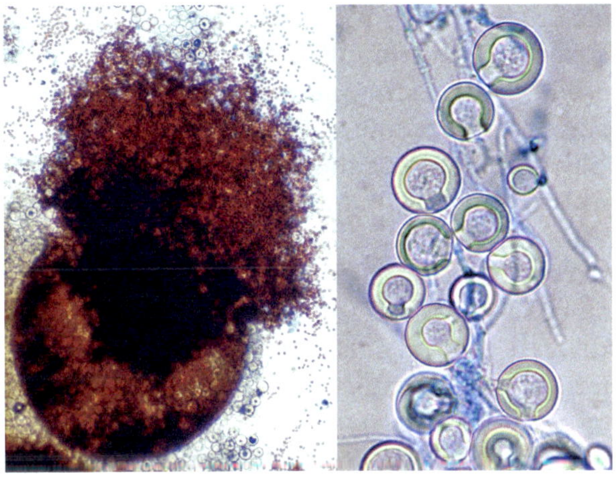

Figure 1.19. Certain species within the genus *Aspergillus*, such as *Aspergillus nidulans*, have been extensively studied for their complex regulatory mechanisms governing sporulation.

Source: https://www.adelaide.edu.au/mycology/sites/default/files/media/images/2021-09/asp-nid-micro1.jpg.

This survival is facilitated by the ability to support not only their existence but also shows the immense impact fungi have on human health and business, further showing how vital they are in the fungus community (Lachance et al., 2018). In addition to ecological and reproductive processes, metabolic flexibility in fungi emphasizes their unique evolutionary processes. Fungi are marked by the ability to break down complex organic matter, a feature that makes them central players in the nutrient cycle in ecosystems. Their enzymatic processes, particularly in lignin and cellulose breakdown, allow them to break down plant material for the sake of ecosystem sustainability. This adaptability not only enhances the quality of the soil but also assists in the growth of other organisms within their environment. Furthermore, some fungi have developed symbiotic relationships, such as mycorrhizae, that give plants more nutrient uptake in exchange for carbohydrates. These reliance illustrate the intricate adaptations that fungi have developed to maximize their ecological roles and show their significance in the facilitation of ecological balance (Chen et al., 2018) (Figure 1.19).

1.5.3. Geographic Distribution of Fungi

Geographic distribution of fungi is a complex tapestry, a rich brocade of numerous ecological, climatic, and anthropogenic influences. Fungi inhabit innumerable environments, from ocean bottom to mountaintops, an extraordinary degree of versatility. Current evidence emphasizes that some species of fungi are not randomly distributed; instead, they have varying appetites for particular ecosystems. For instance, the pathogen *Calonectria pauciramosa* illustrates the point by infecting thousands of plant hosts globally. In studies of this fungus, geographically diverse isolates have exhibited unique morphological and genetic traits, and therefore various cryptic species across various regions have been found (Altschul et al., 2010). This indicates how localized the conditions are to mold fungal diversity and distribution. Interpreting these patterns is significant in mycology because they affect biodiversity conservation and plant pathology, ultimately mirroring the intricate interactions between fungi and their environments. In geographic distribution, scientists also employ molecular methods to separate fungal species and their relationships. Phylogenetic investigations on fungi not just aid in following their evolutionary history but also show how geographical barriers restrict gene flow and impact rates of speciation. To provide an example, research on *Calonectria pauciramosa* identified three new species—*Ca. colombiana* sp. nov., *Ca. polizzii* sp. nov., and *Ca. zuluensis* sp. nov.—through comprehensive genetic testing. This research aims to put more emphasis on the need for broad geographic distribution and robust phylogenetic backbones in understanding fungal classification (Altschul et al., 2010). The discovery of the cryptic species underscores the importance of considering both morphological traits and molecular data in taxonomic studies. Such methods allow mycologists to gain a better understanding of how geographic distribution contributes to fungal diversity and ecological roles in various habitats. Besides, the procedure for adding new genera to mycology indicates the significance of rigorous scientific procedure in the documentation of fungal diversity. New recognized taxa must be monophyletic, and their phylogenetic trees should be highly supported statistically. This rigorous protocol ensures that geographic location, number of species collected, and genetic evidence are adequately covered. As scientists venture into the geographic distribution of fungi, adhering to these standards will ensure an improved knowledge of their world diversity. In the case of conservation and ecosystem maintenance, a knowledge of the interrelationships and spreads of fungi can be critical to preserving biodiversity. Through all-encompassing research techniques, mycologists can contribute valuable information to the role fungi play in their ecosystems and the overall biosphere (Figure 1.20).

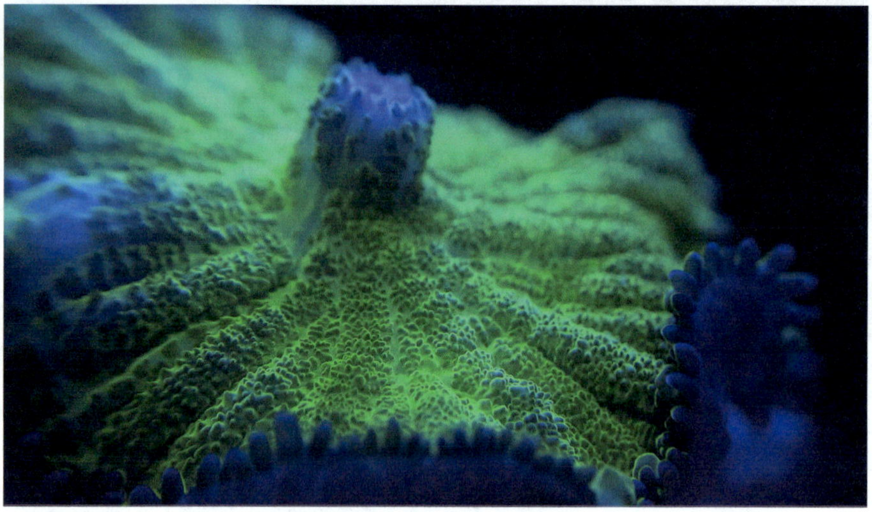

Figure 1.20. Fungi inhabit myriad environments, ranging from the deepest oceans to the highest mountains, showcasing extraordinary adaptability.

Source: https://gumlet.assettype.com/downtoearth%2F2025-01-06%2Fb5ht521v%2FFungi?format=auto.

SUMMARY

Mycology, the science of fungi, includes a great field of biological sciences, namely understanding biodiversity and ecosystem processes. One fundamental fact in this science is a sensing regularly overlooked diversity of fungi. Advanced innovations in molecular analysis have made visible the discrepancies between morphological classifications and genetic data. Specifically, studies have shown that traditional methods tend to underreport the diversity of fungal species to be encountered in various environments, showing the pressing need for DNA-based identification methods. This change of outlook points to the importance of quantifying fungal diversity accurately because DNA sequence data can enable more efficient taxonomic solutions valuable in ecological and conservation applications (Abarenkov et al., 2014). Improving our understanding of the diversity of fungi is the foundation of many applications ranging from agriculture to medicine, illustrating mycology's broader contribution to society. In addition, the addition of molecular information to the study of fungi has profoundly transformed methods across the field. The last two decades have witnessed rapid growth in the use of DNA sequencing technology in fungal systematics, taxonomy, and ecology (Abarenkov et al., 2013). This development is a departure from the traditional morphological studies in which scientists were able to conduct more rigorous and precise classifications. The taxonomic process currently comprises extensive stages like taxon sampling, lab training, and data analysis, all of which considerably influence research findings and interpretation. Using molecular techniques, mycologists are able to uncover genetic relationships that account for evolutionary processes and ecological patterns among fungi. This transition towards molecular approaches assists in standardizing the taxonomy practices, thereby contributing to a more unified approach towards comprehension of fungal kingdoms and their roles in the environment. With further progress in the field of mycology, the need for high standards and well-curated reference databases continues to increase. Availability of good-quality DNA sequence data continues to remain imperative, especially as the discipline is witnessing increased interfacing with molecular ecology and microbiome research. Development of quality-controlled databases, such as the RefSeq Targeted Loci (RTL) database, is a manifestation of efforts extended to improve the identification processes of fungi to provide robust reference sequences assembled from type specimens (Abarenkov et al., 2014). Moreover, development of standards for improved quality data needs to be done to ensure effective species assignments in subsequent research. This ongoing commitment to advancing taxonomic approaches, as well as value for molecular approaches, equips new scientists with the information and seasoned scientists with the instruments needed to advance the field of mycology, and thus improve comprehensive knowledge of fungal diversity and its relevance to ecology (Abarenkov et al., 2013).

A CLOSER LOOK

TAXONOMY

Taxonomy is the scientific procedure for classifying living organisms into a series of hierarchical groups based on shared characteristics and evolutionary relationships. Taxonomy helps scientists assemble and interpret the incredibly rich variety of life on Earth. The main ranks used in taxonomy are domain, kingdom, phylum, class, order, family, genus, and species. Taxonomy was devised by Carl Linnaeus and uses the system of binomial nomenclature, where each species has a two-word Latin name (genus and species). Taxonomy plays a crucial role in biology, ecology, and conservation as it provides a shared terminology for the identification and description of organisms.

REFERENCES

1. Aanderud, Z. T., Kurbessoian, T., Lewis, L. A., Pombubpa, R., et al. (2019). Reproduction and dispersal of biological soil crust organisms. https://core.ac.uk/download/250588058.pdf (accessed on 27th June 2025).
2. Aaronson, M., Abdel-Azeem, A., Adhikari, A., Adhikari, B., Adl, S., Afyon, A., Al-Naama, M., et al. (2016). The numbers behind mushroom biodiversity. https://core.ac.uk/download/153416631.pdf (accessed on 27th June 2025).
3. Abarenkov, K., Aime, M. C., Ariyawansa, H. A., Bidartondo, M. I., et al. (2014). Finding needles in haystacks: Linking scientific names, reference specimens and molecular data for *Fungi*. https://core.ac.uk/download/77019459.pdf (accessed on 27th June 2025).
4. Abarenkov, K., Bertrand, Y. J. K., Hartmann, M., Hyde, K. D., et al. (2013). Incorporating molecular data in fungal systematics: A guide for aspiring researchers. https://arxiv.org/abs/1302.3244 (accessed on 27th June 2025).
5. Abdel-Wahab, M. A., Abdollahzadeh, J., Abeywickrama, P. D., Absalan, F., et al. (2023). Global consortium for the classification of fungi and fungus-like taxa. https://core.ac.uk/download/614350379.pdf (accessed on 27th June 2025).
6. Aguilar-Trigueros, C. A., Bielčik, M., Jeltsch, F., Lakovic, M., et al. (2019). The role of active movement in fungal ecology and community assembly. https://core.ac.uk/download/288114255.pdf (accessed on 27th June 2025).
7. Alastruey-Izquierdo, A., Giraldo, A., Alper, B., Altschul, S., de Azevedo Melo, A. S., Nishikaku, A. S., Normand, A. C., et al. (2015). International Society of Human and Animal Mycology (ISHAM)-ITS reference DNA barcoding database–The quality controlled standard tool for routine identification of human and animal pathogenic fungi. https://core.ac.uk/download/154274446.pdf (accessed on 27th June 2025).
8. Alder-Rangel, A., Bailão, A. M., Bertolini, M. C., Bonatto, D., et al. (2018). The second International Symposium on Fungal Stress: ISFUS. https://core.ac.uk/download/155786971.pdf (accessed on 27th June 2025).
9. Altschul, S. F., Wingfield, M. J., Carbone, I., Crous, P. W., Crous, J. W., Crous, M. J., Crous, A. J., et al. (2010). Multigene phylogeny and mating tests reveal three cryptic species related to *Calonectria pauciramosa*. https://core.ac.uk/download/pdf/29241912.pdf (accessed on 27th June 2025).
10. Ammirati, J. F., Desjardin, D. E., Halling, R. E., Justo, A., et al. (2015). Six simple guidelines for introducing new genera of fungi. https://core.ac.uk/download/55848430.pdf (accessed on 27th June 2025).
11. Amor, A., Ben Daoud, S., Brouwer, C., Cardinali, G., et al. (2013). MycoBank gearing up for new horizons. https://core.ac.uk/download/323080827.pdf (accessed on 27th June 2025).
12. Andrews, A. A., Arnold, A. E., Arnold, R. J., Monzón, A., Askary, H., Audoin, B., et al. (2009). Fungal entomopathogens: New insights on their ecology. https://core.ac.uk/download/47433.pdf (accessed on 27th June 2025).
13. Arastehfar, A., Boekhout, T., Buda De Cesare, G., Butler, G., et al. (2019). Recent trends in molecular diagnostics of yeast infections: From PCR to NGS. https://core.ac.uk/download/286086540.pdf (accessed on 27th June 2025).

14. Barron, E. S., Boddy, L., Dahlberg, A., Griffith, G. W., et al. (2014). A fungal perspective on conservation biology. https://core.ac.uk/download/326666479.pdf (accessed on 27th June 2025).

15. Beker, H. J., Eberhardt, U., Ronikier, A., Schütz, N., et al. (2015). The genus *Hebeloma* in the alpine belt of the Carpathians including two new species. https://core.ac.uk/download/55765041.pdf (accessed on 27th June 2025).

16. Boswell, D. L., Carlile, M. J., Daniel, J. M., Deacon, J. W., Deak, T., Falconer, J., Feldmann, H., et al. (2017). Introduction to fungal physiology. https://core.ac.uk/download/228177974.pdf (accessed on 27th June 2025).

17. Ceci, A., Maggi, O., Persiani, A. M., Pinzari, F., et al. (2017). Saprotrophic soil fungi to improve phosphorus solubilization and release. *In vitro* abilities of several species. https://core.ac.uk/download/98345967.pdf (accessed on 27th June 2025).

18. Chen, W., Cánovas López, D., Dyer, P. S., Eagle, C. E., et al. (2018). Evolution of asexual and sexual reproduction in the *aspergilli*. https://core.ac.uk/download/185608248.pdf (accessed on 27th June 2025).

19. Chotirmall, S. H., Greene, C. M., & McElvaney, N. G. (2010). *Candida* species in cystic fibrosis: A road less travelled. https://core.ac.uk/download/pdf/60775446.pdf (accessed on 27th June 2025).

20. Dominici, L., Irga, P. J., & Torpy, F. R. (2020). The mycological social network: A way forward for conservation of fungal biodiversity. https://opus.lib.uts.edu.au/bitstream/10453/144033/2/b9f2b85e-8206-483b-a3b5-3502c8df5ef6.pdf (accessed on 27th June 2025).

21. Felitti, S. A., García Lemos, A., Gil Cardeza, M. L., Gomez, M. A., et al. (2017). Fungal endophytes in species of *Paspalum* and *Bromus*, occurrence and *in vitro* antagonistic activity assessment. https://core.ac.uk/download/224999098.pdf (accessed on 27th June 2025).

22. Fonseca, M. I., Levin, L. N., Sadañoski, M. A., Velázquez, M. S., et al. (2018). Assessing the ability of white-rot fungi to tolerate polychlorinated biphenyls using predictive mycology. https://core.ac.uk/download/287882473.pdf (accessed on 27th June 2025).

23. Homei, A., & Worboys, M. (2020). Chapter introduction. https://core.ac.uk/download/478128193.pdf (accessed on 27th June 2025).

24. Lachance, M. A., & Walker, G. M. (2018). *Yeasts*. https://core.ac.uk/download/237029612.pdf (accessed on 27th June 2025).

25. Mjaika, N. E. (2022). A systematic review of biodiversity and conservation of indigenous mushrooms (*Basidiomycotina, Ascomycotina*) of Central Africa countryside: Uses, distribution and checklists. https://core.ac.uk/download/524153452.pdf (accessed on 27th June 2025).

26. Ndoro, J. (2023). Mycotoxigenic fungi and multimycotoxin contamination in medicinal plants sold in the Free State Province, South Africa. https://core.ac.uk/download/616422430.pdf (accessed on 27th June 2025).

27. Nozawa, Y. (2025). Structure and functions of fungal cell surfaces. https://core.ac.uk/download/pdf/42846845.pdf (accessed on 27th June 2025).

28. O'Callahan, D. R. (2012). Isolation and characterization of bacterial metabolites as potential wood preservatives. https://core.ac.uk/download/29199753.pdf (accessed on 27th June 2025).

29. Rajendran, R., Ramage, G., Sherry, L., Williams, C., et al. (2012). Fungal biofilm resistance. https://core.ac.uk/download/9650980.pdf (accessed on 27th June 2025).

30. Sánchez Castro, I., & Wijayawardene, N. N. (2021). Current insight into culture-dependent and culture-independent methods in discovering ascomycetous taxa. https://core.ac.uk/download/483743957.pdf (accessed on 27th June 2025).

31. Simmons, E. G. (2010). The International Mycological Association: Its history in brief with summaries of its International Mycological Congresses and diverse international relationships. https://core.ac.uk/download/pdf/8722428.pdf (accessed on 27th June 2025).

32. Victoroff, C. (2020). Response of ectomycorrhizal fungal fruiting to nitrogen and phosphorus additions in Bartlett Experimental Forest, New Hampshire. https://core.ac.uk/download/389009727.pdf (accessed on 27th June 2025).

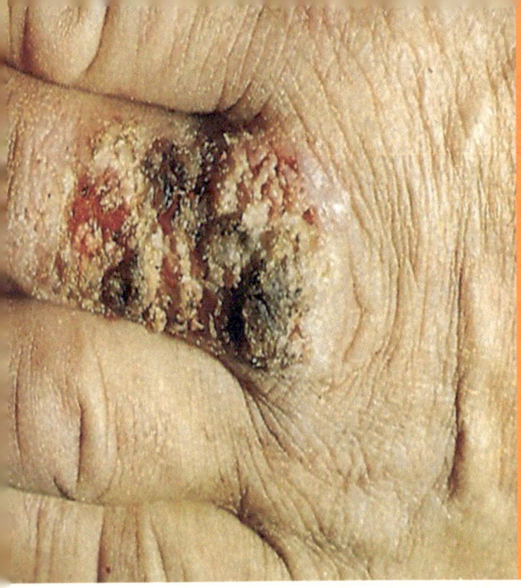

Chapter 2

LABORATORY DIAGNOSIS OF FUNGAL INFECTION

Contents

Introduction

The increased frequency of fungal infections has emerged as a significant public health concern, with the emphasis especially being on accurate laboratory diagnosis. Fungi that were once considered to be non-pathogenic opportunistic pathogens have now become leading causes of morbidity and mortality, most notably in immunocompromised individuals. The challenges in diagnosing these infections lead to mismanagement and ineffective therapy, primarily in resource-constrained regions where common syndromes like fever are often misdiagnosed. For instance, studies documented that malaria was profoundly over-diagnosed in febrile patients, but fungal infections, among other invasive infections, were under-estimated and mostly overlooked during the workup of patients (Bouley et al., 2013). Thus, extensive laboratory testing and advanced diagnostic modalities are required for early identification of fungal pathogens and appropriate therapeutic measures. In the growth of the science of fungal diagnosis, the use of molecular technologies has significantly enhanced the detection and identification of the exact species of fungus. The older methods, while helpful, may be less specific or sensitive and consequently result in an important percentage of undiagnosed infections. More contemporary research employing advanced techniques, such as quantitative polymerase chain reaction (QPCR), enables accurate detection of fungi from clinical samples, thereby their clinical importance in disease pathology (Goldberg et al., 2006). Apart from improved diagnostic sensitivity, these techniques also provide a better understanding of the clinical importance of various fungal species.

Such innovations mean that laboratories have to develop and incorporate newer diagnostic equipment and techniques to meet the growing challenge of managing fungal infections and significantly better patient outcomes. In addition, knowing the clinical significance of fungal infections involves more than just identification; it includes the realization of their effect on patient quality of life. The relationship of fungal presence to disease severity is still an active area of investigation, with research demonstrating that chronic fungal illness can have a detrimental impact on individual health (Goldberg et al., 2006).

Most recent evidence points towards patients with chronic rhinosinusitis having a significant difference in quality-of-life measurements compared with controls, while the direct cause-and-effect relationships for certain fungal species are yet to be investigated (Goldberg et al., 2006). Thus, laboratory diagnosis must not just aim to identify the pathogen but also remember the overall background of health implications determined by these infections. A multi-faceted approach that combines accurate diagnostics with understanding of clinical connotations will play a pivotal role in combating the swelling tide of fungal infections across various populations (Figure 2.1).

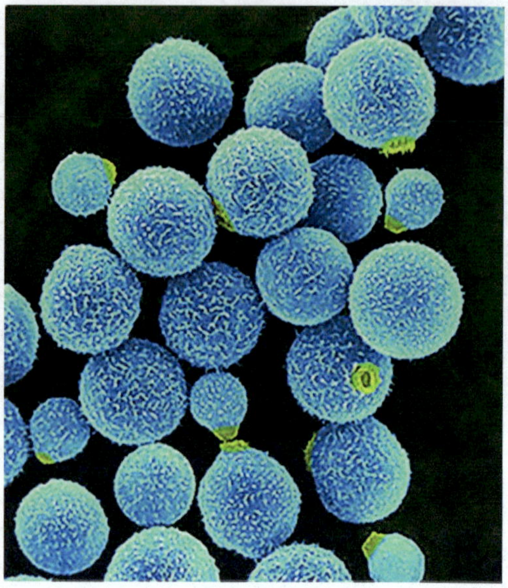

Figure 2.1. The correlation between fungal presence and disease severity remains an area of active research, with studies indicating that chronic fungal diseases can negatively affect individual well-being.

Source: https://www.ncbi.nlm.nih.gov/books/NBK549988/bin/AAMCol.18Oct.2017.fig09.jpg.

2.1. Types of Fungal Infections

Fungal infections are classified into various categories based largely on the route of infection and pathotype. The four most frequent are superficial, cutaneous, subcutaneous, and systemic infections. Super fungal infections, such as those due to *Candida* or *Malassezia,* primarily affect the skin, hair, and mucous membrane and include conditions like athletes foot or thrush. These infections, while irritating, can frequently be successfully treated with topical antifungals. Cutaneous infections, on the other hand, invade deeper into the dermal tissue, typically the fungi such as Dermatophytes, leading to more invasive dermatologic symptomatology and typically necessitating systemic therapy. Determination of the infection nature is significant in the establishment of laboratory diagnosis and follow-up treatment. Subcutaneous mycoses are due to the invasion of fungi into the skin following injury or trauma. The fungi involved, such as *Sporothrix* and *Coccidioides*, are capable of producing chronic localized infection and therefore necessitate early diagnosis. Diagnosis of subcutaneous infection is done in the laboratory using culture and histopathology of infected tissue. The challenge lies in the differentiation of subcutaneous infection from bacterial infections, which present similarly. Diagnostic methods, including serological and imaging diagnostic tests, can augment the traditional culture techniques and facilitate better detection of specific fungal pathogens. Better laboratory practices can make a significant contribution to treatment, and thus the need for rapid identification of pathogens in clinical practice is essential. Systemic infections caused by fungi, as compared to their subcutaneous and superficial counterparts, are a grave threat, particularly to immunocompromised individuals. Pathogens such as *Aspergillus* and Histoplasma may disseminate throughout the body, causing widespread complications in a majority of instances and requiring aggressive treatment. Diagnostic challenges are the norm, as standard culture methods are not always capable of yielding timely information, as evidenced by research that has assessed the value of biomarkers such as cerebrospinal fluid (CSF) (1,3)-β-d-glucan for diagnosing Histoplasma meningitis, where sensitivity and specificity in clinical decision-making are of the utmost importance (Albers et al., 2018). Moreover, the advent of opportunistic yeasts indicates towards an inevitable need for better laboratory diagnostic techniques. Evolution in technologies like high-throughput sequencing and proteomics is expected to offer windows for the rapid identification and susceptibility profiling of fungal pathogens (Arastehfar et al., 2019). Such advancements are imperative in controlling the rising threat of systemic fungal infections and delivering better patient care in a clinical setting (Figure 2.2).

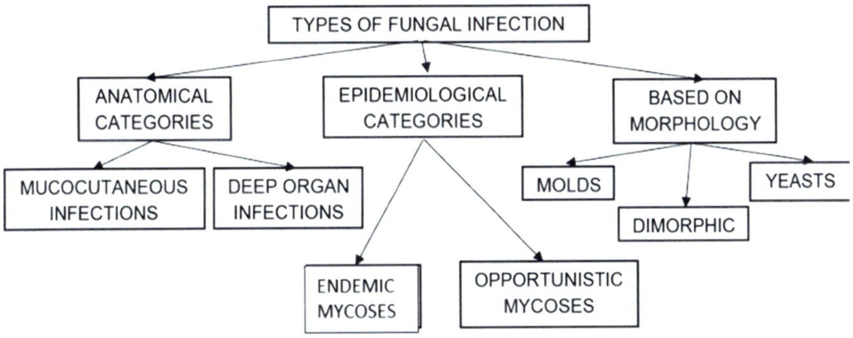

Figure 2.2. Fungal infections are classified into several categories, primarily based on the route of transmission and the nature of the pathogens involved.

Source: https://www.ncbi.nlm.nih.gov/sites/books/NBK572246/bin/trop_fungi_endo_dys-Image001.jpg.

2.1.1. Superficial Fungal Infections

Superficial mycoses, involving mostly the skin, hair, and nails, constitute a significant part of cutaneous conditions that need specific laboratory diagnosis to ensure therapeutic success. Dermatophytes, yeasts, and non-dermatophyte molds are the most common etiological agents for such infections with examples including tinea pedis, onychomycosis, and candidiasis. Because of the variety of fungal causes, clinical findings alone may not be sufficient to establish a diagnosis with certainty. Long-term diagnostic approaches are in order since overlap of symptoms among various fungi can lead to suboptimal treatment in the event of misdiagnosis. The impact of such infections extends beyond physical discomfort since they have an immense effect on the quality of life as well as on the psychological status of individuals, hence the need for quick and accurate laboratory identification of the causative fungal pathogens (Arabatzis et al., 2019). Traditional direct microscopy and culture remain the gold standards for the diagnosis of superficial fungal infections in the conventional sense. Microscopic visualization allows the identification of fungal elements in clinical specimens, facilitating early diagnosis and proper therapy. Even though culture methods provide final species identification, these take time and involve special environmental controls for fungal growth. Recent advances in molecular diagnostic techniques have further transformed the area of mycological diagnostics. These methods yield high-specificity, rapid identification of fungal species and allow clinicians to accurately tailor their treatment regimens accordingly. Such advancements notwithstanding, accessibility could vary with different practices in that molecular methods are not equally accessible to all medical personnel. The variability in practice in diagnosis underscores the necessity for continuous education and distribution of resources in order to deliver comprehensive mycological care (Pietro et al., 2014). The shift of laboratory methods to clinic practice has revealed different preferences among dermatologists for diagnostic approaches of superficial fungal infections. A study of specialists in recent years indicated that a vast majority stress the use of direct microscopy with clinical examinations while diagnosing and treating fungal illnesses. This is a reflection of the assumed efficacy of traditional methods coupled with contemporary practice, a validation of the value of a multidisciplinary diagnosis. Dermatologists attach great importance to the requirement for a mycological diagnosis before the institution of systemic antifungal therapy, especially in the context of the risk of antifungal resistance and varying sensitivities of various groups of fungi. Such meticulous attention to the diagnostic process not only enhances the effectiveness of treatment but also with the eventual goal of minimizing patient suffering from superficial fungal infections (Arabatzis et al., 2019) (Figure 2.3).

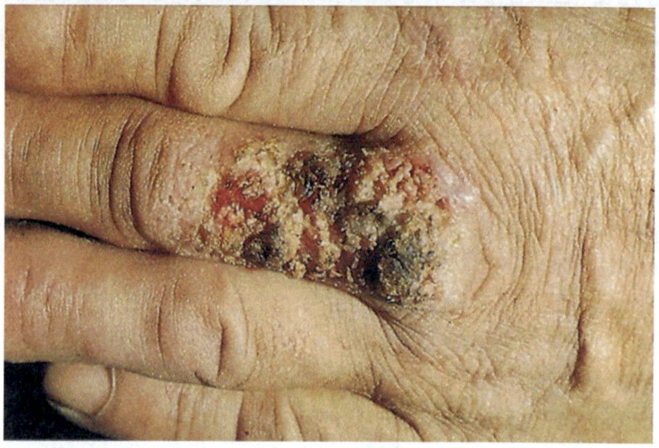

Figure 2.3. Superficial fungal infections, which primarily affect the skin, hair, and nails, represent a significant aspect of dermatological conditions that necessitate accurate laboratory diagnosis for effective treatment.

Source: https://media.springernature.com/lw685/springer-static/image/chp%3A10.1007%2F978-3-662-63709-8_16/MediaObjects/479707_4_En_16_Fig29_HTML.jpg.

2.1.2. Systemic Fungal Infections

The establishment of systemic mycotic infections is a prevalent issue in clinical microbiology, particularly in immunocompromised populations. They most commonly occur with opportunistic pathogens such as *Candida* species, *Aspergillus* species, and *Cryptococcus neoformans*, which can thrive in hosts whose immune defenses are compromised due to underlying disease or treatment. Such infections are diagnosed with heightened suspicion for clinical findings, patient history, and laboratory findings. Laboratory diagnosis plays an important role in the diagnosis, with different techniques like culture, serology, and molecular techniques being employed to detect these fungi. The identification has to be accurate since misdiagnosis might lead to inappropriate treatment, which would aggravate the patient's condition. Laboratory diagnosis for other systemic fungal infections has become advanced with advanced molecular techniques being used, enhancing efficiency and accuracy in the detection of pathogens. Methods such as polymerase chain reaction (PCR) and next-generation sequencing (NGS) enable rapid identification of fungal species from clinical specimens. Not only do these reduce the time to result but also enable one to observe the mechanisms of antifungal resistance, which results in more personalized treatment strategies. In addition, serological assays for single antigens or antibodies play an essential role in diagnosing infections like histoplasmosis and coccidioidomycosis, thus also showing the multi-faceted laboratory methods used in the management of systemic fungal infections. The application of these diagnostic technologies together is essential in improving patient outcomes and lowering morbidity from these infections. The systematic analysis and risk factors of systemic fungal infections should be known in order to implement effective diagnostic methods. Certain populations of patients, including those undergoing hematopoietic stem cell transplantation or major trauma, are particularly at risk for invasive fungal infections. Identification of these risk factors aids in early diagnosis and prompts the clinician to request suitable diagnostic workup, thereby reducing the incidence of major complications. Furthermore, allocation of resources to laboratory diagnosis in endemic areas is significant, as observed by rising post-traumatic invasive fungal infections, particularly in the military and civilian populations. More surveillance and investigation, as noted by recent studies, underscore the importance of realizing the different character of these infections and modifying laboratory techniques correspondingly in an effort to improve the diagnostic process for systemic fungal infections (Bochicchio et al., 2017; Pietro et al., 2014) (Figure 2.4).

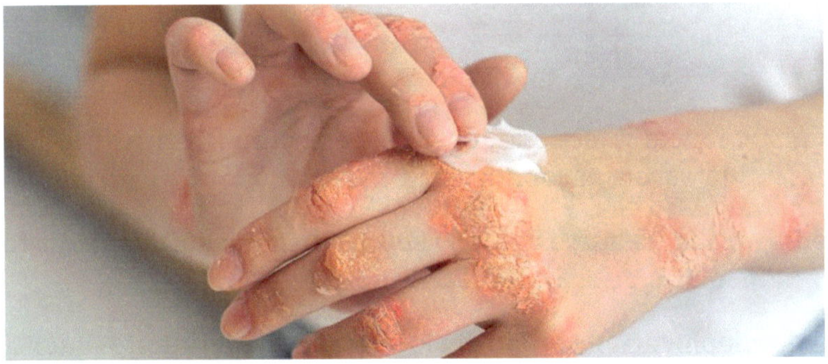

Figure 2.4. Systemic fungal infections.

Source: https://max-website20-images.s3.ap-south-1.amazonaws.com/Fungal_Infections_d0e2344c5a.jpg.

2.1.3. Opportunistic Fungal Infections

Opportunistic fungal infections have dire risk to immunocompromised hosts and often lead to extreme morbidity and mortality. Opportunistic infections result primarily from pathogens that do not typically infect healthy individuals with intact immune systems, such as *Candida*, *Aspergillus*, and *Cryptococcus* species. The increased prevalence of such infections may be attributed to a variety of factors, including the number of patients exposed to immunosuppressive therapy, the number of patients infected with HIV/AIDS, and advances in transplant medicine. Complexity in diagnosing opportunistic fungal infections arises from the diversity and variety of pathogenic species, and this complicates the process of interpreting laboratory results. Hence, it is necessary that the healthcare professionals are vigilant and well-equipped with proper diagnostic techniques so that proper and timely care can be delivered to infected patients. Traditional diagnosis of opportunistic fungal infections relies primarily on culture-based tests, which, although widely practiced, may take time and are usually less sensitive or specific. Organism culture typically involves prior identification of the offending species, which may result in delays in clinical decision-making and therapy.

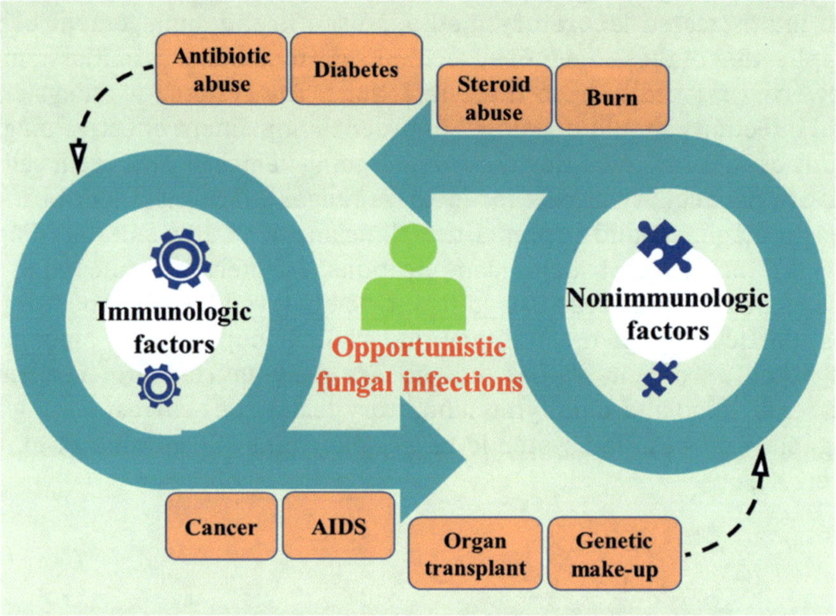

Figure 2.5. Opportunistic fungal infections represent a significant threat to immunocompromised individuals, often leading to severe morbidity and mortality.

Source: https://media.springernature.com/lw1200/springer-static/image/art%3A10.1007%2Fs12010-022-03979-5/MediaObjects/12010_2022_3979_Fig1_HTML.png.

Recent technological developments in the lab, including next-generation sequencing and proteomics, are promising alternatives to conventional diagnostics. These high-throughput methods should be capable of detecting more accurately and quickly fungal pathogens with the potential to initiate treatment earlier. Moreover, they also have the ability to screen the infecting strains for drug susceptibility simultaneously—a feature that grows more significant since antifungal resistance is fast becoming a more pressing concern in the clinic. Progress in these domains is, therefore, central to improving patient outcomes and combat the rising trend in opportunistic infections (Arastehfar et al., 2019). Although promising progress has been reported in diagnostic technologies, significant challenges remain to realize the transition of these methods from bench to bedside. The accompanying cost of more sophisticated laboratory techniques, such as the need for specialized facilities and training, can be a point of limitation towards widespread usage. Moreover, variation in performance in tests among laboratories has the potential to create disparities between diagnosis and diagnostic results, further making clinical management complicated. Having standardized protocols that integrate new diagnostic tools into routine laboratory protocols is crucial to their solution. Ongoing research efforts aimed at streamlining such methodologies and ensuring their dependability will be critical to the fine-tuning of early detection and treatment of opportunistic fungal infections. As the science increases, the future will be predominantly based on collaboration between clinical microbiologists, immunologists, and healthcare clinicians to raise our awareness and management of such potentially life-threatening infections in vulnerable populations (Pietro et al., 2014) (Figure 2.5).

2.2. Common Fungal Pathogens

The fungal pathogen community is wide, comprising an array of species that have the ability to cause serious infections in predominantly immunocompromised individuals. Among the most common is *Candida* spp., a genus that possesses opportunistic infections, the majority of them being mucosal or in the bloodstream. *Aspergillus* spp. is another critical one, its diseases being aspergillosis, where it is found in immunocompromised individuals or those with pulmonary chronic illnesses. The increase in these fungal infections is mirroring growing numbers of vulnerable populations, including individuals with organ transplants or unknown HIV infection. With growing rates of these infections, so does the demand for accurate laboratory diagnosis since knowing the etiologic agent is critical to formulate proper treatment and counteract rising trends of antifungal resistance. Over the past few years, advances in technology have revolutionized laboratory diagnosis of fungal infections, and notably with incorporation of molecular techniques. Conventional diagnostic techniques, based mainly on culture techniques, tend to produce delayed turnaround times and are also known to be unsuccessful in detecting some pathogens owing to their slow growth or unusual presentations. Sophisticated high-throughput technologies such as next-generation sequencing (NGS) are now invaluable tools with their ability to deliver rapid and accurate identification of a wide range of fungal pathogens directly from clinical specimens. Clinical metagenomic next-generation sequencing (mNGS) makes it possible for comprehensive searching of microbial but also host genetic material, significantly increasing the diagnostic capabilities of clinical laboratories. Though these methods have great potential, challenges are still faced regarding implementation, validation, and integration into existing diagnostics protocols that need to be addressed in order to enhance their use in clinical practice for identification of fungal pathogens (Chiu et al., 2019). Beyond molecular methods, the need to detect rapid antifungal resistance profiles is becoming more urgent as resistant strains continue to gain prominence among common fungal pathogens. Specifically, patterns of resistance in some such species as *Candida auris* and certain *Aspergillus* spp. have rung alarm bells in the healthcare industry. Conventional susceptibility testing can be sluggish with the necessity for other methods for immediate results. Innovative methods that track gene markers for resistance and create new phenotypic assays are the mainstay to staying ahead of this burgeoning requirement. High-throughput technologies, as reviewed in some recent reviews, are paving the way for greater sensitivity, precision, and pace in the detection of pathogens and susceptibility testing (Arastehfar et al., 2019). This shift in diagnostic paradigms not only allows for better patient outcomes but also affects broader public health concerns of emerging resistance in fungi (Figure 2.6).

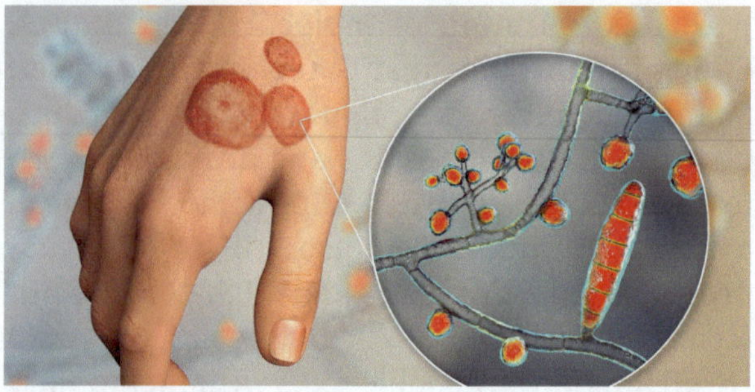

Figure 2.6. Common fungal pathogens.

Source: https://images.theconversation.com/files/533284/original/file-20230621-19-utzvta.jpg?ixlib=rb-4.1.0&rect=0%2C422%2C7234%2C3611&q=45&auto=format&w=1356&h=668&fit=crop.

2.2.1. Candida Species

The *Candida* genus comprises various species of yeasts, and among them, some are human pathogens. The most commonly known organism of them is *Candida albicans*, but *Candida glabrata* and *Candida tropicalis* are progressively being implicated in clinical infections. The diversity table of the species in the *Candida* genus compels diagnosis and treatment to be challenging because not all species respond similarly to antifungal treatments.

The development of opportunistic infections by these yeasts has, in some measure, been caused by improvements in medical technology, particularly in the case of immunocompromised individuals. Expertise in absolutely deciding on the specific *Candida* species involved in an infection is a dependence upon a variety of laboratory techniques that can lead to inconsistency in diagnostic findings. Laboratory scientists must get around the fine pathology of fungal diagnosis, seeking precision in the identification of the etiologic agent in an effort to guide effective management. Contemporary laboratory diagnosis of *Candida* infection is hampered by the traditional methods of culture and biochemical identification, which are time-consuming and not typically specific. Current diagnostic methods may entail prolonged culturing processes that delay timely treatment, thus allowing the infections to progress and make it difficult to manage patients. Rapid diagnostic tests are needed due to the dynamic change in resistance patterns among the *Candida* species, especially with rising instances of antifungal resistance as cited in contemporary literature. For example, most of the *Candida* species have been found to be differentially sensitive to antifungal drugs, which has a significant impact on the treatment. As (Arastehfar et al., 2019) showcases, advancements in high-throughput technologies such as next-generation sequencing and proteomics provide promising lines of enhancing sensitivity and specificity in diagnosis. However, the adoption of such sophisticated methods into routine clinical practice remains daunting logistical and technical challenges. In addition to species identification, antifungal susceptibility testing is also critical in the successful management of *Candida* infection. Heterogeneity in antifungal resistance among species necessitates routine susceptibility testing. As a case in point, as can be observed with the case of *C. tropicalis* infection previously treated with voriconazole, early therapeutic outcome may fail due to the occurrence of resistant strains and biofilm development resulting in treatment failure (Brunetti et al., 2016). This shows the need for ongoing surveillance of antifungal susceptibility, particularly when biofilms are suspected of disrupting treatment efficacy. Furthermore, laboratory markers like 1,3-β-D-glucan can also serve as adjuvant diagnostic and prognostic tools in fungal infection. The interaction between correct diagnosis and proper treatment highlights the critical function that laboratory diagnostics have in the management of invasive candidiasis, and thus timely identification and susceptibility testing as key components of successful patient care (Figure 2.7).

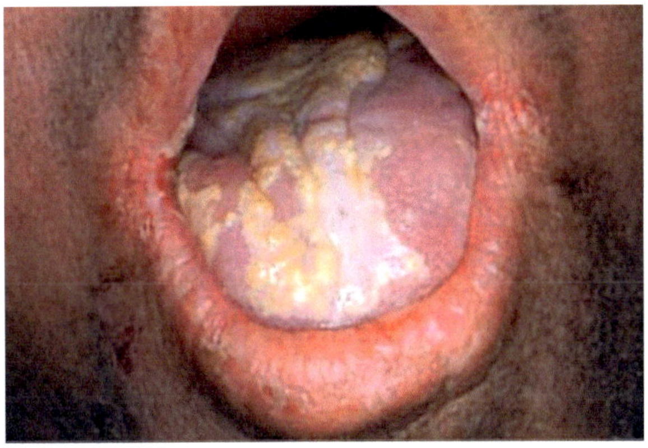

Figure 2.7. *Candida* infections.

Source: https://oralcancerfoundation.org/wp-content/uploads/2016/09/Candida1.jpg.

2.2.2. Aspergillus Species

Aspergillus is a diverse group of fungal organisms, some of which are significant pathogens in humans, particularly the immunocompromised. Of the many species, *Aspergillus fumigatus* is most commonly linked with pulmonary infections in view of its ubiquitous occurrence in the environment. *Aspergillus* spp. are opportunistic pathogens, and they take advantage of compromised host defense, so laboratory diagnosis of infection by these fungi is necessary. Earliest recognition and appropriate classification of *Aspergillus* spp. are required in the guiding of therapeutic approaches and improvement in patient outcomes. Traditional practices, such as microscopy and culture, remain normative; however, technological advancements in molecular diagnostics and imaging techniques are enabling more precise identification and better understanding of the pathogens clinical significance. The importance of early diagnosis of *Aspergillus* infection cannot be overstated, particularly among susceptible populations, such as recipients of stem cell transplants or patients with hematologic malignancy. Proven, probable, and possible invasive fungal disease is an organizing scheme that is the foundation for grading the severity and extent of infection and to support intervention. Specifically, likely invasive disease has been extended to encompass a broader array of clinical settings, and potentially has been defined with reference to the importance of clinical context when a diagnosis is made. These shifts are particularly important to be aware of in individuals who do not fit neatly into prior categories, once again emphasizing the importance of vigilance in monitoring for fungal infections in high-risk populations (Akan et al., 2019).

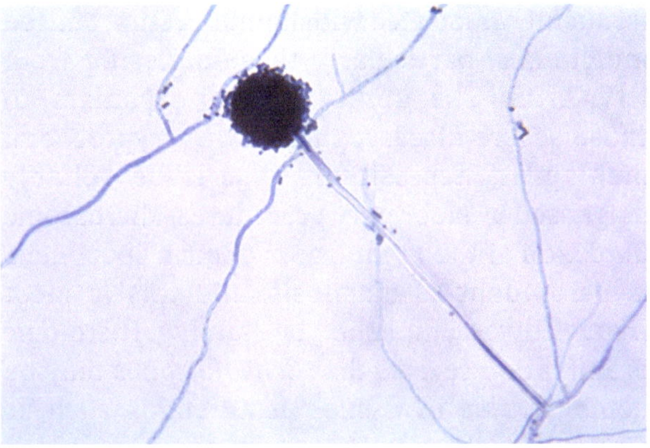

Figure 2.8. *Aspergillus* species are opportunistic pathogens that take advantage of weakened host defenses, making the laboratory diagnosis of infections caused by these fungi critical.

Source: https://upload.wikimedia.org/wikipedia/commons/7/74/*Aspergillus*_niger_01.jpg.

For liver transplant, the risk of invasive aspergillosis underscores the utmost significance of meticulous laboratory diagnosis. In the literature, it is reported that invasive aspergillosis in liver transplant recipients most commonly presents as pulmonary infections and that early diagnosis by culture or serology has significant implications on the management of the patient. Notably, factors such as elevated creatinine values and use of immunosuppressive therapy (e.g., OKT3) have been associated with the risk of invasive disease. The aforementioned association underscores the importance of integrating clinical data and laboratory results in order to accurately establish the risk of invasive aspergillosis (Fung et al., 1992). Ultimately, an effective diagnostic strategy bringing together traditional and modern techniques will facilitate timely and effective interventions, enhancing clinical outcomes among susceptible populations (Figure 2.8).

2.2.3. Cryptococcus neoformans

Cryptococcus neoformans is a serious opportunistic fungal pathogen which is most frequently associated with immunocompromised individuals, particularly those suffering from HIV/AIDS. The ability of the organism to cause severe disease, particularly cryptococcal meningitis, necessitates that it be reliably diagnosed by laboratory procedures. Microscopic detection of the organism in clinical specimens is paramount to diagnosis, and this is most frequently accomplished by staining. Histologic examination reveals that *C. neoformans* may be demonstrated in tissues using stains such as Gomoris methenamine silver method, which stains the yeast cell wall, and mucicarmine, specifically staining the thick capsule of the yeast cells. This capsule is one of the important virulence factors, not only assisting in phagocytic evasion but also in histological detection, which leads to increased diagnostic accuracy and timely treatment of infection caused by this agent (Inohara et al., 1959). Further, laboratory detection of *C. neoformans* extends beyond that of routine microscopy and may include more advanced techniques, e.g., antigen detection assays. The cryptococcal antigen test (CrAg) is a useful diagnostic reagent, enabling rapid screening for cryptococcal infection in high-risk groups. It detects polysaccharide antigens in serum or CSF and has high sensitivity and specificity. The ability to detect cases even before clinical presentation—and in patients who may not present with characteristic symptoms—underscores its value in clinical practice and public health surveillance. With the recent redefinition of invasive fungal diseases (IFDs) that included broadening the context and scope of use of the criteria employed for diagnosis, there is increased emphasis on early laboratory diagnosis to improve patient outcomes (Akan et al., 2019). Aside from direct detection and antigenic detection, culture techniques remain a central part of diagnosing *C. neoformans*.

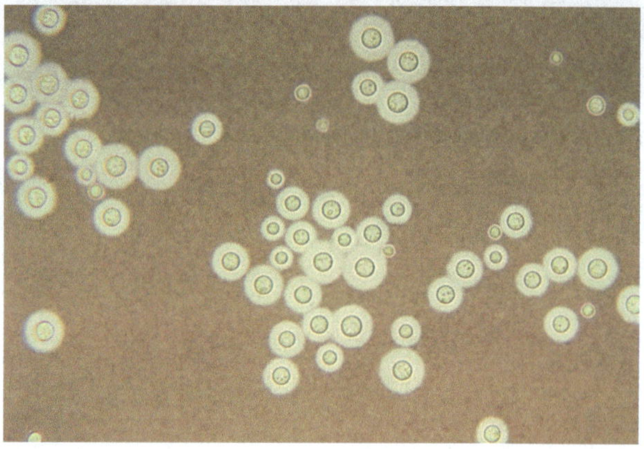

Figure 2.9. *Cryptococcus neoformans*, a significant opportunistic fungal pathogen, is predominantly associated with immunocompromised individuals, notably those with HIV/AIDS.

Source: https://upload.wikimedia.org/wikipedia/commons/6/6f/Cryptococcus_neoformans_using_a_light_India_ink_staining_preparation_PHIL_3771_lores.jpg.

The cultivation and identification of the yeast are made possible by growing the organism on selective media, characteristically identified as mucoid colonies in the form of its encapsulated state. The specific differentiation of *C. neoformans* from other fungal pathogens is important, since its improper identification can lead to ineffective treatment and patient outcome. Laboratories must employ a multi-modal approach, including microscopy, antigen tests, and culture techniques in order to make a confirmed diagnosis. This master plan not only assists in the determination of the presence of *C. neoformans*, but also yields details about the organisms' resistance patterns, enabling clinicians to implement the best antifungal regimen for their patients. It is essential to emphasize such lab practices to enhance the overall management and treatment of cryptococcosis (Figure 2.9).

2.3. Laboratory Techniques for Diagnosis

In laboratory diagnosis of fungal infection, there are several methods that have a vital role in effective identification and treatment. One of these is direct microscopy, which is the elementary one and allows rapid visualization of the fungal constituents in clinical specimens. It is a particularly useful method because it is fast and cost-effective to apply, hence being applicable in various healthcare settings. However, while microscopic diagnosis yields immediate results, its sensitivity is very variable and often necessitates confirmatory investigations with culture or molecular methods. The combination of the two modalities not only enhances diagnostic specificity but also facilitates clinicians in the selection of appropriate antifungal treatments and thus ultimately improves patient outcomes in the case of invasive fungal infections (Akan et al., 2019). Cultural methods, while time-consuming compared to microscopy, play a crucial role in microbial isolation and identification of the fungal pathogens. By growing the specimens on specific media, the laboratories are able to obtain pure fungal cultures that facilitate phenotypic description and antifungal susceptibility testing. The conventional culture technique remains a gold standard in microbiology, but results take several days or even weeks depending on the rate of growth of the organism. The function of early diagnosis is unequivocally central in invasive fungal infections, where early treatment is absolutely indispensable to control morbidity and mortality rates. Therefore, the synergy of culture and rapid molecular techniques such as panfungal PCR is an appealing strategy to enhance diagnostic efficiency and deliver adequate treatment to high-risk patients (Ala-Houhala et al., 2018). Molecular diagnostics, particularly the polymerase chain reaction (PCR), have now become valuable laboratory reagents for the diagnosis of fungal infections. Panfungal PCR, in fact, is a highly effective technique for the detection of many fungal pathogens from deep tissue samples and hence for early and specific diagnosis. The clinical utility of this approach was demonstrated in a study where 16% of the 307 samples were positive, demonstrating the sensitivity and specificity of the techniques. Not only is PCR a faster substitute for culture, but it is also extremely concordant with other laboratory procedures, further solidifying its role in diagnosing invasive fungal infections. With the combination of molecular techniques and microscopy and culture, clinicians can enhance diagnostic expertise and modify treatment protocols in response to the threat posed by fungal infections among vulnerable patient populations (Akan et al., 2019; Ala-Houhala et al., 2018) (Figure 2.10).

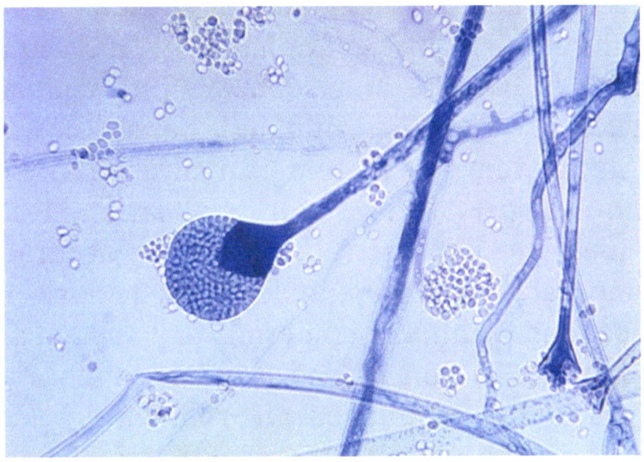

Figure 2.10. Cultural methods, though time-consuming compared to microscopy, play a critical role in isolating and identifying fungal pathogens.

Source: https://www.ncbi.nlm.nih.gov/books/NBK549988/bin/AAMCol.18Oct.2017.fig12.jpg.

2.3.1. Microscopy

In fungal infection diagnosis in the lab, microscopy is an essential tool no laboratory can function without that makes detecting pathogens more precise and faster. Through various microscopy techniques, particularly light and fluorescence microscopy, clinical practitioners can visualize morphological features of fungal organisms upon direct examination of clinical specimens. This initial examination, especially when done with KOH preparations, allows visualization of the cell walls of the fungi, hyphae, and spores, allowing for differentiation of pathogenic fungi from non-pathogenic types. Most importantly, the resolution capability of the microscope provides a major advantage, particularly in the identification of characters that are critical in diagnosis. Due to its ability to deliver instantaneous analysis of the fungal morphology, microscopy aids conventional culture methods in providing quick and efficient identification, which is key in the effective treatment of fungal infections. Apart from conventional microscopy, reflectance confocal microscopy (RCM) is a recent technique whose role in the diagnosis of cutaneous fungal infection has been demonstrated. RCM has a noninvasive, high-resolution imaging technique which is capable of visualizing fine cellular structures to represent fungi, parasites, and inflammatory dermatological alterations in skin lesions. With proper application, RCM is found to demonstrate diagnostic accuracy comparable to histopathology, particularly in infections within the epidermis and superficial dermis. Aside from diagnosis, RCM can monitor therapeutic responses in real-time, thus avoiding unwarranted therapeutic maneuvers. The capacity to view fungal components without invasive methods is a testament to RCMs promise to revolutionize our method of diagnosing cutaneous fungal infections and, by extension, improve the outcomes of patients in dermatological clinics (Arzberger et al., 2020). In spite of newer microscopy technologies, it remains challenging to diagnose opportunistic yeast infections, whose incidence has increased with growing diversity in species and drug resistance. Standard diagnostic procedures frequently employ culture methodologies that are time-consuming, potentially exposing patients to delayed therapy. However, new generation high-throughput technologies like next-generation sequencing and proteomics hold the promise of more sensitive and effective yeast pathogen detection. These novel technologies are under investigation and consideration for incorporation into clinical practice to address the limitations of traditional microscopy and culture methodologies. With their potential to enhance the diagnostic context, these technologies could be used to significantly improve characterization and detection of fungal infections as well as assessment of drug resistance profiles (Arastehfar et al., 2019) (Figure 2.11).

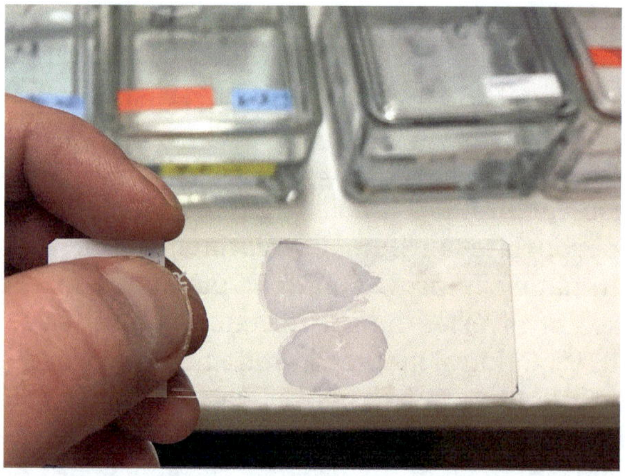

Figure 2.11. Utilizing various microscopy techniques, particularly light and fluorescence microscopy, clinicians can observe morphological characteristics of fungal organisms directly from clinical samples.

Source: https://upload.wikimedia.org/wikipedia/commons/thumb/4/47/Stained_microscope_slide.jpg/1200px-Stained_microscope_slide.jpg.

2.3.2. Culture Methods

The role of culture techniques to the laboratory diagnosis of fungal infections is of utmost significance as they provide valuable information on the existence and the causative fungi. Fungi may grow when clinical samples, such as blood, tissue, or body fluids, are cultured on selective media, hence making them identifiable and characterizable. The use of culture methods allows clinicians not only to identify the infecting organism but also identify its antifungal susceptibility, which is crucial in creating a proper treatment schedule. This is particularly important because of the rising incidence of antifungal-resistant cases among certain fungi, which has been highlighted in the recent literature (Bouley et al., 2013). Moreover, culture methods can offer data on the epidemiology of fungal infections, i.e., their distribution and rates of prevalence in various populations. The data enhance interventions in public health and guide clinical management plans in order to respond to fungal outbreaks. Despite having numerous advantages, culture methods are accompanied by a series of challenges while making laboratory diagnosis of fungal infections. Firstly, the time it will take for cultivation can result in a delay before antifungal treatment is initiated, since some fungi will only grow in days or weeks. Secondly, much of the media employed for culture may lack specificity to enable growth of all fungal species and may result in under-detection. Further, as has been demonstrated through literature, conventional diagnostic tests have revealed too low sensitivity and specificity, particularly in resource-limited countries where more sophisticated laboratory testing may not be accessible (Bouley et al., 2013). This emphasizes the paramount requirement for rapid and precise diagnostic techniques supplementing culture-based methods, such as molecular methods and next-generation high-throughput strategies. Perception of these imperatives is essential to continue advancing diagnostic techniques and enable early management of the patient. New advances in culture methods point to the potential of improved diagnostics with fungal infection. Enriched culture media and inclusion of antibiotics in the growth medium are some of the approaches that may help in the recovery of organisms otherwise recalcitrant for growth. Furthermore, high-throughput technologies like next-generation sequencing and proteomics are being developed to enable quicker and more trustworthy detection of fungal pathogens and their drug resistance patterns (Arastehfar et al., 2019). Such developments are expected to reduce the gap between traditional culture methods and the dynamic nature of clinical diagnosis. However, the context of integrating such new technologies into regular clinical practice faces several challenging obstacles, such as cost, availability, and provision for training the medical professionals. While the potential of the traditional culture techniques is being challenged with the promotion of advanced molecular techniques, a synergistic strategy that allies conventional culture methods with state-of-the-art molecular techniques will prove imperative in the fight against the spread of fungal infection in clinical practice (Figure 2.12).

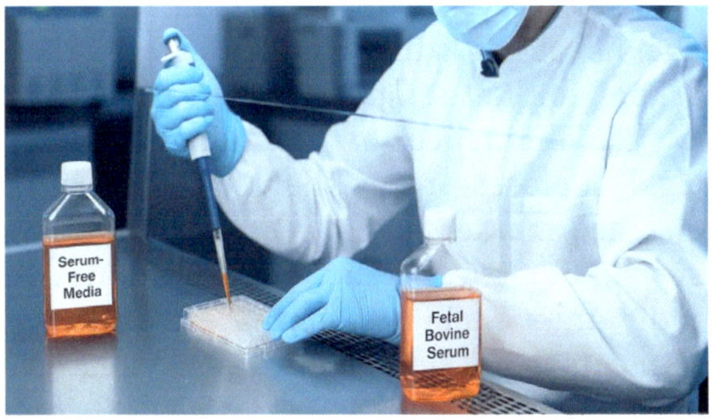

Figure 2.12. When clinical specimens, such as blood, tissue, or bodily fluids, are cultured on specific media, fungi can proliferate, enabling their identification and characterization.

Source: https://www.atlantisbioscience.com/wp-content/uploads/2025/05/Commercial-Benefits-of-Serum-Free-Media-in-Cell-Therapy-Blog-cover.webp.

2.3.3. Molecular Techniques

The advent of molecular techniques has revolutionized laboratory diagnosis of fungal infections with significant advantages compared to traditional methods. Traditional culture-based methods, although significant, have long incubation periods and are not able to effectively address the range of fungal agents that cause infections. Molecular techniques such as polymerase chain reaction (PCR), next-generation sequencing (NGS), and whole-genome sequencing compare favorably with speed and sensitivity towards detecting pathogenic fungus. These strategies bypass many culturing-based limitations, enabling researchers and clinicians to diagnose species-specific infections and presumptive resistance patterns more accurately and quickly. The application of molecular techniques has been proven through research to enhance diagnostic sensitivity and specificity, enhancing therapeutic outcomes as well as patient management in clinical settings, particularly among patients with immunocompromised disease or severe fungal infection presentation (Arastehfar et al., 2019). One of the most important features of employing molecular techniques in diagnosing fungal infections is that they can detect genetic markers for antifungal resistance. With the growing incidence of multidrug-resistant fungal isolates, early detection of these resistance markers is now critical. Molecular tests can detect resistance genes or mutations rapidly, thus enabling appropriate antifungal treatments to be selected and delayed treatment with their side effects to be avoided. Of note, technologies for high-throughput sequencing allow profiling of the entire genome of fungi. Apart from making detection of causative organisms possible, this aspect also aids surveillance programs aimed at tracking antifungal resistance patterns in the fungal population. Integration of these technologies with clinical diagnosis allows laboratories to enhance the quality of treatment provided to patients while simultaneously informing public health programs against antifungal resistance (Arastehfar et al., 2019). Despite their perceived advantages, the implementation of molecular techniques in the clinical environment is not problem-free. Standardization of the test procedures, the necessity of trained personnel, and the exorbitant cost of costly technologies have prevented general application. Moreover, while molecular tests give immediate feedback, working with the advanced genomic data requires extensive understanding of the biology and epidemiology of fungi. Studies still conquer these challenges, including making diagnostic platforms easy to use and streamlined workflow that can make molecular testing more feasible for clinical laboratories. The future of fungal infection diagnosis hangs on the conquest of these challenges, with the promise of a future where molecular techniques become commonplace, eventually improving patient outcomes and our understanding of fungal pathogens (Figure 2.13).

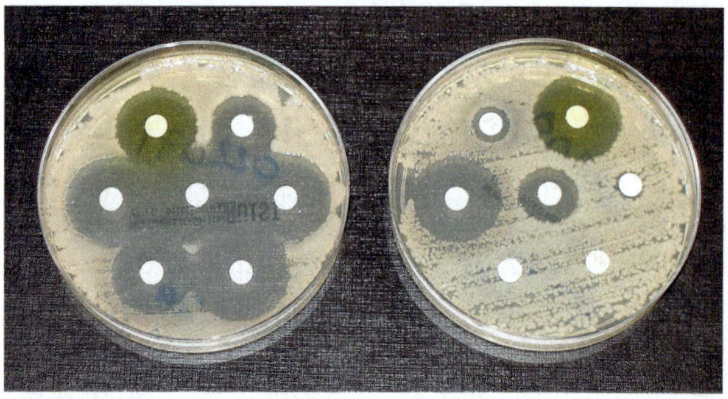

Figure 2.13. Molecular assays can pinpoint resistance genes or mutations rapidly, facilitating the selection of appropriate antifungal therapies and minimizing the risks associated with treatment delays.

Source: https://upload.wikimedia.org/wikipedia/commons/thumb/a/ab/Antibiotic_sensitivity_and_resistance.jpg/1200px-Antibiotic_sensitivity_and_resistance.jpg.

2.4. Role of Serological Tests

The application of serological tests in the diagnosis of fungal infections is increasingly being appreciated as a valuable addition to traditional diagnostic modalities. These tests, which measure host antibodies or antigens to specific fungal pathogens, provide a clear window into the bodys immunocompetence and burden of pathogen. This is particularly beneficial with invasive fungal infections, where rapid and precise diagnosis can determine the outcome for the patient. For example, although serological assays can identify antibodies in cryptococcosis or histoplasmosis, they require meticulous interpretation to prevent cross-reactivity and differing sensitivities from clouding the outcomes.

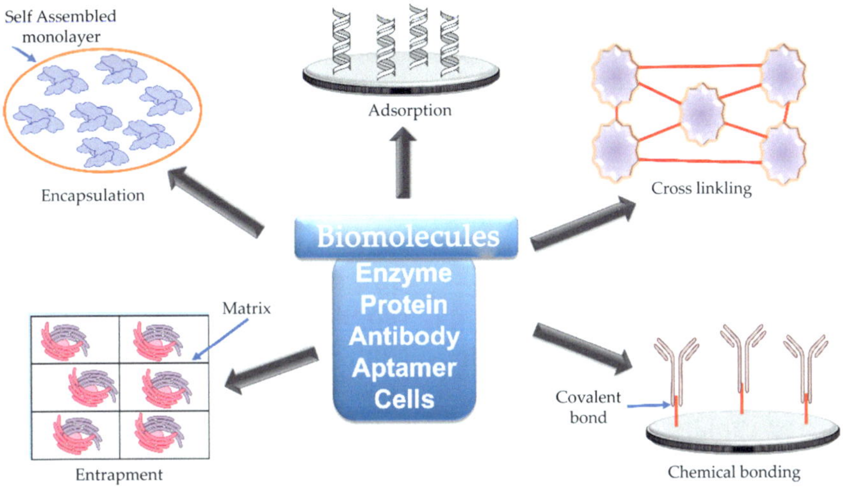

Figure 2.14. The role of serological tests in diagnosing fungal infections is increasingly recognized as a vital adjunct to traditional diagnostic modalities.

Source: https://www.mdpi.com/jof/jof-06-00349/article_deploy/html/images/jof-06-00349-g004.png.

As a whole, the incorporation of serological assays into routine diagnostic schemes improves diagnostic precision for the clinician faced with the variant presentations of fungal infections, leading to enhanced patient management plans. Serology assays are especially beneficial in low-resource settings, where advanced diagnostic equipment is not readily accessible. Excessive diagnosis of malaria in patients who have fever underscores the importance of accurate diagnostic procedures so that mismanagement and complications may be avoided. In northern Tanzania, research indicates that invasive fungal infections are held accountable for significant morbidity but tend to become misidentified or overlooked when compared to more prevalent diseases like malaria (Bouley et al., 2013). Through serological tests, medical practitioners can differentiate among these conditions effectively and consequently administer appropriate treatments to patients. Hence, serology not only facilitates confirmation of the diagnosis of fungal infections, but it also aids in epidemiological surveillance, in guiding public health intervention and resource allocation within these risk groups. However, despite their potential, the use of serological tests for fungal infections does face some challenges, including the defined parameters for use in assays and the need for clinicians to be educated. Serological diagnosis, particularly through emerging technologies such as clinical metagenomic next-generation sequencing (mNGS), is transforming the diagnosis of fungal infections by analyzing both microbial and host genetic material (Chiu et al., 2019). The new approach has the potential to raise the detection rate of challenging pathogens and improve patient care through earlier detection of resistant strains or co-infections in the clinical setting. As the methods shift, it is important for laboratories and health professionals to adapt towards utilizing serological tests effectively. Overcoming the limiting factors of application will enhance increased uptake, eventually resulting in better diagnostic outcomes and public health responses to fungal infections (Figure 2.14).

2.4.1. Antigen Detection

Antigen detection in laboratory diagnosis of fungal infections is a significant development in medical mycology. Antigen detection speeds up the diagnosis and makes it more specific, enabling clinicians to rapidly diagnose fungal pathogens compared to standard culture methods, which could take a day or weeks. Antigen detection relies on the identification of fungal components, such as polysaccharides and proteins, in patient specimens, typically serum or other bodily fluids.

This not only aids in the detection of the organism but also provides insight into the host immunological response. To illustrate, certain tests, i.e., galactomannan or beta-D-glucan tests, are specifically useful in diagnosing invasive aspergillosis and candidemia, respectively. As fungal infections can masquerade as bacterial or viral infections, antigen detection is a great asset in the differentiation of these diseases, which will eventually translate to appropriate therapeutic actions. Moreover, the application of antigen detection is strongly congruent with the urgent need for rapid diagnostic tools in the context of mounting rates of fungal infection, particularly among immunocompromised patients. Recent studies have illustrated how antigen-based tests can significantly reduce pathologic misdiagnosis and consequent treatment delay due to over-diagnosis of disease like malaria among febrile patients residing in endemic regions, as validated by northern Tanzanian studies. Few of the patients who were feverous had malaria in this study, and this underlines the potential for increased diagnostic accuracy through the use of antigen detection technologies. Through the use of these tests, clinicians are better positioned to make more precise decisions that lead to timely and effective treatment regimens, thereby improving patient outcomes for a population increasingly vulnerable to opportunistic infection.

Despite the optimistic promises of antigen detection, there remain challenges to overcome in rendering them universally accurate and applicable. The spread of drug-resistant strains only adds to complications in diagnosis and treatment and calls for ongoing adaptation of detection techniques. Today's antigen tests are quite varied in sensitivity and specificity, and while some have outstanding promise in the lab, their applications to the clinic are frequently hindered.

High-throughput tools like next-generation sequencing hold promise to transform fungal diagnosis with the ability to provide a complete image of the pathogen's resistance profile, but key technical and logistic barriers are still in front of such methods from being utilized routinely within clinical practice.

It appears critical that a multidisciplinary strategy of robust research endeavors accompanied by clinical validation studies is needed to refine antigen detection methods and enhance their application in fungal infection laboratory diagnosis, particularly as it relates to heightened susceptibility to antifungal resistance (Bouley et al., 2013; Arastehfar et al., 2019) (Figure 2.15).

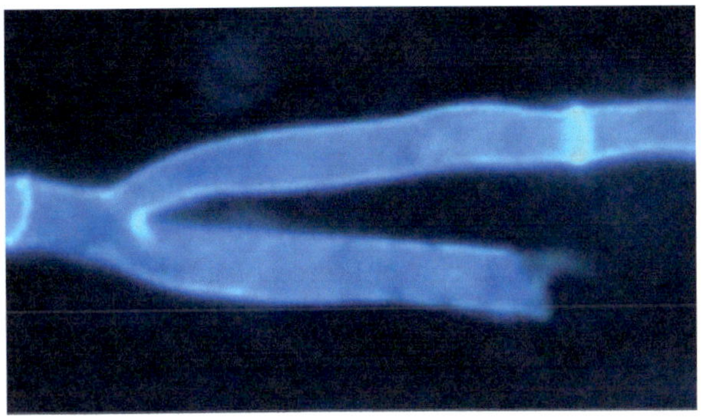

Figure 2.15. The use of antigen detection in the laboratory diagnosis of fungal infections represents a significant advancement in medical mycology.

Source: https://www.thelancet.com/cms/10.1016/S1473-3099(15)70006-X/asset/1346527a-a147-4413-9a5a-0eeaeae3eae5/main.assets/gr1_lrg.jpg.

2.4.2. Antibody Detection

Antibody detection is a significant function in laboratory diagnosis of the fungal infections, particularly in opportunistic fungi whose causation of severe morbidity in immunocompromised hosts makes diagnosis crucial. Antibodies indicate the bodys immune response to certain fungal pathogens. By analyzing serological specimens, professionals can establish the presence of such antibodies, thereby enabling earlier and more accurate identification of the causative agent. Antibody detection can also differentiate between recent infection and past exposure, and this is particularly valuable in the management of chronic fungal infections and in the direction of therapy. To illustrate, in cases where usual culture methods may be slow or inadequate with challenges such as the low fungal burden, serological tests can provide a useful adjunct diagnostic test that helps clinicians react accordingly to avert the toxic effect of invasive fungal diseases. But detection efficacy with antibodies is not unchallengeable, primarily as a result of immune response heterogeneity among different patient populations. Patients with varying degrees of immune competence or patients undergoing immunomodulating therapy may produce different patterns of antibody response. Cross-reactions of antibodies elicited in response to different fungi can also lead to false-positive identification, rendering accurate identification of the causative pathogen difficult. The limitations of current serological tests therefore highlight the importance of ongoing research and development of more robust approaches.

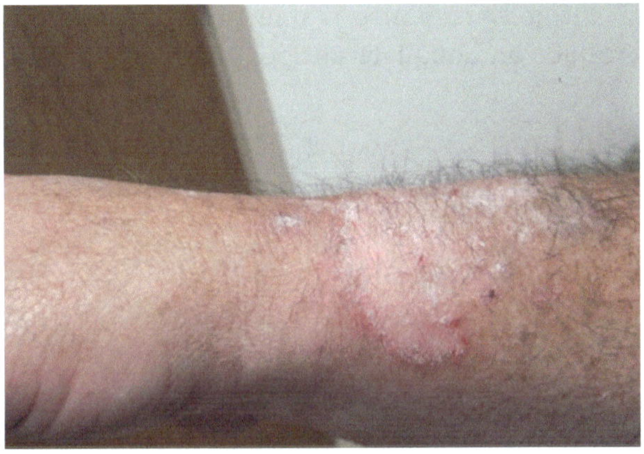

Figure 2.16. Antibody detection can also help differentiate between active infection and past exposure, which is particularly beneficial in managing chronic fungal infections and informing treatment decisions.

Source: https://www.tandfonline.com/cms/asset/1ecb71e6-7fa7-4bbe-8885-3465673cf2e0/ierz_a_960849_f0003_b.jpg.

Emerging technologies such as proteomics and next-generation sequencing have the potential for better sensitivity and specificity in diagnosis of fungal infections and could bridge the gaps identified by traditional antibody detection methods (Arastehfar et al., 2019). In addition, laboratory diagnosis of antibody response also plays a crucial role in guiding public health interventions for control of fungal infections, especially in resource-poor populations. In these environments, misdiagnosis leads to wrong intervention and exacerbation of the burden of fungal disease. For example, a study from northern Tanzania depicted the discrepancy between clinical diagnosis and actual etiology of fever, wherein malaria was grossly over-diagnosed and bacterial and fungal infections were under-estimated (Bouley et al., 2013). This depicts the urgent need for accurate antibody detection techniques that can reliably confirm the presence of fungal infections so that the risk of mismanagement will be minimized. By developing diagnostic capabilities, particularly by combining serological diagnosis with other advanced diagnostic methods, health care professionals can enhance patient outcomes and establish specific prevention strategies against emerging fungal pathogens (Figure 2.16).

2.4.3. Limitations of Serological Tests

Serology has assumed a critical role in laboratory diagnosis of fungal infections but has substantial limitations that can affect clinical outcome and diagnostic accuracy. Patient-to-patient variation in antibody response is one such limitation. Immunocompromised individuals may be unable to produce an adequate antibody response, leading to false-negative test results.

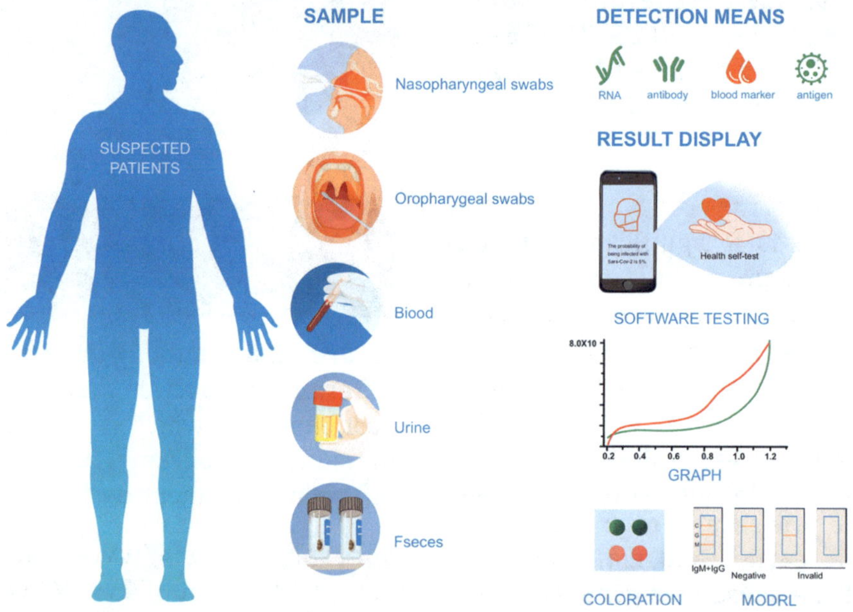

Figure 2.17. Serological tests have gained prominence in the laboratory diagnosis of fungal infections, yet they exhibit notable limitations that can affect diagnostic accuracy and clinical outcomes.

Source: https://media.springernature.com/full/springer-static/image/art%3A10.1038%2Fs41392-021-00731-z/MediaObjects/41392_2021_731_Fig1_HTML.png.

This creates a challenge, particularly in diagnosing infections such as paracoccidioidomycosis, in which there are some patients who present with low titers or non-specific antibodies but are infected. Furthermore, the presence of cross-reactive antibodies from previous infections also complicates the interpretation and leads to misdiagnosis or inappropriate treatment. These points underscore the importance of adequate evaluation of serological data in correlation with clinical data and other modalities to optimize the precision of diagnoses of fungal infections. In addition to variation in immune reactivity, serological tests typically also suffer from issues with specificity, so they may produce cross-reactivity with other pathogens. For instance, in the case of paracoccidioidomycosis, serology tests can be positive due to antibodies developed against other fungal infections, making the diagnosis doubtful. Such cross-reactivity lowers the value of serological tests, especially when individual closely related species of fungi need to be identified separately. The implications in clinical practice of such an inability are serious in that an erroneous diagnosis would lead not only to inappropriate treatment but also to the progression of the causative infection itself. Thus, while serology can be useful in diagnosing individual fungal infections, there is a need for clinicians to exercise caution regarding the appropriateness of the environment in which serology is used, seeking adjunctive diagnostic methods or molecular methods for demonstrating the presence of certain pathogens with greater accuracy. Furthermore, the advances of the last several years in technology toward diagnostic techniques pose additional challenges to the validity of serological tests within the clinical setting. As new molecular and antigen-based diagnostic tests are developed, serological tests can easily fall behind in specificity and sensitivity, further losing their utility as a diagnostic. With the possible delay in results from serological tests and the test's limitations inherent to timing, health care workers must keep abreast of the latest diagnostic modalities to be used for diagnosing fungal disease. For example, even though the gp43-SLPs serological test for paracoccidioidomycosis is very sensitive and specific, not every serological test can be as much, so there is a requirement of more serious familiarity with using them in clinical practice. Considering these aspects, constant investment in research has to be carried out to enhance serological methods and integrate them effectively into comprehensive diagnostic strategies for fungal infections, ultimately bridging the gaps and enhancing patient care (Jourdan et al., 2015; Burger et al., 2015) (Figure 2.17).

2.5. Importance of Sample Collection

Adequate collection of sample is a critical initial step in laboratory diagnosis of fungal infections, enabling proper detection and identification of the pathogen. Integrity of the sample is most critical since contamination or mishandling will lead to false results and delay appropriate therapy. For instance, in hospitals where the patients with fever are being evaluated, one research highlighted the necessity of complete diagnostic testing beyond common assumptions, for instance, overestimation of malaria diagnosis. Within research settings like these, samples must be collected accurately to fully ascertain the presence of less frequent pathogens, for instance, fungi that may be accountable for causing febrile illness. Thus, an appreciation of the complexity of infectious diseases and the fact that good sampling procedures can work wonders in enhancing clinical results by allowing the patients to get best and timely care for their diseases, including invasive fungal diseases (Bouley et al., 2013), is essential. The collection methods employed using sampling techniques are also crucial to the overall efficacy of the diagnostic tests. Various methods, including aspiration, swabbing, and tissue biopsies, each have specific guidelines that are appropriate to the nature of the suspected fungal infection. For instance, the deeper tissues may require special targeting schemes for sampling to obtain the maximum yield of the fungal organism. Advanced techniques like clinical metagenomic next-generation sequencing (mNGS) are also becoming powerful laboratory tools, analyzing genetic material from the sample to give general results for a vast number of infections, including fungal ones. The utilization of mNGS is not without its challenges, particularly in being able to preserve the optimal sample quality and the best representative of the microbial flora involved. Following the technology advancement of mNGS, practice application demands sophisticated sample collection techniques to improve its diagnostic potential (Chiu et al., 2019). Moreover, the technological advancement of diagnostic instruments emphasizes the significance of sample collection not just in the identification of pathogens but also in establishing their epidemiology. Adequate sample collection enables larger epidemiological studies that facilitate health authorities to effectively monitor the spread and prevalence of fungal infections. For instance, detection of host and environmental determinants that expose humans to infections can be boosted by quality-collected samples from diverse populations. Given that research reveals shifting trends among fungal infections as well as resistance profiles, quality samples play a significant role in developing useful public health plans and interventions. This is a holistic view that acknowledges the interrelatedness of good sample collection, laboratory diagnosis, and public health presentation in broader terms, and reiterates the preeminence of good practices in the laboratory diagnosis of fungal infections (Bouley et al., 2013) (Figure 2.18).

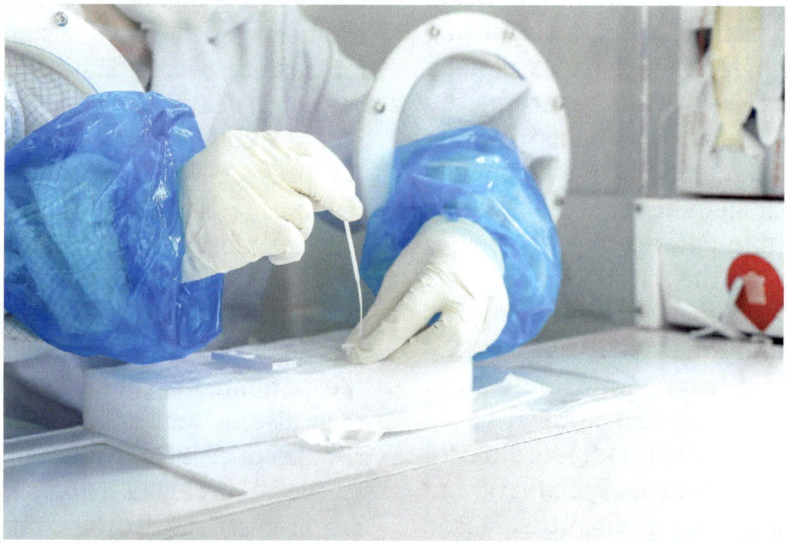

Figure 2.18. Effective sample collection is a critical initial step in the laboratory diagnosis of fungal infections, facilitating accurate detection and identification of pathogens.

Source: https://resourcewebsite.singoo.cc/attached/20240328083407_15654.jpg.

2.5.1. Types of Samples (e.g., Blood, Tissue, Swabs)

In laboratory diagnosis of fungal infections, a selection of the appropriate type of sample is crucial for accurate identification and treatment. Blood samples are utilized frequently, mainly in systemic infection like candidiasis or aspergillosis. The samples can show the presence of fungemia, which plays a critical role in diagnosis, most importantly in immunocompromised patients. Also, various serological tests are employed in the identification of specific antibodies or antigens present in blood to aid in identification of the fungal pathogen. Sensitivity in blood culture can be varied and a negative result does not exclude a fungal infection, hence important to obtain several types of samples for enhanced diagnostic accuracy. Tissue samples represent another significant type of specimen utilized in diagnosing fungal infections. Biopsy samples collected from infected tissues, such as the skin, lungs, or other organs, may provide direct evidence for fungal structures through histopathological examination. Tissue samples, for instance, may produce granulomatous inflammation typical of certain fungal infections. Laboratory special staining techniques can aid in the visibility of fungi, thus allowing for the final diagnosis. The acquisition of such samples is typically performed during the conduct of surgical procedures or by using minimally invasive techniques.

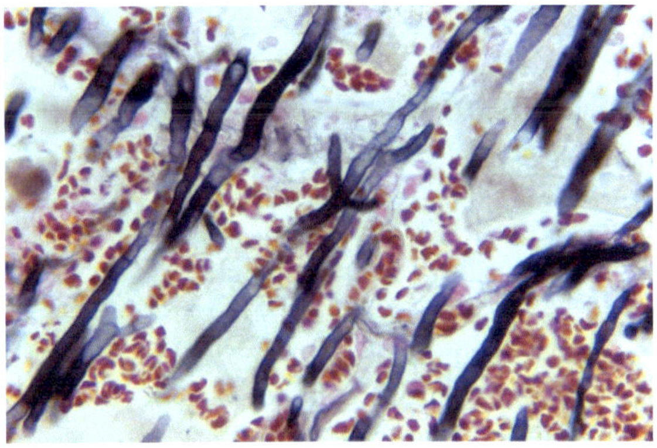

Figure 2.19. Blood samples are frequently utilized, especially in cases of systemic fungal infections like candidiasis or aspergillosis.

Source: https://img.mlo-online.com/files/base/ebm/mlo/image/2021/02/CDC_21199_Aspergillosis.602d7e9b82822.png?auto=format,compress&fit=max&q=45&w=640&width=640.

The integration of tissue sampling with potent histological evaluations can therefore enhance diagnostic effectiveness and guide effective therapeutic measures. Swabs, particularly oropharyngeal or nasal swabs, are particularly helpful to employ when diagnosing shallow mycotic infections, particularly for oral thrush or dermatophyte infection. Swabs are used for quick and painless specimen collection and, as such, are suitable for initial testing. The swabs taken can be grown to allow for isolation and characterization of the causative agent. In addition, molecular techniques such as polymerase chain reaction (PCR) can be applied in swab samples for quick detection and typing of fungal DNA. This method has the impact of shortening diagnosis time significantly and helping infection control measure management. The integration of swab sampling in diagnosis thus emphasizes its value as a way of efficiently and effectively detecting localized fungal infection (Figure 2.19).

2.5.2. Proper Collection Techniques

The diagnostic accuracy of the fungal infections relies in part on correct collection procedures utilized in obtaining the sample. That medical professionals observe rigid guidelines so as not to contaminate and integrity of the specimen being analyzed is paramount. This begins with appropriate choice of material and container, which should be sterilized and suitably designed for fungal cultures. In addition, how and when the specimens are collected is crucial; they should be collected during acute stages of infection because it increases the chances of isolating the pathogen. Proper handling and storage shortly after collection are also essential, because latency or poor conditions will spoil the sample and render diagnostic less trustworthy. Using these procedures enhances the accuracy of laboratory results, but also impacts tremendously on effective treatment and management of fungal infections. In addition, the specific type of specimen collected may vary depending on the suspected fungal infection, which impacts its diagnostic significance. For instance, respiratory specimens such as sputum or bronchoalveolar lavage fluid are frequently used in pulmonary infections, while skin lesions would have to be scraped or biopsied and seen under the microscope. There is a collection of various specimen types with corresponding collection procedures that must be followed. There are special procedures, for instance, correct decontamination of the skin before sampling a lesion, which minimize the risk of contamination. In resource-poor settings, such as in third-world nations, the lack of ability to perform multiple tests emphasizes the importance of precise and diligent collection procedures for the first sample. This supports the necessity for why proper education in and utilization of the proper collection procedures are the keystone in the realm of fungal infection diagnosis. In addition to the physical aspect of collection, proper education and training of personnel handling specimens are key factors in obtaining successful diagnostic outcomes. Ongoing professional development of personnel guarantees that the staff keeps abreast of best practices in specimen collection and transport to the laboratory.

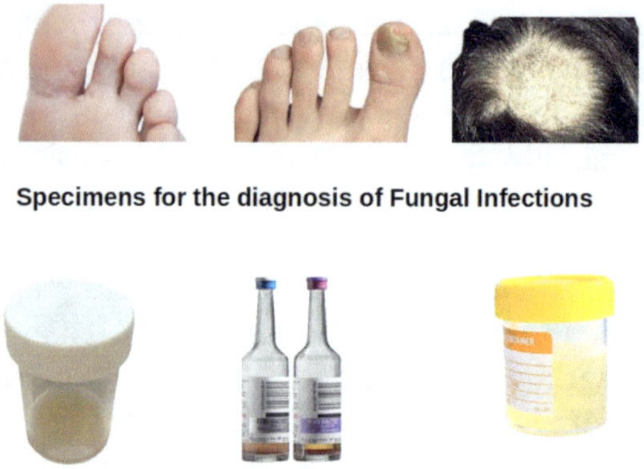

Figure 2.20. The successful diagnosis of fungal infections hinges significantly on the proper collection techniques employed during sample acquisition.

Source: https://microbeonline.com/wp-content/uploads/2021/04/specimen-for-fungal-diagnosis.png.

Acknowledging the significance of varied collection protocols, coupled with the innovation in the rapid diagnostic procedures, enhances the overall efficiency in laboratory diagnosis. For example, innovative techniques, highlighted by the studies on mycolic acids, signal potential to increase diagnostic efficacy in similar diseases (Janiszewska-Drobinska et al., 2013). As the sector evolves, ongoing emphasis on proper collection practices will remain pivotal to securing timely and accurate diagnoses for fungal disease. Such a program is complementary to the general goal of improving patient outcomes through the provision of quality laboratory practice, which eventually translates into improved public health responses against fungal infections (Warris et al., 2018) (Figure 2.20).

2.5.3. Impact of Sample Quality on Diagnosis

Maintaining integrity of the sample received for the diagnosis of fungal infection is very crucial so as to achieve accurate laboratory results. Samples, when contaminated or not properly handled, lead to false positives or negatives and thus complicate the clinical picture. Integrity of the sample is more critical, particularly invasive fungal infection, where the clinical situation can worsen very quickly. Such patients have severe comorbidities and typical patterns of injury, and it is important to incorporate these in the diagnostic workup. For instance, accurate identification of the causative pathogenic fungal agent is compromised by suboptimal samples, leading to misdiagnosis or delayed treatment. This underscores the requirement for rigorous procedures concerning sample collection, transport, and processing for minimizing contamination and preservation of the viability of fungal organisms present in the sample, as the outcomes on patient health are dire, including increased risk of amputation and death associated with inappropriate management of infection (Bochicchio et al., 2017). In the recent years, improvements in diagnostic technologies such as clinical metagenomic next-generation sequencing (mNGS) have been safe bets towards making diagnosis of fungal infections more accurate. Through direct analysis of microbial and host DNA in patient samples, mNGS allows for detection of a broader range of pathogens, some of which can be challenging or impossible to cultivate using standard culture methods. The quality of the sample depends greatly on these techniques. Quality specimens are required to minimize background noise and maximize detection of specific pathogens. Poor-quality biological material can lead to inconclusive results, necessitate retesting, and may prolong time to effective treatment. Taking this into consideration, sample quality standards should be coordinated with these new approaches to fully exploit their diagnostic capacity and improve patient management results in fungal infections (Chiu et al., 2019).

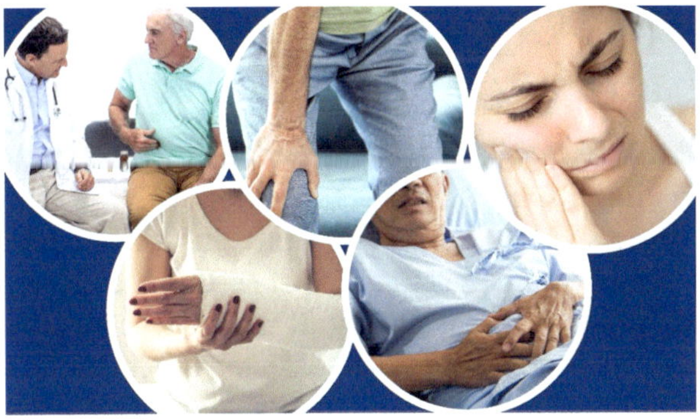

Figure 2.21. Patients suffering from such infections often present with severe comorbidities and specific injury patterns, which are crucial to factor into the diagnostic process.

Source: https://effectivehealthcare.ahrq.gov/sites/default/files/styles/product_hero_desktop/public/images/acute-pain-collage_blue.jpg?itok=m3TtPj2J.

Other than the implications of diagnosis, sample quality also affects treatment for fungal infection. Inadequate samples can lead clinicians to administer inappropriate or ineffective treatment, complicate patients' conditions, and postpone appropriate treatment. As explained in invasive fungal infection research, accurate and swift diagnosis is crucial; delay has the potential to result in increased morbidity and mortality. Moreover, as the level of complexity of fungal pathogens and resistance also grows, the clinicians rely more and more on precise diagnostic information in order to guide antifungal treatment. This thus establishes beyond doubt that the interaction between sample quality and right diagnosis extends beyond the laboratory and forms a critical component of the general management of fungal infections. Keeping the quality samples thus is not just a laboratory challenge but a key factor in maximizing patient care and minimizing adverse results (Bochicchio et al., 2017; Chiu et al., 2019) (Figure 2.21).

2.6. Interpretation of Laboratory Results

The interpretation of laboratory results is certainly at the forefront of laboratory diagnosis of fungal infections. Identification of the causative fungal pathogen with precision is essential for the appropriate therapeutic interventions. Techniques such as culture, serological assays, and molecular diagnostic techniques can provide various bits of information regarding the presence and nature of fungal infection with results to be interpreted carefully. For instance, the isolation of a fungal isolate from clinical specimens must be accompanied by the patient's clinical syndrome and other laboratory findings; culture alone would not do. Further, markers like 1,3-β-D-glucan (BDG) might indirectly detect fungal infections. The reappearance or intensification of BDG in cerebrospinal fluid, as emphasized in recent studies, has been linked with treatment failure, indicating the complexity of interpreting lab findings in conjunction with clinical outcomes (Brunetti et al., 2016). Fungal infection diagnostic techniques usually need multi-dimensional approaches. Invasive tests such as bronchoscopy can be applied when less invasive tests remain ambiguous. However, interpretation of such data requires an advanced understanding of the etiologic bases underlying and patient immunocompromised status. Identification of species such as *Aspergillus fumigatus*, often isolated in acute fungal infections, also requires not just microbiologic assessment but consideration of patient demographics and clinical background.

With the development of various assays for fungal pathogens, distinction between invasion and colonization in infection increases the complexity of laboratory diagnosis, as indicated by evidence from studies of intensive care unit patients (Blasco-Navalpotro et al., 2015). Laboratory results are thus complemented by clinical experience to draw conclusion-based treatment.

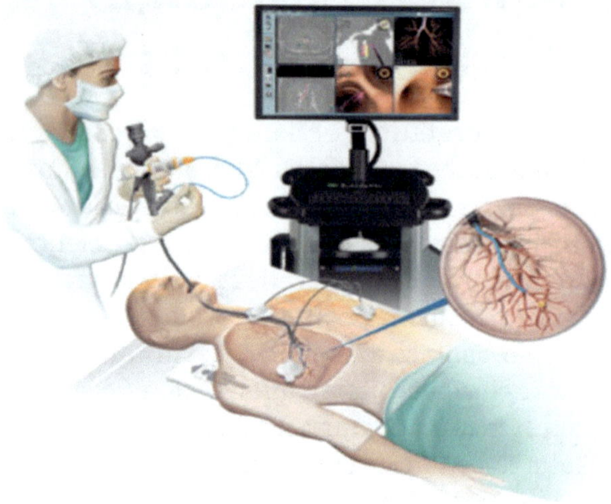

Figure 2.22. Invasive techniques such as bronchoscopy may be employed when non-invasive methods yield inconclusive results.

Source: https://delhichestspecialist.com/wp-content/uploads/2023/12/bronchoscopy-procedure-768x604.jpg.

Finally, interpretation of laboratory results is inherently linked to therapeutic decision-making. Understanding the antifungal susceptibility patterns of the pathogens in isolation is essential to aid in deciding on effective management strategies, particularly in the case of drug-resistant infections. For example, diminution of voriconazole susceptibility in *Candida tropicalis*, as described in single case reports, demonstrates the necessity for active monitoring of antifungal resistance patterns (Brunetti et al., 2016). Besides, in patients who have invasive aspergillosis diagnosis, particularly critically ill patients, risk factors such as age and history of medical procedures must be included in the interpretation of laboratory findings to anticipate potential complications as well as inform therapy. Laboratory diagnosis of fungal infections is therefore not merely results but their interpretations, requiring a concerted effort among clinicians, microbiologists, and infectious disease specialists to achieve the best possible outcomes in patients (Figure 2.22).

2.6.1. Understanding Test Sensitivity and Specificity

In diagnostic testing for infections in the laboratory setting, information about test sensitivity and specificity is of essential concern. Sensitivity, or the ability of a test to correctly identify infected persons, directly affects patient outcomes through the timely start of proper treatment. A sensitive test reduces the risk of false negative results and therefore allows for early treatment of potentially life-threatening fungal infections. Conversely, specificity refers to the test's capacity to correctly identify those who are not infected, minimizing false positives. Non-specific tests could lead to unwarranted treatments, worry, and excessive healthcare costs. Sensitivity and specificity characteristics are of utmost relevance since these are vital parameters determining the usefulness of test diagnosis, highlighting the importance of never-ending advances in the diagnostic method. The development of highly sensitive and specific diagnostic tests has been significantly influenced by advances in technology. Time-consuming and unpredictable culture-based detection methods for fungal pathogens are based on incubating conditions as well as organism growth patterns. Furthermore, due to the rising prevalence of opportunistic fungal infections, diagnosis must become more efficient. Cutting-edge techniques, including next-generation sequencing and proteomics, promise great potential in addressing this issue by allowing rapid and dependable detection of the fungal species and their drug susceptibility profiles.

Yet, while these technologies promise enormous potential, they must overcome obstacles such as the integration into routine clinical practice, to meet the needs of both sensitivity and specificity, ultimately leading to enhanced patient care in fungal infections (Arastehfar et al., 2019). Furthermore, the journey from laboratory to clinic is beset with challenges that must be surmounted in order to provide the maximum benefit from next-generation diagnostic methods. High-throughput methodologies may have potential for increasing sensitivity and specificity in fungal diagnosis, but the variability in the types of pathogens and modes of resistance presents yet another layer of complexity. As reaffirmed in current literature, ongoing research is necessary to continue evolving these approaches so that they can be effectively used within a clinical setting. Continued reflection on contemporary methodologies against future technologies will allow for productive debate about their relative strengths and weaknesses. Significantly, encouraging collaboration among clinicians and researchers can help construct inclusive diagnostic methods that are both clinically significant and geared towards the evolving context of fungal infections (Groll et al., 2012) (Figure 2.23).

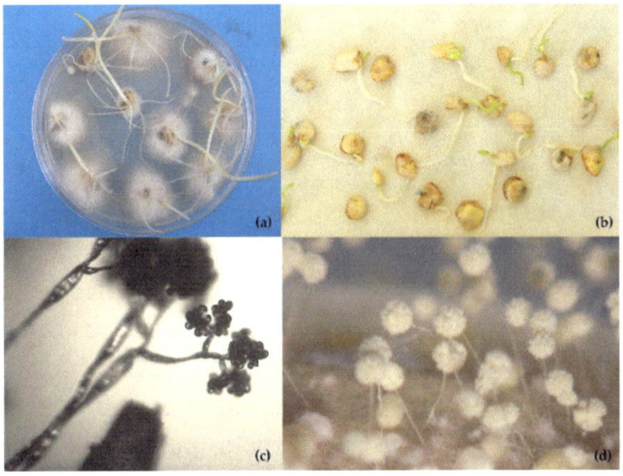

Figure 2.23. Traditional culture methods for identifying fungal pathogens often require time-consuming processes and may produce variable results depending on the incubating conditions and the organisms growth characteristics.

Source: https://www.mdpi.com/plants/plants-11-03167/article_deploy/html/images/plants-11-03167-g001.png.

2.6.2. Correlation with Clinical Findings

The interrelationship between laboratory findings and clinical presentations lies at the heart of the early diagnosis of fungal infections, particularly in immunocompromised hosts. Awareness of the association between some biological markers and clinical signs can enhance diagnostic accuracy significantly. For instance, patients undergoing procedures such as liver transplantation exhibit typical laboratory profiles that can predispose them to invasive fungal infections. Risk indicators including widespread use of nonprophylactic intravenous antibiotics, overall operative time, and certain hematologic abnormalities like thrombocytopenia and reduced T lymphocyte levels have been determined (Dummer et al., 1988). Detection of these correlations allows clinicians to recognize risk patients so that an aggressive surveillance approach can be initiated, improving patient outcomes by intervening earlier. The diagnostic dilemma of pulmonary fungal infections

(PFI) is the finest example of the requirement for integral interpretation of clinical data in the context of laboratory findings. The EORTC-MSG criteria are the standard guideline for defining PFI; however, they risk a lack of sensitivity in the diagnosis based on radiological heterogeneity. A study evaluated various pulmonary infiltrates in patients with acute myeloid leukemia and observed that a large proportion didn't fit under strict guidelines due to a specific radiologic findings observed at initial tests (Ascioglu et al., 2016).

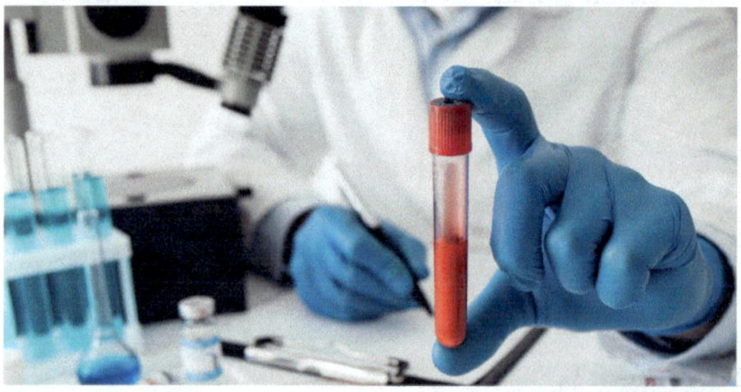

Figure 2.24. Understanding the relationship between specific biological markers and clinical indicators can significantly enhance diagnostic accuracy.

Source: https://bitesizebio.com/wp-content/uploads/2024/02/BsB-Article-What-is-a-Biomarker-Promo.jpg.

This proves the importance of not strictly using diagnostic criteria but rather taking converging clinical and microbiological data to broaden the spectrum of diagnosis. This approach enables healthcare providers to re-evaluate suspected cases so that severe infections are not overlooked and treatment may be initiated early. The integration of clinical data in laboratory diagnosis of fungal infections provides a holistic strategy for patient disease onset and health. For example, laboratory findings such as positive serum galactomannan tests can be a valuable addition to clinical assessment, affecting therapeutic decisions and monitoring to antifungal therapy. Moreover, alterations in radiological information as well as microbiological parameters provide the ability to improve diagnostic protocols. By adopting more relaxed imaging criteria based on laboratory findings, medical practitioners can maximize sensitivity in the detection of PFI, especially among high-risk patients, as was shown in the evaluation of the patients in the above study (Ascioglu et al., 2016). By bringing together laboratory and clinical findings, therefore, not only is detection of fungal infections maximized but also therapy strategies are optimized, with better outcomes for patients (Figure 2.24).

2.6.3. Challenges in Result Interpretation

The interpretive challenges in laboratory identification of fungal infections are significantly enhanced by the biological diversity and complexity of pathogenic fungi. The sheer number of varieties of fungi, including numerous opportunistic pathogens, renders accurate identification for effective treatment to be elusive. It is a characteristic of most laboratory tests, particularly culture-based methods, that they produce nonspecific results due to co-culture of the non-pathogenic and the pathogen. As noted by the literature, such uncertainty can lead to misdiagnosis, inappropriate treatment, or delayed therapy, resulting in poor outcomes for patients. The increasing resistance of antifungals as observed among the majority of fungal strains makes identification in addition to correct drug susceptibility determination a task that existing diagnostic techniques tend to carry out unsuccessfully, calling for enhanced fungal diagnosis (Arastehfar et al., 2019). The other major challenge of interpreting findings comes from the limitations of today's diagnostic techniques, namely their sensitivity and specificity. Traditional methods rely on the culturing of microorganisms, which may be slow and labor-intensive, resulting in delays that have a detrimental effect on patient care. Additionally, some rapid diagnostic tests do not have complete coverage for the species implicated or for resistance patterns, resulting in knowledge gaps in clinical practice.

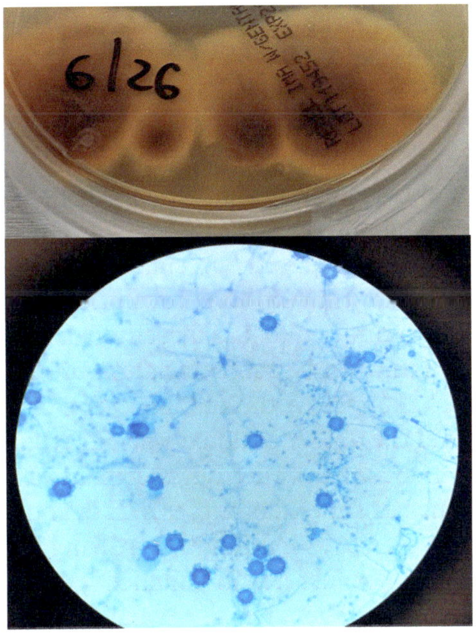

Figure 2.25. Many laboratory methods, particularly those dependent on culture techniques, often yield nonspecific results due to the co-culture of non-pathogenic and pathogenic species.

Source: https://labmedicineblog.com/wp-content/uploads/2025/01/histo1.png.

The arrival of next-generation sequencing technologies presents an exciting horizon, adding to the diagnostic armory with increased sensitivity and turnaround of results. However, as the clinician enters this new arsenal, so too do they encounter new challenges in making sense of the vast data sets produced, raising questions about the integration of such data into routine clinical decision-making (Chiu et al., 2019). Moreover, the clinician's use of advanced techniques such as metagenomic next-generation sequencing (mNGS) introduces additional interpretive challenges that must be addressed by medical staff. While mNGS offers complete pathogen identification independent of upfront culturing, its relevant information is overwhelming and may include numerous genetic pieces of pathogenic as well as commensal microbes. The problem lies in distinguishing clinically significant pathogens from benign flora, and determining the clinical relevance of genetic information for resistance to antifungal agents. These problems will necessitate establishing robust bioinformatics methodologies and clinical guidelines to facilitate supporting clinicians with proper interpretation, so that benefits of these novel technologies are brought to real effects on patient care and outcomes (Chiu et al., 2019) (Figure 2.25).

SUMMARY

The laboratory diagnosis of fungal infections is a sophisticated discipline that is rapidly evolving with the rise in cases of fungal diseases as well as the intricacy in their identification and treatment. One thing to note here is the increased incidence of opportunistic fungal infections, particularly in immunocompromised patients. The high variety of fungi responsible for these infections complicates identification and was further aggravated by the emergence of antifungal resistance. All these underscore the need for prompt detection methods that are capable of detecting the causative species reliably and establishing their drug susceptibility patterns so as to ensure the best treatment and improved patient outcomes (Arastehfar et al., 2019). Technological advancements are instrumental in enhancing the diagnostic situation for fungal infections. Traditional methods, relying on labor-intensive culture procedures, are failing to address the urgency required for clinical application. Technologies such as metagenomic next-generation sequencing (mNGS) are revolutionizing the diagnostic process by allowing global analysis of microbial genomic material directly from clinical specimens, thus facilitating quicker and better detection of pathogens. Such translation of research to clinical application is accompanied by opportunities and challenges, with the integration of mNGS into the laboratory process calling for sensitivity, precision, and the ability to detect various resistance patterns in fungal pathogens (Chiu et al., 2019). Besides, the implication of such advancements extends beyond recognition; it involves broader public health issues, such as surveillance of trends in antifungal resistance. With labs adopting new technology like mNGS, the efforts of fighting the growing menace of resistant fungal organisms are aided considerably. The focus not just lies in enhancing diagnostic capability but also in gaining knowledge about the epidemiology and genetics of the pathogens. With incorporation of prompt identification methods and resistance profile expertise, physicians are able to make treatment regimens more precisely tailored, ultimately improving patient care and managing the public health dimensions of fungal infection (Arastehfar et al., 2019; Chiu et al., 2019).

A CLOSER LOOK

METAGENOMIC NEXT-GENERATION SEQUENCING

Metagenomic next-generation sequencing, or mNGS, is an advanced technique to analyze the genetic material of every microbe present in a sample, without initially culturing them. Unlike more traditional approaches that focus on specific microbes, mNGS provides a general, unbiased description of the entire microbial community—such as bacteria, viruses, fungi, and parasites. It involves extraction of DNA or RNA from a sample (e.g., blood, fecal matter, or environmental sample), high-throughput next-generation sequencing, and bioinformatics interpretation to identify known and hitherto unknown organisms. mNGS is especially beneficial in clinical diagnostics, outbreaks, environmental microbiology, and the study of complex microbial ecosystems. It offers rapid, accurate pathogen identification even when standard testing is unavailable but requires advanced bioinformatics software and interpretation.

REFERENCES

1. Akan, H., Alexander, B. D., Andes, D., Azoulay, E., et al. (2019). Revision and update of the consensus definitions of invasive fungal disease from the European Organization for Research and Treatment of Cancer and the Mycoses Study Group Education and Research Consortium. https://core.ac.uk/download/287649722.pdf (accessed on 27th June 2025).
2. Ala-Houhala, M., Antikainen, J., Anttila, V. J., Kirveskari, J., et al. (2018). Clinical use of fungal PCR from deep tissue samples in the diagnosis of invasive fungal diseases: A retrospective observational study. https://core.ac.uk/download/157587682.pdf (accessed on 27th June 2025).
3. Albers, A., Bloch, K. C., Chow, F. C., Davis, J. A., et al. (2018). Detection of (1,3)-β-d-glucan in cerebrospinal fluid in *Histoplasma* meningitis. https://core.ac.uk/download/227054295.pdf (accessed on 27th June 2025).
4. Arabatzis, M., Emtestam, L., Faergemann, J., Hay, R. J., Lecerf, P., Nenoff, P., Nowicki, R. J., et al. (2019). A survey among dermatologists: Diagnostics of superficial fungal infections–What is used and what is needed to initiate therapy and assess efficacy? https://core.ac.uk/download/287184089.pdf (accessed on 27th June 2025).
5. Arastehfar, A., Boekhout, T., Buda De Cesare, G., Butler, G., et al. (2019). Recent trends in molecular diagnostics of yeast infections: From PCR to NGS. https://core.ac.uk/download/286086540.pdf (accessed on 27th June 2025).
6. Arzberger, E., Bastos, P. M., Ferreira, J., Leal-Filipe, J., et al. (2020). Reflectance confocal microscopy for the diagnosis of skin infections and infestations. https://core.ac.uk/download/322493878.pdf (accessed on 27th June 2025).
7. Ascioglu, S., Chamilos, G., De Pauw, B., Duarte, R., Even, G., Girmenia, C., Girmenia, C., et al. (2016). Pulmonary fungal infections in patients with acute myeloid leukemia: Is it the time to revise the radiological diagnostic criteria? https://core.ac.uk/download/54529664.pdf (accessed on 27th June 2025).
8. Athanasiou, L. V., Papaioannou, N., & Psemmas, D. E. (2018). Conjunctival cytology assessment in dogs and cats: Sampling, diagnostic techniques and findings. https://core.ac.uk/download/518119044.pdf (accessed on 27th June 2025).
9. Barnes, H. J., Basher, H. A., Fonnesbech Vogel, B., Gitter, M., Ivanics, E., Lucas, A., McDiarmid, A., et al. (2015). Outbreak of encephalitic listeriosis in red-legged partridges (*Alectoris rufa*). https://core.ac.uk/download/36778157.pdf (accessed on 27th June 2025).
10. Blackburn, B. G., Chiu, C. Y., DeRisi, J. L., Eckburg, P. B., et al. (2006). Microarray detection of human *parainfluenza virus 4* infections associated with respiratory failure in an immunocompetent adult. https://core.ac.uk/download/323072700.pdf (accessed on 27th June 2025).
11. Blasco-Navalpotro, M., Blot, S. I., Bulpa, P., Cardoso, T., et al. (2015). Epidemiology of invasive aspergillosis in critically ill patients: Clinical presentation, underlying conditions, and outcome. https://core.ac.uk/download/55762158.pdf (accessed on 27th June 2025).
12. Bochicchio, G., Bochicchio, K., Kronen, R., Liang, S., et al. (2017). Invasive fungal infections secondary to traumatic injury. https://core.ac.uk/download/129069519.pdf (accessed on 27th June 2025).

13. Bouley, A. J., Morrissey, A. B., Nadjm, B., Nadjm, B., Pastorino, B., Greenwood, B. M., Petti, C. A., et al. (2013). Etiology of severe non-malaria febrile illness in northern Tanzania: A prospective cohort study. https://core.ac.uk/download/pdf/16666813.pdf (accessed on 27th June 2025).

14. Brunetti, G., Ceccarelli, G., Fallani, S., Ghezzi, D., et al. (2016). Voriconazole treatment of *Candida tropicalis* meningitis: Persistence of (1,3)-β-d-glucan in the cerebrospinal fluid is a marker of clinical and microbiological failure. https://core.ac.uk/download/74321348.pdf (accessed on 27th June 2025).

15. Burger, E., Camargo, Z. P., Fernandes, G. F., Rodrigues, A. M., et al. (2015). Immunodiagnostic of Para coccidioidomycosis due to *Paracoccidioides brasiliensis* using a latex test: Detection of specific antibody anti-gp43 and specific antigen gp43. https://core.ac.uk/download/37741973.pdf (accessed on 27th June 2025).

16. Chiu, C. Y., & Miller, S. A. (2019). Clinical metagenomics. https://core.ac.uk/download/323062552.pdf (accessed on 27th June 2025).

17. Di Pietro, A., Reuben, A., Martinez-Rocha, A. L., Di Pietro, A., Musher, B., de Pauw, B. E., Foster, C. S., et al. (2014). Murine model for *Fusarium oxysporum* invasive fusariosis reveals organ-specific structures for dissemination and long-term persistence. https://core.ac.uk/download/20115566.pdf (accessed on 27th June 2025).

18. Dummer, J. S., Esquivel, C., Ho, M., Kusne, S., et al. (1988). Fungal infections after liver transplantation. https://core.ac.uk/download/12204282.pdf (accessed on 27th June 2025).

19. Fung, J., Irish, W., Kusne, S., Martin, M., et al. (1992). Factors associated with invasive lung aspergillosis and the significance of positive *Aspergillus* culture after liver transplantation. https://core.ac.uk/download/12204865.pdf (accessed on 27th June 2025).

20. Goldberg, A. N., Murr, A. H., & Vesper, S. (2006). Fungal speciation using quantitative polymerase chain reaction (qPCR) in patients with and without chronic rhinosinusitis. https://core.ac.uk/download/323072535.pdf (accessed on 27th June 2025).

21. Groll, A. H., Pham, A. S., De Pauw, B., Costa, C., Girmenia, C., Halliday, C., Mengoli, C., et al. (2012). A MIQE-compliant real-time PCR assay for *Aspergillus* detection. https://core.ac.uk/download/30696634.pdf (accessed on 27th June 2025).

22. Inohara, T., Kanamoto, A., Kuroda, K., Murase, K., et al. (1959). *Cryptococcus*, pathological observations of five autopsy cases and one biopsy case. https://core.ac.uk/download/12548640.pdf (accessed on 27th June 2025).

23. Janiszewska-Drobinska, B., Behr, M., Beukes, M., Brennan, J., Butler, R., Centers for Disease Control & Prevention (CDC), Chang, K., et al. (2013). Rapid method for *Mycobacterium tuberculosis* identification using electrospray ionization tandem mass spectrometry analysis of mycolic acids. https://core.ac.uk/download/71976389.pdf (accessed on 27th June 2025).

24. Jourdan, P. M., & Lamberton, P. H. L. (2015). Human ascariasis: Diagnostics update. https://core.ac.uk/download/46559165.pdf (accessed on 27th June 2025).

25. Sabino, R., Simões, D., Simões, H., Veríssimo, C., et al. (2019). Dermatophytes' identification by matrix-assisted laser desorption ionization-time of flight mass spectrometry (MALDI-TOF MS)–The experience of a clinical laboratory. https://core.ac.uk/download/323276238.pdf (accessed on 27th June 2025).

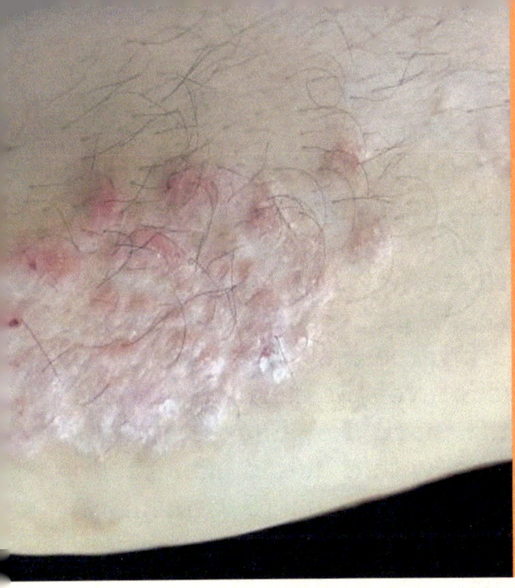

Chapter 3
DERMATOPHYTOSIS

Contents

Introduction

Ringworm or dermatophytosis is a widespread dermatologic condition caused by a set of fungi called the dermatophytes. The pathogens thrive in a keratinous environment and cause infections involving primarily the skin, hair, and nails. The epidemiology of dermatophytosis is that it has a global distribution and occurs in individuals of all ages and regions. Transmission usually takes place by direct contact with infected people, animals, or contaminated objects, making public health interventions an integral part. In addition, public awareness campaigns are also necessary since most cases are undiagnosed or mismanaged because of misinformation regarding the illness. As more cases of dermatophytosis are on the rise, knowing its etiology and implications is vital in formulating effective means to manage and avert this fungal infection. Diagnostic technology has significantly enhanced the treatment of dermatophytosis. Previously, clinical presentation and culture formed the basis of diagnosis but with technological advances, non-invasive and real-time imaging through techniques such as reflectance confocal microscopy (RCM) has been introduced. RCM has proven useful in outlining skin infections, offering the capability to see fungal architecture in the epidermis and superficial dermis. The technique offers diagnostic specificity comparable to that of histopathology with minimal patient discomfort and consumption of resources.

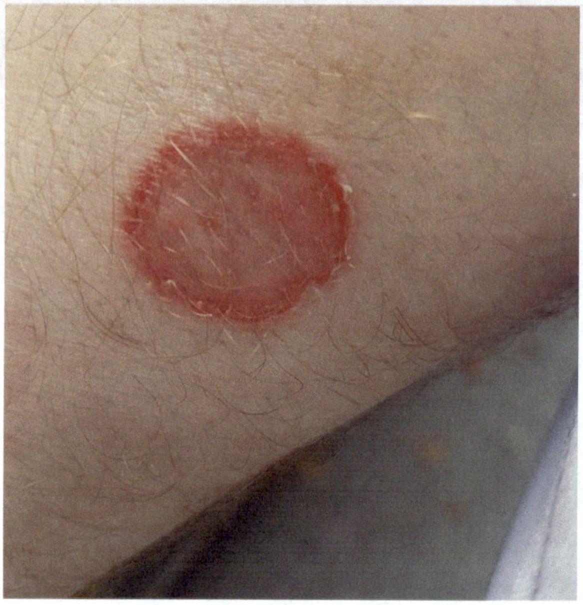

Figure 3.1. Dermatophytosis.

Source: https://static.wixstatic.com/media/acc226_e51a5b1794024ab985039dac8a00bc73~mv2.jpg/v1/fill/w_1000,h_1000,al_c,q_85,usm_0.66_1.00_0.01/acc226_e51a5b1794024ab985039dac8a00bc73~mv2.jpg.

Moreover, the higher resolution of RCM enables clinicians to make a good assessment of treatment responses, hence reducing unnecessary treatments and maximizing patient outcomes. These developments bring to the fore the importance of integrating advanced diagnostic tools into clinical practice for effective management of dermatophytosis and skin conditions in general, ultimately improving patient care in dermatology. Together with advancements in diagnostic technology, epidemiological studies highlight the varied presentation and impact of dermatophytosis across populations. In one study of dromedary camels in Morocco, there were high infection rates with dermatophytes, highlighting the zoonotic nature of the pathogens. This research indicated that a high percentage of the cases of skin disease involved dermatophytes, emphasizing the need for understanding animal reservoirs within the dynamics of dermatophytosis transmission (Bengoumi et al., 2019). Such evidence calls for an expanded scope of understanding, with consideration of the veterinary and human health relationship in regulating fungal infections. By understanding dermatophyte epidemiology and ecology, public health programs can be more narrowly targeted to reduce the occurrence of dermatophytosis, and thus control an important aspect of dermatologic health globally (Figure 3.1).

3.1. Causes of Dermatophytosis

The pathogenesis of dermatophytosis owes its origin primarily to various environmental as well as biological factors favorable for the growth of dermatophyte fungi. Key causative agents of this infection are the species of the genera *Trichophyton, Microsporum*, and *Epidermophyton* that thrive in their ideal habitats in keratin-rich environments such as skin, hair, and nails. The disease occurs when such fungi infect the outer skin layers and produce various forms of tinea or ringworm. Dermatophytosis is exacerbated by poor levels of hygiene, a key risk factor identified in some studies. For instance, a study in Kashmir found that the poorly cared-for individuals were disproportionately affected by dermatophyte infestations, particularly among the population aged 18–32 years, illustrating the correlation between environmental conditions and rates of incidence (Farhana et al., 2021). Age is another major determinant of prevalence of dermatophytosis. Evidence indicates that adolescents comprise a large percentage of victims, as their immune systems may be immature or they may come into closer contact with dermatophyte reservoirs, such as domestic pets. For example, research with Van cats demonstrated seasonality of dermatophyte occurrence, particularly in younger cats, which would suggest that age is a factor for susceptibility to infection with dermatophytes (Akkan et al., 2016).

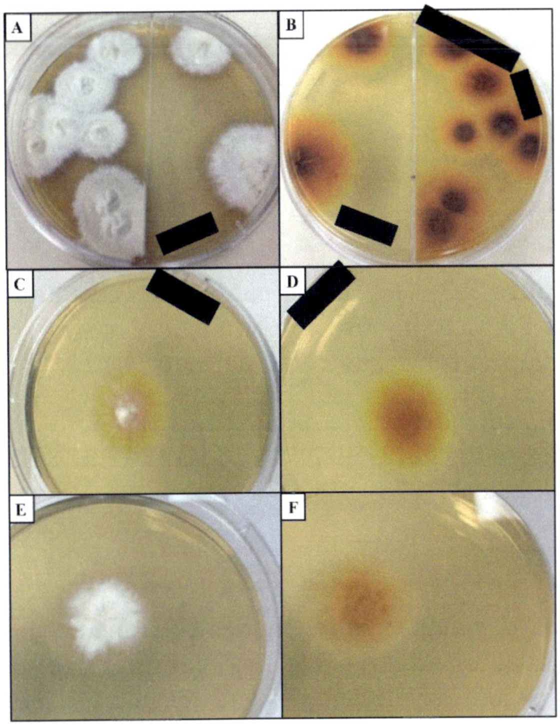

Figure 3.2. The onset of dermatophytosis is primarily linked to a variety of environmental and biological factors conducive to the proliferation of dermatophyte fungi.

Source: https://pub.mdpi-res.com/pathogens/pathogens-11-00957/article_deploy/html/images/pathogens-11-00957-g004.png?1662537509.

Furthermore, demographic factors such as socioeconomic status also have a significant role to play; people from lower socioeconomic status communities are more prone to dermatophytosis. Lack of access to proper healthcare and education increases the likelihood of the patient contracting fungal infections since individuals are not aware of how they can be prevented, and this is a continuation of ill health particularly in vulnerable age groups. Secondly, host-pathogen interaction is also a vital factor in the etiology of dermatophytosis. Individual susceptibility based on immune status, health states, and comorbidities can promote or suppress fungal colonization. In diabetes or HIV/AIDS patients with compromised immunity, for instance, dermatophyte infections are particularly susceptible because the body is not very capable of mounting an effective defense. Additionally, long-term skin conditions like eczema compromise normal skin barriers, presenting simple entry points for dermatophytes into living tissues. Consequently, understanding the intricate aetiologies of dermatophytosis not only aids in infection diagnosis and management but also places the necessity for ongoing prevention measures directed towards susceptible individuals in perspective as a way of controlling the incidence of this infectious skin condition (Figure 3.2).

3.1.1. Fungal Pathogens Responsible

The infections caused by fungi that result in dermatophytosis are best characterized by a subgroup of fungi known as dermatophytes. These fungi infect keratinized tissues selectively, such as skin, hair, and nails. *Trichophyton rubrum*, *Trichophyton interdigitale*, and *Microsporum canis* are some of the most prevalent species. *T. rubrum* is most frequently associated with both superficial and invasive disease and is a predominant pathogen in clinics. The ability of the organism to survive under varying environmental conditions, as well as its pathogenicity, has the effect of emphasizing the importance of understanding its mechanisms of infection. Additionally, recent taxonomic reclassifications of dermatophytes have the effect of making identification processes more complex, given that most clinical laboratories still employ phenotypic methods, which are not always accurate for distinguishing among closely related species. Its significance to effective diagnosis and treatment provides the necessity of possessing complete identification strategies. Effective management of dermatophytosis is highly dependent upon correct identification of the etiologic fungal pathogens. The traditional methods of diagnosis, which are generally macroscopic and microscopic morphology examination based, can lead to misidentifications. This becomes a valid issue with the high level of variation within the dermatophyte species and morphological similarity. The integration of molecular techniques, such as MALDI-TOF MS and genetic marker sequencing, offers a more uniform species identification method. Research employing MALDI-TOF has been shown to be of high accuracy in the identification of isolates, with rare cases of exceptions existing, necessitating the incorporation of a variety of methods to achieve correct classification (Bengoumi et al., 2019). A layered approach enhances specificity in capability to accurately target specific pathogens, leading to opportunities for personalized therapeutic interventions. The prevalence and impact of dermatophytes are not exclusive to human infections but affect animals as well, with the dromedary camel being among the affected animals. In a study on dermatological disease among Moroccan camels, infection by dermatophytes was a leading causative agent and accounted for 30% of reported infections as well as bacterial and viral infections (Bengoumi et al., 2019). The widespread nature of such fungal infections is due to factors such as environmental conditions as well as the art of taking care of animals. Of interest is the fact that the recidivism of dermatosis, even in treatable cases, raises issues regarding veterinary care and preventive work. These findings not only highlight the fascinating interface between animal health and human dermatophytosis but also the requirement for an integrative management approach that accounts for both human and animal dermatophyte infestations, highlighting the broader implications of fungal pathogens on our environment (Figure 3.3).

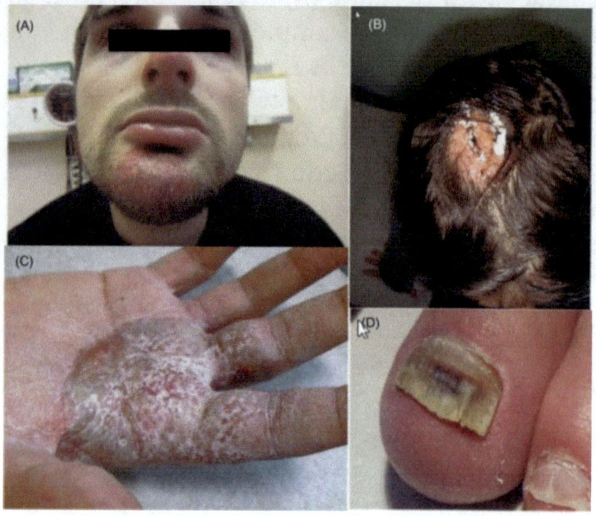

Figure 3.3. The fungal pathogens responsible for dermatophytosis predominantly belong to a group of fungi known as dermatophytes.

Source: https://ars.els-cdn.com/content/image/3-s2.0-B9780128187319002317-f00231-01-9780128187319.jpg.

3.1.2. Modes of Transmission

The dermatophytosis modes of transmission, characteristically a very common fungal infection, may be complex and demand extensive knowledge in order to stem the infections effectively. Here, dermatophytes get transmitted primarily through direct association with infected persons or animals, due to which intimate contact is significant in detecting probable cases. *Microsporum canis*, for example, a very common dermatophyte that infects both cats and humans, depicts this transmission mechanism. Infection can be developed following skin-to-skin contact or indirectly through contaminated surfaces that the spores occupy. This method of transmission emphasizes people's role in practicing hygiene and watchfulness, particularly in crowded populations. Furthermore, studies show that environmental factors play a role in making dermatophyte spores viable, thus making infection control efforts challenging because the spores can survive in the environment for decades (Moskaluk et al., 2022). Besides contact, zoonotic transmission also plays a significant mode of dermatophytosis, presenting challenges to both the veterinary and human healthcare fields. Since both pet owners and veterinarians often interact with infected animals, awareness plays a central role in preventing the spread of the fungi. Due to the intrinsic asymptomatic character of most zoonotic diseases, such as those caused by dermatophytes, there is a need for careful monitoring and preventive activities among animal populations. Additionally, in areas where close human-animal contact is prevalent, extreme caution must be exercised to prevent transmission. Education initiatives directed to pet owners and veterinarians can have a strong impact on safety culture, facilitating better communication about zoonoses and encouraging preventative measures. This education focus is essential for lowering risk and improving overall public health through active prevention. Environmental transmission also deserves special attention as a significant mode of transmission for dermatophytosis. Dermatophytes can survive in high heat and humidity and remain infectious for extended periods on equipment such as grooming, clothes, and furniture. This resilience is what renders the fungus easily transferable from host to host, even at times without direct animal contact. Social areas where people congregate, such as gyms or communal swimming pools, provide fertile ground for potential outbreaks. Implementing stringent sanitation practices in these environments can reduce transmission risk. Furthermore, ongoing research into emerging diagnostic techniques and treatment strategies is crucial to enhance knowledge and control of dermatophyte transmission dynamics and, consequently, public health impact from this widespread and concerning infection (Moskaluk et al., 2022) (Figure 3.4).

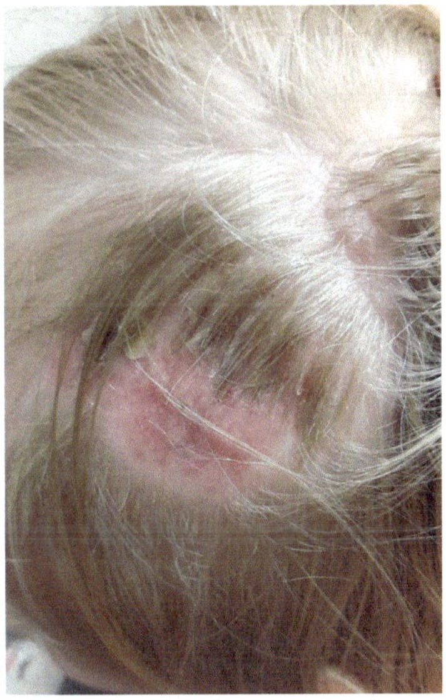

Figure 3.4. *Microsporum canis*, a common dermatophyte affecting both cats and humans, illustrates this transmission dynamic.

Source: https://pub.mdpi-res.com/jof/jof-10-00244/article_deploy/html/images/jof-10-00244-g002.png?1711275223.

3.1.3. Risk Factors for Infection

Concerning dermatophytosis, the risk factors for infection are multifaceted in nature and contribute greatly towards determining the prevalence of the fungal infection. Some of the most important risk factors include setting that favors the growth of the dermatophytes and their transmission. Fungi tend to grow predominantly in warm and moist conditions, and thus environments such as shared baths, swimming pools, and locker rooms are hotbeds for infection. Patients treated in these environments, such as sports individuals or those in direct contact with infected patients, are at greater risk. Additionally, hygienic practices of individuals play a similar role in prevention from exposure; inadequate washing of clothing and failure to dry body skin well raises susceptibility to infection. Identification of these environmental and behavioral risk factors is most crucial for formulating effective prevention strategies among individuals at risk of dermatophytosis. Yet another of the key risk factors for dermatophytosis is the immunocompromised state of the individuals as a result of multiple underlying medical conditions or therapies. Diabetes mellitus, HIV/AIDS, and cancer are some of the conditions that decrease the immune response, thus predisposing individuals to opportunistic infections such as dermatophyte infections. Further, immunosuppressive therapies, like corticosteroids or chemotherapy, also decrease the immune response of the host. In such a situation, heightened vigilance is essential for the diagnosis and control of such skin infections in these risk populations. The epidemiologic insight into these immunological determinants underscores the need for targeted interventions and education so that healthcare providers can enhance detection of manifestations of dermatophytosis and direct appropriate treatment efforts. Demographic factors like age, gender, and occupational risk might also influence the risk of dermatophytosis. Age-related susceptibility is particularly self-evident, with children having perhaps more exposure to dermatophytes due to play and group activities. Older individuals may observe declining skin barrier function or have pre-existing conditions that make them at higher risk. Gender has also been observed to have a significant influence on susceptibility, as certain studies indicate that females are more likely to exhibit higher occurrences of dermatophytosis compared to males, presumably due to variations in personal hygiene practices or exposures at work. Understanding these demographic factors, in addition to lessons learned on investigation in livestock such as the dromedary camel, where infection was prevalent due to a lack of proper treatment and systemic monitoring, illustrates the importance of comprehensive actions within disease risk management pertaining to dermatophytosis (Bengoumi et al., 2019). Also, technology like Reflectance Confocal Microscopy (RCM) presents promising horizons for treatment and diagnosis, enabling more advanced interpretation of fungal infection and assisting in monitoring the response to treatment, thereby impacting risk assessment strategy (Arzberger et al., 2020) (Figure 3.5).

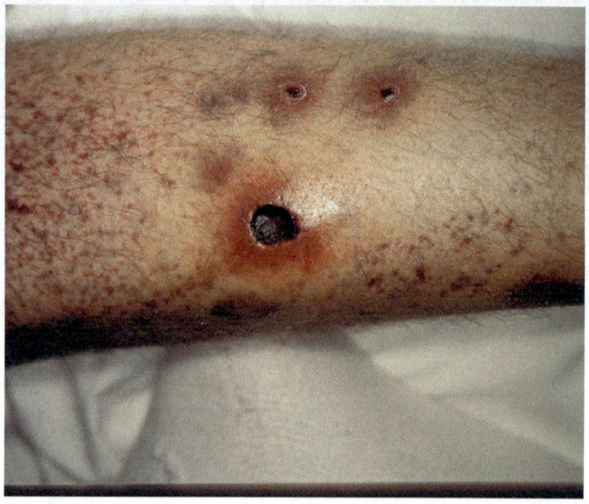

Figure 3.5. Conditions such as diabetes mellitus, HIV/AIDS, and cancer can diminish the immune response, thereby facilitating opportunistic infections including dermatophyte infections.

Source: https://www.cidjournal.com/cms/10.1016/j.clindermatol.2012.01.011/asset/7071fc54-3a67-4887-a1aa-131b0a0307f8/main.assets/gr10_lrg.jpg.

3.2. Symptoms and Diagnosis

It is necessary to know the signs of dermatophytosis for effective and early diagnosis so that doctors can take suitable action. This fungal infection, also known as ringworm, is experienced through various signs in the form of circular, red, and scratchy rashes with central clearing on the body. Scaling, crusting, and hair loss may be observed in the infected areas, particularly in more advanced cases. Besides this, patients may experience inflammation and pain, significantly impairing their quality of life. The variability in the character of the symptomatology also leads to misdiagnosis, emphasizing the importance of an accurate clinical evaluation. As dermatophyte infection may simulate other dermatoses such as eczema or psoriasis, it is important to distinguish between them for the choice of the most appropriate treatment regimen. The diagnostic methods for dermatophytosis are both clinical examination and laboratory diagnosis. Final diagnosis is typically reliant on KOH (potassium hydroxide) microscopy, which reveals fungal spores and hyphae directly from skin scrapings. Culture on particular media can also confirm the presence of dermatophytes, though this takes a few weeks for confirmation. Physicians can also employ Woods lamp examination, where particular dermatophytes show a characteristic fluorescence when subjected to ultraviolet light. Accurate diagnosis serves in that it enables one to develop an appropriate treatment plan according to the dermatophyte species involved. For instance, both diagnosis and symptomology need to guide antifungal therapy decisions because therapeutic differences can exist depending on the etiologic agent. Finally, understanding the epidemiology of dermatophytosis across different populations is critical because it can even make symptoms and diagnosis complex. In regions such as south Morocco, studies illustrate how dermatophytosis affects a variety of animal species, including dromedary camels, with infection rates determining herd management. Such findings point to the necessity of information and education regarding dermatophyte infections both in humans and animals since the infections are easily treatable but remain rife due to the absence of preventive measures. The overall discourse is that identification of signs and application of appropriate diagnostic methods allow for appropriate treatment, which ultimately reduces the rate of recurrence of the infection in both human and veterinary medicine (Bengoumi et al., 2019; Antoine et al., 2014) (Figure 3.6).

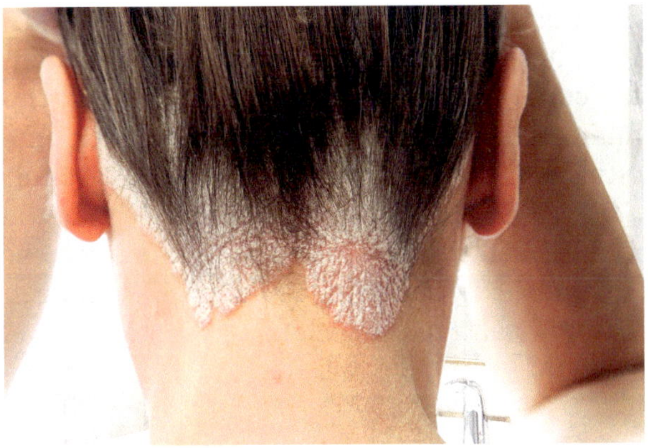

Figure 3.6. Infected areas may exhibit scaling, crusting, and hair loss, particularly in more severe cases.

Source: https://img.lb.wbmdstatic.com/vim/live/webmd/consumer_assets/site_images/article_thumbnails/reference_guide/scalp_psoriasis_ref_guide/1800x1200_scalp_psoriasis_ref_guide_alt.jpg.

3.2.1. Common Clinical Manifestations

Dermatophytosis, or ringworm, is associated with a range of clinical presentations that can significantly impact the quality of life for the patient. The major features are well-defined, pruritic, erythematous lesions that typically have a ring appearance. The lesions can be quite different depending upon the location of the infection; tinea corporis appears on the trunk and extremities, and tinea capitis appears on the scalp and hair follicles. Apart from the external expressions of the disease on the skin, the patients may also present with accompanying symptoms of secondary bacterial infection, scaling, and pustules in some cases that worsen the clinical presentation. The presentation is therefore not only dermatological but also likely to cause psychological discomfort due to the cosmetic concerns, so the management and treatment must be comprehensive. The occurrence of dermatophytosis is influenced by a number of factors, including environmental and host variables such as immune status. Dermatophytosis seems to be more virulent in certain populations, including the immunocompromised. Interestingly, in patients with HIV, there was found to be a greater incidence of dermatophytosis, as 41.07% of the patients had this infection among their regular skin infections, indicating a relationship between general health and dermatological status.

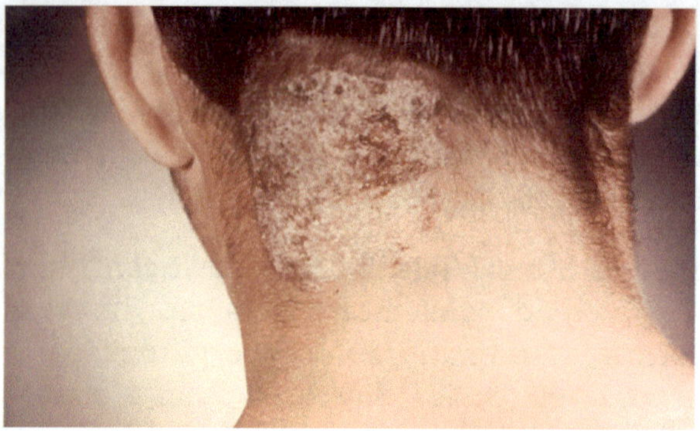

Figure 3.7. Heightened susceptibility to dermatophyte infections is often observed in individuals with compromised immune systems, where overlapping clinical manifestations of various dermatological ailments can occur.

Source: https://www.mdpi.com/jof/jof-10-00357/article_deploy/html/images/jof-10-00357-g001.png.

Skin disease such as this can be the first indicator of overall health issues, leading to further comprehensive clinical evaluations and system-wide infection screenings, including HIV. Early detection of dermatophytosis is important, as in some research, not just to heal the skin infection but also to gain an understanding of the overall implications for the patient's health so that a more proactive, integrated approach to patient care can be taken. In addition to the traditional manifestations of dermatophytosis, secondary fungal infections may complicate the clinical picture. For instance, enhanced susceptibility to infection by dermatophytes is frequently observed in patients with compromised immune status, where there may be overlapping clinical manifestation of varying dermatoses. In a dromedary camel experiment, dermatophyte-caused infections constituted a high proportion of skin diseases observed, highlighting the ecological and zoonotic nature of dermatophytosis. The recurrence of skin ailments to reappear time and again, particularly in untreated cases, highlights the significance of effective management programs considering preventive as well as curative strategies. This dual focus is necessary in limiting the impacts of dermatophytosis and providing proper patient education and awareness, thereby improving long-term health outcomes for those suffering from this disease (Figure 3.7).

3.2.2. Diagnostic Methods Used

The diagnosis of dermatophytosis, which is caused by a range of fungi that infect keratinized tissues, necessitates an approach that is multidimensional. An example is the microscopic examination of potassium hydroxide (KOH)-treated skin, hair, or nail scrapings, where keratin is dissolved and the fungal elements rendered more visible. The relative low cost and rapidity of the procedure render it highly useful for preliminary assessments. Its credibility is also affected because false negatives can be produced in the event of errors in specimen collection or presence of non-dermatophyte mold. These inaccuracies call for further diagnostic tests in an effort to confirm the presence of dermatophytes and identify the best appropriate treatment, thereby highlighting the primary significance of credible diagnostic tests to the treatment of dermatophytosis. Cultures remain the cornerstone of dermatophytosis diagnosis, since they allow absolute specification of pathogenic species. Samples collected from affected sites are cultured on special media, which favors fungal growth and inhibits bacteria. Even though culture method has a more lagged time than microscopy, it provides a certain method of specification, since fungal colony morphology may give some hints for species determination. These recent developments have also introduced molecular approaches, such as polymerase chain reaction (PCR), which have enhanced diagnostic sensitivity and specificity. In particular, the application of real-time PCR, as demonstrated in recent studies, has been useful.

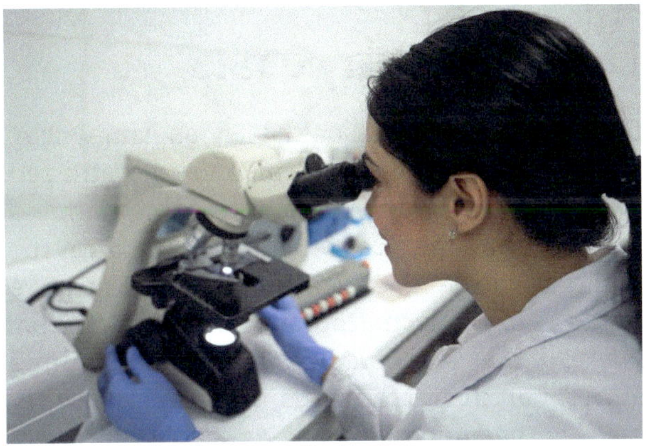

Figure 3.8. A common method involves the microscopic examination of skin, hair, or nail samples treated with potassium hydroxide (KOH), which helps to dissolve keratin and renders the fungal elements more visible.

Source: https://cdn-prod.medicalnewstoday.com/content/images/articles/322/322331/person-using-a-microscope-testing-for-skin-lesion-koh-exam.jpg.

For instance, *Trichophyton* verrucosum, one of the common dermatophytes in bovine dermatophytosis, is presently diagnosed directly from infected hairs by SYBR-Green real-time PCR, which is a faster and more reliable alternative to traditional methods (Araujo et al., 2023). Aside from microscopy and culture, recent non-invasive imaging techniques have emerged as new diagnostic tools in dermatophytosis. Reflectance confocal microscopy (RCM) is a valuable new technology that may be applied to image skin lesions in real-time, at high resolution. RCM can generate well-resolved images of the epidermis and upper dermis, where dermatophyte infection changes can be nicely shown. Since RCM is noninvasive, it may be used to aid diagnosis and longitudinally monitor treatment response. This possibility can reduce the need for invasive biopsy methods and attendant complications. The adoption of RCM into clinical practice therefore highlights how technology is transforming diagnostic practice in dermatophytosis by marrying traditional means with new techniques to improve patient care (Arzberger et al., 2020) (Figure 3.8).

3.2.3. Differential Diagnosis

In clinical dermatophytosis diagnosis, differential diagnosis cannot be overemphasized. Dermatophytosis may occur through a variety of presentations that can be mistaken for other skin diseases, including psoriasis, eczema, or bacterial infections. Proper identification is crucial as misidentification of dermatophytosis could lead to inappropriate treatment that exacerbates the patient's condition. Initial assessments are predominantly performed using clinical inspection; however, because of overlapping of signs and symptoms, further laboratory studies such as potassium hydroxide (KOH) mounts and fungal culture to identify the presence of dermatophytes are needed. Definitive testing for early diagnosis allows personalized therapeutic interventions to enhance patient overall management and avoid chronic infection or relapse (Jayanthi et al., 2016). The epidemiological determinants of dermatophytosis also complicate differentiation from other conditions. In particular, age, gender, and environmental determinants play a critical role in identifying those groups at highest risk. Recent studies suggest a higher incidence in males and the 21st to 30th year age group with factors exacerbating conditions by warm climate and lifestyle, e.g., occlusive footwear. Besides, common comorbidities like malnourishment or endocrinal illness like Cushing syndrome put certain patients at risk of dermatophyte infection and need to be kept in mind while making a differential diagnosis. Practitioners are thus prompted to include a patient history in their evaluation because it can reveal a subclinical condition that can camouflage the clinical picture and require an altered diagnostic approach (Jayanthi et al., 2016). Treatment of dermatophytosis relies heavily on proper diagnosis by differential diagnosis because it is determined by the causative fungal organism and the disease severity.

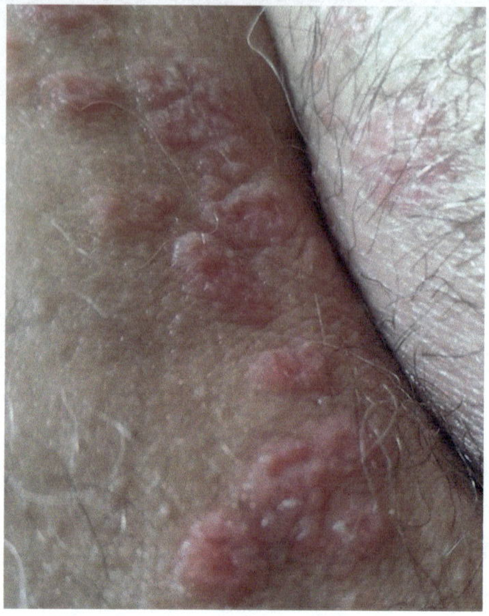

Figure 3.9. Establishing an accurate diagnosis is crucial, as misidentifying dermatophytosis could lead to inappropriate treatments that exacerbate the patient's condition.

Source: https://pub.mdpi-res.com/jcm/jcm-13-03267/article_deploy/html/images/jcm-13-03267-g005.png?1717660962.

Recommendations now call for the use of topical antifungals like miconazole and clotrimazole for localized dermatophytosis and the use of systemic treatment with terbinafine or itraconazole for disseminated infection. Understanding the distinctive characteristics of dermatophytosis against other skin diseases, particularly from laboratory confirmations, allows clinicians to deliver effective therapeutic treatments. Therefore, the integration of differential diagnosis into practice is essential so that dermatophytosis can be efficiently and in a timely manner treated, as witnessed in evidence declaring a high rate of response to effective antifungal treatment (Jayanthi et al., 2016) (Figure 3.9).

3.3. Types of Dermatophytosis

Dermatophytosis, also known as ringworm, is a fungal infection that involves keratinized tissues of the body such as the skin, hair, and nails. Dermatophytes, which are fungi with the ability to digest keratin, are the major causative organisms of dermatophytosis. *Trichophyton*, *Microsporum*, and *Epidermophyton* are the three genera of dermatophytes with over twenty species that infect animals as well as humans. Understanding the types of dermatophytosis is crucial in order to effectively diagnose and manage them since different species present with different clinical presentations. The condition is highly infective, and it is transmitted by direct contact with the lesions or indirect contact with infected surfaces through clothing and hair equipment, thus the need for public awareness and the need to observe proper hygiene (Abdulla et al., 2024). The dermatophytoses can be differentiated based on the location of the body and the fungus. Tinea capitis, for example, is infection of the scalp commonly due to *Microsporum canis*, more so in children and household pets. Another common variety is tinea corporis, affecting body skin and typically occurring as round patches of red color with a lighter-colored center. Tinea pedis, or athletes foot, affects the feet most and is predominantly caused by *Trichophyton rubrum*. Each of the types has distinct symptoms and needs unique management for cure, such as antifungal medication and topical creams. The typology helps healthcare professionals to learn possible risks and arrange appropriate management plans, enhancing patient outcomes (Moskaluk et al., 2022). In addition to the commonly recognized types of dermatophytosis, emerging studies have broadened the field in respect to related fungi and their status within dermatological well-being. Genetic research into *Microsporum canis,* for instance, has shown evolving classifications and characteristics that are possibly decisive with respect to clinical outcome. Besides, new-emerging species, like *Arthroderma,* highlight the demand for continuous research and development of diagnostic techniques, especially since these fungi possess a potential pathogenicity that is yet to be reported. Taxonomy of dermatophytes and mounting evidence on fungal virulence and behavior create the demand for epidemiological studies as well as development of molecular diagnostic tools (Abdulla et al., 2024; Moskaluk et al., 2022). This data not only enhances clinical practice but also highlights measures of prevention against outbreaks of dermatophytosis (Figure 3.10).

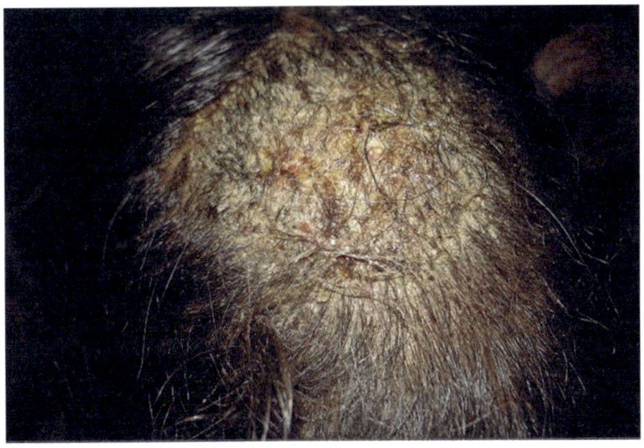

Figure 3.10. Tinea capitis.

Source: https://www.odermatol.com/wp-content/uploads/image/2013%202/3_tinea/Fig_1j.jpg.

3.3.1. Tinea corporis (Ringworm)

Ringworm or tinea corporis is a superficial dermatophyte infection of the skin, primarily of the keratinized tissues. It is due to infection by various species of the *Trichophyton* genus, which are keratin-dependent. The infection presents as oval or round erythematous plaques with well-defined margins, typically on the trunk and extremities. Risk for infection is heightened in the tropics and among individuals who have more physical activity and sweating. Measurement and monitoring of this condition are very important since approximately 25% of the world's population is susceptible to dermatophytosis. These interruptions to the integrity of the skin by environmental factors, such as friction and water, raise the risk of infection with dermatophytes further, which calls for an effective public health intervention aimed at avoiding its transmission and alleviating symptoms of Tinea corporis (Susanto et al., 2022). Clinical evaluation typically follows diagnosis of Tinea corporis, where health practitioners establish typical presentations as well as patient history. The presence of scaling lesions with or without central clearing is suggestive of this diagnosis, although laboratory findings, such as KOH microscopy or culture for fungus, are necessary to confirm this. Numerous effective treatments exist, and topical therapy with agents such as clotrimazole, ketoconazole, and terbinafine is the treatment of choice for limited infection. For more widespread or systemic infection, oral therapy with agents such as itraconazole or fluconazole may be required. Early treatment is not only required to alleviate symptoms but also to prevent the development of antibiotic resistance and recurrence of the disorder. Thus, it is significant to comprehend both the clinical presentation and the optimal modalities of therapy in the successful management of this disorder (Susanto et al., 2022). Public education is a critical aspect of Tinea corporis management, particularly regarding understanding routes of transmission and preventive measures. The disease is described as most commonly being transferred directly from one individual to another, indirectly through dirty objects such as clothes or surfaces, or through infected animals. Thus, stepping up cleanliness and using personal accessories correctly can significantly reduce transmission rates. Further, making individuals aware of the necessity of early recognition of symptoms can lead to early treatment, reducing the chances of large outbreaks. Better knowledge of dermatophyte epidemiology is necessary to guide appropriate public health action. As research continues to reveal the nuances of fungal biology and the environmental determinants for infection prevalence, community health education campaigns can then be tailored to meet the specific needs of the target population at risk and thus yield healthier skin and lower prevalence of dermatophytosis (Abdulla et al., 2024) (Figure 3.11).

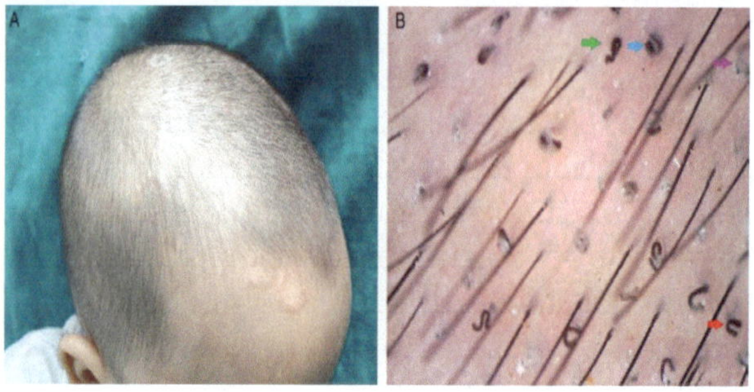

Figure 3.11. Diagnosis of Tinea corporis typically follows a clinical evaluation, where healthcare practitioners assess characteristic symptoms alongside patient history.

Source: https://images.squarespace-cdn.com/content/v1/5243dccde4b08fd9e4fc92ef/1649250842349-KG6WXO98NW2UKVF5RGNY/tinea+capitis.

3.3.2. Tinea pedis (Athlete's Foot)

Tinea pedis, or colloquially as athletes foot, is a frequent dermatological condition caused by a fungal infection but by the family *Trichophyton*. The development of the disease is typically accompanied by itching, redness, and peeling or cracking of the foot skin on the soles and the interdigital space between the toes. Although commonly found among athletes because of the warm, humid conditions of athletic shoes, tinea pedis can occur among individuals across all demographics, such as those who reside in humid environments or participate in a range of activities that encourage moisture buildup on the feet. Knowing the pathogenesis of tinea pedis is important to treat and prevent, especially because its symptoms tend to negatively impact daily functioning and overall well-being. The treatment of tinea pedis has been revolutionized with the advent of topical and systemic antifungal medications. Among those, terbinafine, an allylamine derivative with excellent antifungal activity, has proven to be very effective in curing athletes foot.

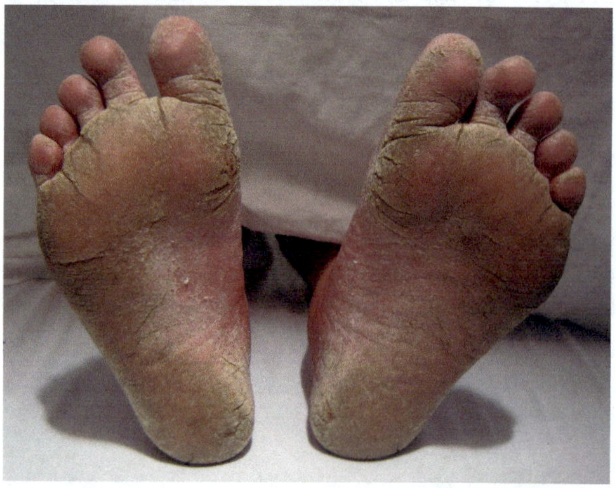

Figure 3.12. Tinea pedis, commonly known as athletes foot, represents a prevalent dermatological condition caused by a fungal infection, particularly from the genus *Trichophyton*.

Source: https://upload.wikimedia.org/wikipedia/commons/c/c0/FeetFungal.JPG.

The medication is available both in the form of creams and oral drug and hence provides diversity based on the intensity of the infection. Of significance, research indicates that terbinafine not only treats tinea pedis symptoms effectively but is also of high safety margin and thus a clinician's preference. This is especially significant as there is also a possibility of the infection spreading to the nails and inducing onychomycosis, which requires more intensive treatment modalities (Ptak et al., 2024). Further, the epidemiology of tinea pedis is influenced by a number of socio-economic determinants and concomitant underlying medical conditions. A study in Kenya, for instance, observed that persons of undetermined HIV status had a greater prevalence of superficial mycoses, including tinea pedis, which represents the interplay between system health and fungal infection (Adungo et al., 2019). Such a co-morbid association highlights the need for careful health assessment in patients with dermatophyte infection, especially where there is a high prevalence of HIV. Hence, such socio-economic and health-related determinants become the key to target not only for controlling tinea pedis but also for broader public health measures towards stemming superficial fungal infections in vulnerable population segments (Figure 3.12).

3.3.3. Tinea capitis (Scalp Infection)

Scalp ringworm or tinea capitis is a prevalent form of dermatophytosis that usually affects children but can affect individuals of all ages. It is due to infection by dermatophytes that infect hair follicles and keratinized scalp tissues preferentially. These fungi occur optimally in warm humid environments and are communicated by direct contact with the affected individual or indirectly using infected objects such as hats, combs, or pillows. Various species, such as *Trichophyton tonsurans* and *Microsporum canis*, have been identified as primary etiologic agents, each yielding unique clinical presentations. The condition may occur as scaly lesions, hair loss, and, in more severe cases, pyoderma type lesions that will result in secondary bacterial infections. There is more need to raise awareness of the condition, given its potential to interfere with both professional and social lives of individuals that have it. The epidemiology of tinea capitis yields a lot of information regarding its prevalence as well as species prevalence. As observed in a major study conducted in São Paulo, Brazil, various dermatophytes were grown, of which *T. rubrum* was most common, with *M. canis* and *T. tonsurans* following closely behind. The research found that tinea capitis accounted for almost 27.5% of the total cases of dermatophytosis noted, thus being among the major fungal infections. Careful scrutiny of these epidemiologic patterns can inform public health policy to contain outbreaks, particularly in densely populated areas such as schools and daycares where transmission is more probable.

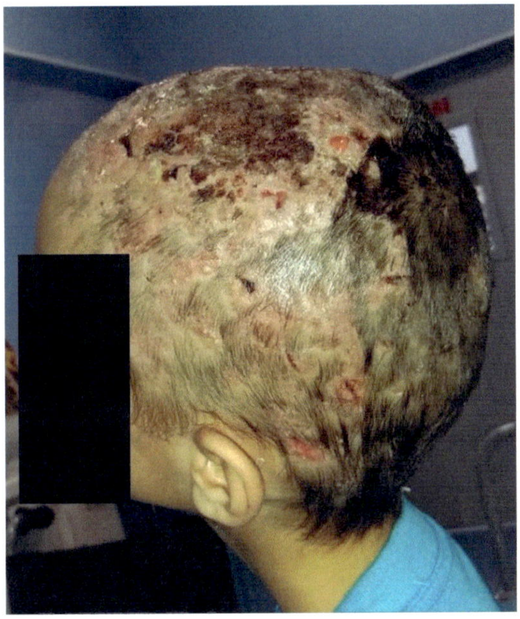

Figure 3.13. *Tinea capitis*, commonly known as scalp ringworm, is a prevalent form of dermatophytosis affecting primarily children, although it can occur in individuals of any age.

Source: https://www.mdpi.com/jcm/jcm-13-00376/article_deploy/html/images/jcm-13-00376-g006.png.

Understanding the disparity in prevalence and distribution of species also underscores the need for targeted therapeutic regimens against specific fungal pathogens responsible for tinea capitis. Tinea capitis is treated with the application of antifungals and with preventative interventions. Oral antifungal agents such as terbinafine and griseofulvin are typically required due to the site of infection at the hair follicles, necessitating systemic therapy. Local medication by itself is typically insufficient when managing this particular infection. In addition to pharmacological management, health education regarding hygiene and avoidance of shared personal items is the mainstay in breaking transmission. Health education campaigns, especially where the incidence rates are high, play a great role in reducing incidence in tinea capitis. Also, continuous research is needed to develop treatment modalities further and to study the evolving patterns of resistance of dermatophytes, which are important for effective management. A proper perception of these parameters is required for clinical practice as well as for public health programs to reduce the impact of dermatophytosis, particularly tinea capitis (Figure 3.13).

3.4. Treatment Options

The management of dermatophytosis has advanced significantly with various antifungal agents employed in the treatment of this prevalent fungal infection. Topical forms remain the drug of choice for localized infections, especially owing to their effectiveness and lesser chances of adverse systemic effects. Commonly employed topical antifungals are clotrimazole, miconazole, and luliconazole that inhibit the development of fungi and lead to faster healing of lesions. These medications are often administered along with supportive therapy such as hygienic care and environmental disinfection, which is a key factor in relapse prevention. The therapeutic area is continually investigated for efficacy; e.g., studies highlight the superiority of newer agents that could provide improved results over the standard therapies. In more disseminated or refractory dermatophytosis cases, systemic antifungal therapy can be employed. Medications like terbinafine and itraconazole are the medications usually prescribed, particularly for infections of larger body surface areas or those with severe symptoms. Terbinafine was reportedly the most commonly prescribed systemic medication with notable efficacy in combating dermatophytosis in a recent report (Badar et al., 2023). The strategy is usually accompanied by surveillance for potential side effects, ensuring the safety of the patient while maintaining therapeutic efficacy.

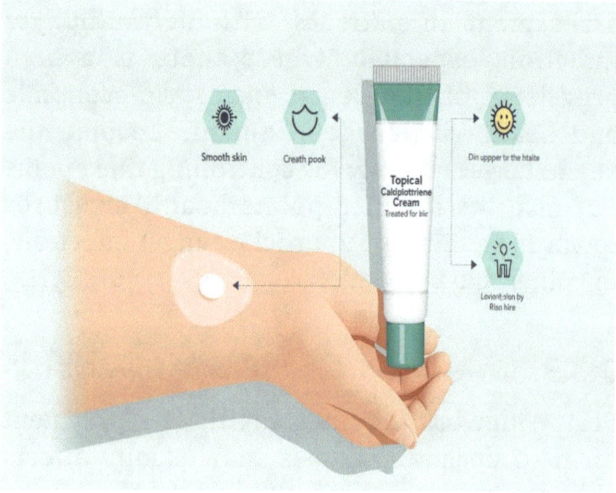

Figure 3.14. Topical therapies remain the first-line approach for localized cases, especially given their efficacy and reduced risk of systemic side effects.

Source: https://www.kaya.in/media/mageplaza/blog/post/t/o/topical-calcipotriene.jpg.

Therefore, treating with topical or systemic therapy is determined by the severity of the infection, overall patient health, and if there are any other conditions that may complicate recovery. Rational drug utilization studies are essential in enhancing treatment procedures for dermatophytosis. Research has revealed disparate prescribing habits across various populations, making it essential to critically analyze the trends (Badar et al., 2023). These types of studies facilitate better understanding of drug utilization and make it possible to optimize treatment programs and uniformity in prescribing antifungals. Prevention and teaching regarding the form of dermatophytosis are also essential in reducing the rate of occurrence. Through continued education and strategic treatment planning, health workers can potentially teach patients about the need to adhere to prescribed therapies, thereby reducing the disease burden of dermatophytosis among populations (Figure 3.14).

3.4.1. Antifungal Medications

Therapy for dermatophytosis is primarily dependent on the use of antifungal medications, and these can further be categorized into topical and systemic medications. Topical antifungals such as clotrimazole and terbinafine are usually suitable for localized disease, targeting the dermatophyte pathogens locally where the local infection exists. Systemic antifungals such as itraconazole and fluconazole would be required for widespread or recalcitrant infections in an attempt to exert optimal therapeutic effects. Choice of the antifungal medication is based on the dermatophyte species that is involved, severity and duration of the infection, and overall health condition of the patient. It is critical to make sure that the effective yet tolerable drug therapy is used, as it may affect the compliance with the drug regimen and the eventual success of the treatment (Bagchi et al., 2021). It has been observed from studies that adherence to treatments is crucial for successful treatment of dermatophytosis, particularly when a combination of topical and systemic antifungal treatments is employed. In one study on the assessment of 60 patients who were reporting with various forms of dermatophytosis, high drug compliance was observed at 96.66%, where oral itraconazole, luliconazole cream, and antihistamines were administered primarily as a combined regimen. The efficacy of this dual treatment resulted in a significant reduction of both pruritus and overall skin discomfort, as measured by standardized indices such as the Dermatology Life Quality Index (DLQI) (Bagchi et al., 2021). This finding emphasizes both the relevance of the pharmacological action of the antifungals and also the improvement in quality of life for patients with dermatophyte infection, which can make a significant difference to psychological as well as physical well-being. While classical antifungal agents are the cornerstone of the treatment of dermatophytosis, other therapeutic approaches have been under the limelight due to increasing numbers of treatment-resistant dermatophyte infections. Numerous studies have evaluated the efficacy of herbal, homeopathic, and Ayurvedic drugs, and most have reported beneficial effects in controlling superficial fungal infections. These alternatives may be attributed as adjunct therapy, particularly for the patients who may be refractory to standard antifungal drugs or are faced with severe side effects. As dermatophytosis continues to better be understood, integrating complementary therapies with standard antifungal therapy is an intriguing possibility for maximizing patient outcomes, thereby possibly setting the stage for better treatment modalities and improved quality of life amidst ongoing challenges in dermatophyte infections (Figure 3.15).

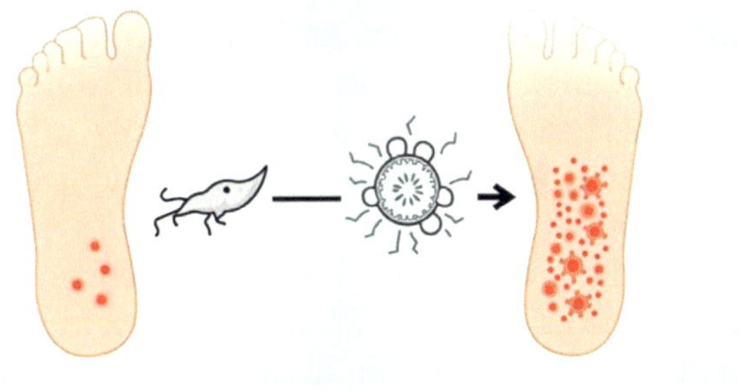

Figure 3.15. Topical antifungals, such as clotrimazole and terbinafine, are typically effective for localized infections, targeting the dermatophyte pathogens directly at the infection site.

Source: https://www.kaya.in/media/mageplaza/blog/post/c/l/clotrimazole-fungal-skin-infections-treatment-guide.jpg.

3.4.2. Topical vs. Systemic Treatments

For dermatophytosis, treatment measures usually revolve around the issue of whether or not to apply topical or systemic medication. Topical medications, for instance, azoles and terbinafine cream, would typically be applied for localized infections, where antifungal agents are directly applied to the infected area. These types of drugs would be most effective against superficial infections due to localized action and limited absorption into the system. They cannot be used, however, for extensive or generalized infection, where systemic medication is the drug of choice. The treatment must be selected therefore by the size and site of the infection as well as patient factors like co-morbidities and subjective tolerance to therapy. More extensive dermatophyte infections are treated with systemic therapy like oral antifungals griseofulvin, terbinafine, and itraconazole. These drugs possess the advantage of systemic absorption, which gives wider fungal clearance, especially in extensive tinea capitis or onychomycosis. There has been evidence to show that a combination of systemic antifungals and topical therapy can give synergistic activity, enhancing clinical response. For instance, the interaction of a topical and an oral medication can enhance clinical as well as microbiologic cure, which would be of considerable interest to clinicians who have to handle tough cases. Moreover, a choice between topical and systemic treatment is largely a function of the correctness of diagnosis, as brought out by a recent paper that illustrated the impact of improper initial treatment. Many of the patients, at the time of presentation, had already been exposed to ineffective therapy, which not only wasted time but also prolonged the healing phase and increased costs (Calabrò et al., 2015). This gives importance to proper mycological assessment before treatment since improper management prolongs the length of systemic therapy. Therefore, an in-depth appreciation of the pathogen's nature, patient history, and potential treatment interactions can guide clinicians to the most rewarding therapeutic alternatives in dermatophytosis treatment (Figure 3.16).

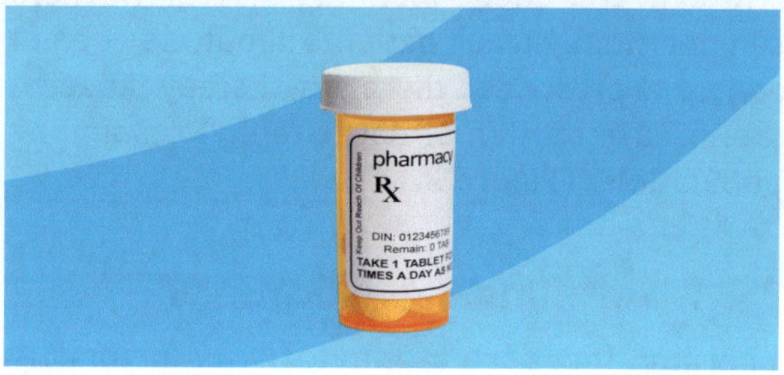

Figure 3.16. Systemic treatments, including oral antifungals like griseofulvin, terbinafine, and itraconazole, are indicated for more pervasive dermatophyte infections.

Source: https://www.singlecare.com/blog/wp-content/uploads/2025/05/terbinafine-for-toenail-fungus-1884x1060.png.

3.4.3. Home Remedies and Alternative Therapies

The growing popularity of home remedies and alternative therapies for the treatment of dermatophytosis is one aspect of a broader societal shift towards natural and integrative health treatments. These therapies are employed in cases where conventional therapies do not work or cause undesirable side effects. Essential oils, for example, have gained attention for their antifungal properties, providing an adjunct or alternative to conventional antifungal medications. Research indicates that plant secondary metabolites possess multiple antibacterial and antifungal activities and are therefore of interest in infection treatments, for example, dermatophytosis. Although in vitro research is positive, further work on field application of essential oils in clinical settings to establish their efficacy and safety in the therapeutic treatment of skin fungal infections is needed (Ebani et al., 2020). Integration of ethnobotanical data into modern therapeutics also serves to underscore the significance of home remedies in combating dermatophytosis. Traditional medicine plants have for centuries been employed in regions such as the Eastern Cape Province of South Africa by indigenous communities to manage a range of health conditions.

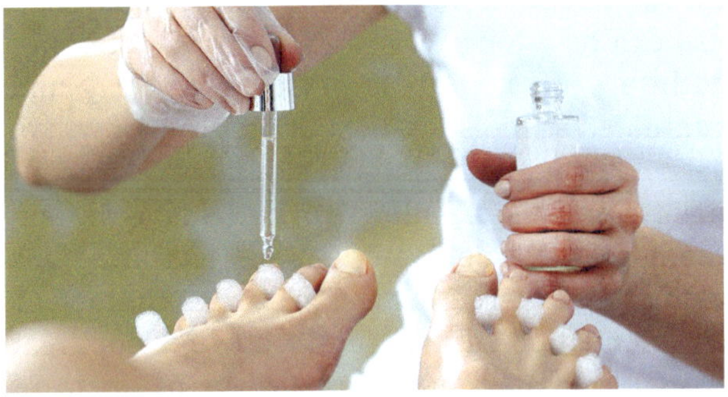

Figure 3.17. Essential oils, for example, have garnered attention for their antifungal properties, presenting a potential adjunct or alternative to traditional antifungal medications.

Source: https://media.post.rvohealth.io/wp-content/uploads/2020/08/5790-Toe_and_nail_fungus-1200x628-Facebook-1200x628.jpg.

A survey of the plants *Arctotis arctotoides* and *Pittosporum viridiflorum,* which were traditionally used to cure opportunistic fungal infections, suggests that such plants are likely to exert antifungal activity. This paper invites empirical investigation of the pharmacological activities of such plant species in an effort to find out if such plant species have potential as drugs in the treatment of dermatophytosis. By combining ancient knowledge and scientific research, we may be able to find new remedies that are effective yet culturally acceptable (Mbeng et al., 2013). While the potential of home remedies and complementary remedies in the management of dermatophytosis is high, one has to approach these methods with caution. One of the issues is the lack of standard dosage and variability in the composition of natural products, thus the therapeutic outcome varies. Most herbal remedies are also not yet subjected to sufficient research on their toxicity, and well-designed scientific studies become crucial. Practitioners should conduct controlled studies to ascertain their safety profile and efficacy against dermatophytes. In conclusion, even as home remedies have the potential to complement conventional therapy for dermatophytosis, careful consideration and assessment are important in defining their role in combined patient management (Figure 3.17).

3.5. Prevention Strategies

Effective preventive measures play a key role in arresting the spread of dermatophytosis, particularly where a person is subjected to higher exposure, such as in animal shelters or farms. The enforcement of rigorous hygiene practices, via frequent cleaning and disinfection of work and living environments, is crucial. Increased education and communication between the public and shelter workers were found in most studies, including those studying the association of veterinary practice with public health, to significantly improve awareness in relation to the transmission of dermatophyte infections. Such preventive measures not only secure the health of animals that reside in such environments but also secure the safety of adopters and visitors, emphasizing the requirement for infection prevention strategy at a broader level (Davic et al. 2025). Moreover, familiarity with the specific conditions that bring about dermatophytosis outbreaks among specific populations enhances preventative measures. As a case in point, an epidemiological survey conducted among farmed rabbits revealed significant associations with environmental conditions and clinical presentation, such as concomitant infection and lesion patterns. Using logistic regression models, scientists were able to detect risk factors for dermatophyte isolation, hence gaining important information in the management of the disease (Coelho et al., 2012). Strategic interventions can then be modified on the basis of this epidemiological data to create site-specific prevention guidelines to counteract the specific difficulties being faced in household as well as farm settings. Last, public education and education of individuals in contact with animals regarding the signs and symptoms of dermatophytosis is an important component of prevention. Public education programs can help equip individuals with information to detect early signs, thereby enhancing timely intervention and reducing secondary transmission. Collaboration with local vets to help disseminate information and materials can ensure greater involvement of the community. Finally, early detection and treatment of infected animals will be in a position to end the transmission cycle, contributing greatly towards the overall reduction of dermatophyte cases. While complemented by systematic data collection and analysis, such measures form a composite system sufficiently addressing the multiaxiality of dermatophytosis prevention (Figure 3.18).

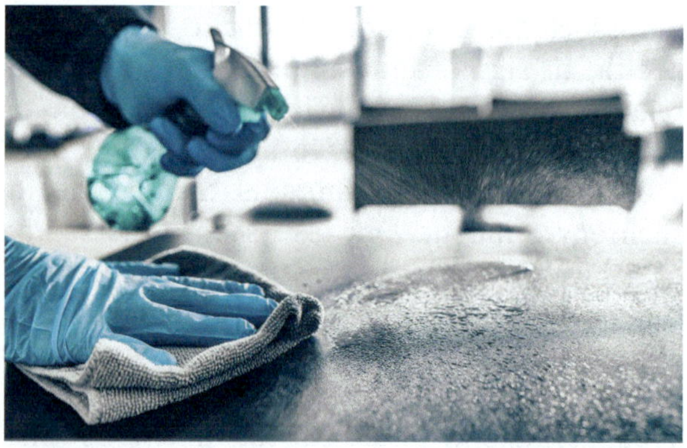

Figure 3.18. Implementing rigorous hygiene practices, including frequent cleaning and disinfection of living and working areas, plays a vital role.

Source: https://www.bbcleaningservice.com/wp-content/uploads/2024/06/office-desinfection.jpg.

3.5.1. Personal Hygiene Practices

Personal hygiene practices are highly significant in the control and prevention of dermatophytosis, a very common fungal infection of hair, skin, and nails. The dermatophyte fungi thrive in warm, moist conditions, which can be aggravated by poor hygiene. Maintaining one's cleanliness through regular bathing and antifungal soap use can be a long way in avoiding infection. In addition, affected areas must be kept dry and ventilated as moisture encourages the growth of such fungi. Individuals must also be careful about maintaining the cleanliness of individuals around them because dermatophytosis is contagious and can be spread through direct contact or an infected object. Therefore, the development of habitual personal hygiene in the form of repeated daily washing of the body becomes not only an individual obligation but also a social one, aimed at halting the spread of dermatophyte infections. Of special significance is also the role of clothing and footwear in personal hygiene in dermatophytosis. Individuals should use air-permeable clothing and ensure that clothing is clean so that sweat and moisture cannot have any opportunity to get accumulated. Antifungal powders professional in nature can also be used to prevent the growth of fungi as well, particularly in regions where sweating happens most, such as the feet. Personal items such as towels, socks, and shoes should be avoided being shared as it leads to direct transmission of fungal spores. In settings such as swimming pools or a gym, where the dermatophytes will be provided with an environment to grow, the proper footwear and individual mats can act as a barrier against infection. Overall, cautious attention to cleanliness of the footwear and garments is a step that will effectively minimize the ill impacts of dermatophytosis (Muhammad et al., 2023). The inclusion of personal hygiene habits in daily practices can go beyond mere cleanliness and clothes maintenance, focusing on the care of the skin. Those with health conditions that weaken their skin barrier, like eczema or psoriasis, should take extra care in maintaining their skin to avoid any secondary infections, such as dermatophytosis. This can include using moisturizers as part of regular practice to help maintain the hydration and integrity of the skin. Further, laborers engaged in occupations that expose them to potential sources of fungi—such as agriculture, veterinary work, or even outdoor sports—should undertake proactive measures like protective clothing and prompt washing of clothes after exposure to animals or soil. These preventive measures, accompanied by general personal hygiene practices, are the secrets behind reducing the frequency of dermatophytosis among individuals (Figure 3.19).

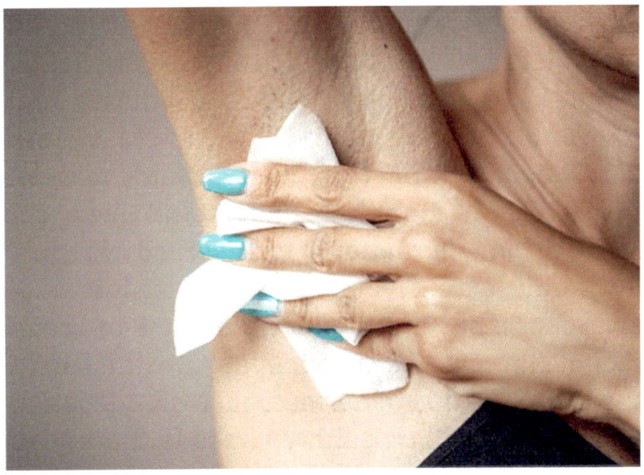

Figure 3.19. Personal hygiene practices play a crucial role in the prevention and management of dermatophytosis, a common fungal infection affecting the skin, hair, and nails.

Source: https://media.post.rvohealth.io/wp-content/uploads/2021/02/woman-wipes-armpit-732x549-thumbnail.jpg.

3.5.2. Environmental Control Measures

Implementation of efficient environmental control measures plays a critical role in the prevention of dermatophytosis, particularly where animals are kept or reared in close confinement. These encompass various practices that are designed to restrain the contact of both animals and humans with dermatophyte fungi, which can thrive well in contaminated environments. Some of the major practices include stern cleaning and disinfection processes for animal housing facilities, in addition to effective ventilation that limits humidity levels favorable to fungal growth. Regular inspection and monitoring of the health of the animals can also lead to early detection of outbreaks to facilitate timely intervention. Thus, the use of effective environmental control measures not only guarantees animal welfare but also public health by reducing the risk of transmission to people who are exposed to such facilities, as highlighted through the association between veterinary medicine and public health in animal shelters (Davic et al. 2025). Aiding further the efficacy of environmental control measures is the understanding of epidemiological data pertaining to dermatophyte spread across different animal populations. A study on farmed rabbits in Northern and Central Portugal has revealed a high 82.7% prevalence of dermatophyte species, primarily *Trichophyton mentagrophytes* and *Microsporum canis* (Coelho et al., 2012). This underscores the importance of tailoring interventions to the conditions and demographic variables on animal farms. It is by examining such variables as breed, age, and concomitant infection that effective control can be devised. Development of risk factors through studies becomes central to the development of targeted environmental interventions that can adequately reduce the prevalence of dermatophytosis among animals and individuals who come into contact with infected groups. Community education and partnership further highlight the importance of using environmental control measures in the management of dermatophytosis. Education programs for pet owners, breeders, and veterinary staff can increase awareness on how to recognize early signs of infection and become aware of the environmental conditions that facilitate the growth of dermatophytes. By fostering an active participation strategy, communities can become more accountable for the health of their animal population, ensuring that they adhere to best hygiene practices and surveillance. Coordination with local animal shelters and public health departments can also help amplify the effectiveness of such measures, as represented by the collaboration between veterinarian roles and public health activity (Davic et al. 2025). Ultimately, support of these educational measures in combination with rigorous environmental controls represents a multi-faceted protective measure against dermatophytosis, exerting a significant influence towards its prevention and control in various contexts (Figure 3.20).

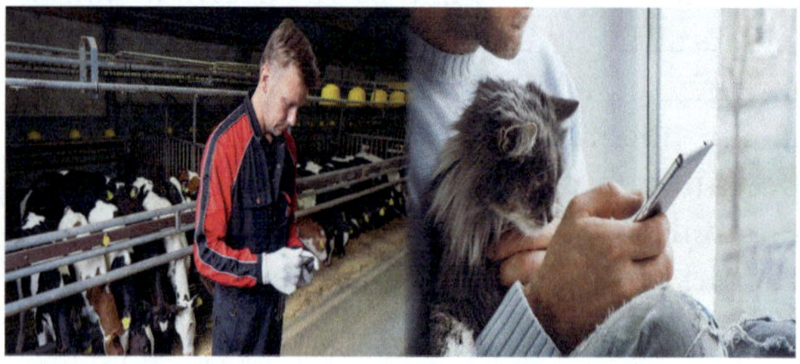

Figure 3.20. Regular inspections and monitoring of animal health can also lead to early detection of outbreaks, allowing for swift intervention measures.

Source: https://healthforanimals.org/wp-content/uploads/2022/01/06559-digital-revolution-banner_02-scaled.jpg.

3.5.3. Education and Awareness

Education and sensitization are key in preventing and managing dermatophytosis, a fungal infection with the highest tendency to infect the skin, hair, and nails. Effective education can provide individuals with knowledge on the causation, symptoms, and control of the diseases, hence reducing the susceptibility to infection. For instance, initiatives targeting at-risk groups, such as sportsmen and individuals with communal lifestyles, can promote behaviors such as the utilization of sanitary habits and non-sharing of individual possessions. Through dissemination of such information via workshops, seminars, and web-available resources, public health agencies can significantly enhance awareness among people, which will culminate in better outcomes in the fight against dermatophytosis. Furthermore, public awareness should extend to the environmental factors of dermatophytosis transmission. Swimming pools, gyms, and locker rooms are common locations where fungal spores can find a habitat, thus increasing infection rates. Understanding environmental persistence of the dermatophytes allows people to take preventive action such as the utilization of sandals or flip-flops at public showers and drying skin regions with a high likelihood of moisture retention. Through specifically targeted education, including educational pamphlets and peer-to-peer classroom discussions within community health classes, the public can more fully understand their part in preventing dermatophytosis spread. Not only does this extensive system boost individual awareness, but it also creates a sense of group responsibility toward community health. Lastly, the incorporation of dermatophytosis education into larger public health courses is the key to building an educated healthcare workforce. As observed in studies that evaluate levels of awareness in medical students, most are not adequately educated about proper disposal of drug wastes and impacts of inappropriateness in the practice of medicine (Beck et al., 2020). Incorporating dermatophytosis lessons in medical and paramedical schools allows students to appreciate prevention, diagnosis, and proper management of dermatophyte infections. Moreover, bridging the knowledge gap with extensive training can lead to improved practice in healthcare, and, as a consequence, have beneficial effects on patients and the population at large. Increased sensitivity in the healthcare setting puts more focus on hygiene, health education, and application of effective therapies for dermatophytosis, in line with public health objectives (Davic et al. 2025) (Figure 3.21).

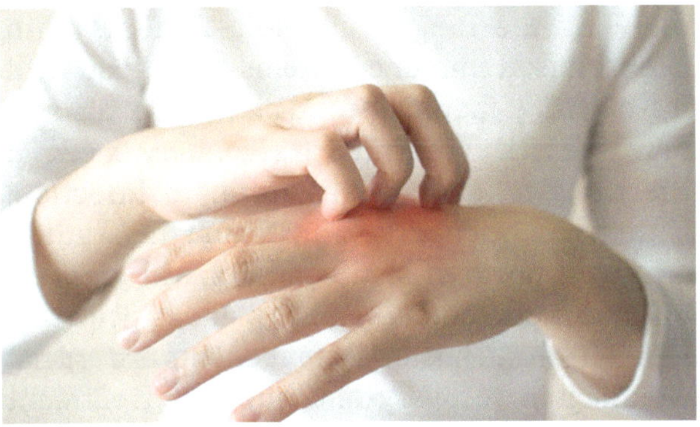

Figure 3.21. Education and awareness play a pivotal role in the management and prevention of dermatophytosis, a fungal infection commonly affecting the skin, hair, and nails.

Source: https://d502jbuhuh9wk.cloudfront.net/articles/63ec9fcde4b0d9900d16302b/ij82timage59.png.

3.6. Complications and Long-Term Effects

The sequelae to dermatophytosis extend beyond immediate clinical presentation and are potentially capable of having a very dramatic effect on patients quality of life. Maybe the most common complaint of tinea infections is one of chronic pruritus, or itching, which has the potential for secondary bacterial infection and skin destruction as a result of excessive scratching. The psychosocial impact of having a chronic cutaneous disease may be staggering, inducing withdrawal from society and lower self-esteem. Reports indicate that not only does dermatophytosis hinder physical comfort but also causes a psychological load in the sense that patients become ashamed or embarrassed because of lesion visibility. Therefore, it is not just a matter of curing such infections with proper antifungal therapy but also resolving the related psychosocial complications that may occur due to recurrent skin involvement and associated symptoms. Long-term effects of dermatophytosis are common in the form of treatment complications, particularly if chronic treatment is necessary for repeated infections. The patients are normally faced with a high economic burden through the uncertain prices of antifungal agents, particularly if generics or cheaper options are not available. Research determines that the variability in costs of commonly prescribed antifungal medications is high, with variations of up to 237.5% in certain oral preparations of itraconazole (Dumra et al., 2023).

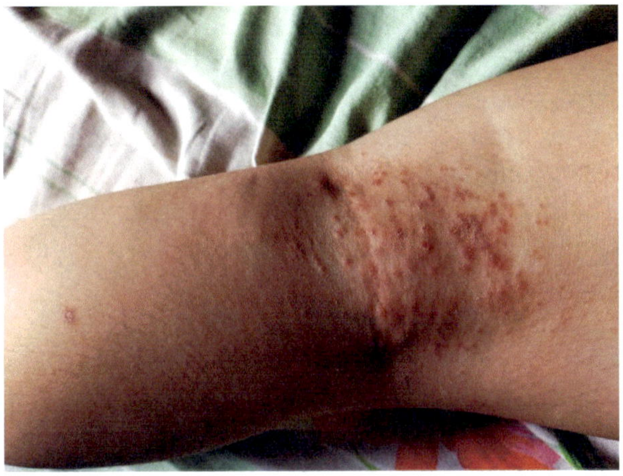

Figure 3.22. One of the most common issues associated with tinea infections is the persistent pruritus, or itching, which can lead to secondary bacterial infections and skin damage due to excessive scratching.

Source: https://www.news-medical.net/images/Article_Images/ImageForArticle_22961_16596010963361695.jpg.

This financial burden could lead to poor patient compliance with treatment guidelines, increasing the risk of failure and recurrence of dermatophytosis. Moreover, the necessity of chronic antifungal therapy increases the risk of adverse effects and drug interactions, which make patient management difficult and highlight the importance of careful drug selection and monitoring. The long-term consequences of dermatophytosis can be systemic disease in susceptible patients, particularly those who are immunocompromised. Conditions such as erythroderma, an inflammation of the skin in a diffuse pattern, can be caused by a systemic response to uncontrolled dermatophyte infection (Patel et al., 2025). It can complicate the clinical presentation, and its treatment is more challenging due to the risk of acquiring secondary infections. In severe cases, systemic involvement can lead to fatal outcomes such as sepsis. It is here that early detection and treatment are crucial, as prompt identification of the fungus and treatment can prevent further complications. Understanding the broader implications of dermatophytosis allows healthcare professionals to adopt holistic treatment approaches that encompass both the physical and psychosocial aspects of care, resulting in improved patient outcomes (Figure 3.22).

3.6.1. Secondary Bacterial Infections

The relationship between dermatophytosis and secondary bacterial infection induced subsequently is a relevant factor in dermatologic health. Dermatophytosis, which is due primarily to fungal pathogens, compromises the skin barrier, thereby increasing its vulnerability to bacterial colonization. When the skin is compromised by fungal infection, such as tinea, it allows the perfect environment for opportunistic bacteria to invade. This event typically leads to secondary infections, which can aggravate the clinical presentation of dermatophytosis and complicate therapeutic efforts. Consequently, the management of dermatophytosis must consider the event of such bacterial overlapping's, as they could drastically influence patient outcomes. Research indicates that secondary infections typically happen in cases where infections caused by dermatophytes are not treated or are insufficiently treated. For instance, bacterial infections have been found to be prevalent in dermatophytosis patients, particularly where inflammation is severe and there is pruritus following the fungal infection. Patients with compromised immune systems and those with pre-existing medical conditions are also at increased risk of contracting secondary bacterial infections following dermatophyte infection. With the evidence demonstrated in studies, such as reports of skin conditions in animals, it is evident that management plans anticipating both fungal and bacterial components are crucial in aiding in recovery and effective treatment (Bengoumi et al., 2019).

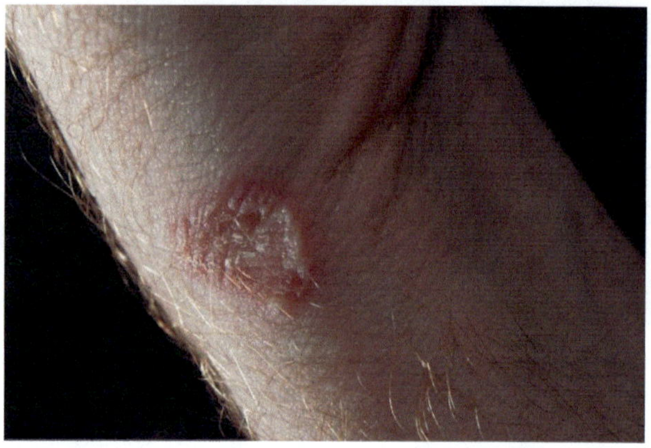

Figure 3.23. When the skin is disrupted by fungal infections, such as tinea, it creates a conducive environment for opportunistic bacteria to invade.

Source: https://i0.wp.com/cdn-prod.medicalnewstoday.com/content/images/articles/158/158134/ringworm-is-a-fungal-infection.jpg?w=1155&h=974.

In veterinary medicine, the same has been documented for dermatophytosis and its complications in a number of animal species, especially in dromedary camels and domestic cats. For example, research has indicated series of dermatological disease reports with respect to both bacterial and fungal infections, in which findings indicate the prevalence of high bacterial infections in addition to dermatophyte diseases. Surprisingly, secondary bacterial infection was observed in higher frequency among the infected animals that were not offered systematic treatment or prophylactic management. This interaction highlights the significance of elaborate assessment and harmonized treatment protocols incorporating dermatophytosis alongside secondary bacterial infection. By recognizing and managing these interconnected issues, clinicians can optimize treatment outcomes and promote healthier skin healing in human and animal medicine (Alautaish et al., 2024) (Figure 3.23).

3.6.2. Chronic Dermatophytosis

Chronic dermatophytosis is a common issue in the dermatology field with chronic fungal infections that are not responsive to conventional treatment. An infection with such disabling presentations is primarily due to dermatophytes, which are fungi that inhabit keratin-containing tissues like skin, hair, and nails. Failure of chronic infections to respond to conventional antifungal treatments highlights the need for knowing the diseases pathophysiology in detail. Factors such as host immunity, related skin disorders, and external barriers are the cause of chronicity of such infections. Chronic dermatophytosis has been proven by studies to not only affect the physical health of the patients but also their mind, since chronic skin disorders have been found to result in social withdrawal and diminished quality of life. Determinants of the occurrence of chronic dermatophytosis vary significantly geographically as well as among populations. Where certain animals, such as the dromedary camel, are widespread within a region, dermatophyte infection may become endemic due to their wide transmission rates within herds. A study conducted in southern Morocco revealed that dermatophyte infections accounted for approximately 30% of the skin diseases among camels, which suggests possible cross-species infection and environmental impacts on human health (Bengoumi et al., 2019). Moreover, this data shows the importance of identifying dermatophytosis not only as a problem for animals but as a complex public health element. Greater awareness and preventive treatment can reduce the risk of chronic dermatophytosis, emphasizing animal health's interdependence with human health. The treatment regimen for chronic dermatophytosis is controversial in nature, sometimes needing an integrated strategy.

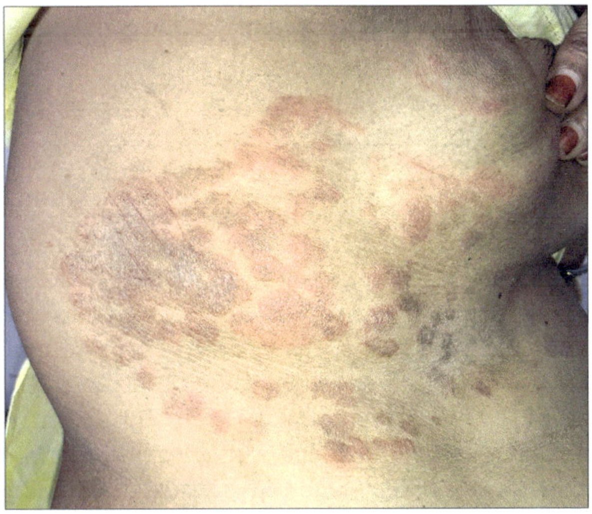

Figure 3.24. Chronic dermatophytosis represents a pervasive challenge in the field of dermatology, characterized by persistent fungal infections that resist conventional treatment.

Source: https://ijdvl.com/content/126/2021/87/2/img/IJDVL-87-154-g019.png.

Conventional antifungal drugs often provide suboptimal outcomes, resulting in lifelong recurrences of the infection. As such, there has been increased enthusiasm towards alternative treatment options, such as herbal and homeopathic therapy, which have demonstrated efficacy in controlling recurrent fungal infections. Research indicates that certain herbal medications, together with Siddha and Ayurvedic therapy, might combat dermatophytes better, validating the realization that a combination of standard remedies would yield better results in patients (Bipin raj et al., 2022). This paradigm shift, further, not only indicates greater awareness regarding integrated health but also encourages more personalized practices of therapy that target the unique ailment of patients who are battling long-term dermatophytosis (Figure 3.24).

3.6.3. Impact on Quality of Life

The effect of dermatophytosis on quality of life (QoL) is very significant, and it affects patients of all age groups. At a large tertiary care center, investigations showed that an astounding 98.7% of patients had an increase in QoL due to this fungal infection. The findings indicate that not just are people burdened with the physical unpleasantness of itch and pain but also felt psychologically through social withdrawal and loss of esteem. The mean Dermatology Life Quality Index (DLQI) values of 13.4 ± 7.3 indicate that dermatophytosis significantly affects day-to-day functioning, verifying that skin diseases go beyond the physical dimension to encompass overall well-being (Khoso et al., 2022). The connection between therapeutic efficacy and QoL amelioration serves to further highlight the complex interaction between dermatophytosis and the life of the infected patients. A prospective observational study had previously demonstrated improvement in QoL parameters post-prescribed therapy, as measured by the DLQI and 5D-itch scale, with indication of direct correlation between successful control of infection and enhanced quality of life. Specifically, the average scores of DLQI were noticed to significantly improve following treatment for six weeks, reflecting the effectiveness of certain interventions to overcome the harmful effects generated due to this condition (Bagchi et al., 2021). This improvement underscores the necessity of healthcare professionals to ensure not just the eradication of the fungal agents but also patients' restoration of daily activities and psychological well-being. In addition, the socioeconomic impact implicated in dermatophytosis contributes significantly to its quality-of-life burden. Less educated patients suffer a higher degree of anxiety and stigma that coincides with their capacity to seek healthcare services. The majority of the patients included in the study did not have an education, representative of the likelihood that less educated patients are subjected to the psychosocial impacts of dermatophytosis. In addition, dermatophytosis occurrence among young adults aged 16-30 is a generational risk since this age group is most susceptible to social pressures and body image issues that enhance their disease burden on QoL. Multidisciplinary interventions are required to manage such multi-faceted issues with education, access to medical care, and psychological guidance in an effort to enhance the quality of life for dermatophytosis patients (Khoso et al., 2022) (Figure 3.25).

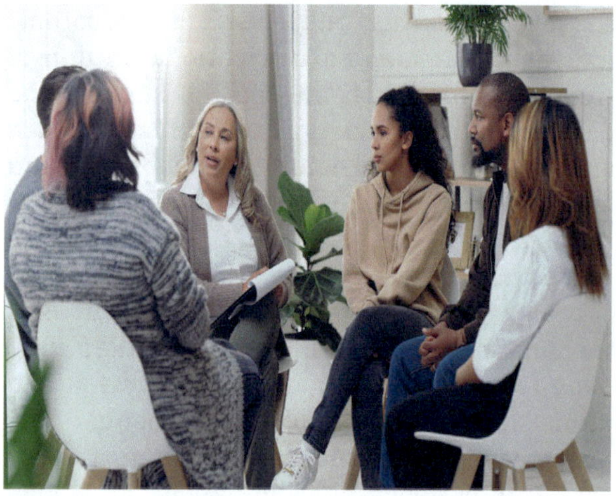

Figure 3.25. Patients from lower educational backgrounds often experience a heightened sense of anxiety and stigma, which intersects with their access to healthcare resources.

Source: https://publichealth.tulane.edu/wp-content/uploads/sites/3/2021/01/Understanding-Mental-Health-as-a-Public-Health-Issue.jpg.

SUMMARY

A complete description of causative agents must be known to understand dermatophytosis, and these agents are primarily dermatophytes, a group of fungi that parasitize keratin-containing tissue. Not only can such pathogenic fungi infect skin but also produce growth on hair and nails and cause a variety of superficial infections in animals and humans. Notably, the taxonomy of these fungi is shifting with gene-level analysis, with significant implications for clinical diagnosis and therapy. Current studies have underscored the plasticity of certain species, such as *Microsporum canis*, which is becoming increasingly pertinent in that it may be facing extinction of one of its mating types, thus influencing its epidemiological trends and future infection prospects (Moskaluk et al., 2022). The impact of dermatophytosis extends beyond the clinical picture, associating with the public health dimensions. The infections pose an important risk, especially in urban areas where the transmission is bound to rise. An examination of the epidemiology of fungal infections demonstrates that the dermatophytes are responsible for a substantial proportion of dermatologic diseases globally, highlighting the need for prompt and accurate diagnostic processes (Klimas et al., 2025). The advancement in molecular diagnostics, including the identification of keratin metabolites that are formed during fungal development, offers promising solutions to increasing diagnostic sensitivity and early treatment in infected patients. This new reality highlights the imperatives of continued research aimed at understanding the dynamics of dermatophyte infections and maximizing clinical outcomes through effective management. Outside the clinical arena, the genetic characteristics of dermatophytes like *M. canis* emphasizes the complexity of treatment and prevention strategies. Recent studies have shown how specific genes, such as those controlling keratin adhesion, play a key role in the virulence of these fungi. Furthermore, the identification of new species within the *Arthroderma* genus indicates an expanding spectrum of potential pathogens that need to be recognized and understood in clinical practice. Recent research not only contributes to the development of effective therapies but also to the increase in knowledge concerning infection mechanisms and host interaction, finally resulting in effective public health campaigns against dermatophytosis (Moskaluk et al., 2022).

A CLOSER LOOK

MICROSPORUM CANIS

Microsporum canis is the species of fungus that primarily causes dermatophytosis, or more commonly ringworm, in man and animals. It is a zoophilous dermatophyte that, in primary, infects animals—most commonly cats and dogs—but can be transmitted to human beings by direct contact with the infected animals or fomites.

*M. c*anis infects keratinized tissues such as skin, hair, and nails and causes round, pruritic red papules with a scale border. In animals, it causes patchy shedding of hair. It can be diagnosed by Wood's lamp examination, microscopy, or fungal culture. It can be treated with topical antifungals or with systemic therapy in advanced cases. Hygiene must be assured and infected animals need to be treated in order to prevent transmission.

REFERENCES

1. Abdulla, S. N., Abdullah, B. A., Farhan, M. S., Mamdwooh, A., et al. (2024). Review of the clinical types of dermatophytes. https://core.ac.uk/download/613199118.pdf (accessed on 27th June 2025).
2. Adebiyi, A. I., & Oluwayelu, D. O. (2019). Zoonotic fungal diseases and animal ownership in Nigeria. https://core.ac.uk/download/478436841.pdf (accessed on 27th June 2025).
3. Adungo, F., Bii, C., Makwaga, O., Matiru, V., et al. (2019). Factors associated with superficial mycoses in patients visiting Alupe Clinic and its environs in Busia, western Kenya. https://core.ac.uk/download/478368623.pdf (accessed on 27th June 2025).
4. Akkan, H. A., Ekin, I. H., Ilhan, Z., Karaca, M., et al. (2016). Detection of seasonal asymptomatic dermatophytes in Van cats. https://core.ac.uk/download/pdf/82806476.pdf (accessed on 27th June 2025).
5. Alautaish, H. H. N., Naji, H. A., & Saud, Z. A. H. (2024). Clinical study of common bacterial, fungal and parasitic skin diseases in cats. https://core.ac.uk/download/616936536.pdf (accessed on 27th June 2025).
6. Antoine, N., Bagut, L. T., Cambier, L., Defaweux, D., et al. (2014). Assessment of the cutaneous immune response during *Arthroderma benhamiae* and *Arthroderma vanbreuseghemii* infection using an experimental mouse model. http://orbi.ulg.ac.be/bitstream/2268/164151/1/bjd12673.pdf (accessed on 27th June 2025).
7. Araujo, R. P., Ferreiro, L., Franceschi, N. T., Ravazzolo, A., et al. (2023). Bovine ringworm: Detection of *Trichophyton verrucosum* by SYBR-Green real-time PCR. https://core.ac.uk/download/576871391.pdf (accessed on 27th June 2025).
8. Arzberger, E., Bastos, P. M., Ferreira, J., Leal-Filipe, J., et al. (2020). Reflectance confocal microscopy for the diagnosis of skin infections and infestations. https://core.ac.uk/download/322493878.pdf (accessed on 27th June 2025).
9. Badar, V. A., Chavan, R., Gaikwad, P., Pradhan, S., et al. (2023). Drug utilization study of patients with dermatophytosis attending dermatology outpatient department in tertiary care teaching hospital in Central India. https://core.ac.uk/download/570905516.pdf (accessed on 27th June 2025).
10. Bagchi, C., Chatterjee, K., Das, A., Tripathi, K., et al. (2021). An OPD-based prospective exploratory study of dermatophytosis–Focus on treatment outcomes, medication adherence, and quality of life. https://core.ac.uk/download/477856245.pdf (accessed on 27th June 2025).
11. Beck, R. K., Kachhap, S., Kumar, U., Singh, A., et al. (2020). A study to assess the knowledge and awareness regarding safe disposal of pharmaceutical wastes among 2nd year medical and para-medical students in a tertiary care teaching hospital in North India. https://core.ac.uk/download/539897823.pdf (accessed on 27th June 2025).
12. Bengoumi, M., Faye, B., Kamili, A., Tligui, N., et al. (2019). Invited review: Camel skin diseases survey in Morocco. https://core.ac.uk/download/288641826.pdf (accessed on 27th June 2025).
13. Bii, C., Chepchirchir, A., & Ndinya-Achola, J. O. (2009). Dermatophyte infections in primary school children in Kibera slums of Nairobi. https://core.ac.uk/download/478296421.pdf (accessed on 27th June 2025).

14. Boulware, L. E., Harvey, V. M., & Paul, J. (2016). Racial and ethnic disparities in dermatology office visits among insured patients, 2005–2010. https://digitalscholarship.unlv.edu/cgi/viewcontent.cgi?article=1388&context=jhdrp (accessed on 27th June 2025).
15. Calabrò, G., Fiammenghi, E., Lo Conte, V., Patalano, C., et al. (2015). Cost analysis of inappropriate treatments for suspected dermatomycoses. https://core.ac.uk/download/349833829.pdf (accessed on 27th June 2025).
16. Campelo, M. B. Z., Costa, G. da C., Nascimento, B. K. F., Oliveira, M. L., et al. (2023). The role of pacas of captivity as a potential reservoir of zoonotic fungi in Acre, Western Amazon, Brazil. https://core.ac.uk/download/588294305.pdf (accessed on 27th June 2025).
17. Chimelli, P. A. V., Martins, J. E. da C., Nunes, R. S., Sofiatti, C., et al. (2003). Agents de dermatofitoses an Cicada de São Paulo no period de 1992 e 2002. https://core.ac.uk/download/268293306.pdf (accessed on 27th June 2025).
18. Coelho, A. C., Coelho, A. M., Miranda, A., Monteiro, A., et al. (2012). Epidemiological survey of dermatophytosis in meat rabbits with alopecia in Portugal. https://core.ac.uk/download/641675074.pdf (accessed on 27th June 2025).
19. Davic, B. (2025). Aligning public health and shelter medicine: The connection between a veterinarian and the public. https://core.ac.uk/download/153432898.pdf (accessed on 27th June 2025).
20. Dumra, G. H., & Modi, R. D. (2023). Drug utilization pattern evaluation and cost variation analysis of anti-fungal agents in tinea-infected patients in dermatology department of a tertiary care teaching hospital. https://core.ac.uk/download/596247077.pdf (accessed on 27th June 2025).
21. Ebani, V. V., & Mancianti, F. (2020). Use of essential oils in veterinary medicine to combat bacterial and fungal infections. https://core.ac.uk/download/534218794.pdf (accessed on 27th June 2025).
22. Farhana, A., Jahan, T., & Kanth, F. (2021). Prevalence and spectrum of dermatophytes in patients attending a tertiary care hospital, Srinagar, Kashmir. https://core.ac.uk/download/539911860.pdf (accessed on 27th June 2025).
23. Jayanthi, S., Lavanya, M., Nagamani, R., Rao, K., et al. (2016). A clinical, epidemiological and therapeutic scenario of dermatophytosis in a tertiary care hospital in the state of Telangana, India. https://core.ac.uk/download/539913480.pdf (accessed on 27th June 2025).
24. Khoso, B. K., Uddin, F., Hussain, W., Dashti, M. O., et al. (2022). Impact of dermatophytosis on the quality of life in patients attending a tertiary care hospital, Karachi. https://core.ac.uk/download/544153923.pdf (accessed on 27th June 2025).
25. Klimas, F., Pawłowski, B., Potoczek, A., Pudełko, M., et al. (2025). Fungal infections: Epidemiology, clinical challenges, and advances in diagnosis and treatment–A review. https://core.ac.uk/download/646079891.pdf (accessed on 27th June 2025).
26. Mbeng, W. O. (2013). Antifungal evaluation and phytochemical analysis of selected medicinal plants used in the treatment of fungal diseases associated with HIV infection in the Eastern Cape Province, South Africa. https://core.ac.uk/download/327278941.pdf (accessed on 27th June 2025).

27. Moskaluk, A. E. (2022). Novel approaches to characterizing feline-associated dermatophytic fungi. https://core.ac.uk/download/553287495.pdf (accessed on 27th June 2025).

28. Muhammad, M. I. (2023). Almajiri health: A scoping review on disease, health literacy and space for participatory research. https://core.ac.uk/download/571283472.pdf (accessed on 27th June 2025).

29. Patel, N., Patel, S., & Joshi, R. (2025). A comprehensive study on erythroderma: Etiologies, clinical features, and histopathological insights. https://core.ac.uk/download/640070619.pdf (accessed on 27th June 2025).

30. Ptak, A., & Szyc, M. (2024). Athlete's foot: A common fungal infection in athletes and beyond. The use of terbinafine in treating *Tinea pedis* and *Onychomycosis*. https://core.ac.uk/download/636385508.pdf (accessed on 27th June 2025).

31. Rahim, G. F. (1940). Eczematoid dermatoses of the hands with special reference to mycotic infection. https://core.ac.uk/download/429727921.pdf (accessed on 27th June 2025).

32. Raj, B., & Chetan, H. K. N. (2022). Dermatophytosis and antifungal therapies in various systems with special emphasis on homoeopathy: A narrative review. https://core.ac.uk/download/543112181.pdf (accessed on 27th June 2025).

33. Rajagopalan, R., & Vedhanayagam, M. (2017). Prevalence of mucocutaneous manifestations in human immunodeficiency infection–Learning from a rural center in Tamil Nadu, India. https://core.ac.uk/download/543136416.pdf (accessed on 27th June 2025).

34. Sabino, R., Simões, D., Simões, H., Veríssimo, C., et al. (2019). Dermatophytes' identification by matrix-assisted laser desorption ionization-time of flight mass spectrometry (MALDI-TOF MS)–The experience of a clinical laboratory. https://core.ac.uk/download/323276238.pdf (accessed on 27th June 2025).

35. Susanto, I. K. (2022). *Tinea corporis* therapy. https://core.ac.uk/download/543014253.pdf (accessed on 27th June 2025).

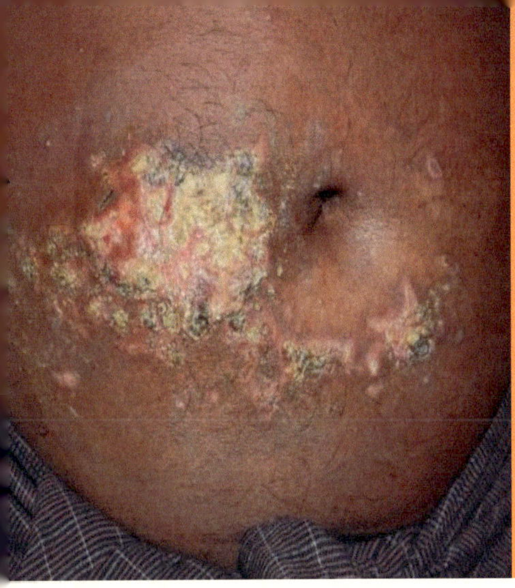

Chapter 4
SUPERFICIAL CANDIDIASIS

Contents

Introduction

Candidiasis, a frequent fungal infection, is primarily caused by the overgrowth of *Candida* species, the most common of which is superficial candidiasis. The infection takes place at various locations, such as the skin, oral cavity, and mucous membranes, and most commonly presents pain and clinical complications without treatment.

It is important to understand the pathophysiology of superficial candidiasis because infections caused by candida are usually encountered when the hosts immune system is down or when there is a local environment conducive to fungal growth. Evidence shows that causative factors like the use of antibiotics, diabetes, and immunosuppression raise susceptibility greatly to such infections, making effective management imperative. Since (Arora et al., 2022) enlightens, the usual treatment protocol involves antifungal drugs; however, drug resistance proves challenge to therapeutic outcomes. A detailed review of superficial candidiasis reveals its impact on the quality of life and puts a stress on early diagnosis and comprehensive treatment protocols, further discussed in subsequent sections of this chapter.

4.1. Understanding Candida Species

Species of *Candida* are a diverse group of yeasts not only omnipresent as commensals in human flora but also as significant opportunistic pathogens. The most significant species, *Candida albicans*, has for long been the prime focus of research; however, infection cases caused by non-albicans species such as *Candida glabrata* and *Candida tropicalis* have begun to emerge in increasing numbers, reflecting a shift in candidiasis pathology (Albertson et al., 2017).

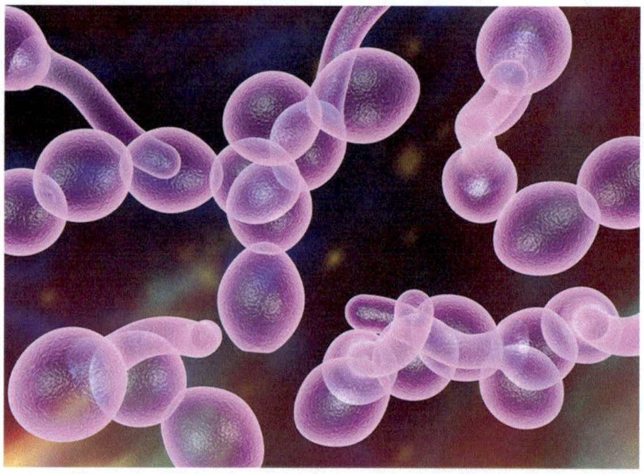

Figure 4.1. *Candida* species encompass a diverse group of yeasts that are not only prevalent as commensals in human microbiota but also significant opportunistic pathogens.

Source: https://cdn.the-scientist.com/assets/articleNo/71368/aImg/50968/fungus-tug-of-war-1-l.jpg.

Most notably, these species have variable levels of resistance to antifungals, complicating treatment and necessitating the utilization of rapid diagnostic methods to manage them effectively (Arastehfar et al., 2019). Among the most significant facts about *Candida* species is their ability to form biofilms, which contribute significantly to their resistance against antifungal agents. The complexity of biofilm formation, along with factors like starvation and intrinsic resistance mechanisms, emphasizes the very need for improving research on diagnostic as well as treatment measures to adequately manage superficial candidiasis (Figure 4.1).

4.1.1. Classification of Candida Species

The classification of *Candida* species is important to the understanding of superficial candidiasis and optimal therapy establishment. The *Candida* genus comprises over 200 known species, and only a few of them are etiologic agents of infections in human beings, the most prevalent being *Candida albicans*. However, increased recognition of non-albicans species such as *Candida glabrata* and *Candida tropicalis* necessitates an advanced system of classification.

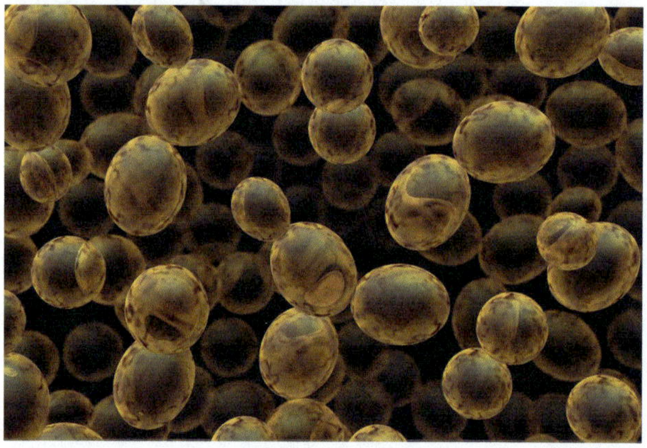

Figure 4.2. *Candida glabrata.*

Source: https://www.drhagmeyer.com/wp-content/uploads/2021/09/what-is-candida-glabrata-how-is-it-treated-3.jpeg.

Recent research has pointed to the importance of molecular methods, including multilocus sequence typing (MLST), in the discrimination of these species and the evaluation of their epidemiology in various environments, particularly in clinical settings (Vikholt et al., 2014). In other groups, including liver transplant patients, *Candida* species caused a significant proportion of invasive fungal disease, highlighting the need for correct identification and classification (Camargo et al., 2011). Thus, a good understanding of *Candida* species classification is vital to improve clinical success and tailor antifungal strategies to superficial candidiasis (Figure 4.2).

4.1.2. Common Types of Candida Causing Infections

Superficial candidiasis is caused predominantly by several different *Candida* species, but *Candida albicans* is the most prevalent. The yeast opportunistically colonizes mucosal surfaces and produces infections such as oral thrush and vaginitis. Vaginal candidiasis in particular is noteworthy, involving millions of healthcare contacts annually, highlighting the significant distress as well as expense of the infection; it has been estimated that over a billion dollars are spent yearly on self-treatment as well as consultations to a healthcare provider(Galea et al., 2013). Additionally, *Candida glabrata* is now a major non-*Candida albicans* pathogen of superficial infections with treatment challenges because it is resistant to antifungals that are used routinely. The heterogeneity of the species of *Candida* involved in superficial infections highlights the need for accurate diagnosis and tailored treatment regimens, which are most important in managing this common and widespread public health problem(Vikholt et al., 2014) (Figure 4.3).

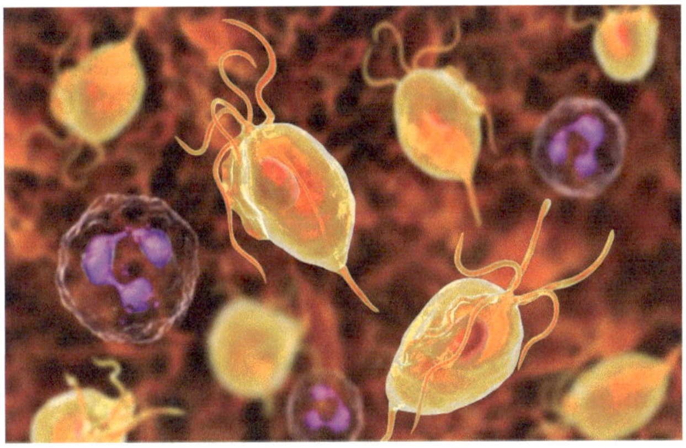

Figure 4.3. Vaginal candidiasis is particularly significant, accounting for millions of healthcare visits annually.

Source: https://clpmag.com/wp-content/uploads/2018/11/STI_Trichomonas-vaginalis_crop3500x2052p-scaled.jpg.

4.1.3. Characteristics of Candida albicans

Candida albicans is a dimorphic fungus that is commensal in nature as an organism within the human microbiota but also as a leading pathogen responsible for causing superficial candidiasis. The organism has numerous properties that contribute to its pathogenicity, including its ability to form biofilms and its adhesive property, which plays a significant role in colonization of host tissues. Research has also shown that *Candida albicans* strains have different levels of adhesiveness, with approximately 51.37% being nonadherent and a negligible 17.12% highly adhesive, serving to illustrate a complex interaction with the host surface to influence infection outcomes (Kushnirenko et al., 2016). Moreover, the presence of proteins such as mp58, a fibrinogen-binding protein, indicates a sophisticated mechanism of immune evasion and infection establishment with diversity among clinical isolates (Murgui et al., 2010). It should be appreciated so as to develop therapeutic strategies for superficial candidiasis (Figure 4.4).

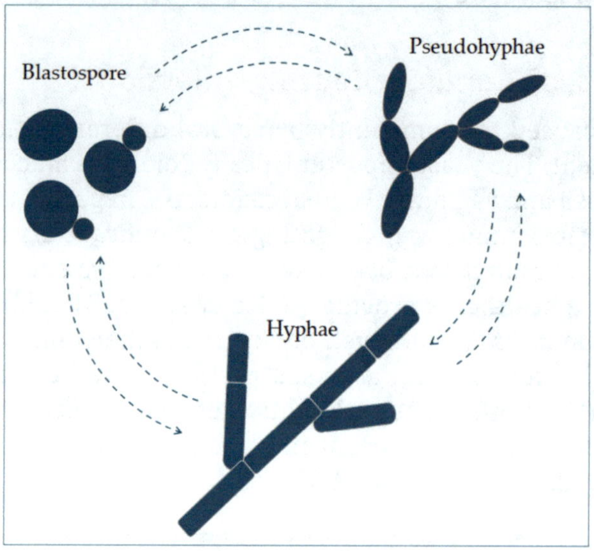

Figure 4.4. *Candida albicans* is a dimorphic fungus recognized for its role as a commensal organism in the human microbiota, yet it is also a significant pathogen responsible for superficial candidiasis.

Source: https://www.mdpi.com/jof/jof-07-00079/article_deploy/html/images/jof-07-00079-g001.png.

4.1.4. Role of Candida in Human Microbiota

The role of *Candida* in the human microbiota is multifarious and complex, particularly in superficial candidiasis. *Candida* is a commensal inhabitant of various human niches such as the oral cavity, gastrointestinal tract, and vaginal area where it usually maintains a harmonious coexistence with the other microbiota members. However, certain conditions—e.g., antibiotic treatment, immune suppression, or pH changes—interrupt this homeostasis, leading to opportunistic infection. For instance, excessive growth of *Candida* species, particularly *Candida albicans*, will cause superficial infections with manifestations of inflammation and itching. This disruption calls for studying host-pathogen interaction in order to be able to develop effective antifungal treatments, such as with the latest discoveries regarding understanding fungal transcriptomes and how they interact with the host (Coucke et al., 2019). Additionally, *Candidas* presence in oral microbiomes is notable, as it is most frequently associated with diseases of dental infection and other skin conditions (Hare et al., 2013).

4.1.5. Factors Causing Candida Overgrowth

Determinants of *Candida* overgrowth are multifactorial and often interactive, exerting a significant impact on the epidemiology of superficial candidiasis.

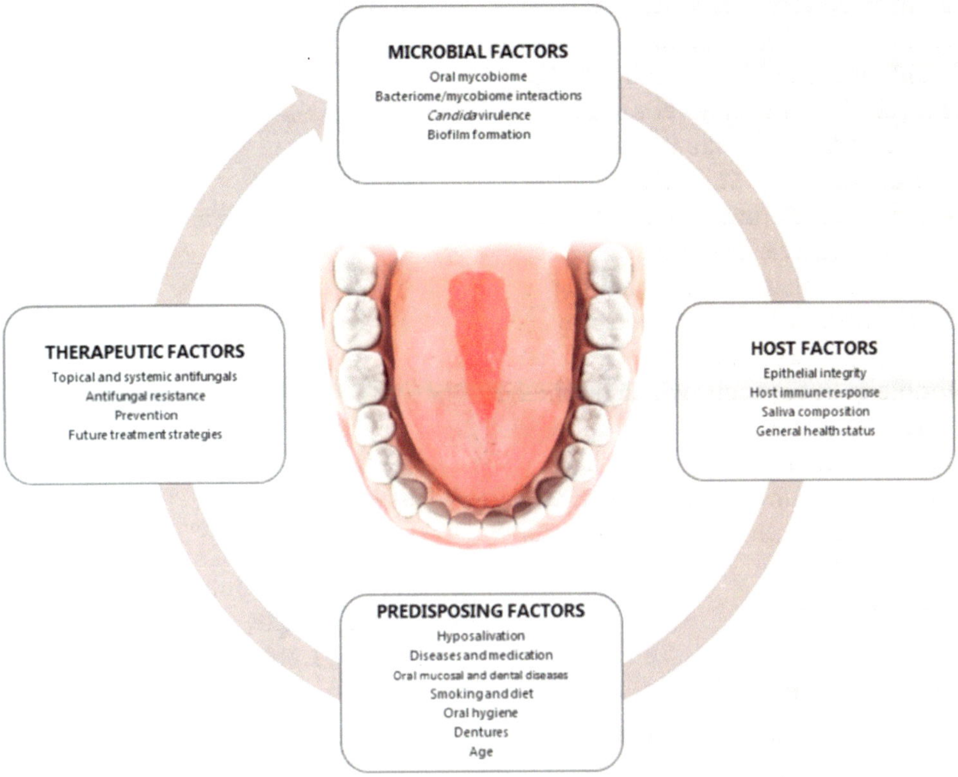

Figure 4.5. Factors leading to *Candida* overgrowth are multifaceted and often interlinked, significantly impacting the prevalence of superficial candidiasis.

Source: https://onlinelibrary.wiley.com/cms/asset/a2dc7f22-68f8-4d4c-b53c-fb0c4b5f4769/apm13412-fig-0001-m.jpg.

Host immunocompetence is one of the predisposing conditions; individuals with compromised immunity, such as those with HIV infection or on immunosuppressive therapy, are characterized by increased susceptibility to *Candida* infection. This is aggravated by predisposing environmental conditions that enable the growth of the fungus, such as the administration of antibiotics, which can interfere with the normal microbial flora and create ecological niches for *Candida* (RA et al., 2011). The presence of systemic inflammation and *Candida*'s capacity to generate immunomodulatory oxylipins, which regulate the immune response of the host, also contributed to overgrowth. The studies have shown that these oxylipins inhibit protective Th1 responses, leading to uncontrolled fungal growth (Kundu et al., 2010). Hence, these factors play a crucial role in controlling and preventing superficial candidiasis (Figure 4.5).

4.1.6. Pathogenic Mechanisms of Candida

Understanding the mechanisms of pathogenicity is important for the control of superficial candidiasis. The opportunistic fungus employs numerous mechanisms to promote survival and pathogenicity in host settings. Adhesion to epithelial surfaces is the initial step in infection, where studies have shown that close to 51.37% of *Candida* strains are non-adherent, but only 17.12% exhibit high adhesiveness levels (Kushnirenko et al., 2016). This adhesion is critical for tissue invasion and colonization. Additionally, *Candida*'s ability to switch between yeast and hyphal phases bestows increased invasiveness and resistance to host defense mechanisms. Additionally, the antifungal susceptibility patterns employed prove that as high as 97.8% of *Candida* isolates remain susceptible to fluconazole, which implies a potential therapeutic therapy to manage superficial infections (Alonso-Monge et al., 2013). These pathological mechanisms emphasize the need for continual research directed towards developing effective prevention and treatment strategies for candidiasis.

4.1.7. Environmental Factors Influencing Growth of Candida

The environmental factors influencing the growth of *Candida* play a major role in the etiology of superficial candidiasis. Temperature, pH, and humidity can greatly enhance the growth of this yeast, particularly in warm, moist areas of the body where the fungus grows optimally. High humidity favors the formation of biofilms, one of the characteristics in persistent infections because *Candida albicans* biofilm has the ability to initiate new infection or re-activate latent infection, accounting for about 40% of disseminated candidiasis (Ayodeji et al., 2015). Besides, host immune status is another important parameter; host weakening of immunity can lead to overgrowth of *Candida* species and increase the subject's susceptibility to clinical presentation of candidiasis (Lewis et al., 2017). Thus, information in regards to these environmental factors is required to formulate efficient prevention regimens and treatment modalities in the treatment of superficial candidiasis (Figure 4.6).

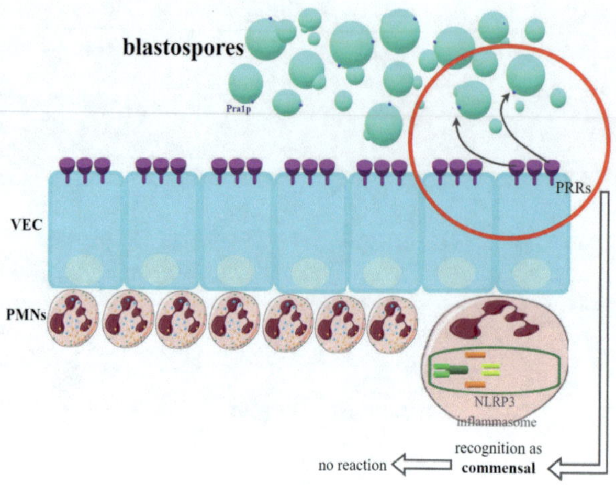

Figure 4.6. The environmental factors influencing the growth of *Candida* play a crucial role in the development of superficial candidiasis.

Source: https://pub.mdpi-res.com/ijms/ijms-23-05895/article_deploy/html/images/ijms-23-05895-g001.png?1653460102.

4.1.8. Genetic Variations Among Candida Species

The genetic variation among *Candida* species plays a significant role in understanding superficial candidiasis, as the variation significantly affects pathogenicity and therapeutic outcome. Research has established that variations in genetic composition between species, for instance, *Candida albicans* and *Candida parapsilosis*, can provide significant variations in antifungal susceptibility as well as virulence determinants. For instance, although *C. albicans* is most often the most common pathogen involved in superficial infections, *C. parapsilasis* has also been increasingly identified in opportunistic infections, particularly in immunocompromised patients. The evolution of such strains as *Candida glabrata* has also raised alarm with its multidrug resistance, complicating treatment (Vikholt et al., 2014). More importantly, studies have shown that there are distinct minimum inhibitory concentrations (MIC) among different *Candida* species, which means that special therapeutic strategies may be needed in a bid to effectively treat such infections. Understanding these genetic differences therefore becomes important in developing enhanced prevention and treatment plans against superficial candidiasis (Figure 4.7).

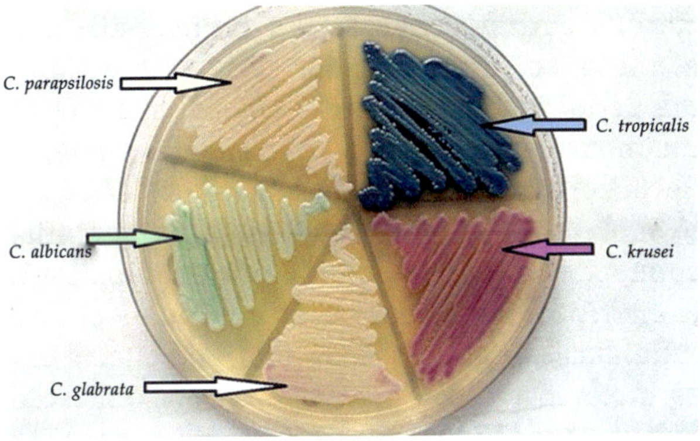

Figure 4.7. *Candida glabrata.*

Source: https://microbenotes.com/wp-content/uploads/2020/05/Laboratory-Diagnosis-of-*Candida*-glabrata.jpg.

4.1.9. Antifungal Resistance in Candida

The emergence of resistance to antifungal agents among *Candida* species is a heavy burden in the therapy of superficial candidiasis. Recent studies indicate that while the majority of *Candida* species remains sensitive to fluconazole, a significant proportion are resistant or partially resistant to antifungal agents.

In a large study involving samples drawn from HIV patients, 97.8% were found to be susceptible to fluconazole but 24.4% were moderately resistant to itraconazole, indicating a startling pattern of resistance to antifungals in some strains (Kushnirenko et al., 2016). This resistance is not only dependent on previous antifungal therapy but is also being exacerbated by other causes such as the failure of the mucosal barrier, one of the causes of the pathogenicity of *Candida* species (Alonso-Monge et al., 2013). Thus, understanding resistance mechanisms is required for effective therapeutic regimens that can counteract the increasing prevalence of superficial candidiasis.

4.2. Clinical Presentation of Superficial Candidiasis

The clinical manifestation of superficial candidiasis is limited largely to the skin and mucosal surfaces upon which the opportunistic fungus *Candida albicans* would be able to exist under certain circumstances. Superficial candidiasis most commonly presents as erythematous, pruritic rashes usually with a characteristic whitish exudate, especially in warm, moist environments such as intertriginous areas—skin fold areas where heat and moisture create conditions for fungal growth. They will also have characteristic oral manifestations, such as thrush, where there are white patches of the mucous membranes and it may be painful or uncomfortable on swallowing. Surprisingly, these manifestations are excellent markers for early diagnosis and treatment, particularly in immunocompromised individuals. Besides, this is information medical professionals must have since early diagnosis can dramatically enhance the success of therapy and overall quality of life of superficial candidiasis patients, uncovering latent autoimmune diseases or justifying further immunological assessment (Agarwala et al., 2017; Bossù et al., 2018).

4.2.1. Types of Superficial Candidiasis

Superficial candidiasis encompasses several discrete forms with each having distinct clinical characteristics and anatomical sites involved. Oral candidiasis is the most common form and tends to be caused by *Candida albicans*, which occurs as white plaques on oral mucosa and can affect individuals with compromised immunity or those on broad-spectrum antibiotics. In addition, cutaneous candidiasis is most often found in warm, moist areas of the body, such as the intertriginous areas, where *Candida* can grow due to moisture and friction. Clinical diagnosis is primarily the means of diagnosis in these conditions, but microbiological techniques can verify suspected cases in order to exclude other illnesses, particularly in complex cases with drug resistance (Castellote et al., 2013). Prevention and therapy interventions typically rely on the recognition of predisposing factors and adopting antifungal treatment based on the distinctive characteristics of the implicated *Candida* species (El-garhy et al., 2015). Recognition of the various superficial candidiasis forms is thus critical for effective control (Figure 4.8).

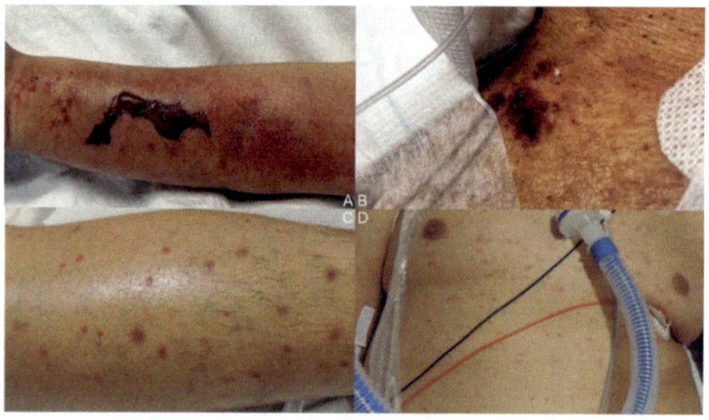

Figure 4.8. Superficial candidiasis encompasses several distinct forms, each characterized by its specific clinical manifestations and affected anatomical sites.

Source: https://media.springernature.com/lw685/springer-static/image/art%3A10.1007%2Fs12281-024-00485-5/MediaObjects/12281_2024_485_Fig1_HTML.jpg.

4.2.2. Symptoms of Oral Candidiasis

Oral candidiasis, or thrush, presents with a multitude of signs and symptoms that are significantly impacting the quality of life. Patients primarily present with white lesions on the inner cheeks and tongue that may also affect the roof of the mouth, gums, and tonsils, forming a cottage cheese-like appearance. The lesions may be tender and uncomfortable, particularly with eating or swallowing, and therefore compromising nutrition. Additionally, an individual may exhibit symptoms such as cottonmouth, taste loss, and redness or pain in the affected area. Under serious infections, the condition may lead to corner cracking at the mouth, also referred to as angular cheilitis. Because conditions of the oral cavity can lead to more serious problems—such as potential connections to systemic health problems—it is of critical importance that symptoms of oral candidiasis be addressed rapidly and effectively, as dictated by existing research of connected health conditions like those discussed in Agarwala et al., (2017) and Galea et al., (2013).

4.2.3. Cutaneous Candidiasis Symptoms

Cutaneous candidiasis symptoms are varied and may have a significant effect on the life quality of an infected person. It tends to occur in hot, moist areas on the human body, such as skin folds and intertriginous areas, as a red, itching rash that is often accompanied by white patches or pustules. Redness and itching may be present, particularly in localized regions where the yeast grows. This infection can occur in a great variety of populations, such as immunocompromised individuals and patients with diseases such as diabetes or obesity, which further illustrates its opportunistic nature. Secondary infection will complicate the clinical picture and cause misdiagnosis if not accurately evaluated. Effective treatment of cutaneous candidiasis relies on timely detection of symptoms and antifungal therapy directed specifically against the condition, illustrating the value of raising awareness for this common yet significant skin condition (Agarwala et al., 2017; Adaskevich et al., 2014) (Figure 4.9).

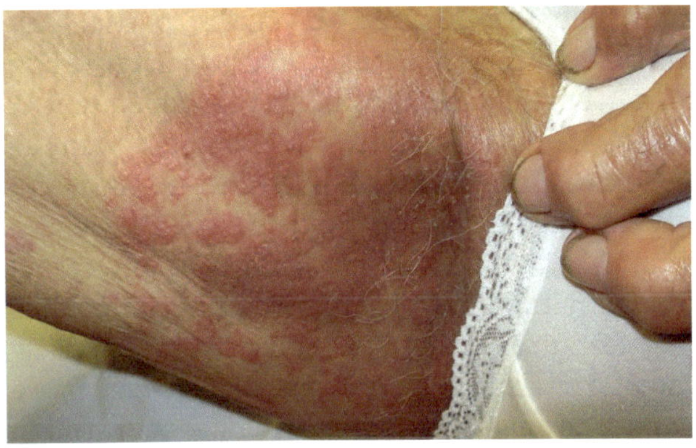

Figure 4.9. Typically occurring in warm, moist areas of the body, such as skin folds and intertriginous zones, this condition presents as a red, itchy rash often accompanied by white patches or pustules.

Source: https://i0.wp.com/post.healthline.com/wp-content/uploads/2019/02/Intertrigo_due_to_candida_infection-1296x728-gallery_slide1.jpg?w=1155.

4.2.4. Symptoms of Vaginal Candidiasis

The symptoms of vaginal candidiasis are generally characterized by hallmark physical discomfort and emotional distress. Women may experience profuse itching, vulval swelling, and redness, together with a thick white discharge resembling cottage cheese. These are detrimental to regular living, resulting in painful sex as well as heightened feelings of self-consciousness that can weigh heavily upon social interaction and total wellness. Not only is vaginal candidiasis a health issue, it's also a cause of psychological distress for most, representing significant healthcare visits; vaginitis is said to be responsible for nearly 6 million consultations each year due to related symptoms that have a negative effect on self-worth and performance at the workplace (Galea et al., 2013). Thus, timely diagnosis and treatment are necessary in order to alleviate such symptoms and improve the quality of life for patients with this commonly occurring condition (Alonso-Monge et al., 2013).

4.2.5. Esophageal Candidiasis Symptoms

Esophageal candidiasis, often caused by an overgrowth of *Candida* species, is characterized by a variety of varying symptoms that go on to complicate the clinical syndrome. Dysphagia, the primary symptom, causes severe swallowing difficulty, particularly with solids.

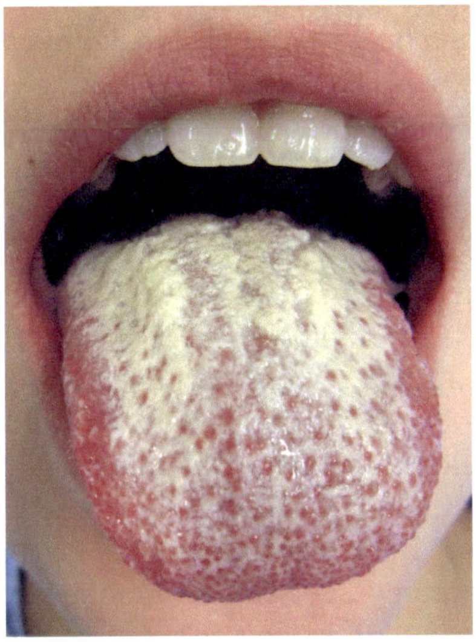

Figure 4.10. Esophageal candidiasis, often resulting from an overgrowth of *Candida* species, manifests through a variety of distinct symptoms that often complicate the clinical picture.

Source: https://upload.wikimedia.org/wikipedia/commons/a/a0/Human_tongue_infected_with_oral_candidiasis.jpg.

The symptom may advance to odynophagia, or painful swallowing, which complicates the patient's discomfort and may impede the intake of food, hence putting nutrition insufficiencies at risk. In some cases, patients will present with pain in the chest or throat fullness, along with oral thrush signs (Contreras et al., 2014). As the condition advances, immunocompetent patients may remain asymptomatic and most will present with no overt infection signs (Contreras et al., 2014). But patients with underlying immunocompromised conditions—

i.e., neoplasms—are significantly more likely to present with hyper-responsive symptoms, and the double-edged role of immunocompetence within the esophageal candidiasis pathology is thereby highlighted (Contreras et al., 2014) (Figure 4.10).

4.2.6. Impact on Quality of Life

The impact of superficial candidiasis on quality of life can be substantial, affecting physical, psychological, and social well-being. Patients typically experience distressing signs and symptoms such as itch, pain, and observable lesions, which may result in decreased self-esteem and disturbance of body image. The symptoms not only affect normal functioning but can also lead to anxiety and depression, as the patients have difficulty with the long-term nature of infection. Studies indicate that the development of fungal infection growths, including those of candidiasis, are widespread and have been approximated to occur in approximately 25% of the global population (Coucke et al., 2019). Furthermore, complications arising from superficial candidiasis may render social interactions and work assignments difficult, leading to subsequent isolation and emotional distress. Consequently, resolution of these multifaceted effects is of critical significance to the overall care of the patient, underscoring the urgent necessity of sound practice management to improve the overall quality of life of the patient with this condition (Agarwala et al., 2017).

4.2.7. Complications Associated with Untreated Candidiasis

The implications of untreated candidiasis extend beyond the realm of mere superficial irritation and discomfort and may result in severe complications that undermine the overall health of the individual. In situations where infection with candida is not well managed, patients may develop worsening symptoms that can contribute to systemic involvement, particularly among immunocompromised hosts. Such advancement often includes the development of invasive candidiasis, where the fungus becomes imbedded deep within tissues and organs, causing extreme disease such as sepsis, which is potentially deadly if left untreated. Further, untreated oral and vaginal candidiasis may lead to chronic inflammation and secondary infections making the treatment process more complicated. It has been established through research that chronic fungal infection can also be associated with negative effects on host immune responses, exacerbating predisposed conditions and posing risks for subsequent infections (AAP et al., 2014). As discussed in current studies, improving antifungal strategies is imperative owing to the complexity attributed to drug resistance and interactions with the host (Fahmitha et al., 2024) (Figure 4.11).

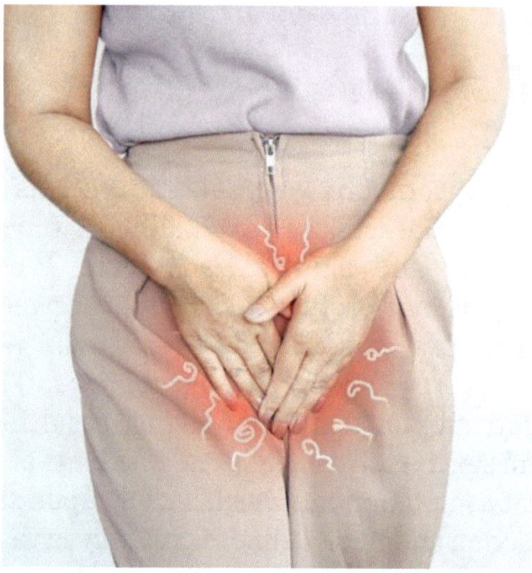

Figure 4.11. Untreated oral and vaginal candidiasis can lead to chronic inflammation and secondary infections that complicate treatment outcomes.

Source: https://cdn-ilcpcol.nitrocdn.com/cZQGwpmIRbxvVwNPEGnuMlfBMhmqrSWv/assets/images/optimized/rev-b2a0f50/ezraclinic.sg/wp-content/uploads/8342c10f-2187-40cb-96c1-4aa87d342e61-768x512.jpeg.

4.2.8. Differential Diagnosis of Candidiasis

Understanding the differential diagnosis of candidiasis is crucial for accurate identification and treatment, particularly in the context of superficial candidiasis. Clinicians must differentiate between various forms of candidiasis, including oral and esophageal candidiasis, as the presentations can overlap with other conditions. For instance, oral candidiasis may mimic other mucosal disorders, necessitating a comprehensive evaluation to avoid misdiagnosis. Besides, esophageal candidiasis is also usually asymptomatic in immunocompetent hosts and can occur insidiously in conditions where there are associated malignancies to mask the clinical presentation (Abdullah et al., 2006). Molecular epidemiology of *Candida* species such as *Candida glabrata* is also significant for this differential diagnosis since various species can have varying patterns of resistance as well as virulence factors affecting clinical outcomes (Vikholt et al., 2014). Therefore, accurate diagnosis and effective intervention require a critical analysis that considers both laboratory and clinical information.

4.2.9. Importance of Early Identification

The importance of early diagnosis in superficial candidiasis cannot be overestimated since timely diagnosis and treatment are highly effective in the prevention of complications and in attaining a favorable outcome among patients. Superficial candidiasis frequently occurs among immunocompromised hosts like diabetic and chronic patients, hence the need for health workers to be vigilant in observing early warning signs. If the condition is not detected in time, it may lead to more morbidity as delayed treatment may allow for the progression of the infection and even transmission. Significantly, the interaction between superficial candidiasis and other opportunistic pathogens such as *Streptococcus agalactiae* underlies the complexity of co-infection and how it undermines treatment success (Patenaude et al., 2023). Subsequently, timely diagnosis not only facilitates the implementation of effective antifungal therapy but also enables clinicians to evaluate potential synergistic interactions of co-infections, for example, *Candida auris*, that further complicate the clinical scenario (Brown et al., 2020). Vigilance and rapid action are thus paramount to successful control of this prevalent fungal infection (Figure 4.12).

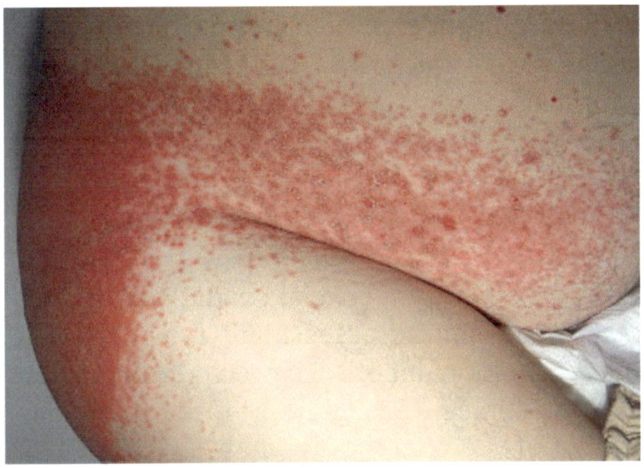

Figure 4.12. Superficial candidiasis often manifests in immunocompromised populations, including those with diabetes and chronic illnesses.

Source: https://ars.els-cdn.com/content/image/3-s2.0-B9780124055469000406-f40-10-9780124055469.jpg.

4.3. Diagnosis of Superficial Candidiasis

Diagnosis of superficial candidiasis is primarily clinical based on thorough assessment and patient history. Practitioners can generally diagnose the disease through observation of common symptoms such as itching, erythema, and lesions on affected areas. As in more recent literature, microbiological methods can be utilized to verify clinical suspicion, especially in cases of resistance to antifungal therapy or in instances when differential diagnosis is warranted (Castellote et al., 2013). KOH staining and cultures on specialty media such as Sabouraud dextrose agar are common practices for isolating *Candida* species. Moreover, advanced techniques such as multilocus sequence typing (MLST) allow for accurate epidemiological analysis and determination of individual *Candida* strains (Vikholt et al., 2014). Lastly, a merge of clinical information with microbiological findings ensures a comprehensive strategy to accurate superficial candidiasis diagnosis, allowing for timely and sufficient therapeutic approaches.

4.3.1. Clinical Evaluation and History Taking

While assessing superficial candidiasis, history taking and clinical assessment are the key to the recognition of both the precipitating factors and the clinical presentation of the infection.

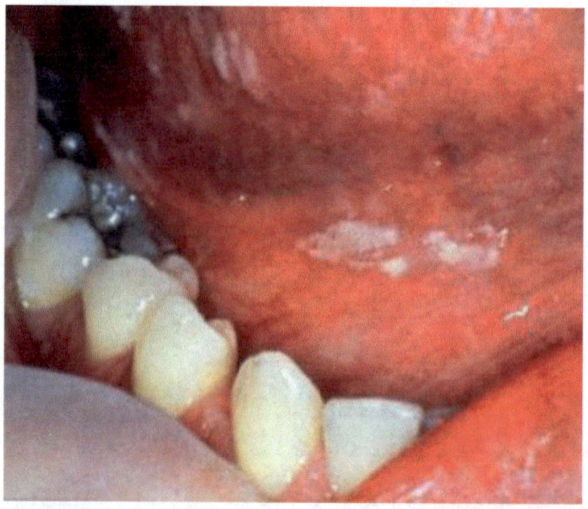

Figure 4.13. During physical examination, clinicians often observe characteristic lesions that assist in confirming the diagnosis of oral candidiasis and differentiating it from other mucosal conditions.

Source: https://img.medscapestatic.com/pi/meds/ckb/18/44418tn.jpg.

A clear medical history can reveal important predisposing factors such as immunosuppression, diabetes mellitus, or the use of broad-spectrum antibiotics, which may compromise host immunity against *Candida* species, with particular focus on *Candida albicans*, the most common species recovered in such infections (Lewis et al., 2017). On examination, clinicians can identify characteristic lesions that aid in making the diagnosis of oral candidiasis and differentiating it from other mucosal conditions (Vikholt et al., 2014). In effect, this holistic process not only facilitates proper diagnosis but also lays the groundwork for a focused treatment plan that involves intervention for any risk factors noted and the need for antifungal treatment, so taking history is a critical part of treating superficial candidiasis (Figure 4.13).

4.3.2. Laboratory Tests for Diagnosis

Laboratory tests are also critical in the clinical diagnosis and treatment of superficial candidiasis. Initial tests typically involve a full oral exam consisting of an examination of the oral cavity for erythema or white lesions indicative of candidiasis and a complete medical history to establish risk factors and symptomatology (Burgess et al., 2017).

Additionally, laboratory results such as culture and serological tests can provide valuable information; culture can verify the presence of *Candida* species while serology can be used to test for immune reaction to infection. Importantly, studies have identified the significance of specific mannoproteins, e.g., mp58, in candidiasis. In particular, mp58 was detected in tissue from patients with systemic candidiasis, suggesting potential diagnostic utility, and antibodies to the antigen were not detected in superficial infections (Murgui et al., 2010). This underscores the necessity for specific laboratory tests in determining between forms of infection.

4.3.3. Microscopic Examination Techniques

Microscopic diagnostic methods are of significant importance in the management and diagnosis of superficial candidiasis because they help distinguish between commensal and pathogenic organisms in the oral environment. The most frequently used techniques are 10% KOH smear preparations, which effectively lyse debris and allow visualization of fungal morphology, and culture on specific media like Sabouraud dextrose agar, that can allow the growth of *Candida* species (Castellote et al., 2013). Secondly, reflectance confocal microscopy (RCM) is a sophisticated noninvasive instrument that facilitates real-time imaging of the skin and mucosal surfaces, facilitating recognition of parasites and fungi with good accuracy. RCM not only facilitates diagnosis but also facilitates evaluation of response to treatment, thereby improving outcomes of patients in superficial candidiasis (Arzberger et al., 2020). This broad strategy highlights the importance of microscopic techniques in the augmentation of clinical efficacy in candidiasis control (Figure 4.14).

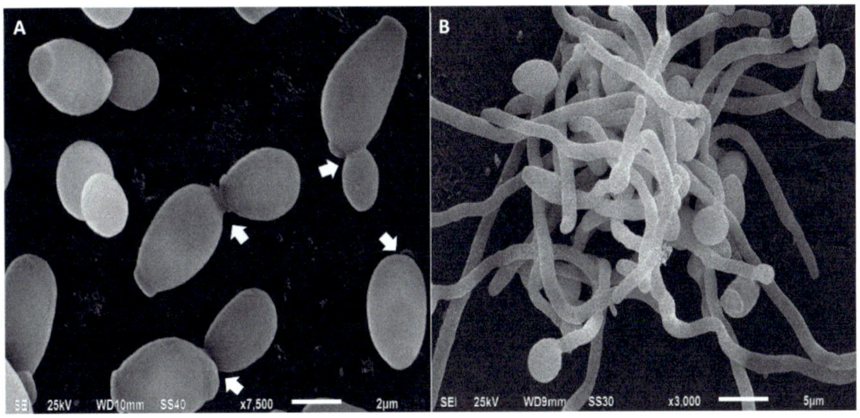

Figure 4.14. Microscopic examination techniques play a crucial role in the diagnosis and management of superficial candidiasis, as they enable clinicians to distinguish between commensal and pathogenic organisms within the oral cavity.

Source: https://static.elsevier.es/multimedia/03257541/0000005500000002/v1_202306160952/S0325754122000840/v1_202306160952/en/main.assets/gr1.jpeg.

4.3.4. Culture Methods for Candida

Isolation of *Candida* spp. is required for the diagnosis of superficial candidiasis and involves different methodologies for isolation and identification of the causative pathogen. The most common methods of cultivation include the use of Sabouraud dextrose agar, which favors fungal growth but inhibits bacterial growth. Furthermore, chromogenic media have also gained significance with its ability to facilitate identification of specific *Candida* species based on differential colors of colony appearance. These culture methods can function quite differently depending on the strain and growth conditions, as evidenced by research into the cell wall-associated fibrinogen binding mannoprotein (mp58) of *Candida albicans*, which has not only been detected in clinical isolates but also has differing expression patterns with various culture conditions (Murgui et al., 2010). Appreciation of these cultural intricacies is critical for successful clinical diagnosis. and treatment of superficial candidiasis in light of differences in pathogenicity between *Candida* species (Vikholt et al., 2014).

4.3.5. Molecular Diagnostic Techniques

Molecular diagnostic techniques have made it easier to detect and identify superficial candidiasis, a ubiquitous fungal infection. Traditional diagnostics, while appropriate for superficial infections, prove to be insensitive in infections that are more deep-seated. Nucleic acid amplification and proteomic characterization by MALDI-TOF have been recognized as effective tools to enhance the efficiency of diagnosis. These approaches allow for the identification of *Candida* species by analyzing genetic material, circumventing the limitations posed by the immunological response of the hosts (Marot et al., 2013). Also, the enrichment of fungal nucleic acids, which are derived from targeted lysis strategies, enables a more extensive exploration of fungal transcriptional profiles in clinical specimens (Coucke et al., 2019). As a result, the use of such molecular diagnostics not only allows prompt treatment of superficial candidiasis but also advances our knowledge of its pathophysiology, improving patient outcomes and informing successful antifungal therapies (Figure 4.15).

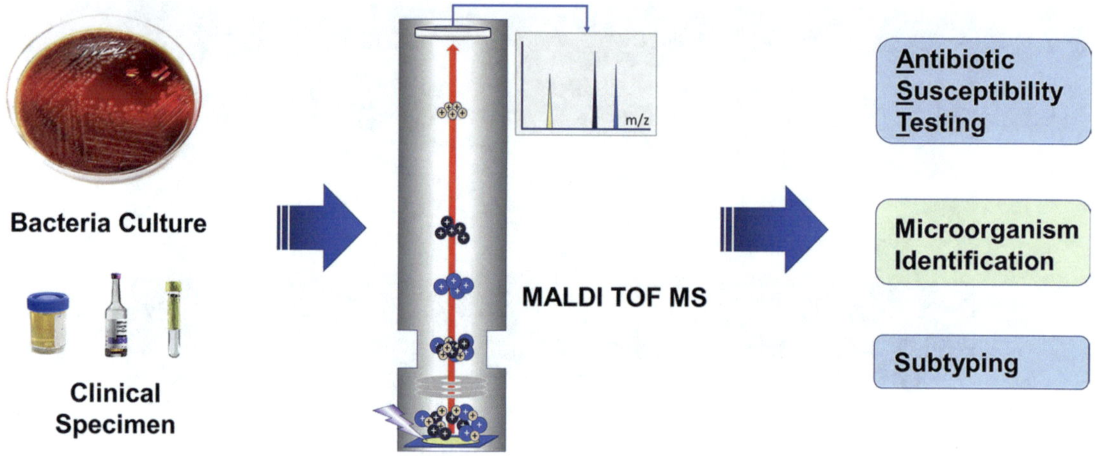

Figure 4.15. Molecular approaches, such as the amplification of nucleic acids and proteomic analysis via MALDI-TOF, have emerged as promising tools to enhance diagnostic accuracy.

Source: https://ars.els-cdn.com/content/image/1-s2.0-S1021949819300146-fx1.jpg.

4.3.6. Role of Serological Tests

Application of serological tests in diagnosing superficial candidiasis has gained attention due to the limitations in the application of classical culture techniques. The tests allow for the identification of specific antibodies to *Candida* species that can be critical in separating superficial and systemic infections. While promising, serological tests have been found to be inconsistently specific, e.g., positive detection of antibody in healthy carriers with *Candida* as a commensal (Burges et al., 1982). In addition, the intrinsically complex antigenic structure of *Candida* poses difficulties towards inducing adequate serological responses, which leads to inconsistent results in routine tests such as agglutination or complement fixation tests (Fraser et al., 1971). Technique developments, such as quantitative immunofluorescence and Ouchterlony gel-diffusion, have the potential to enhance diagnostic accuracy by offering greater specificity for the identification of immune responses present with superficial candidiasis, improving clinical decision-making and patient management.

4.3.7. Challenges in Diagnosing Candidiasis

Diagnosis of candidiasis follows a series of significant barriers that disrupt timely and effective treatment. One key hindrance is that laboratory diagnosis is reliant upon it, and these tests cannot always yield definitive results; the majority of non-culture tests, with the exception of histological tests, lack the capability to identify various species of fungi and are not accessible in developing nations, such as India (Choudhary et al., 2019).

Additionally, some patient populations, particularly those who are immunocompromised, may have atypical clinical presentations that blur the lines of normal candidiasis symptoms, complicating diagnosis (Govender et al., 2009). Intrapersonal variation in clinical presentation can also lead to misdiagnosis or a delay in diagnosis, ultimately affecting patient outcomes. Thus, a knowledge of the limitations of the diagnostic techniques and the complexity in patient presentations is essential to increase the understanding and management of superficial candidiasis (Figure 4.16).

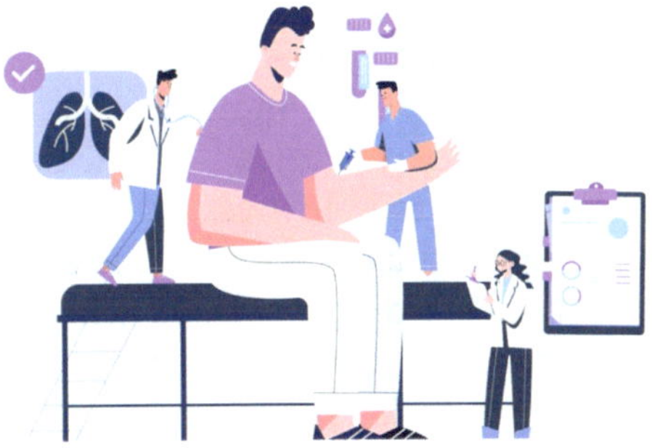

Figure 4.16. The variability in clinical manifestations among different individuals can also lead to misdiagnosis or delayed diagnosis, ultimately affecting patient outcomes.

Source: https://rapidlaboratory.in/wp-content/uploads/2024/03/Diagnostic-and-Medical-Care-1.png.

4.3.8. Importance of Accurate Diagnosis

Accurate diagnosis plays a critical role in the management of cutaneous candidiasis because inappropriate identification will lead to unsuccessful treatment and serious complications. The diagnostic process is often compromised by the diversity of *Candida* species and their variable susceptibility to antifungal agents. Therefore, early and correct identification becomes necessary to facilitate the right therapy regimens. New technologies for diagnostic tools such as next-generation sequencing and immunological assays have great potential to further enhance diagnostic correctness. Notably, the detection of *Candida albicans* germ-tube-specific antibodies has proved to distinguish between colonization and invasive infection, underpinning the value of diagnostic criteria specificity (Aranzazu Sáez-Rosón et al., 2014). Moreover, long-standing issues with sensitivity and standardization of such methods call for continued research in order to arrive at trusted conclusions (Arastehfar et al., 2019). Consequently, improving procedures of diagnosis is crucial for effective treatment, as well as for curbing the rising number of cases of antifungal resistance, in a bid to attain better patient outcomes in superficial candidiasis.

4.3.9. Guidelines of Healthcare Providers

During treatment of superficial candidiasis, medical professionals must adhere to guidelines involving proper assessment and treatment protocol. This starts with a good physical examination and history, as these allow practitioners to identify risk factors and background conditions that put patients at risk for developing candidiasis. As per (Burgess et al., 2017), it is essential to conduct systemic intraoral examination so that the practitioner can spot oral lesions and other features of this illness. Moreover, the World Health Organization highlights that oral health must be treated as a central component of overall health, as has been emphasized in their 2022 report; there are a number of oral disorders that can significantly influence systemic health (Campisi et al., 2024). Hence, it's important that the providers acknowledge and treat candidiasis not merely as a superficial condition but as a part of an integrated treatment of health so that the patients are given holistic care which treats current symptoms as well as preventive measures in the long run (Figure 4.17).

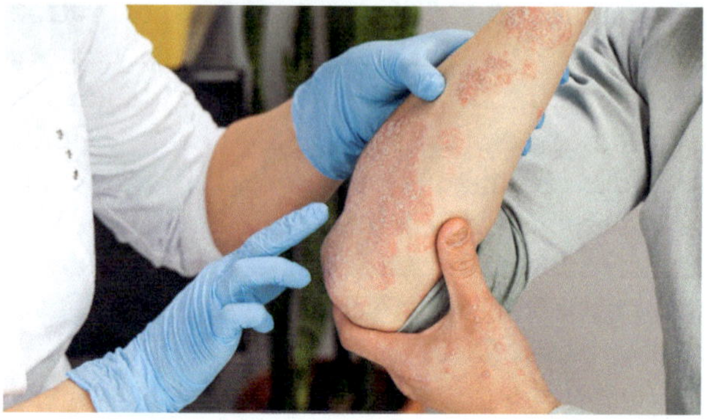

Figure 4.17. Initially, a thorough medical history and physical examination are crucial, as they allow providers to identify risk factors and underlying conditions that predispose patients to candidiasis.

Source: https://www.practicenursing.com/media/mqkn5fnt/adobestock_393573411.jpeg?width=1002&height=564&bgcolor=White&v=1db887b55986fd0.

4.4. Treatment and Management of Superficial Candidiasis

Treatment of superficial candidiasis needs a multidisciplinary approach based on the combination of pharmacological treatment and lifestyle changes. Topical antifungals, such as clotrimazole and miconazole, are typically the first line of treatment and can readily eliminate focal infections, particularly in wet, frictional areas, like the groin and axilla. In more serious or resistant cases, systemic drugs such as fluconazole may be warranted but must be weighed against potential adverse effects and drug interactions. Education of the patient is similarly crucial in preventing recurrence; these include cleansing and drying of the skin and measures for management of underlying conditions like diabetes which predispose to infection. Thus, a treatment strategy that utilizes an effective antifungal regimen combined with aggressive patient management can optimize results in those who are suffering from superficial candidiasis (Alonso-Monge et al., 2013; Brown et al., 2009).

4.4.1. Overview of Antifungal Medications

Antifungal medications play a significant role in the management of superficial candidiasis, which is a yeast mucocutaneous infection due to *Candida* species. Antifungal medications may be classified as topical and systemic medications, and the topical medications are usually utilized as first-line therapy in localized infections. Typical agents among them include clotrimazole and miconazole, which induce cell membrane disruption in fungi and lead to cell death. For more disseminated or persistent infections, systemic drugs such as fluconazole are usually prescribed due to their ability to achieve higher tissue concentrations. Their efficacy is provided by good research, such as the molecular epidemiology of *Candida glabrata*, which illustrates the development of resistant strains among immunocompromised patients (Vikholt et al., 2014). Similarly, pharmacodynamics and drug resistance knowledge is essential in the optimization of treatment in patients, especially given the complicated patient profiles that are usually seen in the clinical setting (Agarwala et al., 2017) (Figure 4.18).

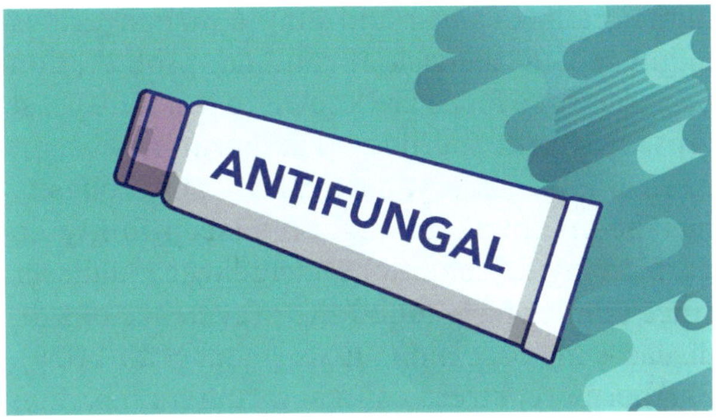

Figure 4.18. Antifungal medications play a crucial role in the management of superficial candidiasis, a common yeast infection caused by various *Candida* species.

Source: https://www.cdc.gov/candidiasis/media/images/2024/03/347136_43_RingwormTreatmentNoRX.png.

4.4.2. Topical Treatments for Candidiasis

Topical treatment of candidiasis is a primary component of the management of this common fungal infection, particularly in superficial candidiasis involving skin and mucosal surfaces. Initial therapy is commonly antifungal agents such as clotrimazole or miconazole that effectively inhibit the proliferation of *Candida* species through disruption of the fungal cell membrane. These treatments are generally well tolerated and can be applied in various forms, including creams, ointments, and powders, thus being suitable for various parts of the body involved. In addition, recurrent infections need to be paired with modifications in lifestyle and, at times, with systemic therapy to optimize results. Although topical antifungals are efficacious, treatment compliance and the management of predisposing factors remain crucial to prevent recurrences of candidiasis and therefore an integrated treatment plan being a necessary tool for effective control (Agarwala et al., 2017; Mészáros Judit et al., 2016).

4.4.3. Systemic Treatments for Severe Cases

Severe forms of superficial candidiasis often necessitate the administration of systemic therapy, particularly in individuals with profound immunocompromise or complicating conditions that increase infection severity. Systemic antifungal agents such as fluconazole and the echinocandins may be employed to effectively treat *Candida* pathogens leading to widespread mucocutaneous disease.

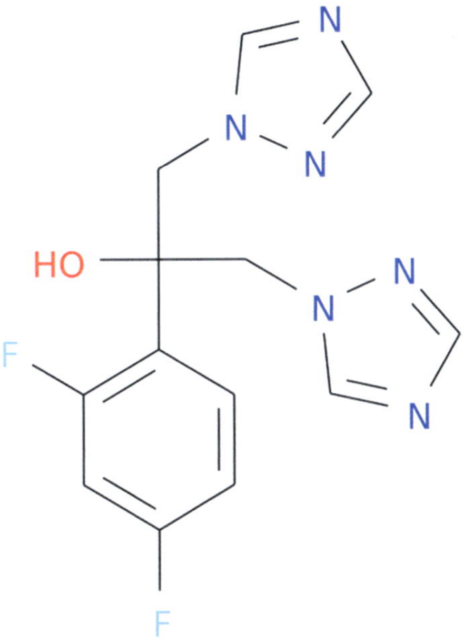

Figure 4.19. Fluconazole.

Source: https://pubchem.ncbi.nlm.nih.gov/image/imgsrv.fcgi?cid=3365&t=l.

Though skin-level presentations of candidiasis are possible in healthy patients, severe infection is more common in critically ill or immunocompromised patients with a greater risk of morbidity and mortality (Bassetti et al., 2025). Notably, recent data are also indicating the emergence of antifungal resistance and new pathogens, which makes treatment regimens more challenging and necessitates an adaptive strategy for management (Bassetti et al., 2025). Therefore, identification of the severity of candidiasis and prompt application of systemic therapies are essential in preventing complications and patient recovery from such incapacitating infections (Figure 4.19).

4.4.4. Role of Probiotics in Management

Treatment of superficial candidiasis can significantly be enhanced by the addition of probiotics in conjunction with routine antifungal therapy. Probiotics, particularly preparations containing species such as *Saccharomyces boulardii* and *Lactobacillus sporogenes*, are likely to enhance the efficacy of vulvovaginal infections, which are often caused by fungal overgrowths such as *Candida*. A patient trial with a combination of antimicrobial medications and probiotics recorded significant decrease in symptoms and rate of recurrence from participants who were on the conventional treatments alone, indicating the function of the probiotics in creating a balanced microbial flora (Patil et al., 2021). Additionally, the increasing prevalence of fungal infection, combined with factors such as immunosuppressive therapy and the administration of broad-spectrum antibiotics, highlights the potential contribution of adjunctive treatments like probiotics towards the reduction of recurrence risk and improvement of patient outcomes (Kuriyama et al., 2012). As such, the addition of probiotics to the treatment protocol for superficial candidiasis provides an effective approach to therapeutic efficacy enhancement.

4.4.5. Lifestyle Changes to Prevent Recurrence

Effective treatment of superficial candidiasis extends beyond antifungal medication and involves significant lifestyle modification in order to avoid recurrence. Key modifications include maintenance of good hygiene, such as a clean and dry skin, since moisture fosters fungal growth. Diet also plays a critical role; reduction in the intake of sugar and simple carbohydrates might reduce the risk of candidal proliferation because these foods are known to facilitate yeast growth within the body. Furthermore, weight control is necessary, particularly since obesity has been linked to higher susceptibility to dermatological conditions, including candidiasis, since studies have found the prevalence of skin diseases in obese individuals (Iqbal et al., 2016). Furthermore, stress control through relaxation may improve immune function, as well as reduce susceptibility to infections. By incorporating these actionable alterations, one can significantly minimize the chances of a recurring superficial candidiasis infection, providing long-term skin wellness and health (Figure 4.20).

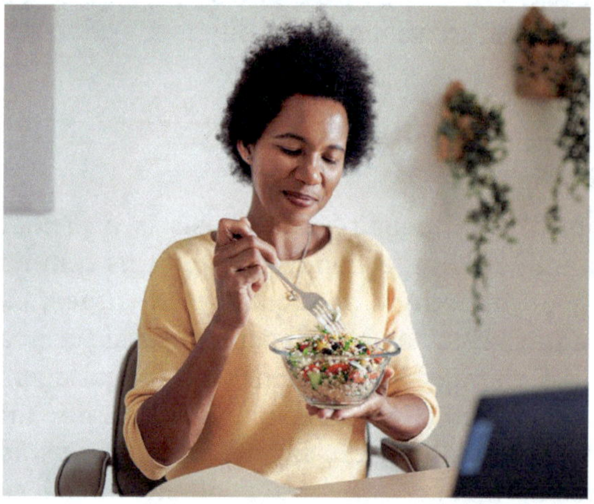

Figure 4.20. Dietary adjustments play a crucial role; reducing sugar and refined carbohydrates can lower the risk of candidal proliferation, as these substances can fuel yeast growth in the body.

Source: https://media.post.rvohealth.io/wp-content/uploads/2024/05/woman-eating-a-quinoa-salad-header.jpg.

4.4.6. Importance of Patient Education

Effective patient education is a significant component of superficial candidiasis care, and being able to educate patients on everything they require to learn about their illness and treatment program. Patient education on the etiology, symptomatology, and prevention of the recurring fungal infection can improve the outcomes of treatment and minimize recurrence risk by healthcare providers. Research has shown that patients with education are prone to embracing healthy proactive life styles, which involve personal hygiene and early recognition of infection symptoms. Beyond that, education regarding the epidemiology of fungal infections, as illustrated in reports of their prevalence and determinants, can inspire patients to see the physician timely, thereby reducing the disease burden in the population (Klimas et al., 2025; Denning et al., 2018). Therefore, patient education promotes not only individual health but also contributes to overall public health efforts in the prevention of superficial candidiasis as well as the quality of overall healthcare.

4.4.7. Monitoring Treatment Effectiveness

Effective monitoring of treatment effectiveness against superficial candidiasis is essential for optimal patient outcomes. Clinicians are now obligated to employ various diagnostic methods for evaluation of response to antifungal therapy such as clinical evaluation, laboratory tests, and imaging tests, if necessary. *Candida* species can acquire differing sensitivities towards antifungal agents over time, and hence follow-up assessments of response to treatment are crucial, particularly in light of emerging resistance to antifungal agents. As noted in recent literature, assessment of microbiological culture results in conjunction with clinical presentation can provide insight into the appropriateness of prescribed treatment and the need for potential modality adjustments. Moreover, the dynamics of interactions among the opportunistic pathogens, as uncovered by research on coexistence of *C. albicans* with bacteria like *Streptococcus agalactiae*, underscore the complexity of treatment effectiveness in co-infections (Klimas et al., 2025; Patenaude et al., 2023). Thus, constant monitoring not only enhances the effectiveness of treatment but also enhances the overall management of superficial candidiasis (Figure 4.21).

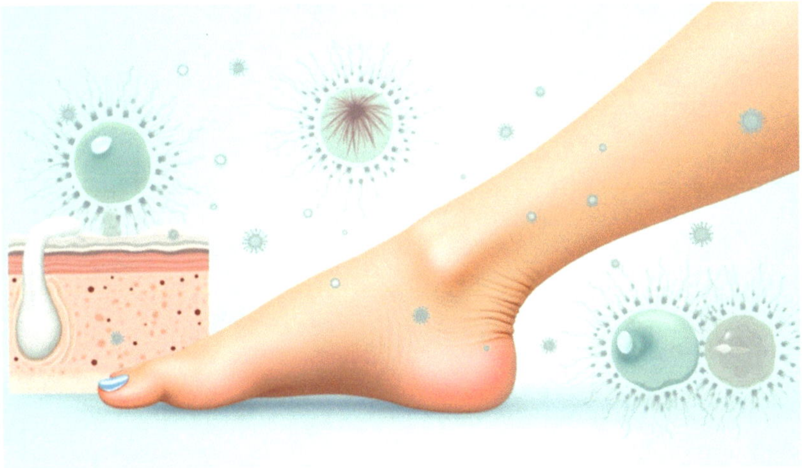

Figure 4.21. Effectively monitoring treatment effectiveness for superficial candidiasis is crucial for optimizing patient outcomes.

Source: https://www.kaya.in/media/mageplaza/blog/post/c/i/ciclopirox-uses-benefits-fungal-infections-guide.jpg.

4.4.8. Addressing Underlying Conditions

The management of superficial candidiasis demands a profound understanding and management of the predisposing conditions responsible for the occurrence of these infections. The factors of immunosuppression, uncontrolled diabetes, and overuse of antibiotics carry significant weight in the promotion of *Candida* growth, suggesting the need for rigorous patient assessments and interventions aimed at minimizing such risk factors. For instance, diabetes patients are not only more susceptible to infection but also experience more severe symptoms when candidiasis does occur because the hyperglycemic environment favors the growth of fungi.(Vikholt et al., 2014) Furthermore, the inappropriate prescription of antibiotics has the ability to disrupt the balance of the normal microbiota, allowing the opportunistic pathogen *Candida* to flourish and thus the importance of appropriate antibiotic stewardship in the clinic. (Alonso-Monge et al., 2013) The treatment of these underlying conditions is very important as it not only eliminates existing infections but also plays a critical role in preventing a return of the infection and generally in enhancing the well-being of the patient.

SUMMARY

The commonality of superficial candidiasis highlights the value of detection of its clinical features and related risk factors, especially in susceptible groups like immunocompromised individuals. The findings in various studies indicate high incidence of oral candidiasis in renal transplant recipients with approximately 60% presenting oral lesions such as candidiasis and leukoplakia, thus demonstrating the immediate need for improved oral hygiene among such patients (Ram et al., 2005). Additionally, the widespread occurrence of candida esophagitis in non-HIV individuals emphasizes the strong correlation of the disease with predisposing conditions of diabetes mellitus and the use of corticosteroids, which necessitates an interdisciplinary treatment and prevention strategy (Abid et al., 2003). Coping with the issues of superficial candidiasis requires ongoing research, effective screening, and patient-specific therapy to mitigate its impact on the victim.

In summary, superficial candidiasis is a critical public health concern, signaled by the ongoing research elucidating its pathophysiology and therapeutic options. One key observation is that IL-17 receptor signaling is instrumental in affording resistance to oropharyngeal candidiasis as shown in studies affirming its integral role in orchestrating immune responses in human and mouse models. Notably, conditional deletion of IL-17RA in oral epithelial cells further increased susceptibility to infection, highlighting the importance of these cells to modulate defense against *Candida* species via antimicrobial peptides like β-defensin 3 (BD3) (Brane et al., 2016). Moreover, the agreement between IL-17-responsive gene expression in human and mouse tissues further validates the translational significance of such findings for optimizing therapeutic strategies (Dereeper et al., 2012). These findings not only enrich our understanding of superficial candidiasis but also set the stage for improved clinical care.

A CLOSER LOOK

LEUKOPLAKIA

Leukoplakia is a clinical term for white plaques or patches that appear on the mucous membranes of the gums, tongue, or mouth and cannot be removed by wiping. Leukoplakia is also a precancerous lesion, meaning that it can become oral cancer, specifically squamous cell carcinoma.

The exact cause of leukoplakia is often debated, but it is strongly associated with chronic irritation, such as caused by tobacco (smoking or chewing), alcohol, ill-fitting dentures, or coarse teeth. The majority of leukoplakia patches are benign, but a few may uncover dysplasia (abnormal growth of cells) on biopsy.

It is diagnosed and proved clinically by biopsy and histopathology. It is managed by the removal of risk factors, monitoring of the lesion periodically, and by surgical excision if dysplasia or cancer features are found.

REFERENCES

1. Abdullah, M. (M.), Atmakusuma, J. (J.), Chen, K. (K.), Syam, A., et al. (2006). Candidiasis in malignancy. https://media.neliti.com/media/publications/65320-EN-candidiasis-in-malignancy.pdf (accessed on 27th June 2025).
2. Abid, S., Hamid, S., Hussainy, A. S., Islam, M., et al. (2003). *Candida* esophagitis: Risk factors in non-HIV population in Pakistan. https://core.ac.uk/download/47259682.pdf (accessed on 27th June 2025).
3. Adaskevich, V. P., Katsina, M. A., & Tsikhanouskaya, I. V. (2014). *Basic Dermatology*. https://core.ac.uk/download/80151520.pdf (accessed on 27th June 2025).
4. Agarwala, S. S., Burgess, J., Cade, J. E., Lynch, M., et al. (2017). Hairy leukoplakia. https://core.ac.uk/download/213072866.pdf (accessed on 27th June 2025).
5. Albertson, D., Baillie, A., Budtz-Jorgensen, E., Chiocchio, F., Fox, R., Goodman, H., et al. (2017). *Candida* species biofilms' antifungal resistance. https://core.ac.uk/download/80557160.pdf (accessed on 27th June 2025).
6. Alonso-Monge, R., Braun, B. R., Csank, C., De Bernardis, F., Diez-Orejas, R., Fonzi, W. A., Hube, B., et al. (2013). *Candida albicans* pathogenicity mechanisms. https://core.ac.uk/download/20327923.pdf (accessed on 27th June 2025).
7. Arastehfar, A., Boekhout, T., Buda De Cesare, G., Butler, G., et al. (2019). Recent trends in molecular diagnostics of yeast infections: From PCR to NGS. https://core.ac.uk/download/286086540.pdf (accessed on 27th June 2025).
8. Arora, M., Kumar, V., Bhatheja, N., Prakash, K., et al. (2022). Fungus disease and its homoeopathic approach using homoeopathic repertories. https://core.ac.uk/download/635338743.pdf (accessed on 27th June 2025).
9. Arzberger, E., Bastos, P. M., Ferreira, J., Leal-Filipe, J., et al. (2020). Reflectance confocal microscopy for the diagnosis of skin infections and infestations. https://core.ac.uk/download/322493878.pdf (accessed on 27th June 2025).
10. Ayodeji, I. O. (2015). Metabolic adaptation of *Candida albicans* biofilms. https://core.ac.uk/download/42953687.pdf (accessed on 27th June 2025).
11. Bassetti, M., Chen, S. C. A., Cornely, O. A., Flörl, L., et al. (2025). Global guideline for the diagnosis and management of candidiasis: An initiative of the ECMM in cooperation with ISHAM and ASM. https://core.ac.uk/download/646830845.pdf (accessed on 27th June 2025).
12. Bossù, M., Di Carlo, G., Giovarruscio, F., Polimeni, A., et al. (2018). Autoimmune diseases and their manifestations on oral cavity: Diagnosis and clinical management. https://core.ac.uk/download/159635803.pdf (accessed on 27th June 2025).
13. Brane, L., Bruno, V. M., Childs, E. E., Coleman, D. C., et al. (2016). IL-17 receptor signaling in oral epithelial cells is critical for protection against oropharyngeal candidiasis. https://core.ac.uk/download/77064960.pdf (accessed on 27th June 2025).
14. Brown, A. J. P., d'Enfert, C., Enjalbert, B., Pietrella, D., et al. (2009). A multifunctional, synthetic *Gaussia princeps* luciferase reporter for live imaging of *Candida albicans* infections. https://core.ac.uk/download/2797164.pdf (accessed on 27th June 2025).

15. Brown, J., Gulmez, D., Kean, R., Ramage, G., et al. (2020). *Candida auris*: A decade of understanding of an enigmatic pathogenic yeast. https://core.ac.uk/download/293868702.pdf (accessed on 27th June 2025).

16. Burges, G. E. (1982). Immunological approaches to the diagnosis of systemic candidiasis. https://core.ac.uk/download/480680001.pdf (accessed on 27th June 2025).

17. Camargo, L. F. A., Colombo, A. L., Ferraz-Neto, B., Zicker, F., et al. (2011). Epidemiology of fungal infections in liver transplant recipients: A six-year study of a large Brazilian liver transplantation center. https://core.ac.uk/download/37709801.pdf (accessed on 27th June 2025).

18. Campisi, G., & Panzarella, V. (2024). Exclusive papers of the editorial board members of *Oral*. https://core.ac.uk/download/621427045.pdf (accessed on 27th June 2025).

19. Carey, B., Hodgson, T., Lambourne, J., Porter, S., et al. (2018). Chronic mucocutaneous candidiasis due to gain-of-function mutation in STAT1. https://core.ac.uk/download/158171133.pdf (accessed on 27th June 2025).

20. Cawson, R. A., Cotter, G., Williams, D., Eyerich, K., Fine, D. H., Hazen, K. C., Hube, B., et al. (2011). Pathogenesis and treatment of oral candidiasis. https://core.ac.uk/download/pdf/8559630.pdf (accessed on 27th June 2025).

21. Choudhary, M., Jandial, R., & Singh, K. (2019). Histomorphology spectrum of fungal infections. https://core.ac.uk/download/539912051.pdf (accessed on 27th June 2025).

22. Contreras, E. M., & Gupta, S. K. (2014). Steroids in pediatric eosinophilic esophagitis. https://core.ac.uk/download/228066172.pdf (accessed on 27th June 2025).

23. Coronado Castellote, L., & Jiménez Soriano, Y. (2013). Clinical and microbiological diagnosis of oral candidiasis. https://core.ac.uk/download/71024308.pdf (accessed on 27th June 2025).

24. Coucke, P., Guillemyn, B., Rodriguez Sánchez, A., Vaneechoutte, M., et al. (2019). Nucleic acids enrichment of fungal pathogens to study host-pathogen interactions. https://core.ac.uk/download/286086547.pdf (accessed on 27th June 2025).

25. Denning, D. W., Hedayati, M. T., Hilmioğlu-Polat, S., Ilkit, M., et al. (2018). Estimated burden of serious human fungal diseases in Turkey. https://core.ac.uk/download/186341631.doc (accessed on 27th June 2025).

26. Dereeper, A., Hartl, A., Hubel, A., Shonhai, A., Walther, A., Yamamoto, A., Sanchez, A. A., et al. (2012). Small but crucial: The novel small heat shock protein Hsp21 mediates stress adaptation and virulence in *Candida albicans*. https://core.ac.uk/download/11303948.pdf (accessed on 27th June 2025).

27. El-Garhy, O. H. (2015). An overview of the azoles of interest. https://core.ac.uk/download/482244134.pdf (accessed on 27th June 2025).

28. Fahmitha, F. H. F., Kaviya, G., Nisha, D., Dhandayuthapani, P., et al. (2024). Global clinical case studies in *Candida* species: A review. https://core.ac.uk/download/621161240.pdf (accessed on 27th June 2025).

29. Fraser, E. W. (1971). Serological studies on twelve species of *Candida*. https://core.ac.uk/download/217400206.pdf (accessed on 27th June 2025).

30. Galea, T. (2013). Epidemiology of mixed vaginitis and its management. https://core.ac.uk/download/46604441.pdf (accessed on 27th June 2025).

31. Govender, N. (2009). HIV-associated opportunistic fungal infections: A guide to using the clinical microbiology laboratory. https://core.ac.uk/download/478383566.pdf (accessed on 27th June 2025).

32. Hare, D. L., Jaarsma, T., Johansson, P., Toukhsati, S. R., et al. (2013). Medical microbiology in dentistry. https://core.ac.uk/download/80150434.pdf (accessed on 27th June 2025).

33. Herrera, D., Alonso, B., de Arriba, L., Santa Cruz, I., Serrano, C., & Sanz, M. (2014). Acute periodontal lesions. *Periodontology 2000, 65*(1), 149–177.

34. Iqbal, S. (2016). A clinical study on the dermatological manifestations of obesity. https://core.ac.uk/download/235662077.pdf (accessed on 27th June 2025).

35. Klimas, F., Pawłowski, B., Potoczek, A., Pudełko, M., et al. (2025). Fungal infections: Epidemiology, clinical challenges, and advances in diagnosis and treatment–A review. https://core.ac.uk/download/646079891.pdf (accessed on 27th June 2025).

36. Kundu, G. (2010). Immunomodulatory effect of host and fungal eicosanoids during host-pathogen interactions with *Candida albicans*. https://core.ac.uk/download/56687157.pdf (accessed on 27th June 2025).

37. Kuriyama, T., Lewis, M. A. O., Malic, S., Silva, A., et al. (2012). *Candida* biofilms and oral candidiasis: Treatment and prevention. https://core.ac.uk/download/55618170.pdf (accessed on 27th June 2025).

38. Kushnirenko, I. (2016). Adhesive properties and sensitivity to antifungal drugs of *Candida albicans*, which are released from patients of gastroenterological profile with candidiasis of the mucosa of the upper part of the digestive tract. https://core.ac.uk/download/322516272.pdf (accessed on 27th June 2025).

39. Lewis, M., & Williams, D. (2017). Diagnosis and management of oral candidiasis. https://core.ac.uk/download/145638202.pdf (accessed on 27th June 2025).

40. Marot, A., & Pihet, M. (2013). Diagnostic biologique des candidoses. https://core.ac.uk/download/52410970.pdf (accessed on 27th June 2025).

41. Mészáros, J., & Zitás, É. (2016). The most common childhood skin diseases. https://core.ac.uk/download/154371673.pdf (accessed on 27th June 2025).

42. Murgui, A., Navarro, D., Cantón, E., López-Ribot, J. L., Martínez, J. P., & Sepúlveda, P. (2010). *Candida albicans* fibrinogen binding mannoprotein: Expression in clinical strains and immunogenicity in patients with candidiasis. https://core.ac.uk/download/159084447.pdf (accessed on 27th June 2025).

43. Patenaude, K. (2023). Interactions between *Streptococcus agalactiae* and *Candida albicans* affect persistence and virulence. https://core.ac.uk/download/604795780.pdf (accessed on 27th June 2025).

44. Patil, N. U., Patil, D., Geetha, S., Shivamurthy, S., et al. (2021). Efficacy of supplementation of probiotics along with antimicrobial agents in vulvovaginal infections in a tertiary care hospital. https://core.ac.uk/download/482238462.pdf (accessed on 27th June 2025).

45. Sáez-Rosón, A., Moragues, M. D., & Sevilla, M. J. (2014). Identification of superficial *Candida albicans* germ tube antigens in a rabbit model of disseminated candidiasis: A proteomic approach. https://core.ac.uk/download/159084627.pdf (accessed on 27th June 2025).

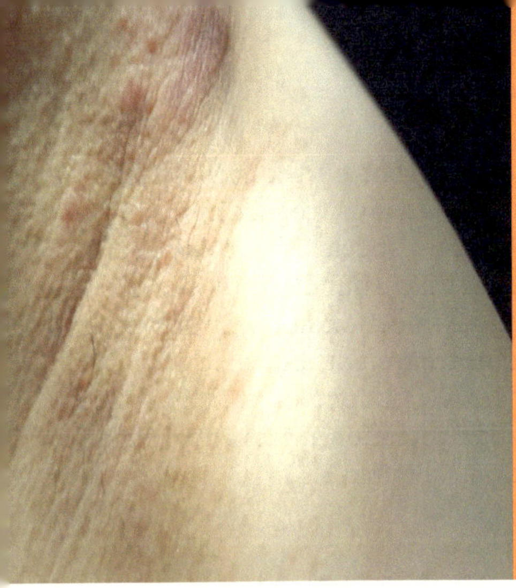

Chapter 5

OTHER CUTANEOUS FUNGAL INFECTIONS

Contents

Introduction

Cutaneous fungal infections have been of great concern in medical and dermatology literature primarily due to their impact on public health. These infections, caused by several fungal species, are capable of infecting individuals from various demographics and statuses of health. While most believe that such infections imply something on the surface and insignificant, the reality is otherwise. Diseases like diabetes, immunosuppression, and chronic disease can worsen the intensity of these infections, turning them into more severe health issues. Among these, certain fungal genera, such as *Fusarium* spp, have been proven to be capable of life-threatening infections primarily in immunocompromised patients, thus it is required that special care and prompt medical intervention be exercised in diagnosis and treatment at the time of diagnosis and management of the various forms of cutaneous fungal infections (Cadden et al., 2014). Further, awareness of cutaneous fungal diseases extends beyond clinical presentation; it encompasses a multitude of etiological factors, which can affect their pathogenesis and prevalence. For instance, patients with chronic autoimmune conditions, such as Systemic Lupus Erythematosus (SLE), are more predisposed to acquiring fungal infections alongside other comorbid diseases such as periodontitis and dental caries.

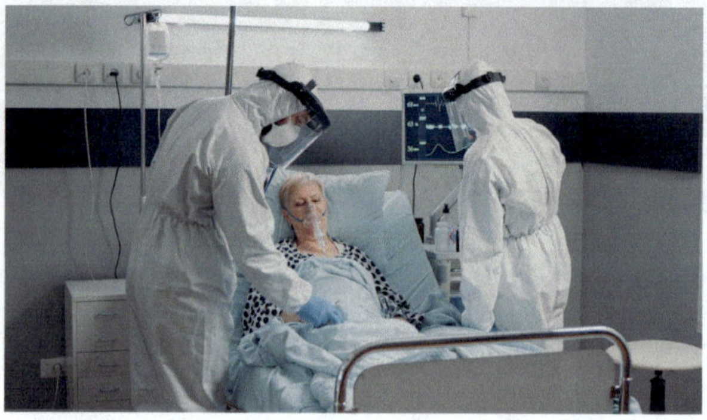

Figure 5.1. Cutaneous fungal infections.

Source: https://biovox.eu/wp-content/uploads/2025/04/Antifungals-scaled.jpg.

The inherently inflammatory nature of SLE itself may predispose to alterations in cutaneous and oral flora, which serve as the nidus for growth of fungi (Brown et al., 2018). As clinicians learn more about these associations, treatment guidelines can be created that are even more effective, addressing not only the infections themselves but also the more systemic ramifications thereof, leading finally to improved patient outcomes. The necessity of a holistic method for the treatment of cutaneous fungal infection highlights the necessity of an interdisciplinary model in health care. It is increasingly expected that practitioners will consider both dermatological and systemic patient information when formulating diagnoses and treatments for such infections because the interaction between dermatological health and systemic illness can significantly affect the success of treatment. Patient education on preventive care and early treatment methods is more important, especially for patients with predisposing risk factors. As research continues to evolve, it is imperative that healthcare providers remain current on the latest trends and treatment guidelines regarding fungal infections so that all aspects of patient health can be addressed. This abundant appreciation of cutaneous fungal infection not only serves to facilitate effective treatment, but also inspires more comprehensive patient care in the face of these prevalent yet often underappreciated medical conditions (Figure 5.1).

5.1. Causes and Risk Factors

Cutaneous fungal infection is due to a variety of causes and risk factors, with environmental causes especially significant. Fungi thrive under warm and moist conditions, and hence such areas as swimming pools, locker rooms, and public showers are hot spots for transmission. Individuals who spend most of their time engaging in activities that expose their skin to humidity or moisture are at higher risk, as the moisture permits the proliferation of fungi. In addition, physical contact with infected individuals or surfaces can transmit pathogenic fungi to susceptible skin. Others, such as the dermatophytes and yeasts, are also more prevalent in warm and humid climates, thus the need to understand about one's environment when preventing diseases. Understanding these risk factors will enable individuals to take precautions, thereby lowering the incidence of these fungal cutaneous infections. Comorbidities are also responsible for increasing the susceptibility to cutaneous fungal infections. A weakened bodys immune system due to diabetes, obesity, and immune deficiency makes it increasingly likely to develop fungal diseases. For instance, individuals with diabetes may experience altered blood flow and skin integrity, which provides a successful environment for fungal growth to colonize. Moreover, individuals who are immunocompromised, such as those undergoing chemotherapy or those with HIV/

AIDS, are also at a greater risk through their compromised immune states, which predispose them to more aggressive forms of fungal infection. It is therefore essential that clinicians and patients have a clear understanding of these predisposing medical conditions.

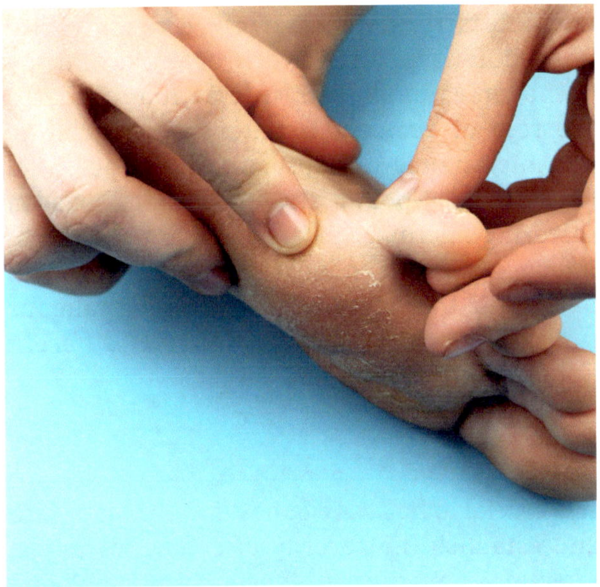

Figure 5.2. Individuals who frequently engage in activities that expose their skin to humidity or wetness are at greater risk, as the moisture facilitates fungal growth.

Source: https://lh5.googleusercontent.com/LdIv2Trp_7qy7JXQ9OknKdfZ9K_WzhXLmnFYLYdvJ_VO9YTPyFpE8KR9BZk9IUEgq1KwsbuToSOmSizvcM7cVXJBmG4uUrQ44Tu8FFAwzmt7oeMbu9pc2Ko-7LyzjidyCFYykWRzXqL-Jq2jl5i4WDQ.

Through treatment of these risk factors, healthcare practitioners can maximize the patients' outcome and develop specific prevention and treatment strategies for fungal infections, particularly those occurring on the skin. Finally, some lifestyle practices and hygiene procedures can decrease or increase the susceptibility to developing cutaneous fungal infections. Poor hygiene, such as not washing well and failure to dry the skin sufficiently after taking a shower, will cause fungi to thrive. Also, tight clothes made from non-porous materials can potentially form a hot, moist microclimate conducive to fungal growth. Risky behavior, such as engaging in athletics or sharing personal care products like towels and razors, also increases the risk. Also, individuals who do not manage pre-existing skin disorders, e.g., eczema or psoriasis, can place themselves at greater risk due to disrupted barriers of the skin. Hence, stressing the right use of personal hygiene and awareness of high-risk situations is essential in preventing other cutaneous fungal infections, providing practical tools for public health interventions as well as for individual educational measures (Figure 5.2).

5.1.1. Environmental Factors

The environmental factors are central to the determination of the incidence and presentation of cutaneous fungal infections. Humidity, temperature, and contact with contaminated surfaces all work together to create a favorable environment for the development of fungi. Increased humidity, particularly, causes maceration of the skin, which can compromise the integrity of the epidermal barrier and facilitate the entry of fungi. Environments like locker rooms and public pools, where there is warm and humid weather, serve as breeding grounds for pathogenic conditions that enable the spread of the disease among individuals. Furthermore, geographical locations with tropical or subtropical climates tend to have high cases of fungal infection, which emphasizes the role of the environment in the disease's etiology. The interplay of such variables and the vulnerability of the skin is crucial in identifying and managing the risk of cutaneous mycoses in various populations. Beyond climatic conditions, individual lifestyle conditions also have a significant role in the development of cutaneous fungal infections. Occupations that require prolonged exposure to damp environments, such as health, agriculture, and outdoor sports, might increase the risk of fungal colonization of the skin. Likewise, both personal hygiene behavior and occlusive clothing use decrease or increase the risk of infection. As an illustration, the use of impermeable or tight clothing, for instance, can keep the skin moist and create a best environment for fungi growth. Additionally, antibiotic exposure lowers microbiome diversity of the cutaneous microbiome, as indicated by recent evidence that hints at the correlation between diversity of the microbiome and healthy skin.

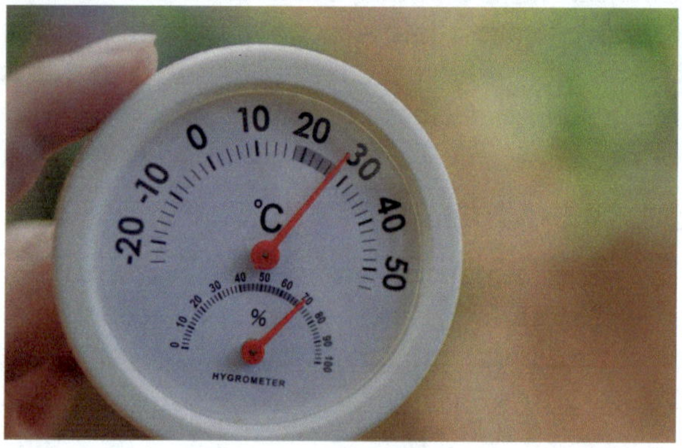

Figure 5.3. Elevated humidity, in particular, contributes to skin maceration, which can compromise the integrity of the epidermal barrier, allowing for easier fungal invasion.

Source: https://geosmatic.com/wp-content/uploads/2023/08/Impact-of-humidity-1080x675.jpg.

By modifying the skin's resident flora, these practices can potentially promote the development of opportunistic fungal pathogens at the expense of the skin's normal flora, eventually leading to the manifestation of cutaneous infections. The delicate balance between environmental factors and the cutaneous microbiome beautifully explains the issues surrounding fungal infections. The skin is a dynamic interface with the external world, teeming with diverse microorganisms that play a crucial role in the preservation of its barrier function. As (Gallo et al., 2019) indicates, harmony in the cutaneous microbiome is vital to ensure that pathogenic organisms do not grow and regulate immune function. Disruptions, often the product of environmental stress, are more likely to render individuals vulnerable to infections. For instance, environmental exposure to some fungal spores can act with resident skin microbiota in a way that could compromise host defenses and allow colonization by pathogenic fungi. This interaction validates the role of ecological contexts in regulating the microbiome and also highlights potential for new therapeutic strategies that focus on restoring microbial diversity to combat fungal infection. Understanding these interactions will be key in treating and preventing cutaneous fungal infections effectively across different populations (Figure 5.3).

5.1.2. Host Factors

It is crucial to be aware of host factors that cause and establish the severity of cutaneous fungal infections in order to effectively prevent and cure them. Host factors are various individual characteristics like genetic susceptibility, immunity competence, and pre-existing diseases. For instance, patients with compromised immune systems such as those suffering from diabetes or HIV/AIDS are susceptible to developing fungal infections. Besides, genetic variability can ascertain the host's ability to mount a successful immune response, influencing the development of infection as well as the inflammation response thereafter. Thus, identification of these host factors can aid in the individualization of prevention and therapy strategies aimed at countering the risk of cutaneous fungal infection. Determinants of environment and lifestyle intersect with host factors in further specifying the risk profile for cutaneous fungal infections. Environmental factors like hot and humid weather could cause a substantial rise in the development of fungi, thereby elevating the risk of infection in vulnerable individuals. Moreover, activities precipitating maceration of skin or the wearing of occlusive footwear can enhance the risk. We notice that in certain geographical points, such as regions within Saudi Arabia, the presence of specific environmental factors interacts with host susceptibility to impact incidence rates of disease prevalence, as reported through heterogeneity of response to various treatment protocols (Acosta-Serrano et al., 2019). Therefore, recognition of these interlinked factors is imperative for the development of effective public health interventions and education campaigns designed to reduce infection rates.

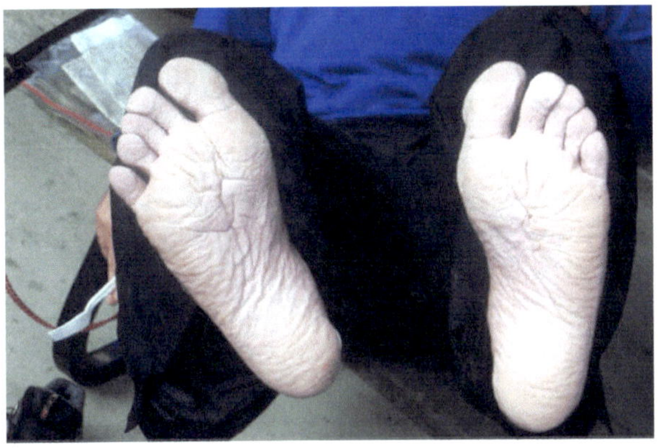

Figure 5.4. Behaviors such as wearing occlusive footwear or engaging in activities that promote skin maceration can exacerbate the risk.

Source: https://www.blister-prevention.com/cdn/shop/files/Macerated_feet.png.

The interplay between host factors and pathogen characteristics is crucial in giving insight into the dynamics of cutaneous fungal infection. For instance, the virulence of different fungal species could be extremely diverse, something that is promoted by host conditions. When certain fungal species are exposed to a susceptible host, particularly one with pre-existing health issues, the infection may be more virulent or immune to conventional treatment. Research indicates that secondary infection may be a key determinant of treatment response, which implies that the host's general state of health plays a key role in clinical outcomes. This is underscored in evidence regarding treatment outcome for specific conditions, substantiating the need for treatment regimens tailored to the individual that address not only host specifics but also the unique properties of the causative fungal agent involved (Brown et al., 2009). An integrative approach in this manner would have a significant impact on patient care and outcome in the treatment of cutaneous fungal infections (Figure 5.4).

5.1.3. Lifestyle Choices

The relationship between lifestyles and the presence of other cutaneous fungal infections is a fascinating area to investigate. Diet, exposures, and personal hygiene all can have a significant influence on an individual's risk for these types of infections. Poor hygiene has a tendency to support a good environment for fungal growth, particularly in hot, moist areas of the body. Additionally, consumption of specific foods can alter an individual's microbiome and could break the balance of skin flora that protects against pathogenic fungi. Further insights into how daily decisions are most likely to affect skin health can contribute to preventative practices and has the potential to facilitate public health results for fungal infections, emphasizing the importance of education concerning lifestyle impact on dermatological disorders. Besides diet and hygiene, other lifestyle practices could include the application of cosmetic products and exercise. Cosmetic products with irritants contained within them will compromise skin barrier function and encourage fungal growth, which implies that people must view their skincare regimes critically. Moreover, habitual physical exercise impacts such functions as sweat production and microcirculation, which can improve or impair the skins defense mechanisms against pathogens. The need for a balanced lifestyle for fitness and care programs is evident because lifestyle decisions help reduce the risk of infection, thereby maintaining skin integrity and overall well-being. Account being taken of such factors is fundamental in giving a solution to the complex problem of cutaneous fungal infections. Lastly, the environmental environment in which individuals work cannot be overlooked when it comes to selecting lifestyle decisions about fungal infection. Urban and rural habitats differ widely because of varied exposures to possible fungal pathogen exposures. For example, where individuals live in humid climatic situations, they potentially expose themselves to mold, and thereby their risk might be increased, suggesting that geographical living options play a major role in fungal pathogen mechanisms. Simultaneously, pet ownership habits, such as managing stray cat populations, also determine the intersection between human and animal health that is again likely to make it even more difficult to detect zoonotic diseases and prevention (Halls et al., 2022). In applying this knowledge in public health policy, it is likely to guide intervention activities that limit fungal infections by bridging an integral understanding of lifestyle and environmental factors with effective interventions in health (Figure 5.5).

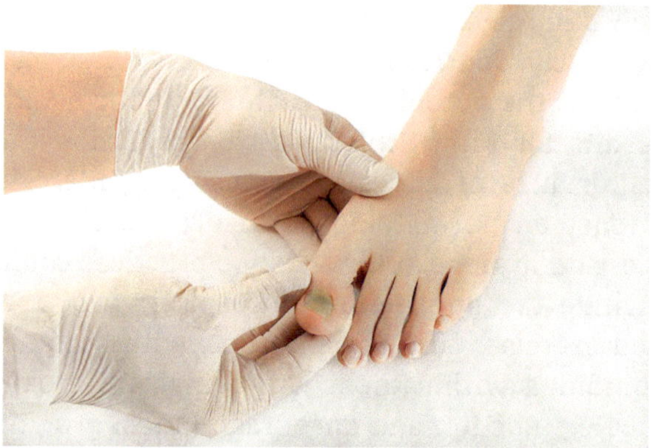

Figure 5.5. Poor hygiene often creates an environment conducive to fungal growth, particularly in warm, moist areas of the body.

Source: https://www.pearlchemistgroup.co.uk/media/magefan_blog/The_Role_of_Hygiene_in_Preventing_Fungal_Infections.jpg.

5.2. Symptoms and Diagnosis

Recognition of cutaneous fungal infection symptoms is highly significant for effective diagnosis and management. Cutaneous fungal infections present in most cases on the skin and are responsible for a variety of clinical presentations that are erythematous, scaly patches, pruritus, or in certain cases, vesicular lesions. Clinical presentation depends largely on the specific fungus involved. For instance, Tinea corporis may be presented with the usual ring-shaped and centrally cleared appearance, whereas candidiasis presents itself as red wet lesions in folds of the body. The identification of such symptom patterns allows clinicians to differentiate between various types of fungal infections and institute the proper corrective measures. Additionally, the visual characteristics of lesions can help clinicians differentiate fungal infections from other skin conditions, thereby increasing diagnostic accuracy and patient outcomes.

Cutaneous fungal infection workup is typically a combination of clinical evaluation and laboratory investigations to corroborate the presence of underlying fungal infections. KOH preparation remains a standard method of detection of fungal elements in skin scrapings, providing a quick and effective means of making a diagnosis. Culture tests are also available to isolate the specific fungal organism so that proper identification and resulting susceptibility testing can be performed. These methods are significant as they rule out misdiagnosis and mistreatment, particularly among patients with atypical presentations or those with compromised immune systems. When dealing with systemic ailments like Systemic Lupus Erythematosus (SLE) in which patients are predisposed to contracting fungal infections, appropriate diagnostic measures are even more important to help guide clinicians to embrace tailor-made treatment strategies that consider the systemic well-being of the patient and associated risks as highlighted in recent literature (King et al., 2017). Outside the realms of clinical and laboratory examination, awareness of the underlying risk factors for fungal infection dictates the process of diagnosis.

History from the patient is essential in identifying those who are at risk, especially the immunosuppressed or those on certain medications for chronic disease. SLE, for example, is a disease characterized by autoimmune response with increased susceptibility to fungal infection, as paraphrased in contemporary research on periodontitis and other oral manifestations (Brown et al., 2018). The association between cutaneous fungal infections and systemic disorders emphasizes the importance of full evaluations with consideration of dermatological presentation and the patient's history. Health practitioners must remain sensitive to the intricate nature of fungal infection, employing an integrated approach that enhances diagnostic capabilities while facilitating enhanced management and treatment for patients suffering with such a condition (Figure 5.6).

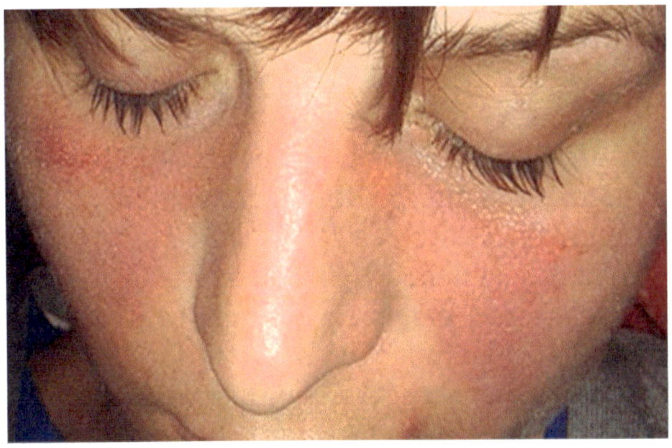

Figure 5.6. Systemic lupus erythematosus (SLE).

Source: https://i0.wp.com/images-prod.healthline.com/hlcmsresource/images/Image-Galleries/Systemic-Lupus/642X361_SLIDE_2_Systemic_Lupus_Erythematosus.jpg?w=1155.

5.2.1. Common Symptoms of Cutaneous Fungal Infections

Cutaneous mycotic infections are characterized by varied symptomatology ranging from local signs and symptoms depending on the etiologic fungus and the host's immune response. Redness, itching, and edema of the skin are frequent signs, which can be accompanied by the appearance of a rash or scaling. Tinea infections, for instance, ringworm, may present as round, raised patches with distinct borders, easily mimicking other dermatoses. Additionally, in the case of candidiasis, the patients usually experience a red rash that is wet, particularly in areas such as the armpits or groin, complicating diagnosis and treatment. These external indicators are crucial for clinicians to use in diagnosing such infections because early detection can avoid further complications arising from such infections. Yet another characteristic feature of cutaneous fungal infections is the development of pustules or vesicles, which may occur as the body reacts to the invading pathogen with inflammation. Such fluid-filled lesions may rupture and become crusted over, leading to secondary bacterial infection that will in turn worsen the initial fungal infection. For example, in athlete's foot, vesicular lesions can occur between the toes, leading to significant pain and risk of infection spread. In addition, chronic fungal infections can result in more long-lasting changes to skin that are more chronic, like hyperkeratosis, where thickened skin impedes movement and function during the day. Detection of early subtle fungal infection signs will enhance patient outcomes and also guide effective therapeutic interventions. Systemic causes are also implicated in the pathogenesis of cutaneous fungal infections and may affect symptomatology. Systemic lupus erythematosus (SLE) enhances susceptibility to oral and cutaneous secondary fungal infections following intrinsic inflammation or immunosuppressive therapy. From a review of the literature, SLE patients generally have increased risks of periodontitis and candidiasis, showing the association between systemic disease and cutaneous disease (Brown et al., 2018). Similarly, patients who receive certain treatments may have compromised skin flora or compromised barriers, which predispose them to infection. Clinicians thus need to pay close attention to patient histories, particularly in immunocompromised patients, and evaluate potential risks so that treatment protocols can be modified accordingly (King et al., 2017) (Figure 5.7).

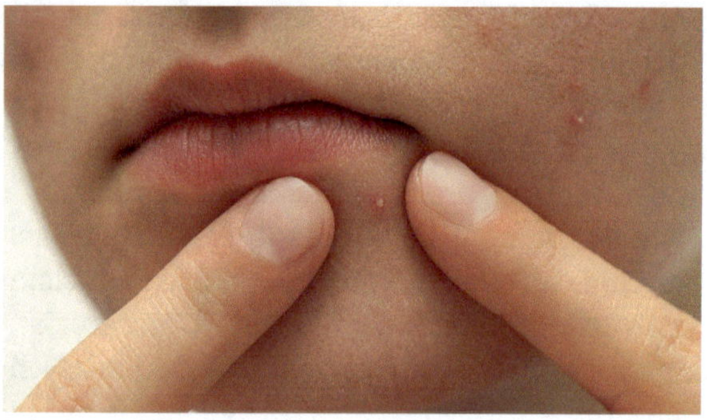

Figure 5.7. Pustules.

Source: https://media.post.rvohealth.io/wp-content/uploads/2024/04/close-up-woman-face-lip-fingers-touching-pimple-acne-1296x728-header.jpg.

5.2.2. Diagnostic Methods

Effective diagnostic methods play a critical role in detecting and treating cutaneous fungal infections due to their diversity of clinical presentations. Traditional procedures such as skin scraping and culture remain simple techniques, allowing for recognition of fungal morphology from infected skin sample directly. These methods, though, require time for the growth of fungi and thus cause delayed diagnosis and treatment. Recent advances in molecular diagnostics, including polymerase chain reaction (PCR) assays, provide rapid and accurate identification of pathogenic fungi with better early detection and intervention. Reflectance confocal microscopy (RCM) is a more sophisticated method for real-time, non-invasive imaging of fungal morphology in the epidermis. Because it offers a real-time diagnosis akin to histopathological inspection, RCM may reduce the reliance on invasive biopsy, making treatment of various cutaneous fungal infections simpler and enabling immediate therapeutic options (Arzberger et al., 2020). Moreover, the diagnostic area is complemented by state-of-the-art technologies that promote accuracy in the clinic. Serological tests and antigen-detecting tests are being researched more and more, particularly for systemic fungal infection with cutaneous involvement. These tests are capable of accelerating the identification of specific fungal pathogens and, as such, ensuring proper management regimes are applied early during the treatment. Imaging techniques, such as high-frequency ultrasound, have also been found to differentiate superficial from invasive infections in localized areas. By integrating such emerging diagnostic technologies, healthcare providers can enhance patient outcomes through etiologic evidence-based decision-making processes guided by precise etiologic intelligence. With such an integrated approach, the utility of adopting diverse diagnostic modalities to effectively address varied complexities with different cutaneous fungal infections comes into prominence (Arzberger et al., 2020). In certain contexts, particularly in immunocompromised individuals or those with severe comorbidities, the threat of invasive fungal infections (IFIs) warrants heightened vigilant diagnostic process. In such cases, diagnosis typically depends on clinical presentation with supporting laboratory evidence. Histological examination of biopsies remains the gold standard for Mucorales pathogens, most commonly implicated in post-traumatic IFIs and posing a serious threat for morbidity and mortality. Early surgical debridement with systemic antifungal therapies is the key to successful management. But to fit the needs of IFIs, changing diagnostic methods have also to change, such as rapid testing and accurate imaging for enabling early detection of invasive infection and prevention of complications such as amputation and prolonged hospitalization (Figure 5.8).

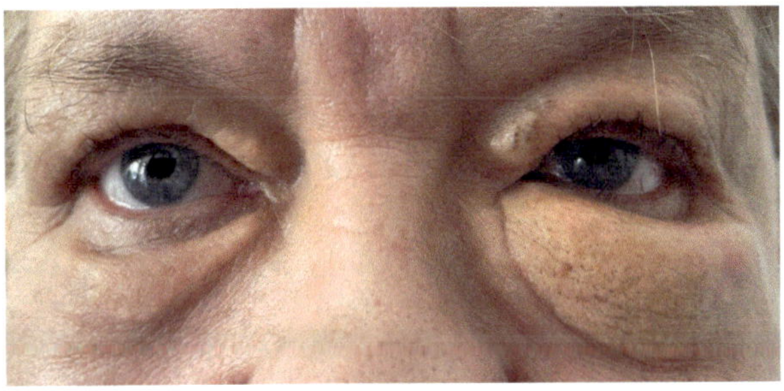

Figure 5.8. Reflectance confocal microscopy (RCM) represents a more progressive method, enabling real-time, non-invasive visualization of fungal elements within the epidermis.

Source: https://pub.mdpi-res.com/jcm/jcm-14-01359/article_deploy/html/images/jcm-14-01359-g001.png?1739882422.

5.2.3. Differential Diagnosis

The skill of differential diagnosis is most crucial in the diagnosis and treatment of cutaneous fungal infections because of their overlapping clinical presentation with a host of other dermatological diseases. Accurate differentiation is only possible through the traditional clinical history, physical examination, and perhaps additional laboratory studies such as skin culture or histopathology. Common fungal infections like tinea corporis and candidiasis typically present as erythematous papular plaques that can mimic other clinical presentations like psoriasis or eczema. Medical practitioners should therefore remain vigilant while differentiating between these conditions on the basis of distinctive features like the presence of scaling or pruritus in order to rule out diagnostic mistakes and the subsequent inappropriate treatment regimens. The subtleties of differential diagnosis highlight the need for a thorough understanding of fungal pathogenicity and morphology in order to facilitate timely, accurate medical intervention for cutaneous-expressed symptoms in patients. Where differential diagnosis is made more complex, such as opportunistic infections in immunocompromised individuals, the risks are extremely high. For example, in infection of the central nervous system, pathogens like *Alternaria* may cause misdiagnosed complications as common pathogens. For example, a rare case of leptomeningitis due to *Alternaria* secondary to cerebral shunt insertion highlights the clinical dilemma of the diagnosis (Chen et al., 2016). Such infections may clinically deteriorate rapidly and therefore must be recognized early and treated.

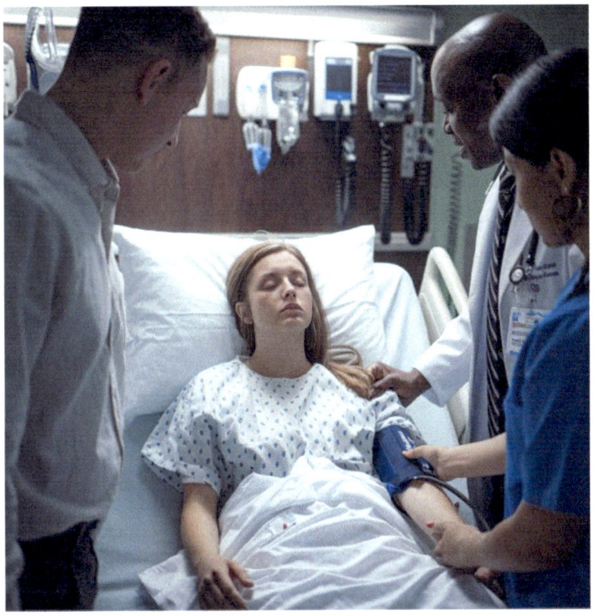

Figure 5.9. Healthcare professionals must remain vigilant in distinguishing these conditions based on distinct features, such as the presence of pruritus or scaling, to avoid misdiagnosis and inappropriate treatment regimens.

Source: https://i0.wp.com/iem-student.org/wp-content/uploads/2024/12/a-photo-of-a-22-year-old-female-patient-with-seizure-the-image-was-produced-by-using-ideogram-2.0.jpeg?fit=656%2C656&ssl=1.

Therefore, precise differentiation not only influences prognoses but also treatment since effective clinical management depends on proper identification of the causal organism involved. Geographical and environmental factors may further obfuscate differential diagnosis of cutaneous mycoses. Certain fungus species have a predilection for specific locations, as seen from the distribution of *Leishmania major* and *L. tropica* in Saudi Arabia endemic areas (Acosta-Serrano et al., 2019). The variability of treatment results across different Leishmania infections also echoes the need for tailored approaches towards diagnosis and treatment. Secondary infection cases may influence the outcome, showing a compounded interaction among environmental, pathogen, and host variables. Given these subtleties, medical practitioners and dermatologists must treat differential diagnosis from a multi-angled viewpoint, involving environmental history and patient demographics in an attempt to optimize clinical practice and patient outcomes under the circumstances of cutaneous fungal infections (Figure 5.9).

5.3. Treatment Options

Treatment options for cutaneous fungal infections are diverse and mostly dependent on the infecting organism, severity of infection, and overall health of the patient. The initial treatment usually includes topical antifungal agents, which are regarded as effective against infection by dermatophytes and yeasts that affects only superficial regions of the body. Clotrimazole, miconazole, and terbinafine are some of the drugs used commonly, which exert their action through interference with the fungal cell membrane and inhibition of cell growth. For dermatophyte infections, treatment is typically successful with topical treatment, leading to successful clearing of the infection in most cases. In situations where the infection is widespread or in an immunocompromised patient, systemic antifungal treatment may be needed, calling for a more global treatment approach for clearing the infection to ensue. For infections caused by more virulent fungi, such as *Fusarium* spp., treatment is typically a combination of pharmacologic and surgical management. Surgical interventions may be needed with the development of an abscess, in which debridement permits better access to the infection and enhanced efficacy of antifungal therapy.

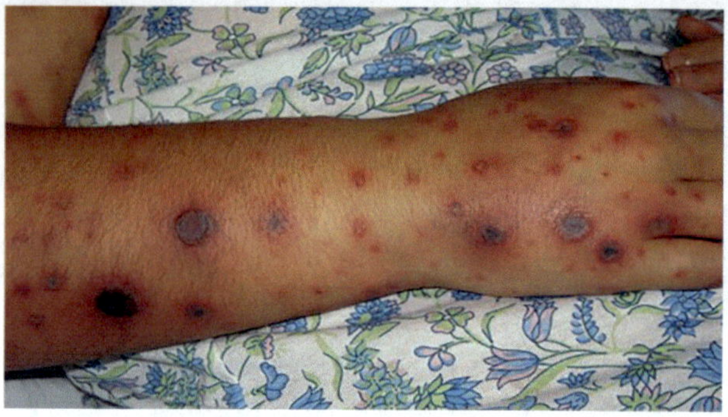

Figure 5.10. *Fusarium* abscess.

Source: https://journals.asm.org/cms/10.1128/cmr.00159-22/asset/4e8b9486-eda0-4978-a254-0d33f1cfd357/assets/images/large/cmr.00159-22.f011.jpg.

Any type of surgical intervention, in turn, will typically need long-term intravenous antifungal therapy to ensure complete eradication of the infection. This is observed in the management of a documented case of an immunocompetent patient with a *Fusarium* abscess, cured by surgical removal and sustained antifungal therapy, showing the potential for recovery despite such complex situations with this particular organism (Cadden et al., 2014). Treatment of invasive fungal infections involves medications like voriconazole, especially in cases caused by *Aspergillus* spp. Due to the extensive morbidity of these infections, early and effective treatment is paramount, particularly in immunocompromised hosts. Voriconazole is employed as first-line treatment due to its broad spectrum of activity against *Aspergillus*.

Yet, clinicians may choose alternative or adjunctive therapy, i.e., polyenes or newer triazole agents or combination therapy with an echinocandin, depending on patient-specific factors, e.g., degree of immunosuppression and drug tolerance (Stewart et al., 2016). The variability of therapeutic options is a reflection of the variability of cutaneous fungal infections and underscores the necessity of individualized therapeutic interventions for optimal patient outcomes (Figure 5.10).

5.3.1. Antifungal Medications

Antifungal medications play a critical role in the management of diverse cutaneous fungal infections, which are predominantly opportunistic and occur in both immunocompetent and immunocompromised individuals. The antifungal medications have diverse modes of action through different mechanisms in fungal cells, disrupting their growth and proliferation. For instance, azoles such as fluconazole and itraconazole act by inhibiting the pathway of sterol synthesis in the fungi and thereby disrupting cell membrane integrity. In addition, systemic drugs such as amphotericin B are particularly vital in treating serious infections, including those due to mucormycosis, a highly virulent type of infection affecting immunocompromised patients (Gopal et al., 2022). Antifungal treatment is frequently dependent on the etiological fungal agent involved and sometimes requires prolonged therapy to avoid inducing resistance. Of all the antifungal agents, amphotericin B stands out in that it possesses a broad-spectrum activity against numerous species of fungi, such as notorious pathogens *Candida* and *Aspergillus*. It is primarily employed in the therapy of severe, systemic infections and exhibits extremely impressive activity against cutaneous lesions that are a feature of invasive fungal infection. Nonetheless, the use of amphotericin B is limited by its harmful side effects, particularly nephrotoxicity and infusion reactions (Anand et al., 2020). Efforts to increase the therapeutic index of amphotericin have guided the formation of new formulations, such as lipid-based and nanoemulsion preparations. These newer agents are designed to maintain the drug's intense antifungal efficacy with no diminishment of its toxicologic effect, thereby optimizing patient outcomes in clinical practice where cutaneous fungal infections are such a formidable challenge.

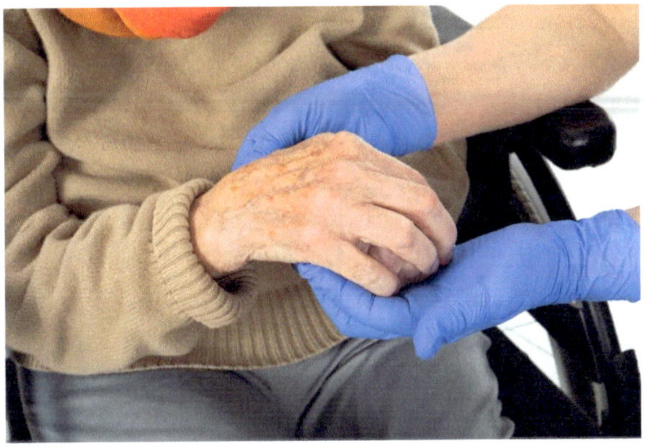

Figure 5.11. Proactive patient education on hygiene practices, the importance of maintaining skin integrity, and awareness of potential sources of infection can significantly mitigate the risk of fungal infections.

Source: https://simplenursing.com/wp-content/uploads/2023/04/iStock-1143268853-1024x683.jpg.

Therapy for cutaneous fungal infection is a multifaceted strategy comprising not just successful antifungal therapy but also adjunctive measures aimed at preventing recurrence and managing risk factors. Preventive patient education about hygiene practices, the importance of maintaining skin integrity, and the recognition of infection sources can prevent fungal infections effectively. Additionally, avoidance of the immunocompromised states caused by diabetes or immunosuppressive treatment remains essential in preventing the onset of infections like mucormycosis. These complex actions, combined with proper use of antifungal agents, form a critical component of effective control of cutaneous fungal infections, thereby improving the overall public health situation. With ongoing development in therapeutic interventions, the future prospects of improving patient outcomes in the management of these infections are quickly emerging (Figure 5.11).

5.3.2. Topical Treatments

Effective cure of cutaneous fungal infections often relies heavily on topical therapy, which has been proved useful in many skin conditions. Terbinafine is perhaps one of the most widely used topical medications, a synthetic allylamine drug with high efficacy against dermatophytes that produce infections such as tinea pedis. Clinical trials demonstrate that only a single week of usage with terbinafine 1% cream can achieve fungal pathogen eradication, and quite frequently, with even superior results than the standard four-week courses of topical azole derivatives. This rapid action is especially useful for patients requiring immediate relief from symptoms and limiting the transmission risk; the concentration gradient generated on the skin surface allows prolonged contact of the drug, allowing optimal utilization. In contrast to the fungicidal action of terbinafine, the majority of topical azoles are predominantly fungistatic in action, which could necessitate longer treatment durations to become effective. This emphasizes the importance of selecting a proper antifungal drug for the infection. Azole drugs are good penetrators of the stratum corneum, but their tendencies to work primarily by inhibiting the growth of the fungus at the cost of directly killing the spores can create issues in the relapsing nature if the treatment is not for sufficient duration. The predicament, therefore, is the combination of treatment efficacy and compliance of patients, making terbinafine a desired option for the majority of patients suffering from infections caused by dermatophytes. They give us an idea of the reasons why topical treatments have remained the norm in treating cutaneous fungal infections. However, although topical treatments like terbinafine are promising for the management of localized fungal infections, they constitute only a portion of the complete picture of addressing fungal infections comprehensively.

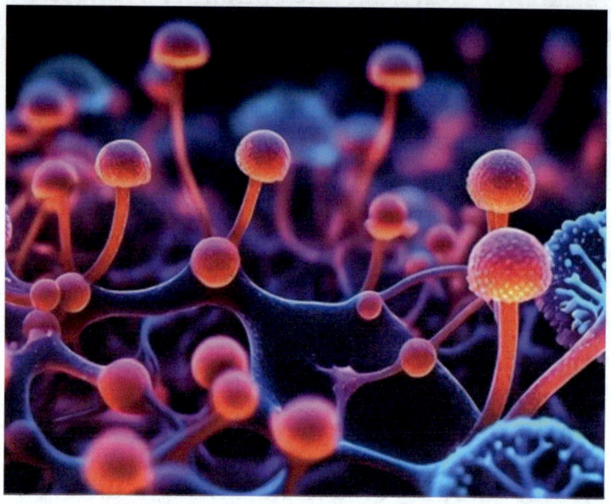

Figure 5.12. Invasive fungal infections (IFIs) have demonstrated that underlying risk factors, such as trauma or compromised immune systems, necessitate careful diagnostic evaluations and tailored treatment regimens.

Source: https://etimg.etb2bimg.com/photo/110147551.cms.

For instance, more critical conditions that require deeper tissue engagement or dissemination at the systemic level would necessitate the employment of more aggressive measures, including systemic antifungals alongside topical formulations. In critical infections, invasive fungal infections (IFIs) have demonstrated that such underlying risk factors as trauma or immunocompromised hosts necessitate comprehensive diagnostic evaluations and tailored treatment regimens. As indicated, post-traumatic IFIs, which are frequently associated with severe injuries, may lead to considerable morbidity and require that treatment must also account for patient-specific aspects (Bochicchio et al., 2017). Therefore, although topical therapy is crucial when managing cutaneous fungal infections, a comprehensive management of the patient must be ensured for optimal health outcomes (Figure 5.12).

5.3.3. Home Remedies and Alternative Therapies

Home therapies and alternative medicines have received a lot of attention in cutaneous fungal infection management, especially considering that they provide inexpensive and readily available alternatives. Most patients suffering from conditions like athletes foot or ringworm resort to such remedies so that they can find relief from the discomfort and minimize the risk of side effects related to standard antifungal drugs. Substances that occur naturally like tea tree oil, garlic, and apple cider vinegar are often listed as having antifungal properties. Not only can these treatments assist in alleviating symptoms, but they may also be used in a more overall health strategy, in that they are less invasive to the body compared to artificial treatment. The integration of these alternative therapies into a treatment regimen is capable of providing an essential complement to the standard path of medical practice, thereby encouraging a more versatile means of treating skin infections. The variety of treatments that is increasing mirrors the significance of learning from disparate therapeutic options in the broader context of fungal infections. It seems that certain plant-based traditional medicines, such as utilized in nations such as Suriname, possess significant antifungal activity. For instance, ethnobotanical studies have looked at the applications of numerous native plants to combat fungal diseases, creating a rich cultural tapestry of alternative medicines used by the indigenous population. These remedies are often steeped in cultural heritage and can be supported by burgeoning phytochemical science that verifies their potential effectiveness against fungi. The exploration of these home remedy and alternative treatments can demonstrate how efficient combinations of new and old therapies present, thereby enhancing overall effectiveness in the treatment of pathogenic fungi-induced diseases like *Candida albicans* (Heredia et al., 2022). Although the application of home remedies and alternative medicine is promising, care should be taken to approach these with a critical perspective, especially when considering whether to introduce them into standard treatment regimens. The efficacy of herbal medicines may be greatly variable, depending on the preparatory methods and patient response. Moreover, excessive dependence on uncontrolled herbal therapy can lead to insufficient control of fungal infections with complications. As would be understood from current work, including in-depth analysis of the antifungal activity of some plants, there is a need to synthesize traditional knowledge with rigorous scientific appraisal. This balance not only governs the safe application of alternative interventions but also allows an environment where integrative healthcare practices can flourish, and ultimately, patient outcomes for the treatment of cutaneous fungal infections are optimized (Figure 5.13).

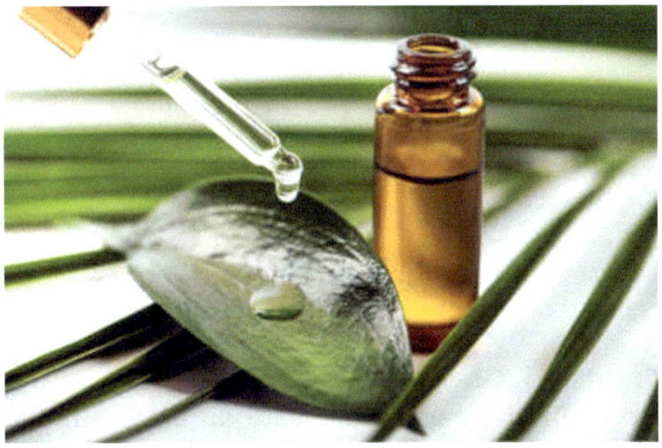

Figure 5.13. Natural substances like tea tree oil, garlic, and apple cider vinegar are often highlighted for their antifungal properties.

Source: https://static.toiimg.com/thumb/msid-114259561,width-400,resizemode-4/114259561.jpg.

5.4. Prevention Strategies

Effective prevention against cutaneous fungal infections is significant in minimizing their frequency and attendant health effects. A central strategy involves imparting knowledge regarding hygiene. Individuals are encouraged to practice clean and dry skin, particularly in areas that tend to become wet, i.e., the groin and feet. Education is especially crucial among high-risk groups, such as athletes and those living in communal living institutions. As per studies, the rate of fungal infections appears to be increasing and thus calls for in-depth awareness campaigns to enlighten members of the general public on risk factors and initial infection signs. Through the promotion of active hygiene measures, such as regular washing and aseptic drying of skin folds, communities can create a protective barrier against these infections, and thus their occurrence and long-term health impacts in both civilian and military populations as documented in recent studies examined in Bochicchio et al., (2017).

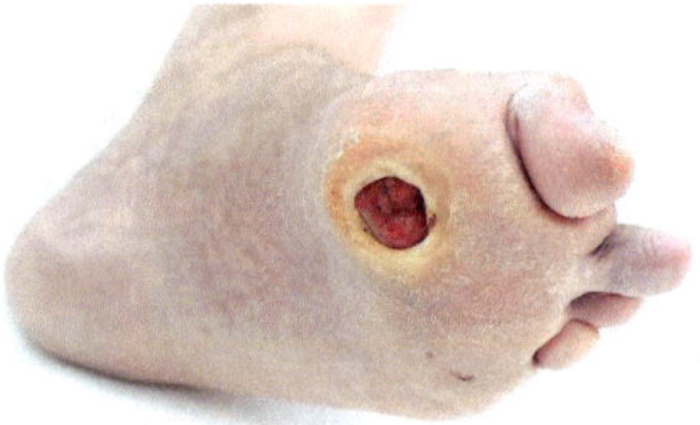

Figure 5.14. Chronic conditions, such as lower limb ulcers, can create an environment conducive to fungal growth, emphasizing the need for healthcare providers to adopt proactive screening practices.

Source: https://assets.technologynetworks.com/production/dynamic/images/content/354250/simplifying-complex-wound-care-with-innovative-medical-technologies-354250-640x360.jpg.

Other than personal hygiene, environmental control is also necessary in the prevention of cutaneous fungal infections. This involves common area management, such as lockers and swimming pools, where spores can survive and multiply. Adding regular cleaning practices in conjunction with antifungal chemicals can reduce transmission risk in these shared areas. Proper ventilation, and the regular disinfection of surfaces, can also limit fungal growth. Public educational programs must focus on highlighting the importance of these environmental factors to reduce risk in communal contact. In cases such as those in the military, where injuries may provide the basis for infections, it is especially important to build a healthier environment, as observed in Bochicchio et al., (2017). Beyond that, timely medical attention cannot be overemphasized in prevention against cutaneous fungal infections. Early diagnosis and treatment of the skin trauma are important in order to prevent secondary infection, which includes fungal infection. Chronic diseases, such as lower limb ulcers, may create the appropriate environment for fungi growth, so it is important that medical professionals use preventive screening. Patients with skin wounds should be provided with thorough examinations to identify risk factors for fungal infection. These procedures can play a vital role in successful treatment. By integrating timely medical care with teaching and environmental interventions, a comprehensive prevention plan for cutaneous fungal infections can be implemented, ultimately improving public health results (Figure 5.14).

5.4.1. Personal Hygiene Practices

Good personal hygiene practices are of prime significance in the prevention of other fungal infections of the skin. Fungal pathogens need to grow within moist, warm, and rich organic environments, and skin hygiene is vital in reducing their transmission. A regular bath, effective drying of folds, and use of antifungal powders will significantly reduce the risk of colonization by fungi. The skin provides the first defense of the body against such infections, and poor hygiene can compromise this barrier to leave lesions such as tinea capitis or tinea corporis. Besides, the correlation between sex, age, and infectious dermatoses prevalence is a pointer to the need for particular hygiene practices, as evidenced by research which revealed the prevalence of such infections being higher in men compared to women (Kalu et al., 2015). Thus, there is a need to promote the practice of personal hygiene in populations with a high level of stringency to help mitigate the risk of cutaneous fungal infection. Within facilities, such as clinics and schools, hygiene is not only an issue of individual conduct but also the cleanliness of the environment. The presence of bacterial and fungal spores on shared surfaces can be blamed for the spread of infections, particularly in high-usage areas. Research has determined that infrequent disinfection practices can lead to increased microbial loads on surfaces, thereby increasing the transmission among users (Kingham et al., 2019). Therefore, stringent hygienic practices in public areas have to be followed to safeguard against cutaneous fungal infection. Proper hygiene through frequent washing with disinfectants and promoting cleanliness on an individual basis among users are part of a successful strategy for maintaining a clean environment. Educational campaigns pointing out the importance of both personal and environmental hygiene have the potential to develop community perception and compliance, ultimately restricting the spread of fungal infections. Moreover, the psychological and social impact of cutaneous fungal infections, exacerbated by personal hygiene, cannot be overlooked. The infections can lead to pain, embarrassment, and social ostracism, particularly among adolescents. As seen in the prevalence of infectious dermatoses among children with various backgrounds, education and sensitization on good hygiene practices are crucial (Kalu et al., 2015). Training programs that involve issues of personal hygiene along with education regarding the impact of fungal infections can allow individuals to adopt preventive habits. Further, having a platform where the topic of hygiene is rendered ubiquitous can help overcome the stigma associated with infection. By integrating robust personal hygiene teaching into community health initiatives, the aggregate prevalence of cutaneous fungal infections can be significantly reduced, emphasizing the often overlooked interaction between health status and hygiene practices (Figure 5.15).

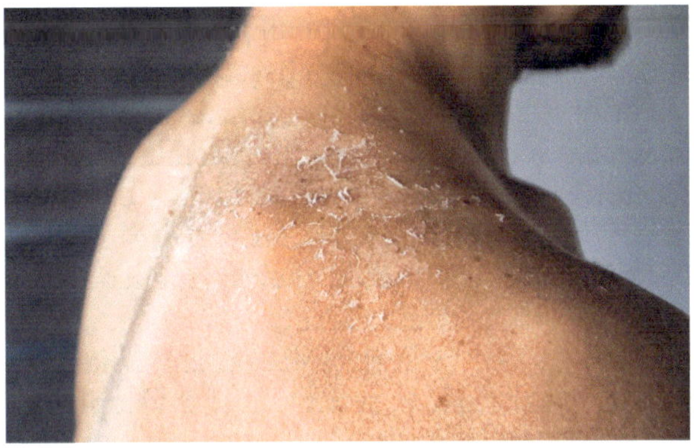

Figure 5.15. Regular bathing, thorough drying of skin folds, and the use of antifungal powders can significantly decrease the risk of fungal colonization.

Source: https://microwinlabs.com/wp-content/uploads/2022/03/Picture1.jpg.

5.4.2. Environmental Control Measures

Efficient measures to control the environment are necessary in minimizing the risk of cutaneous fungal infection, which flourishes under some environmental conditions. Fungi develop well in warm and damp climates, normally due to low hygiene levels.

Therefore, facilities such as the gym, swimming facilities, and communal living spaces must have high cleanliness standards. Regular surface cleaning and disinfection, along with the institution of proper humidity levels, can also reduce fungal load considerably. In addition to this, patient education regarding the importance of personal hygiene, such as drying the skin thoroughly and wearing ventilated clothing, is also essential. As institutions integrate environmental control strategies with promoting personal responsibility, incidence of infections from fungal pathogens can be effectively checked, leading to healthier communities. Environmental-fungal growth interaction is the foundation on which exposure to fungi is prevented proactively, especially where high exposure occurs. Beyond simple hygiene, environmental precautions must address pet ownership as a passive contributing factor to fungal infection spread. As mentioned, pets can serve as carriers for a multitude of zoonotic disease types, such as types of fungal infections like sporotrichosis. Environmental control measures should therefore encompass responsible pet ownership practices. This involves regular veterinary checks and upkeep of pet living spaces to prevent fungal development. Implementation of rigorous sanitation practices at the family level, particularly in settings where pets and humans interact highly, can also help curb threats. Moreover, public awareness campaigns can teach pet owners about the signs of fungal infections in pets and about the necessity of veterinary intervention before onset of transmission. Awareness and prevention can introduce a healthier relationship between pets and their owners, thereby reducing the rate of occurrence of fungal infections. Green environmental design also plays a significant role in reducing the occurrence of cutaneous fungal infections. Planning and design that promote natural light, airflow, and moisture control can render the environment less conducive to fungal growth. For instance, incorporating materials that are resistant to water and planning to provide effective drainage can diminish the waterlogged conditions required for fungal growth. Furthermore, public amenities should be planned with ventilation and cleanliness in consideration, particularly in areas found to be high-risk for acquiring the fungal infection. The integration of green spaces into urban designs not only enhances beauty but also public health in general through the provision of environments less conducive to fungal growth. Thus, an integrated strategy for combining environmental planning and public health interventions can yield significant long-term returns in combating the prevalence of cutaneous fungal disease while addressing both preventive and systemic needs simultaneously (Figure 5.16).

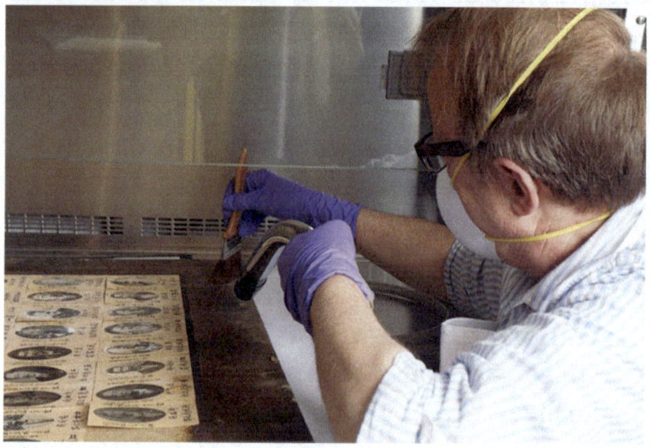

Figure 5.16. Regular cleaning and disinfection of surfaces, as well as the maintenance of appropriate humidity levels, can significantly reduce fungal load.

Source: https://www.canada.ca/content/dam/cci-icc/images/services/conservation-preservation-publications/technical-bulletins/mould-prevention-collection-recovery/figure-15.jpg.

5.4.3. Education and Awareness

Public education about cutaneous fungal infection is crucial for several reasons, including prevention and early intervention. Public health awareness programs can stop the prevalence of infection by educating people about personal hygiene and skin care practices. This is especially the case in high-risk groups, particularly in developing countries, where there is limited access to healthcare facilities and this is related to ignorance. Focused educational efforts can bridge this gap, teaching communities about matters of concern regarding the importance of dry skin and keeping it clean, the wearing of proper shoes, and the treatment of associated conditions that place an individual at risk for infection with fungus. Education is thus a building block for prevention and a way of promoting a culture of health awareness in riskier environments. The role of healthcare professionals in raising awareness and educating the masses cannot be overemphasized. Physicians and dermatologists need to engage themselves in community outreach programs aimed at educating the masses on the symptoms, signs, and risks associated with fungal infections. This may be in the form of workshops, pamphlets, and community health fairs, through which the professionals can pass on evidence-based methods for preventing fungal infections. The significance of creating awareness about the prevalence of such conditions, such as candidemia, particularly in dangerous hospital settings, is crucial, as can be seen from studies that reflect the most common pathogen in such conditions being *C. albicans* (Jain et al., 2021). With collaborative efforts, healthcare systems can better inform patients about risk and prevention strategies, thus leading to better health outcomes. Education in another key area involves removal of myths about cutaneous fungal infections. Misconceptions about the etiology and treatment of such infections have the potential to lead to stigmatization and delayed presentation. For example, some individuals may believe that fungal infection is a result of poor hygiene and therefore fail to access medical care because they do not want to be judged. Such public health interventions therefore need to involve both education and destigmatization to ensure that individuals feel free to access care without fear of social reprimand. Increasing the awareness of how environmental conditions and the health status of a person influence susceptibility to these infections is also important (Amjad et al., 2020). Ultimately, a proper strategy for education and awareness can not only make provision for information but also an improved support network for the victims of fungal infections (Figure 5.17).

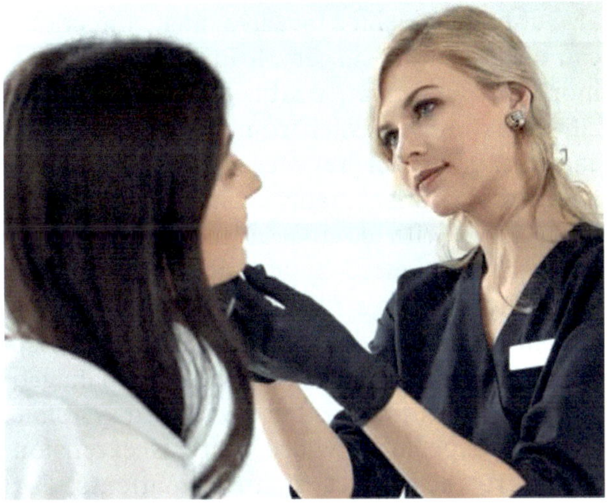

Figure 5.17. Medical practitioners and specialists in dermatology should engage in outreach programs that aim to inform the public about the signs, symptoms, and risks associated with fungal infections.

Source: https://www.healthcert.com/hs-fs/hubfs/2023%20-%20HCE%20course%20page%20refresh%20images/Professional%20Certificate%20of%20General%20Dermatology/PCDTL.webp?width=500&height=400&name=PCDTL.webp.

5.5. Complications and Prognosis

The consequences of skin fungal infections extend beyond immediate symptoms, and even in some instances may lead to severe complications that affect patients quality of life. For instance, such infections' lesions may offer secondary sites for bacterial invasion, which may lead to cellulitis or the formation of abscesses. Additionally, pain and cosmetic effect of extensive fungal infections may lead to psychological distress in terms of anxiety and low self-esteem. In addition, the risk of systemic fungus infections is greatly enhanced in immunocompromised patients with diabetes or HIV. Those admitted to hospital for surgery are also at high risk since invasive fungal infections can develop after surgery, leading to increased morbidity and even death. It is critical that clinicians identify such complications so that early treatment can prevent severe consequences and improve patient management. The prognosis in patients with cutaneous fungal infections is largely influenced by various determinants, including causative fungus, infection severity, and host's health status. A majority of these are self-limiting and can be effectively managed with topical antifungals but some need systemic therapy, especially where there is extension or where they affect high-risk patients. For example, Mucorales infections may lead to invasive fungal disease, which is generally hard to treat and has a very high fatality rate if not treated in time. Indeed, (Bochicchio et al., 2017) points out that patients who are post-trauma may have a greater risk of amputation and other severe sequelae as long-term complications when invasive fungal infections are present. Thus, it is imperative that health care providers develop a strong appreciation of such variables to accurately predict outcomes. There is more evidence to suggest that early diagnosis and management of complications after cutaneous fungal infections will have an impact on patient outcomes. Preventive measures in the form of extensive infection assessments and preemptive antifungal therapy in the high-risk group can reduce morbidity and mortality. There also exists the developing sensitivity that knowledge of potential complications allows intervention to be performed earlier, as noted in Shaw et al., (1985). As a result, an interdisciplinary action by the dermatologists, infectious disease physicians, and primary care practitioners remains the most significant method to deal with the complexities of such infections. Increased research is required to develop evidence-based guidelines to deal with complications and improve the overall prognosis for the infected patients. By means of an expansive comprehension of these dynamics, health systems can better counter the dangers of cutaneous fungal infections and their ensuing complications (Figure 5.18).

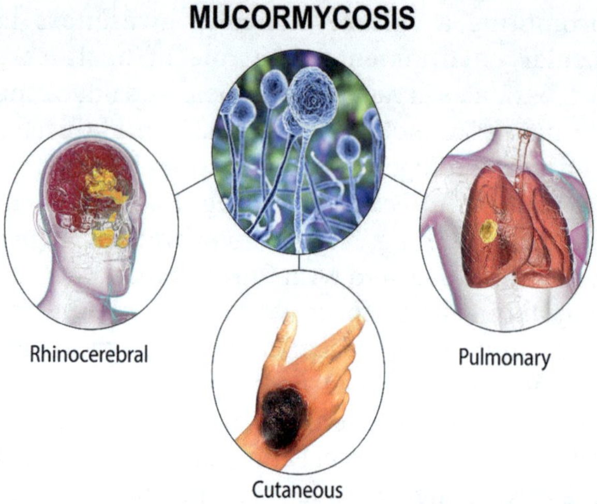

Figure 5.18. Infections linked to Mucorales can lead to invasive fungal disease, which is often challenging to treat and carries a high mortality rate if not addressed promptly and adequately.

Source: https://www.tandfonline.com/cms/asset/bd6651a1-a918-4498-9e22-29ca3990008f/iero_a_2233906_f0001_oc.jpg.

5.5.1. Potential Complications of Untreated Infections

If untreated, cutaneous fungal infections by pathogens like *Candida albicans* can lead to severe complications beyond the surface level. As the infection progresses, it can reach deeper tissues and skin layers and trigger a systemic response. A cutaneous *Candida* infection, for instance, could progress to more severe disease, such as invasive candidiasis, particularly in immunocompromised patients or in the presence of open wounds. The severity of this complication is further indicated by the fact that it is linked to high morbidity and mortality rates, wherein invasive candidiasis causes a staggering 3-23% of severe burn infections with mortality rates ranging from 14 to 70% (Adam et al., 2012). The consequences of an untreated superficial infection can therefore be disastrous and need urgent medical intervention to avoid developing into life-threatening infections. The complexity of complications that develop from untreated infection is enhanced by potential secondary infection. When the skin's protective barrier is compromised, either through the primary fungal infection or trauma, pathogens have the freedom to capitalize on these weaknesses, leading to the complication of cellulitis or sepsis. The synergy of fungal infection with other bacterial pathogens leads to a lethal cycle where it is increasingly more difficult to treat. In particular, biofilm's function in chronic infections makes the therapeutic process cumbersome because it provides a protected niche for microbes, and it is hard for traditional treatments to be effective. Monitoring and creating atypical means to address the multidimensionality of such infections, most importantly among immunocompromised individuals or in postoperative recovery, is therefore imperative. New therapeutic strategies, such as the application of nitric oxide releasing nanoparticles, hold promise for surmounting the obstacle posed by untreated cutaneous fungal infections. The nanoparticles have been proven to possess antifungal activity along with promoting wound healing, in that they reduce the fungal burden and augment immune response modulation (Adam et al., 2012). In addition, technical advancements in sensors of wound exudate that will be able to measure conditions of wounds appropriately are an important development towards managing fungal infection complications. By quantifying the physiological changes in environments within the wounds, for instance, the transformations in urates, medical practitioners will gain insight into the development of infections and adjust treatment in response. In unison, these technologies are paramount to the prevention of potential complications and effective control of cutaneous fungal infections, thus ensuring improved patient outcomes (Figure 5.19).

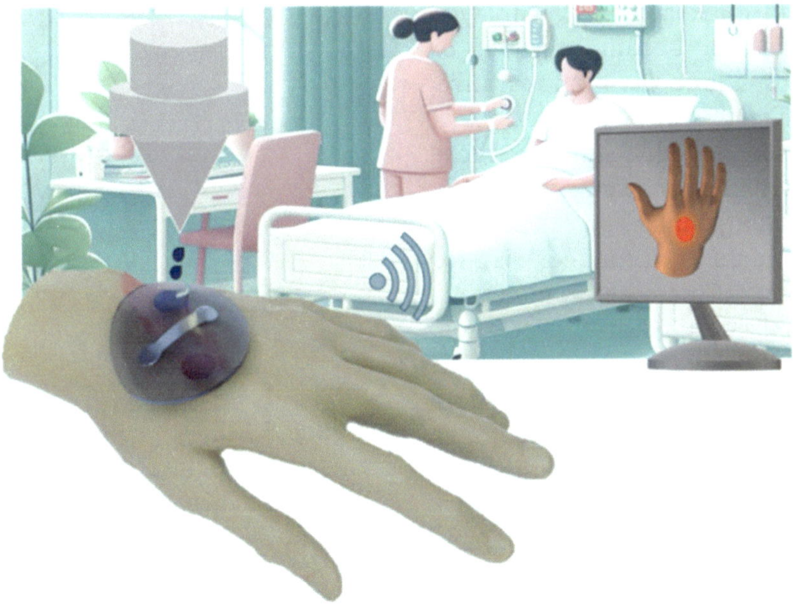

Figure 5.19. By assessing the physiological changes in wound environments, such as urate transformations, medical professionals can gain insights into the infections progression and adapt treatment protocols accordingly.

Source: https://media.springernature.com/m685/springer-static/image/art%3A10.1038%2Fs41528-025-00421-8/MediaObjects/41528_2025_421_Figa_HTML.png.

5.5.2. Long-Term Effects on Skin Health

The long-term effect of cutaneous fungal infections on skin health is complex and multifaceted, as they can lead to recurring skin disease that goes beyond the external manifestations of the infection. For example, infections with fungi such as *Trichophyton rubrum* may lead to various complications like chronic inflammation and hyperpigmentation of the skin even after the initial infection has been cleared successfully.

Patients can develop skin changes that are permanent coloration or texture alterations due to the inflammatory response to infection. Moreover, the psychological impact of visible changes in the skin must not be downplayed because individuals may become nervous or even self-conscious about their appearance, thus affecting their quality of life. In the case of immunocompromised individuals, such as those with chronic underlying conditions, the long-term implication of fungal infection can actually be worse. Such patients are at higher risk for recurrent and severe dermatological infections from their compromised skin barrier protection. A case in point is evidenced through research on *Fusarium* spp infections, where ongoing damage to the integumentary system facilitates conditions that allow secondary infections or complications, such as impaired skin integrity recovery following infection. Extended antifungal therapy and vigilant monitoring thus become essential aspects of patient care that not only ensure the eradication of the current infection but also ensure long-term skin well-being. This necessitates an ever-changing treatment regimen that treats acute and residual impact on dermal well-being. Prophylaxis is also a major component of treating the long-term effect of cutaneous fungal infections. Health education and awareness about proper foot care can prevent diseases like tinea pedis, which is prevalent but diagnosed or treated wrongly or not treated in the first place, as shown through recent literature.

By promoting early diagnosis and appropriate interventions, healthcare providers can ensure the prevention of the occurrence of chronic skin conditions related to fungal infections. Moreover, the application of preventive methods like keeping the skin dry, proper personal hygiene, and antifungal powder or sprays can significantly enhance the strength of the skin. This anticipation is capable of minimizing the risk of recurrent infections and with it, the associated long-term dermatological changes, resulting in improved skin health in the general population as well as in at-risk groups (Cadden et al., 2014) (Figure 5.20).

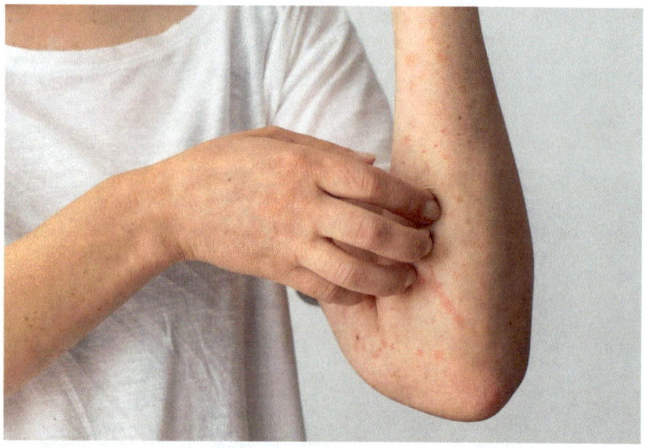

Figure 5.20. By promoting early identification and appropriate interventions, healthcare professionals can help reduce the prevalence of chronic skin issues related to fungal infections.

Source: https://docsmedicalgroup.com/docsurgentcare/wp-content/uploads/sites/2/2023/08/skin-allergy-reaction-persons-arm_23-2149140472-min.jpg.

5.5.3. Prognosis with Timely Treatment

The prognosis of cutaneous fungal infection patients is significantly improved by prompt diagnosis and treatment. Early treatment is essential as most fungal infections can evolve from superficial to more invasive types if left untreated. For instance, the initial onset of superficial dermatophyte or yeast skin lesions may become grave in immunocompromised individuals or those with pre-existing illness. Prompt recognition of such infections generally facilitates more effective pharmacologic therapy, minimizing risk for secondary infection and for illness-related morbidity. Early treatment of the infections by physicians can also yield improved outcomes for patients, illustrating the value of maintaining a high index of suspicion in at-risk groups. Still more so in those whose immune system is weakened, either by HIV infection or immunosuppressive therapies, cannot be overemphasized the need for prompt treatment. Cutaneous presentations in these individuals often serve as important indicators of global health and immune function. A study pointed out that the early detection of cutaneous manifestations among HIV-infected patients may enable early diagnosis and treatment and ultimately improve prognosis considerably. Early treatment can include the prescription of antifungal agents that are specifically targeted against the causative pathogens, thus minimizing the risk of life-threatening systemic infections and optimizing the patient's immune recovery. Such an understanding of early intervention and prognosis is therefore crucial to healthcare practitioners who manage patients with cutaneous fungal infection. Also, the specificity of fungal pathogens necessitates adaptable treatment strategies taking into account the organism at hand and its sensitivity to antifungal agents. In infections like disseminated *Fusarium solani*, where the pathogen is resistant to conventional antifungals, rapid and accurate diagnosis is even more crucial. The timely initiation of targeted therapies has the potential to impact patient outcomes substantially, particularly in such presentations that are neutropenic, where the patient's immune system is significantly weakened. By making sure that the medical profcssionals are adequately skilled to make quick diagnoses and implement appropriate treatment early, the incidence of life-threatening consequences in such frail patients can be decreased to a considerable extent. Thus, a standardized strategy emphasizing early diagnosis and personalized treatment protocols is necessary to improve prognostic outcomes for cutaneous fungal infection patients, ultimately resulting in improved quality of life and survival (Figure 5.21).

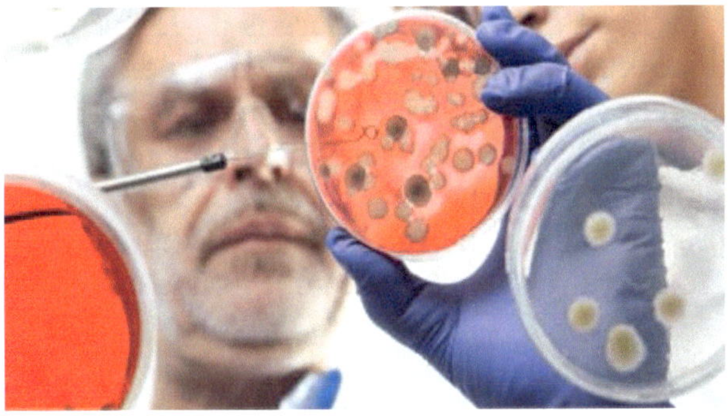

Figure 5.21. The diversity of fungal pathogens necessitates adaptable treatment strategies that take into account the specific organism involved and its susceptibility to antifungal agents.

Source: https://www.ncbi.nlm.nih.gov/books/NBK549988/bin/AAMCol.18Oct.2017.fig04.jpg.

SUMMARY

When discussing exploring the realm of other cutaneous fungal infections, several key points become apparent that do a good job of communicating the seriousness of these diseases. Fungal infections infuse various regions of the skin, and sheer incidence of the conditions attests to the significance of heightened awareness among patients and healthcare professionals alike. Diseases such as tinea pedis, otherwise known as athlete's foot, have widespread influence due to their infectious nature and amplified myths. As seen through the scope for misdiagnosis, this emphasizes the importance of proper education and recognition of polymerization of fungi, with a focus on the importance of timely treatment. Mandatory implementation of the importance of urgent diagnosis ensures the patient receives due treatment to prevent complication, thus expanding overall knowledge about cutaneous mycoses. Recognizing the intricacies of the patient population that is afflicted by cutaneous fungal infections gives insight into specific susceptibility. For instance, systemic disease patients such as those for systemic lupus erythematosus (SLE) patients exhibit an increased predisposition to opportunistic infections, including fungi. According to elaborate research discussions, the immunocompromised condition of SLE patients can result in the exacerbation of oral infections such as angular cheilitis and lichen planus. Furthermore, the chronic inflammation of SLE may predispose to colonization with fungi, loading the oral cavity and skin surfaces with additional complexities. This serves to underscore the importance of clinicians performing a thorough analysis of the medical history and immune status of a patient in evaluating cutaneous fungal infection, and fostering a holistic approach to management of the patient. Consultation on preventive measures as well as treatment regimens constitutes a critical component in the management of cutaneous fungal infections. The massive incidence of tinea pedis, often mistaken for harmless skin conditions, may itself indicate that there is a greater issue of public health education oversight involving the diseases. Prevention would involve educative programs that enumerate risk factors and habits of meticulous foot care and hygiene so that rates of transmission drop. In addition, as implied in the literature, regular examination can prevent fungal skin infection from reaching the advanced stage. Lastly, a combined strategy involving patient education, awareness of systemic condition, and prevention will be required in order to curtail the impact of cutaneous fungal infections among multicultural populations to improve overall health outcomes.

A CLOSER LOOK

SYSTEMIC LUPUS ERYTHEMATOSUS

Systemic lupus erythematosus (SLE) is an autoimmune disorder that has existed for a long time and involves the body's immune system attacking its healthy tissues and organs. It may affect more than one organ system, including the skin, joints, kidneys, heart, lungs, brain, and blood cells. The etiology of SLE is unknown but is presumed to be the result of a combination of genetic, hormonal, and environmental factors. It is more common in women and specifically during the childbearing ages.

The typical symptoms are arthralgia, tiredness, rash on the skin (most prominently the butterfly-shaped rash on the face), fever, and sensitivity to light. Because of heterogeneity of symptoms, diagnosis depends upon a blend of clinical characteristics, laboratory results (such as ANA and anti-dsDNA antibodies), and history of medicine.

SLE cannot be treated, but the symptoms are controlled and flares prevented by the administration of medications like NSAIDs, corticosteroids, antimalarials (hydroxychloroquine), and immunosuppressants. Long-term management depends on close follow-up and lifestyle modifications.

REFERENCES

1. Abdel-Fattah, A., Adámek, M., Agui, J., Atiyeh, B., Ayton, M., Becker, D., Bongaerts, J., et al. (2008). Carbon fiber composites: Integrated electrochemical sensors for wound management. https://core.ac.uk/download/30635566.pdf (accessed on 27th June 2025).
2. Abdolhazadeh, F., & Shakeri Hosseinabad, M. A. (2017). Cutaneous symptoms and rashes in patients with HIV-positive infections (A review article). https://core.ac.uk/download/235570939.pdf (accessed on 27th June 2025).
3. Acosta-Serrano, Á., Al-Salem, W. S., Al-Shahrani, A. M., Alraey, A., et al. (2019). Old World cutaneous leishmaniasis treatment response varies depending on parasite species, geographical location and development of secondary infection. https://core.ac.uk/download/211977505.pdf (accessed on 27th June 2025).
4. Amjad, M., Javed, A., Zahra, G., & Gull, E. (2020). Feet microbial infections. https://core.ac.uk/download/327183357.pdf (accessed on 27th June 2025).
5. Anand, N., Dhawan, R. K., Kaur, L., Kaur, S., et al. (2020). Role of nano emulsion for safe and cost-effective delivery of amphotericin B. https://core.ac.uk/download/482243635.pdf (accessed on 27th June 2025).
6. Arzberger, E., Bastos, P. M., Ferreira, J., Leal-Filipe, J., et al. (2020). Reflectance confocal microscopy for the diagnosis of skin infections and infestations. https://core.ac.uk/download/322493878.pdf (accessed on 27th June 2025).
7. Bansal, M. K., Kumar, M., Kumar, V., Singh, R., et al. (2021). Mucormycosis during second wave of COVID-19 in India: Exploratory analysis from tertiary care center of Uttar Pradesh. https://core.ac.uk/download/586040549.pdf (accessed on 27th June 2025).
8. Bochicchio, G., Bochicchio, K., Kronen, R., Liang, S., et al. (2017). Invasive fungal infections secondary to traumatic injury. https://core.ac.uk/download/129069519.pdf (accessed on 27th June 2025).
9. Brown, A. J. P., d'Enfert, C., Enjalbert, B., Pietrella, D., et al. (2009). A multifunctional, synthetic *Gaussia princeps* luciferase reporter for live imaging of *Candida albicans* infections. https://core.ac.uk/download/2797164.pdf (accessed on 27th June 2025).
10. Brown, B., Simms, M., & Smith, S. C. (2018). Would you recognize lupus? https://core.ac.uk/download/215483268.pdf (accessed on 27th June 2025).
11. Cadden, J., Commins, D., Giannotta, S. L., Lee, K., et al. (2014). Intracranial *Fusarium* fungal abscess in an immunocompetent patient: Case report and review of the literature. https://core.ac.uk/download/323065034.pdf (accessed on 27th June 2025).
12. Calia, C., Capolongo, C., Dalfino, L., Delia, M., et al. (2016). Fusariosis in a patient with acute myeloid leukemia: A case report and review of the literature. https://core.ac.uk/download/54182946.pdf (accessed on 27th June 2025).
13. Chalya, P. L., Gilyoma, J. M., Kidenya, B. R., Mbunda, F., et al. (2012). Experiences with surgical treatment of chronic lower limb ulcers at a tertiary hospital in northwestern Tanzania: A prospective review of 300 cases. https://core.ac.uk/download/pdf/11307793.pdf (accessed on 27th June 2025).

14. Chen, M. Y., Dadwal, S. S., Jandial, R., Tegtmeier, B., et al. (2016). Chronic leptomeninges's and spinal intradural mass secondary to *Alternaria* infection in a patient with ventriculoperitoneal shunt. https://core.ac.uk/download/212868606.pdf (accessed on 27th June 2025).
15. Chomel, B. B. (2014). Emerging and re-emerging zoonoses of dogs and cats. https://core.ac.uk/download/323070120.pdf (accessed on 27th June 2025).
16. Das, S., & Khader, S. (2017). Yin and yang of interleukin-17 in host immunity to infection [version 1; referees: 2 approved]. https://core.ac.uk/download/84911322.pdf (accessed on 27th June 2025).
17. Firinu, D., Serusi, L., Lorrai, M. M., Barca, M. P., Peralta, M., Massidda, O., et al. (2010). Successful treatment of chronic mucocutaneous candidiasis caused by azole-resistant *Candida albicans* with posaconazole. https://core.ac.uk/download/pdf/8500429.pdf (accessed on 27th June 2025).
18. Friedman, A. J., Macherla, C., Sanchez, D. A., Vellozzi, E. M., Nosanchuk, J. D., Martinez, L. R., Martinez, L. R., et al. (2012). Nitric oxide releasing nanoparticles for treatment of *Candida albicans* burn infections. https://core.ac.uk/download/pdf/8737717.pdf (accessed on 27th June 2025).
19. Gall, L. S., & Riely, P. E. (2025). Effect of diet and atmosphere on intestinal and skin flora. *Volume II–Literature Survey.* https://core.ac.uk/download/pdf/85249155.pdf (accessed on 27th June 2025).
20. Gallo, R. L., Irvine, A. D., Kong, H. H., Luger, T., et al. (2019). The microbiome in patients with atopic dermatitis. https://core.ac.uk/download/323064499.pdf (accessed on 27th June 2025).
21. Gopal, M., Parameswaran, S., Pichaivel, M., Samundi, R., et al. (2022). An overview of mucormycosis. https://core.ac.uk/download/542934049.pdf (accessed on 27th June 2025).
22. Halls, V., Kohn, B., Krämer, F., Lappin, M., et al. (2022). Vector-borne and other pathogens of potential relevance disseminated by relocated cats. https://core.ac.uk/download/553570211.pdf (accessed on 27th June 2025).
23. Heredia, D. G. (2022). Tyrosyl production of *Candida* species by plant extracts used for skin treatment remedies. https://core.ac.uk/download/534419841.pdf (accessed on 27th June 2025).
24. Jain, N., Jansone, I., Meisters, J., Obidenova, Y., et al. (2021). Epidemiological characterization of clinical fungal isolates from Pauls Stradins Clinical University Hospital, Latvia: A 4-year surveillance report. https://core.ac.uk/download/487562747.pdf (accessed on 27th June 2025).
25. Kalu, E. I., Nwadike, V. U., Ogbaini-Emovon, E., Ojide, C., et al. (2015). Age and sex prevalence of infectious dermatoses among primary school children in a rural south-eastern Nigerian community. https://core.ac.uk/download/478429205.pdf (accessed on 27th June 2025).
26. King, J., Lehrnbecher, T., Pana, Z. D., Steinbach, W. J., et al. (2017). Recognition and clinical presentation of invasive fungal disease in neonates and children. https://core.ac.uk/download/131024549.pdf (accessed on 27th June 2025).
27. Kingham, M. C. (2019). Monitoring treatment table hygiene in a chiropractic training clinic. https://core.ac.uk/download/323341146.pdf (accessed on 27th June 2025).

28. Korting, H. C., Schäfer-Korting, M., & Schöllmann, C. (2008). Fungicidal activity plus reservoir effect allows short treatment courses with terbinafine in *tinea pedis*. https://core.ac.uk/download/16432245.pdf (accessed on 27th June 2025).

29. Pohly, A. E. (2020). Pathological characterization of natural *Ophidiomyces ophiodiicola* infection in wild-caught Lake Erie water snakes: A standardized approach to documentation of disease. https://core.ac.uk/download/334979870.pdf (accessed on 27th June 2025).

30. Shaw, B. W., Starzl, T. E., & Wood, R. P. (1985). Extrahepatic complications of liver transplantation. https://core.ac.uk/download/12204047.pdf (accessed on 27th June 2025).

31. Sigurgeirsson, B., Paul, C., Dupuy, A., Guberman, D., Korting, H. C., Kerl, H., Hull, P. R., et al. (2004). Chronic dermatomycoses of the foot as risk factors for acute bacterial cellulitis of the leg: A case-control study. https://core.ac.uk/download/16432790.pdf (accessed on 27th June 2025).

32. Stewart, E. R., & Thompson, G. R. (2016). Treatment of primary pulmonary aspergillosis: An assessment of the evidence. https://core.ac.uk/download/323070109.pdf (accessed on 27th June 2025).

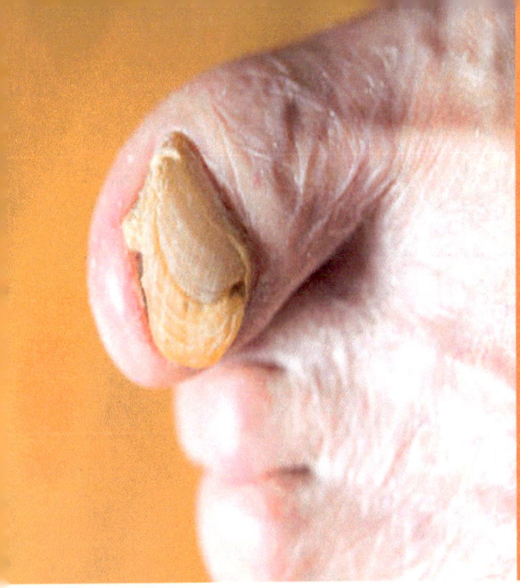

Chapter 6

MOULD INFECTIONS OF NAILS

Contents

Introduction

The prevalence of nail mould infection, particularly onychomycosis, is a significant public health concern that is impacting populations worldwide. Onychomycosis, or fungal infection of the nail bed, has a much higher incidence in toenails than in fingernails. The frequency difference tends to lead to underdiagnosis of cases due to the slow clinical presentation exhibited, particularly for cases of fingernails. With the emergence of various fungi as pathogens, identification of the relevant moulds present and their epidemiological importance becomes a requirement. *Scopulariopsis brevicaulis*, for instance, is one of the most frequently cultured moulds from a nail infection, and familiarity with mould-specific characteristics becomes a prerequisite for effective treatment protocol (Macura et al., 2015). Thus, acceptance of the significance of the same infections is required in order to improve diagnostic performance and patient outcome. Mould nail infections, especially those caused by *Scopulariopsis brevicaulis*, require teamwork in correct diagnoses and treatment. The research indicates that the mould infection is predominantly observed among toenails and can coexist with other fungal agents, making treatment more complicated (Macura et al., 2015). Besides, characteristics of various mould infections can often be alike, calling for both clinical and mycological tests in distinguishing one infection from another.

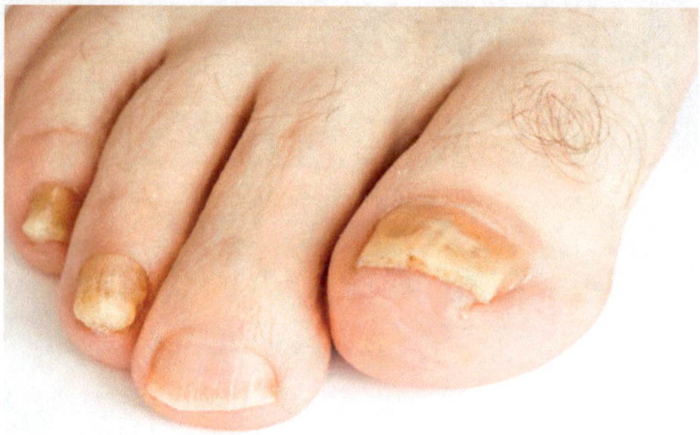

Figure 6.1. Onychomycosis.

Source: https://dermgroup.org/wp-content/uploads/2022/04/Onychomycosis-toes-1200x804.jpg.

Dermatological examination, that is, careful patient history and dermatological examination, plays a crucial role in diagnosing the presentation of appearance such as discoloration, thickening, and nail detachment. Rigorous analysis in the form of culture needs to be done to determine the exact mould responsible for infection and eventually guide proper antifungal treatment. In addition to clinical evaluation, advances in diagnostic methods, such as dermoscopy, have also been found to be helpful in enhancing the diagnosis of onychomycosis. Dermoscopy can detect some specific clinical findings characteristic of certain fungal infections, such as subungual hyperkeratosis and chromonychia, which may assist in distinguishing onychomycosis from other nail diseases. Nevertheless, mycological diagnosis remains the most crucial for the diagnosis because cultural methods have grown to isolate a broad spectrum of fungi that lead to nail infections, from *Trichophyton rubrum* and *Candida* species to *Scopulariopsis brevicaulis*. Hence, a multi-disciplinary approach that brings together clinical expertise and laboratory precision is central to the effective treatment of mould infection of the nails, whereby patients receive the best diagnosis and management available (Figure 6.1).

6.1. Types of Mould Infections

One needs to understand the various types of mould infections in the context of onychomycosis, most importantly as it pertains to nail infection. Some of the most common pathogens are dermatophytes, non-dermatophyte moulds (NDMs), and yeasts. Dermatophytes such as *Trichophyton* species tend to be the most well-known causative organisms in terms of leading to nail infections and account for a significant percentage of cases. However, NDMs have emerged as a similarly noteworthy group, causing around 47.5% of onychomycosis infection, particularly in tropical and subtropical regions where climatic conditions are favorable for their growth (Borah et al., 2018). The clinical relevance of this group is tremendous; different fungi may demonstrate varied sensitivities to antifungal medication, so precise diagnosis and targeted treatment modalities become essential to effectively treat and eradicate the infection. The prevalence of non-dermatophyte moulds is particularly common among certain groups, including workers on farms who would presumably be more vulnerable through occupational contact. The study discussing demographics of nail infection referenced that farmers were the most common group to be affected, with reference to the interaction between environment and sources of infection (Borah et al., 2018). Beyond their origins of cosmetic disruption, these infections can lead to severe complications when not treated. These moulds are often associated with infections that grow in moist environments, and the ability of these moulds to penetrate the tissue of the nail indicates an urgent need for vigilance and preventive measures by susceptible populations. Diagnosis of these infections can come a long way in improving clinical outcomes and the quality of life of affected subjects.

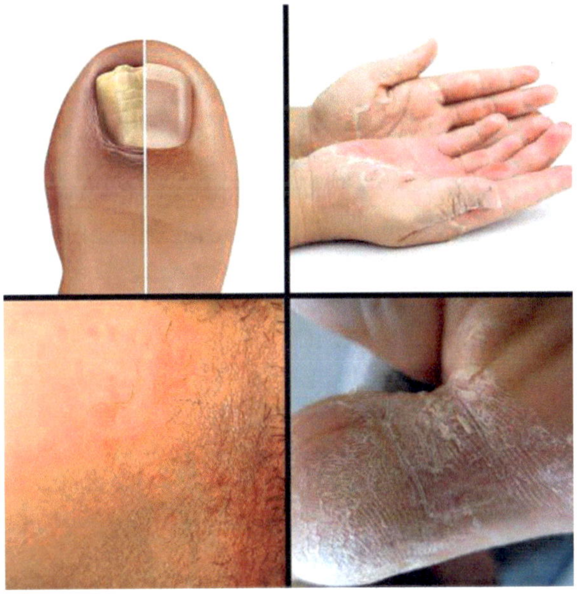

Figure 6.2. Mould infections.

Source: https://www.uniindia.com/cms/gall_content/2024/6/2024_6$largeimg27_Jun_2024_174736557.jpeg.

Yeast forms, another component of mould infections, account for around 33.8% of cases of nail infections. These infections are typical in immunocompromised patients or those with a generalized medical illness, presenting a varied pathophysiologic picture compared to that of dermatophytic infection. The range of yeast infection, like infection by *Candida* species, defines the complexity of nail onychomycosis, which often requires careful clinical evaluation to be differentiated from other fungal infections. Since the research continues to unveil the multifarious etiologic agents, the practitioners have an enhanced ability to use efficient diagnostic methods and interventions. Information regarding the intricacy involved in the diagnosis and management of different types of mould infections is essential, particularly since these infections usually take place concurrently among different patient populations, suggesting the need for comprehensive treatment mechanisms targeting all potential fungal culprits (Figure 6.2).

6.1.1. Dermatophyte Infections

Dermatophyte infection, particularly onychomycosis, is one of the dominant problems of nail disease. It is usually caused by dermatophytes, a group of fungi which are able to survive in keratin-rich environments. Among all forms of onychomycosis, DLSO (distal lateral subungual onychomycosis) is the most frequent clinical presentation, with most cases presenting in toenails. This predilection for the nail matrix is then amplified by risk factors in the guise of trauma and occupational exposure, particularly for workers in agricultural settings. As studies have shown, agricultural workers and agro industry workers are disproportionately affected by these infections, not only lowering quality of life but also compromising labor productivity due to chronic pain and deformity of the nails (Borah et al., 2018). Dermatophyte infections are typically defined by the gender and age distribution of infected persons. A current study indicates a predominance of males, particularly in the 21- to 30-year age group, indicative of the demographic risk factor of these infections. The increasing frequency of dermatophyte onychomycosis demands precise laboratory diagnosis to differentiate such fungal infections from other nail pathology. Application of laboratory techniques such as KOH preparations and fungal cultures remains critical in the identification of the real causative pathogens for onychomycosis. Utilizing correct diagnosis, medical practitioners can apply the best treatment modes using the same, hence preventing conditions such as nail deformation and related pain (Kumar et al., 2018). Correct treatment of dermatophyte infections relies heavily on correct identification and awareness of their epidemiological trends. Case series prove that yeasts and non-dermatophyte moulds also significantly contribute to the onychomycosis spectrum, and thus supporting the role of extensive mycological investigation. Research evidence proves that in certain regions of the world, dermatophytes are not responsible for more than a minority of cases, and thus a broader range of fungal pathogens must be considered in making a diagnosis. Apart from these, the effects of untreated onychomycoses extend beyond direct clinical presentations; long-term infections cause severe psychosocial impairment and socioeconomic burdens. Early screening and treatment, therefore, are required to mitigate the effects of onychomycosis caused by dermatophyte, making it a critical public health concern (Borah et al., 2018) (Figure 6.3).

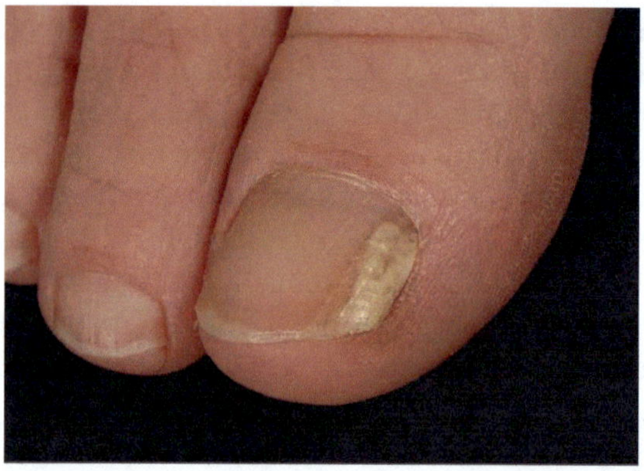

Figure 6.3. Distal lateral subungual onychomycosis (DLSO).

Source: https://www.researchgate.net/profile/Janos-Varga-4/publication/24189865/figure/fig4/AS:668289772552200@1536344106475/Distal-lateral-subungual-onychomycosis-of-the-great-toenail.png.

6.1.2. Non-Dermatophyte Mould Infections

The increasing prevalence of infections by non-dermatophyte moulds highlights the dynamic and complex nature of onychomycosis, a condition primarily distinguished by its fungal causation. Current studies have identified the truth that non-dermatophyte moulds (NDMs) make up a significant majority of cases of onychomycosis, clearly indicating the need for rigorous diagnostic protocols. For instance, under a study in Assam, NDMs have been reported to account for 47.5% of infections, surpassing the traditional dermatophytes at 18.8% (Borah et al., 2018). This shift necessitates the reevaluation of the clinical management of nail infections, particularly among exposed populations, such as farmers and workers, who are continually exposed to environmental fungi. The presence of NDMs makes treatment regimes more complicated, with the emphasis being on causative specific fungal pathogen detection in order to ensure efficacious treatment protocols and avoid chronic nail deformity. In addition to their increased prevalence, non-dermatophyte mould infections also pose special clinical challenges because of their varied pathogenic potential. In contrast to dermatophytes, which are usually limited in their potential for causing infection, NDMs can exhibit a broader range of virulence factors, able potentially to cause more virulent and drug-resistant infections. For example, research conducted in Rajasthan has shown that while *Trichophyton* spp. remains the most frequent cause of onychomycosis, moulds were responsible for 25% of infections, demonstrating a high level of diversity among fungal pathogens (Kumar et al., 2018). This spectrum of moulds can lead to confusion in clinical diagnosis and treatment since most medical professionals get into the habit of treating dermatophyte infections without considering the various profiles and treatment requirements for NDMs. In view of this, early diagnosis and tailored treatment protocols for such infections are paramount in guaranteeing better health outcomes. The management of non-dermatophyte mould infections is also a multidisciplinary approach, considering the socioeconomic determinants which put certain populations at risk for these infections. The agricultural matrix and wet work groups—those exposed more often to trauma, which puts them at risk for fungal penetration—bear higher rates of infection. The same applies to the Assam study, identifying the farmers as a highly impacted group (Borah et al., 2018). Management of conditions underlying these infections extends beyond hospital care; public health initiatives have to be introduced to educate affected populations in prevention and foot care, especially in high-risk occupations. Additionally, inclusion of modern diagnostic tools, such as mycological tests that differentiate between dermatophytes and non-dermatophyte moulds, will enhance accuracy of diagnoses and effectiveness of treatments in such high-risk groups (Figure 6.4).

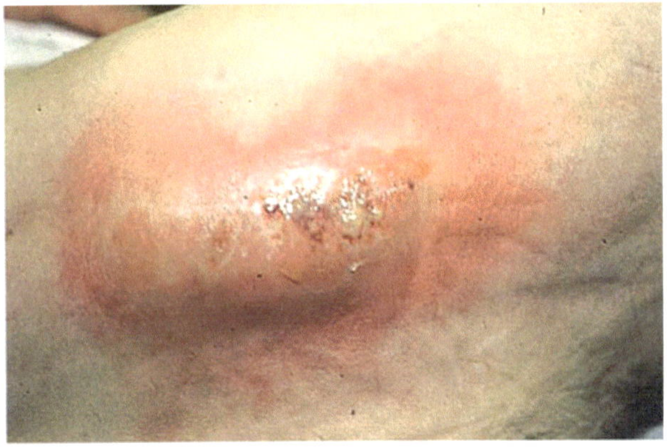

Figure 6.4. The management of non-dermatophyte mould infections also necessitates a multidisciplinary approach, considering the socioeconomic factors that predispose certain groups to these infections.

Source: https://clinicalgate.com/wp-content/uploads/2015/04/image10704.jpeg.

6.1.3. Yeast Infections

Yeast infections are a common but often overlooked form of onychomycosis, particularly as a form of nail infection. The infections, which are due to *Candida* species in the majority of cases, present as a form of nail dystrophy and have various complications like pain and cosmetic concern. Yeast infections of the nails typically manifest in patients with predisposing conditions like immunocompromisation or underlying systemic disorders. Most significantly, the prevalence of yeast infection can be dependent on location, with some groups, like farmers, being more prone due to extensive exposure over long periods to moisture, which is a favorable environment for the growth of yeasts. The ability to identify the type of fungal infection, including yeasts, precisely is relevant in establishing the optimal treatment strategy and preventing further complications, as has been indicated in studies conducted in clinics (Borah et al., 2018). The clinical picture of yeast infection also readily mimics other forms of onychomycosis and hence is more challenging in diagnosis. They present typically with discoloration, thickening, and lifting from the nail bed, either with or without any attendant pain or discomfort. Unlike dermatophyte infections that usually present with a well-delineated pattern, yeast infection presents with a less well-defined and diffuse type, which complicates the diagnosis at an early stage. Studies have demonstrated that among populations affected by onychomycosis, the majority of cases are attributed to moulds and yeasts that are not dermatophytes, thereby complicating treatment protocols further. As highlighted in recent studies, the identification of the causative agent through laboratory tests is important, especially when the clinical presentation differs from that of a common dermatophyte infection (Wilson et al., 1923). Optimal treatment of yeast infections of the nails can best be accomplished through a multidisciplinary strategy involving both topical and systemic therapy. The most common drugs used are antifungal medications such as azoles and polyenes, as reported. The nature of the treatment may change with the extent and severity of infection, along with specific patient conditions. Apart from this, healthcare providers should also consider predisposing factors like diabetes mellitus and immunosuppression, since these could also impact outcomes significantly. Ongoing research still emphasizes the role of tailor-made therapeutic regimes to cure yeast infection effectively, along with the need for carrying out further research to clearly delineate their pathophysiology. This is especially crucial in advancing our information and management of yeast infection in the general context of mould nail infection, so that those infected are cured to their utmost benefit (Borah et al., 2018) (Figure 6.5).

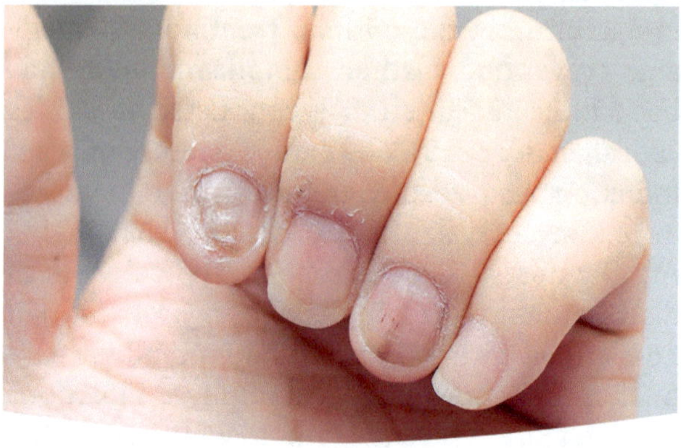

Figure 6.5. Yeast infections represent a significant yet often overlooked category of onychomycosis, particularly in the context of nail infections.

Source: https://www.renaissancederm.com/wp-content/uploads/2023/01/Nail-Problem-Hero-Mobile.jpg.

6.2. Causes and Risk Factors

The aetiology of mould infections of nails, also known as onychomycosis, is multi-factorial, with numerous fungal pathogens involved. Mostly, the infections are caused by dermatophytes, non-dermatophyte moulds, and yeasts. The etiological complexity warrants strong laboratory identification to ascertain the particular causative agent so that appropriate treatment can be initiated. For instance, for diabetic patients, some of the most prevalent pathogens were *Biopolaris hawaiiensis* and *Trichophyton rubrum*, which demonstrate the diversity of fungi that are implicated in onychomycosis. Each pathogen is expected to have different clinical manifestations and implications, highlighting the necessity of accurate diagnosis in order to treat successfully nail infections and avoid potential complications associated with chronic infection (Bii et al., 2012). Risk factors for mould infection of the nails are both intrinsic and extrinsic. Age is one significant risk factor since older persons are more susceptible to such infections due to the natural atrophy of the nails and less effective immune mechanisms.

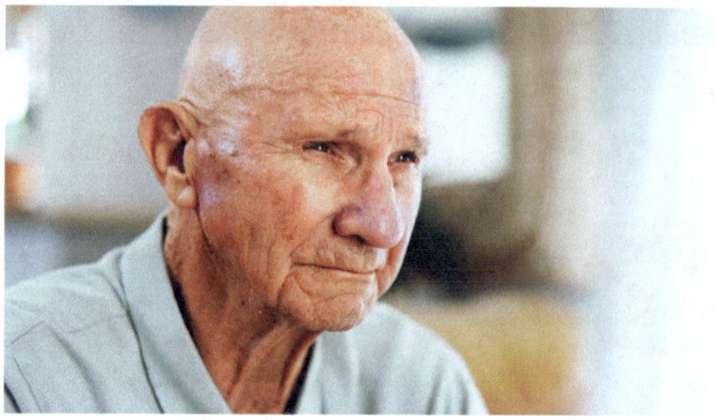

Figure 6.6. Age is a significant risk factor since older adults are more susceptible due to natural nail thinning and reduced immune responses.

Source: https://www.pharmacymagazine.co.uk/images/view/bb106f0043a6b8ae8212f92b228754e5.jpg.

Moreover, employees in some occupations that involve exposure to routine moisture or harsh conditions are at greater risk; an example of such a person is a farmer, who was referenced as an especially high-risk group within an onychomycosis infection study (Borah et al., 2018). Additionally, patients with existing medical conditions such as diabetes are at greater risks as they might have chronic wounds where fungal colonization and infection can thrive. These risk factors necessitate a preventative approach, particularly for high-risk groups. The environment also has a major contributing role to the development of mould infections. Onychomycosis is more prevalent in hot and damp environments, which foster the growth of fungi. In addition, lack of proper foot hygiene and the use of occlusive footwear can be a fungal-promoting environment. Studies have shown that the majority of nail infection occurs in toenails as opposed to fingernails, owing to the moisture inside shoes that is created. In addition, nail injury opens up space for fungi to invade with greater ease, which also raises the chance of infection. With this information on environmental factors, the public will be able to devise the best ways of stopping the occurrence of mould nail infections among at-risk groups (Figure 6.6).

6.2.1. Environmental Factors

Environmental reasons behind mold infections of the nail are multifaceted, with physical and biological components. There's excess humidity, for instance, which creates susceptible environments for fungus to thrive. Warm and wet environments are loved by mold where there is moisture penetration through the nail beds that allows fungi to grow and multiply. This is particularly observed in poorly ventilated and air-circulated environments, e.g., in enclosed footwear, which may create a micro-climate with humid conditions supporting the development of mold. Excess moisture may be induced by various sources such as over-saturation in water during activities such as bathing or swimming and occupation of areas with humid climatic conditions. Combined, these environmental stresses enhance the risk of fungal nail infection, thereby putting maximum emphasis on preventive measures to ensure maximum foot and nail cleanliness. Additionally, the role of malnutrition and its secondary consequence on susceptibility to the environment should not be overlooked. Malnutrition can impair the immune system, rendering the body more vulnerable to infection, even mold infections. According to research, low socio-economic groups often suffer from malnutrition issues since they do not have quality access to food, and this increases susceptibility to infections, including mold infections.

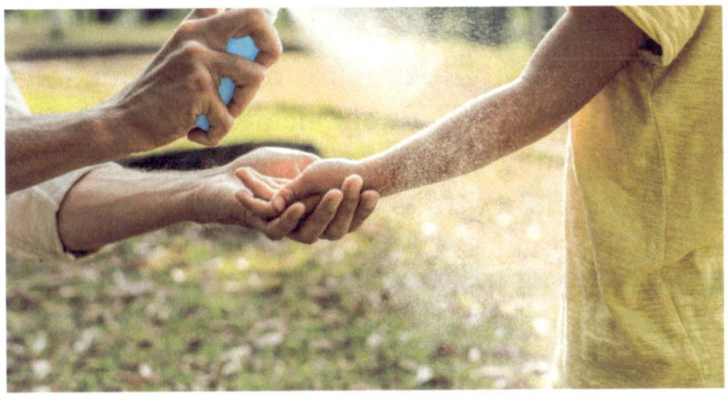

Figure 6.7. Excess moisture can stem from various sources, including prolonged exposure to water during activities such as bathing or swimming, as well as living in regions characterized by humid climatic conditions.

Source: https://www.clinikally.com/cdn/shop/articles/DAILY_BLOG_BANNER_-_IMAGE_vaishnavi_2_b73df256-d31d-4eb6-b328-318def68dfa9.png?v=1688546302.

Children who have ongoing exposure to areas where their nutritional needs are not addressed may exhibit significantly impaired immune response, making them even more susceptible to mold infections. Thus, the regulation of both environmental condition and nutritional value through programs intended to improve exposure to healthy food is important in reducing the incidence of mold infections (Nhlapo et al., 2013). Apart from this, the constructed environment surrounding an individual, for example, the materials used for construction, is also pivotal in supporting the development of mold. For instance, homes constructed from mold-retaining materials or water-damaged homes may have excessive amounts of mold populations that affect the health of occupants. New technologies such as optoelectronic sensors have been developed to monitor real-time mold growth on building materials. The sensors can become important in identifying conditions that favor mold, such as temperature variations and humidity, which have been associated with fungal infections of the nails. Having this knowledge of environmental factors, house owners can implement preventive interventions to combat the growth of mold and thus reduce chances of environmental exposure-related infections (Sauer et al., 2008). Public health interventions to prevent mold and promote awareness among sensitive populations become critical in this context (Figure 6.7).

6.2.2. Personal Hygiene Practices

Maintenance of good personal hygiene practices is crucial in the prevention of mould infections of the nails that can thrive under conditions with excessive moisture and organic loads. Individuals who fail to maintain such simple hygiene practices such as washing their hands regularly, clipping their nails, and drying their hands can unintentionally provide fertile ground for fungi growth. For instance, failure to dry or clean areas prone to accumulating moisture, like between the toes or under fingernails, can create a habitat for fungal colonization. Furthermore, personal hygiene practices like sharing towels or nail clippers without sterilization increase transmission risk of fungal spores. Thus, inculcating the habit of promoting cleanliness will decrease chances of acquiring nail mould infections significantly. Other than hand hygiene, wearing the right footwear is also a crucial step in avoiding mould infections. Footwear that holds moisture, such as synthetic shoes that are not ventilated, is the ideal environment for fungi growth. Wearing footwear made of natural fibers with good ventilation, especially when for long-term use, is advisable. On top of that, socks should be replaced frequently and maintained dry because moist material traps water against the skin. The inclusion of all these habits not only helps an individual feel comfortable but also plays a vital role in preventing fungus infections. Suitable education and understanding of foot hygiene can directly complement individual measures against mould infection to lead to healthier feet and improved overall hygiene. Finally, the role of education in hygiene practice among individuals cannot be overstated, particularly in environments such as in schools or community living where shared spaces intensify exposure to pathogens. Practice training in hygiene practice on a regular basis, for instance, that offered via efforts at increasing food safety in school food practice is critical. These programs typically evaluate the knowledge, attitude, and practice of individuals who are responsible for hygiene, emphasizing regular and effective cleaning practices. It was found that ineffective cleaning techniques in food premises can result in more cases of contamination, which is the main manner in which poor personal hygiene can cause more fungal infections. By promoting proper hygiene education, individuals have a greater opportunity of engaging in practices required to prevent infections, including those pertaining to nail mould. Personal initiative in hygiene not only benefits the personal health of one but also that of the general populace (Nhlapo et al., 2013; Burak et al., 2013) (Figure 6.8).

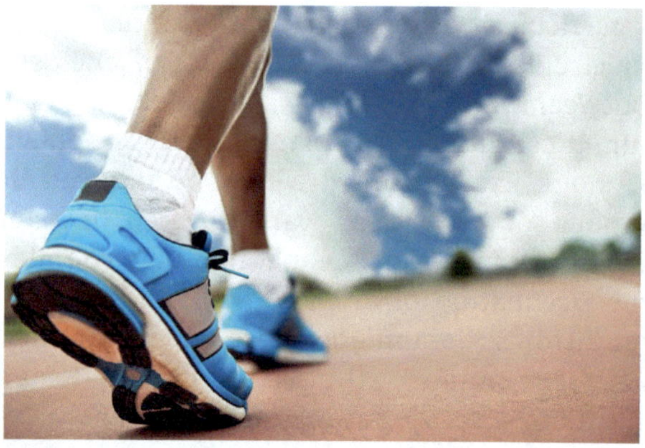

Figure 6.8. Footwear that retains moisture, such as synthetic shoes that lack breathability, creates an environment conducive to fungal growth.

Source: https://feetfirstclinic.com/wp-content/uploads/iStock-508421897.jpg.

6.2.3. Underlying Health Conditions

Underlying medical illnesses are a significant factor in the prevalence and severity of mould infections of the nails, especially among vulnerable populations such as diabetic patients. Studies indicate that onychomycosis infection, a prevalent fungal infection of the nails, is abnormally high among patients with diabetes. This heightened susceptibility could be attributed to factors such as compromised blood flow, immunodeficiency, and neuropathy—factors prevalent among individuals with diabetes. Research indicates that if left untreated, onychomycosis can potentially reveal serious complications in the form of secondary bacterial infection and cellulitis, which further exacerbate the diabetic patient's medical condition (Chitra et al., 2015). It is therefore crucial that these underlying medical conditions are diagnosed at the right time and treated well so that patient outcomes may be enhanced. In addition to diabetes, other predisposing health conditions such as immunosuppression and peripheral vascular disease are likely to cause an enhanced vulnerability to the development of fungal infections of the nails. Individuals with weakened immune systems—after conditions such as HIV/AIDS, chemotherapy for cancer, or organ transplantation—are vulnerable to developing a variety of infections, including fungal infections. Such impaired immune functions limit the ability of the body to completely eliminate fungal pathogens, thereby encouraging the development of infections. Furthermore, peripheral vascular disease can result in reduced blood flow to the extremities, enabling fungal growth and increasing the challenge of treating the infection. Treatment of these concomitant disorders is essential, as this will significantly affect the prognosis and the response to therapy of nail mould infections in infected patients. The emerging role of certain fungal pathogens, particularly in those with co-morbid conditions, has motivated further investigation and surveillance. For instance, *Candida parapsilosis* has been identified as a more common etiology of onychomycosis in diabetic patients. The trend reflects the importance of acquiring the epidemiological characteristics of the fungal etiologies with regard to associated pathology in guiding appropriate therapeutic intervention. Clinicians must remain vigilant, with the fact that non-dermatophytic moulds like *Fusarium* species should not be overlooked upon diagnosis since their presence also indicates more severe underlying conditions (Chitra et al., 2015). Hence, improvement in clinical awareness on how mould infection and overall health are interconnected can enhance preventive activities, early diagnosis, and comprehensive treatment strategies vital to managing such difficult cases (Figure 6.9).

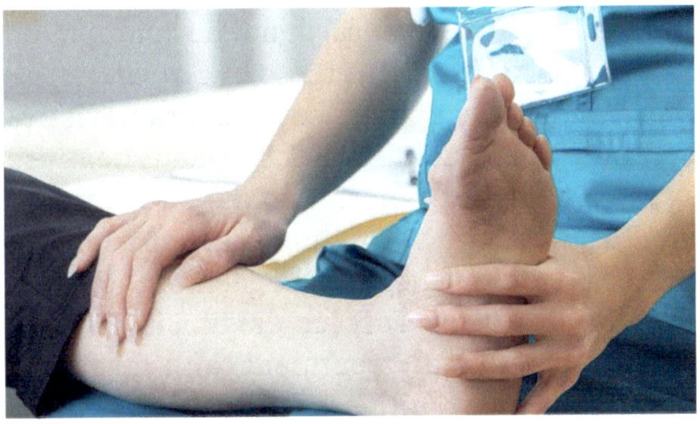

Figure 6.9. Peripheral vascular disease can result in reduced blood flow to extremities, creating an ideal environment for fungal growth and making treatment more challenging.

Source: https://media.post.rvohealth.io/wp-content/uploads/sites/3/2020/02/322182_1100-1100x628.jpg.

6.3. Symptoms and Diagnosis

Mould nail infections, or onychomycosis, typically have a range of symptoms that can significantly impact a person's quality of life. The patients will complain about discoloration of the nails, whether it is yellow, brown, or black, depending on the fungal organism involved. Also being seen are thickening or crumbling of the nail, detachment of the nail from the nail bed, and pain or tenderness in the affected area in more serious cases. Their severity and nature differ exceedingly in their development in individuals, making it important for medical professionals to conduct thorough examinations in order to distinguish among several types of nail infections and other skin conditions. Diagnosis of mould infections begins with a careful clinical assessment, where the medical personnel inquire about the patients' medical histories and investigate the overt signs. Direct microscopy using potassium hydroxide preparations is a fundamental process that allows for a view of fungal structures indicating an infection. For instance, in nondermatophytic mould infections, such as those by *Scopulariopsis brevicaulis*, some diagnostic characteristics become evident. Culture on Sabourauds dextrose agar can further determine the presence of moulds with the result normally presenting characteristic colonies and fungal morphologies. This is crucial as correct diagnosis enables correct antifungal treatment and prevents transmission of the infection to other nails or other individuals. There are approximately 13 reported cases of *S. brevicaulis* onychomycosis diagnosed in Korea, and newly developing cases in older and younger patients, the necessity to diagnose varied presentations of nail infection and to recognize them becomes increasingly necessary. Clinical presentation, predominantly distal and lateral subungual onychomycosis, has been found to be widespread, particularly in men, and indicated by statistics in which the average age of the patients was 46.1 years. This awareness of demographic trends and clinical presentation enables health care professionals to appropriately diagnose and treat mould infections. Early treatment not only alleviates patient distress but also prevents chronic infection, which is why accurate diagnosis and treatment protocols remain important in the management of onychomycosis (Pietro et al., 2014; Arrese et al., 2012) (Figure 6.10).

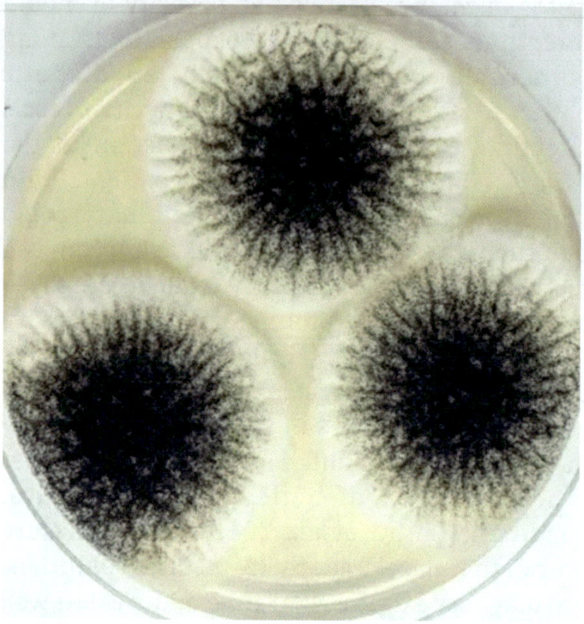

Figure 6.10. Culture tests on Sabourauds dextrose agar can further confirm the presence of moulds, with findings often revealing characteristic colonies and fungal structures.

Source: https://biologynotesonline.com/wp-content/uploads/2024/05/image-275.png.

6.3.1. Common Symptoms of Nail Infections

Nail infections, particularly mould-caused infections, are caused through a variety of extremely frequent symptoms that can have a serious impact on an individual's health and way of life. The initial and most frequent symptom of infection is the colour change of the nails, typically yellow, green, or black in colour, based on the infecting pathogen. Such a discoloration is often accompanied by thickening or crumbling of the nail, which can lead to a roughened texture that is unappealing as well as painful. In severe infection, the nail plate may eventually dislodge from the nail bed, a phenomenon known as onycholysis. These symptoms not only disturb the beauty of one's nails but also make them painful and, in some cases, lead to secondary infections, further worsening the condition. Early detection of these symptoms is necessary for effective treatment and to prevent the spread of infection to the surrounding nails and tissue. Red and painful nail area are typical symptoms that are observed with nail infections. The patients may develop redness and swelling as the body's response to the fungal infection. The inflammation will be very painful and will prevent the patient from engaging in daily functioning as well as lower the quality of life. Further, infections can progress at times, and it is not uncommon for them to become more systemic in character, e.g., fever in advanced cases of disseminated fungal infection, such as those reported in clinical studies on *Fusarium* spp. infections (Arendrup et al., 2004). These extreme reactions only serve to emphasize the need for early medical treatment. Discomfort associated with infected nails can cause those who have them to attempt relief through over-the-counter medication or home treatments, although the latter rarely bring permanent relief and only serve to temporarily mask the condition. Additionally, the presence of an offensive odor from the infected nail area could be a sign of underlying mould infection. The odor would usually be caused by the breakdown of materials by the fungal organism that leads to volatiles and other decay-related compounds. Odors are socially stigmatizing and cause anxiety and avoidant behavior on the part of those who are affected such that they become reluctant participants in social interaction. Recognition of the full spectrum of symptoms is important as they emphasize the need for early evaluation and treatment by medical professionals. Therapeutic interventions for nail infections can vary, but the result is always the same: removal of the infection and healthy nails. Effective control almost prevents the risk of recurrence and completely eliminates the pain and medical repercussions of such infections. Identification of the common symptoms, thus, is an essential step in the treatment and restoration to full health (Pietro et al., 2014) (Figure 6.11).

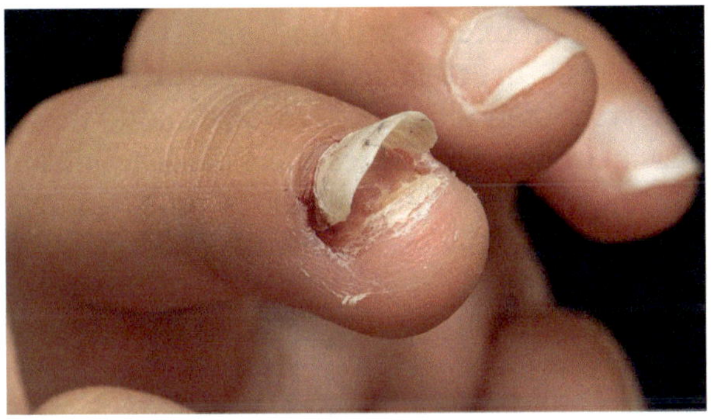

Figure 6.11. Nail infections, particularly those caused by mould, manifest through a variety of common symptoms that can significantly impact an individual's health and quality of life.

Source: https://www.healthdigest.com/img/gallery/nail-fungus-causes-symptoms-treatments-and-prevention/types-of-nail-fungus-1678451661.jpg.

6.3.2. Diagnostic Methods Used by Healthcare Professionals

Diagnostic methods of onychomycosis or fungal infections of the nails utilize a combination of clinical and laboratory methods to diagnose infection by fungal pathogens. Preliminary checks typically involve keen observation of the affected nail, where medical professionals check for visible symptoms such as color alterations, thickening, and brittleness. Clinical inspection forms a crucial platform for diagnosis. Although, sole reliance on visual inspection can lead to misdiagnosis because the same symptoms are caused by non-fungal etiology. Hence, dermatologists emphasize the need for confirmation of clinical findings by mycological laboratory techniques, i.e., microscopy and fungal culture, in order to make accurate diagnoses and modify treatment accordingly, particularly before initiating systemic antifungal treatments (Arabatzis et al., 2019). One of the laboratory techniques used is direct microscopy, which is still a fundamental tool to use for the diagnosis of nail infections. Direct microscopy helps the clinician to quickly establish the existence of fungal components within nail clippings or scrapings. Direct microscopy results are an important step towards decision-making in the treatment approach since the establishment of the fungal genus or species can really matter in treatment outcome. While this older method has been found to be effective, newer molecular diagnostics are becoming increasingly popular.

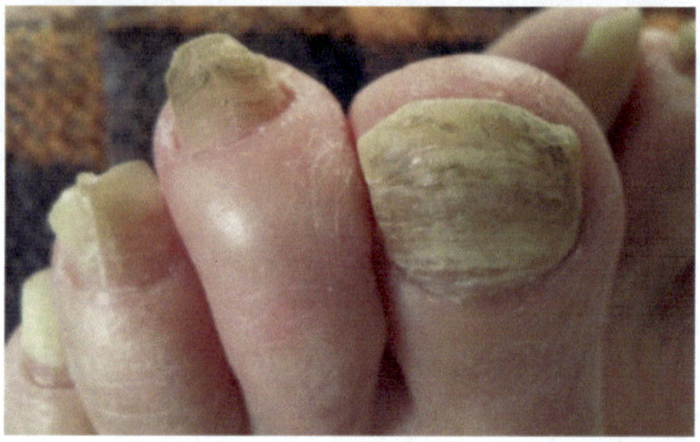

Figure 6.12. As treatment progresses, dermatologists often utilize a combination of clinical assessments and laboratory tests to evaluate the viability of the infecting fungus.

Source: https://ars.els-cdn.com/content/image/3-s2.0-B9780128196403000036-u03-20-9780128196403.jpg.

The new techniques, though not yet standard, have proven to be more sensitive and specific to most fungal pathogens (Arabatzis et al., 2019). With both of these tools utilized simultaneously, clinicians are able to more completely study onychomycosis, which results in more specific treatments. In addition, the importance of correct diagnosis is not confined to the primary treatment; it plays a central role in monitoring therapy effectiveness. Throughout the process of treatment, dermatologists have a tendency to employ a combination of clinical inspection and lab results to evaluate the viability of the infecting fungus. The clinical practice habits of these diagnostic methods in clinical settings can also vary significantly among health professionals, subject to the customary practices of the area and availability of resources (Arabatzis et al., 2019). Furthermore, adherence to hygiene practices, as highlighted in healthcare facility research, could influence diagnostic outcomes and patient safety indirectly. Rendering a hygienic environment reduces the risk of contamination and misinterpretation of test results, emphasizing the imperative necessity for rigorous hygienic practices in medical centers while diagnosing mould infections of nails (Figure 6.12).

6.3.3. Importance of Early Diagnosis

Early detection of nail mould infections is crucial for effective treatment and curbing disease transmission. In dermatophyte infections, the lag in identification has a tendency to aggravate symptoms and help spread infection to adjacent areas, as well as to other individuals. Early diagnosis allows for the use of appropriate antifungal therapy, which can enormously improve the physical condition as well as the psychosocial well-being of patients with these annoying illnesses. Recognition by healthcare professionals of the sophistication of onychomycosis infection, i.e., species identification and presentation, results in better diagnostic practice. There exists an urgent need to learn about causative organisms such as *Epidermophyton* and *Trichophyton* species to guide treatment regimens that are most appropriate for patients (Wilson et al., 1923). Furthermore, timely diagnosis is best for individual health but also in the public health interest. Mould infections may have a wide-ranging economic impact because of higher healthcare costs from longer or failed treatments and lost productivity from individuals missing work due to being infected. Having the knowledge to quickly detect and treat these infections can lower the economic burden on patients and health care facilities. Additionally, early diagnosis minimizes the risk of outbreaks in groups of individuals, where the spread of nail infection can be particularly rampant. As highlighted in some of the clinical findings, e.g., from the cases where respective fungi were isolated from patients, early diagnosis is paramount in establishing an integrative spread prevention management plan and maintaining public health (Pietro et al., 2014). Finally, the importance of early detection in infections of nails by mold cannot be overstressed. Not only does it speed up the healing process of the patient but it is also involved in minimizing potential complications and enhances disease control at the community level. Doctors should remain vigilant in detecting the signs and symptoms of these infections and using advanced diagnostic tools whenever indicated. The inclusion of education and regular screening in primary care settings can also consolidate early identification programs further, leading to improved patient outcomes. Overall, creating a culture that prioritizes early diagnosis is crucial in the fight against nail mould infection effects, eventually creating healthier populations (Wilson et al., 1923) (Figure 6.13).

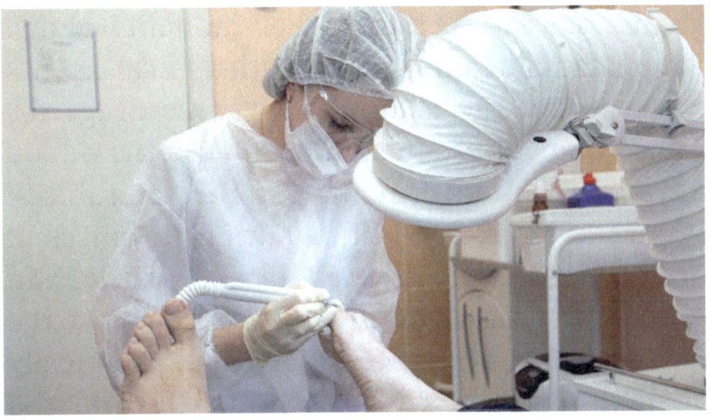

Figure 6.13. Awareness among healthcare professionals regarding the nuances of nail mould infections, including species identification and clinical manifestations, contributes to better diagnostic practices.

Source: https://www.healthdigest.com/img/gallery/nail-fungus-causes-symptoms-treatments-and-prevention/prevalence-of-nail-fungus-1678451661.jpg.

6.4. Treatment Options

Treatment modalities of mould infections of nails are mostly topical and systemic antifungals with each having efficacy and method of administration. Topical antifungal agents such as clotrimazole and terbinafine are commonly prescribed in mild to moderate infections, where the infection is localized to the outer layers of the nail. These agents inhibit the growth of fungi and thereby cure symptoms and preserve nail health. Where topical treatment is not effective or the infection is generalized, systemic antifungal agents like itraconazole or terbinafine are indicated. These agents penetrate deeper into the nail matrix, providing a greater degree of protection against deep penetration infections. The choice between topical and systemic therapy should always be preceded by factors like the severity of the infection, the patient's general health status, and drug-drug interaction, thus requiring individualized treatment. In more recent studies, essential oils have been proven to be potential new alternative treatments for mould infections based on efficacy and safety.

Lavender essential oil, for instance, has been reported to display antifungal activity in research, which hints at its application as an adjunct or alternative treatment to conventional antifungal medications. In laboratory testing, lavender essential oil displayed a significant minimum inhibitory concentration (MIC) against dermatophytes, which suggests that it is effective against mould infections of the nails. Moreover, this oil could prove to be an efficient immunotherapy for patients with compromised immunity or those with chronic diseases because it presents less toxic natural therapy compared to traditional medicine. Incorporation of natural products like lavender oil in the treatment regimens could not only improve patient prognosis but also present a more integrative method to combat nail infection with reduced toxicity (AL-Hattab et al., 2015). Despite the conventional and alternative treatment options having different ways of treating mould-related nail infection, a universal management plan must include both preventive care and proper hygiene. Preventive care and hygiene are part of the recurring infection management, and the patient is ought to be educated on practices such as nail dryness as well as frequent nail clipping. The individual must also be advised on avoiding areas that are likely to become infected, such as damp public places. Preventive measures are particularly relevant in those at higher risk, e.g., those with previous dermatophytic infection or immunosuppressed individuals. On the whole, an integrated approach that includes effective treatment techniques such as systemic antifungals and innovations such as lavender essential oil along with preventive strategies can significantly enhance the management of mould nail infections (Fang et al., 2017) (Figure 6.14).

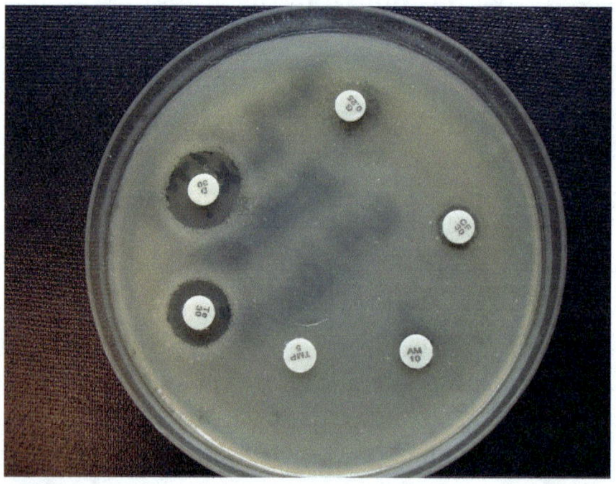

Figure 6.14. Minimum inhibitory concentration (MIC).

Source: https://www.microbiolaboratory.com/wp-content/uploads/2022/09/MIC-1024x768.jpg.

6.4.1. Topical Antifungal Treatments

Topical therapy with antifungals is a key component in the treatment of nail mould infection, especially onychomycosis. Topical treatment of the nail typically entails local application of antifungals to the nail, which allows localized action without undue systemic side effects. Some of the most commonly prescribed topical medications are amorolfine and ciclopirox, which both work to inhibit fungal growth, namely dermatophytes, yeasts, and nondermatophyte moulds that cause nail infection. The efficacy of the drugs is at times optimized by strict adherence to application schedules, with the formulation having to penetrate through the nail plate such that it gains access to the site of infection. Sophisticated formulation techniques have led to improved penetration, improving the rate of success for treatments and increasing patient compliance by reducing treatment duration and side effects (Sudha et al., 2010). Current studies have elucidated the relative effectiveness of topical antifungals compared with systemic therapy for onychomycosis. While systemic agents, such as terbinafine, have been found to be more effective with severe or refractory infections, topical agents remain the first line for mild infections or those that contraindicate systemic therapy. Combination therapy of topical and systemic agents has also emerged as a significant field of research, and these treatments can have a greater cure rate than either modality alone. For instance, combination with topical agents can also aid the action of systemic drugs for rapid removal of infected nails with the added advantage of improving patient tolerability (Conrado et al., 2019). In addition, advances in drug delivery systems, such as nanoparticles and micellar preparations, could further enhance the efficacy of antifungals when applied topically against resistant fungal strains. Despite the guarantee of effective treatment, there are some constraints in the management of nail infections with topical antifungals. One of the significant constraints is the resistance of certain fungal organisms, particularly nondermatophyte moulds like *Fusarium* spp., which are quite resistant to conventional antifungal drugs. There are emerging products on the horizon to fight these resistant infections, such as photodynamic therapy (PDT), with the goal of bringing non-invasive treatments that take advantage of the synergy of light and photosensitizing agents. Research has indicated that PDT is able to achieve significant reductions in fungal burden, providing a second line of treatment for those who fail to respond to traditional treatment (Conrado et al., 2019). However, further clinical trials must be conducted to establish the long-term efficacy and safety of these new therapies, which serves to underscore the ongoing necessity for innovation in the topical antifungal treatment of onychomycoses (Figure 6.15).

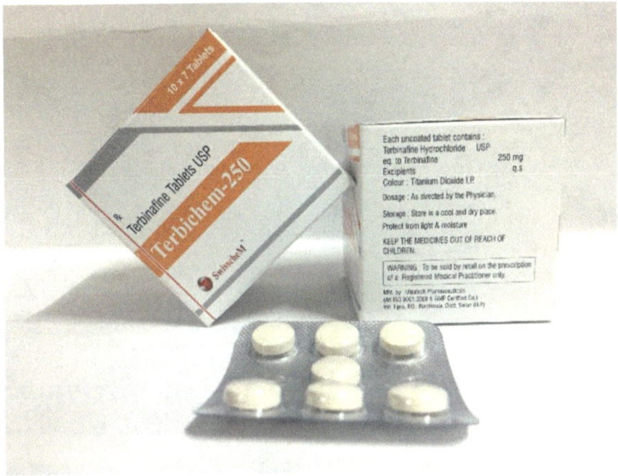

Figure 6.15. Terbinafine.

Source: https://www.swisschem.in/wp-content/uploads/2017/01/Terbinafine-Tablet.jpg.

6.4.2. Oral Antifungal Medications

The use of oral antifungal drugs plays a critical part in treating mould infections of the nails, most importantly in onychomycosis, where the condition is mainly caused by nondermatophyte moulds, dermatophytes, and yeasts. The infections are typically difficult to treat topically since they are not exposed to the surface but instead develop beneath the nail plate, hence the need for more systemic effect. Oral agents like terbinafine and itraconazole are often used in order to attain greater local concentration within the nail matrix, thereby improving treatment effectiveness. Terbinafine, in this context, has been prominent in attracting attention for its good therapeutic profile and being effective not just against dermatophytes but also against some of the nondermatophyte moulds (Sudha et al., 2010). Long-term trials demonstrate that systemic treatment leads to excellent improvement of nail status and recovery rates, underlining the importance of proper antifungal therapy for effective treatment of nail infections. Additionally, the design and implementation of the regimen of therapy with oral antifungal drugs should consider factors depending on the patient, including severity of the infection and side effects of the drugs. These are of great significance as they affect patient compliance and treatment adherence. While terbinafine has been shown to be highly effective, there needs to be watchful monitoring for side effects like liver enzyme elevation for which regular biochemical monitoring must be done during therapy. Furthermore, knowledge about the clinical presentation of onychomycosis and etiologic organisms is essential for a specific oral antifungal therapy (Sudha et al., 2010). Medical practitioners must balance therapeutic effectiveness against safety, thus informing the patient completely about potential risks and benefits inherent. Also, the value of adding traditional and herbal approaches to conventional oral antifungal therapy must be considered as part of a total treatment regimen. Research findings among plant-based traditional medicines reveal that a number of plant alternatives have antifungal properties, providing alternatives for patients who dislike taking systemic medications or are sensitive. For example, medications extracted from specific plants have been found to be effective against diverse fungal pathogens, increasing the therapeutic value in curing nail infections. Incorporating these complementary therapies into treatment protocols may enhance patient outcomes, particularly among populations with unequal access to healthcare and where traditional practice remains dominant. This complementary approach could evolve more appropriate and effective model of care for onychomycosis and expand the range of care beyond medication alone (Figure 6.16).

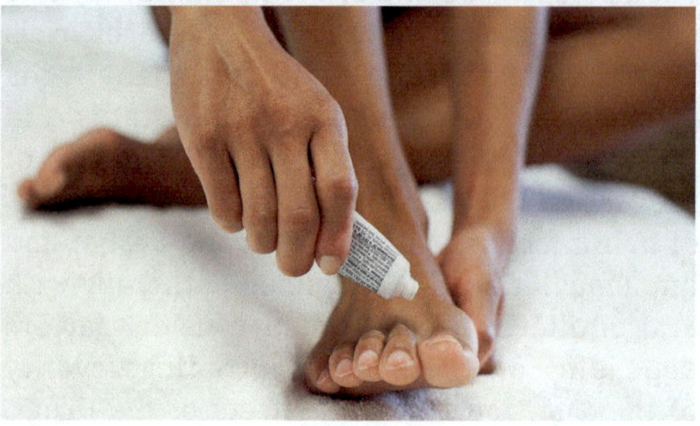

Figure 6.16. While terbinafine has shown a high success rate, it is essential to monitor for side effects like liver enzyme elevations, which require regular biochemical assessments during treatment.

Source: https://media.post.rvohealth.io/wp-content/uploads/2022/08/female-applying-foot-cream-ointment-1200-628-facebook-1200x628.jpg.

6.4.3. Surgical Interventions

Surgical procedures of onychomycosis, or mould infections of the nails as it is also referred to, are used when non-surgical treatment methods, such as antifungal medications, fail to eradicate the infection. Severe cases, especially where the infection has led to significant destruction of the nail plate or has extended to the surrounding tissues of the nail, will need surgery. The primary surgery is nail avulsion or removal of part of the nail. Nail avulsion involves the removal of the entire nail to facilitate direct treatment of the infected nail bed so that antifungal treatment can be directly applied to the infected region. Avulsion can significantly reduce the duration of infection and enhance the effectiveness of subsequent antifungal treatment, allowing for more rapid healing and better outcomes for the patient. There are times, however, where these issues recur or lead to complications. In these instances, more aggressive surgical treatment may be required. Total excision of the nail matrix is one such surgery that targets where nail growth originates in an effort to prevent reformation of the infected nail. Studies have shown that utilization of surgical methods can obtain greater success at eliminating the infection than simply treating by non-surgical methods. ntial (Burak et al., 2013) (Figure 6.17).

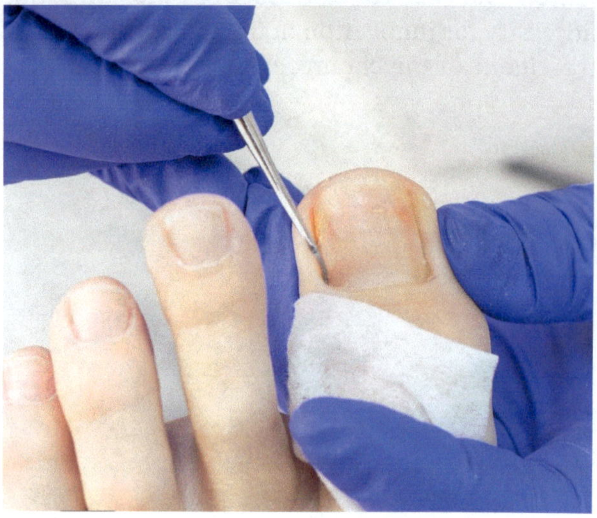

Figure 6.17. Post-surgical care is pivotal in ensuring successful recovery from mould infections of nails.

Source: https://thehouseclinics.co.uk/userfiles/images/Untitled%20design%20(24).jpg.

Besides, studies have shown that about 10% of procedures performed in specialty centers are for the treatment of non-unions due to associated conditions, reflecting the value of surgical intervention in managing fungal nail infection-related complications. In so doing, surgical interventions not only provide a quick remedy but also act as a preventive measure against future complications. Post-operative management is a key for successful recovery from mould nail infections. Proper post-operative wound care and ongoing post-operative antifungal treatment are crucial features of preventing recurrence. Combination of surgical methods with adjunctive focused antifungal treatment offers an effective dual modality strategy addressing both the existing infection and susceptibility. Nail care, the monitoring for signs of re-infection, and the monitoring of healthcare workers are some of the essential surgery patient practices. Given the multifactorial nature of onychomycosis, practitioners should assess each situation individually based on patients overall health, infection severity, and history of response to previous therapies in order to create an entire treatment plan that will ensure the highest probability of long-term healing while lowering recurrence pote

6.5. Prevention Strategies

Effective prevention of nail mould infection is largely a question of maintaining good hygiene and environmental control. Good hand washing and cleanliness of the nails with dryness thereof goes a significant way towards preventing fungal growth. It is crucial to make people cut their nails short and avoid injury, as this creates portals of entry for the fungi. Also, the wearing of breathable shoes and moisture-wicking socks can help keep the feet clean, thereby avoiding the environment that encourages mould growth. Education dissemination matters; educating vulnerable populations, for instance, sportspeople or individuals in humid areas, about these prevention measures can make the creation of a health-promoting culture that discourages mould infections. As X. et al. add, hygienic measures with an actionable quality are imperative foundations of larger prevention regimens aimed at nail mould infections, and thus, they are a full-fledged approach to public health education and self-care. Along with individual preventive measures, removal of the elements in the environment is also of prime importance in restricting mould infection risk. Poor ventilation and high humidity levels in the home can give fungi ideal breeding conditions. Therefore, using measures that allow enhanced airflow within indoor environments is crucial. This can include the use of mechanical ventilation systems with appropriate filters, as evidence regarding the impact of climate change on indoor air health and quality indicates. Policy improvement in building design to prevent moisture from collecting is also critical; for instance, using a mix of moisture-resistant materials can minimize damp conditions under which mould growth occurs. The role of local government agencies in the enforcement of building codes that take into consideration ventilation and moisture control cannot be minimized. Successful indoor environmental regulation takes a multi-factorial measure to the prevention of nail infection, thereby promoting overall public health and safety measures in alignment with the evidence in Chalabi et al., (2015). Health education and intervention by healthcare personnel also has the ability to be effective prevention measures in anti-mould infection of the nails. Public campaigns that raise awareness about symptoms and risks of nail infection can trigger early intervention and treatment, reducing chronic cases. Moreover, healthcare workers need to be provided with the ability to recognize the signs of mould infection and educate patients on effective prevention. Coordination between health care workers and public health managers should facilitate an integrated approach towards implementing community-based prevention programs tailored for high-risk groups. This collaboration is necessary in containing the tide of mould infections and can be supported by programmatic models focused on education and resource distribution. With an extensive network of care around prevention practices, communities are capable of drastically restricting the occurrence of mould infections of the nail, hence contributing to enhanced public health outcomes as debated in environmental health research (Figure 6.18).

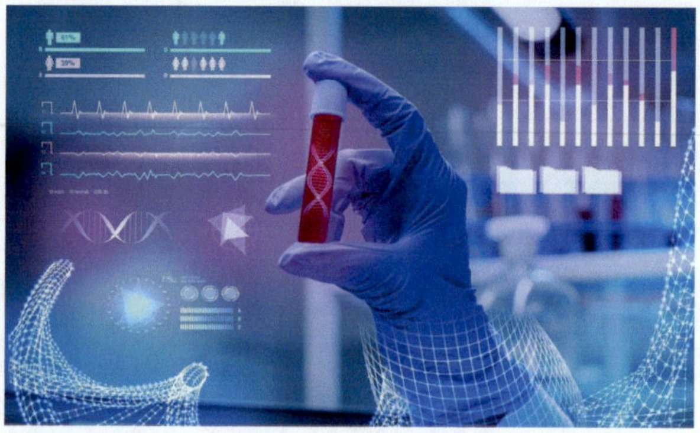

Figure 6.18. Knowledge dissemination plays a crucial role; educating at-risk populations, such as athletes or individuals in high-humidity areas, about these preventive measures can foster a culture of health awareness that diminishes the prevalence of infections.

Source: https://indian-retailer.s3.ap-south-1.amazonaws.com/s3fs-public/2023-09/biotechnology-specialist-laboratory-conducting-experiments%20%281%29.jpg.

6.5.1. Proper Nail Care and Hygiene

Good nail hygiene and care are essential in preventing nail mould infection, which may significantly impair one's general well-being and health. Clean nails not only enhance personal appearance, but also form a vital aspect of preventing the introduction of pathogens into one's body. Soap and water washing regularly is crucial since it removes dirt, bacteria, and potential fungal spores that are likely to grow in unclean surroundings. Furthermore, drying the nails properly is also advisable since moist conditions provide a ground that makes fungi grow. Trimming and shortening nails regularly can also reduce the infection surfaces, hence being a preventive measure against mould growth. The sharing of nail care tools, such as clippers and file tools, also needs to be prevented to minimize cross-contamination and fungal infection exposure. Infection prevention is of paramount importance, particularly in groups where individuals may be immunocompromised or at higher risk for infection. It is a fact that medical settings need to employ strict hygiene practices to prevent hospital-acquired infections (HAIs) resulting from poor nail hygiene, especially in settings like radiology departments where patients of various health status interact. Failure to follow the practice of nail hygiene can lead to common surfaces being contaminated, and as a result, infection-causing organisms are spread.

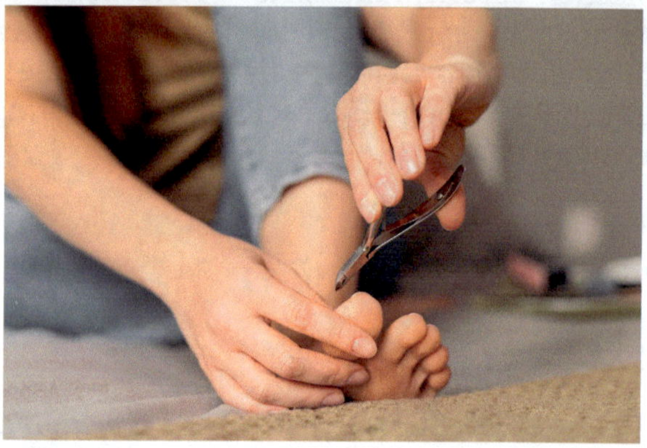

Figure 6.19. Maintaining proper nail care and hygiene is essential in preventing mould infections of the nails, which can significantly impair one's overall health and well-being.

Source: https://kulanispa.com/wp-content/uploads/2023/06/The-Importance-of-Proper-Foot-and-Nail-Hygiene-in-Preventing-Fungal-Infection-04.jpg.

Where the workers do not observe the minimum standards of hygiene, there is great risk of contamination in the case of nail care. As much as avoiding procedures that do not wear jewelry, such as rings and bracelets, which provide an ideal platform for pathogens, reducing the risk of mould infection of nails is critical in the public and private sectors (Palmqvist et al., 2020). Further, understanding the significance of nail care measures in healthcare and community environments has broader implications for public health. Sanitary and ergonomic issues, especially in the building or renovation of medical facilities, are also relevant to preventing airborne transmission of infectious agents, including mold. The creation of building protection barriers during construction can significantly minimize airborne infection agent risk in relation to vulnerable patient populations. Adequate training and communication of healthcare and construction workers about appropriate hygiene practices are essential to ensure a secure environment and prevent the risk of mould infection in patients, particularly invasive procedures or immunocompromised patients (Bassett et al., 2013). In the end, the adoption of rigorous nail hygiene and care processes into everyday life can be a first line of defense in preventing mould infection of the nails, resulting in better health for everyone (Figure 6.19).

6.5.2. Footwear Choices and Practices

Shoes choice has a dramatic effect on foot health, particularly the susceptibility to developing mould infections of the nails. The majority may consider fashion over form, ignoring how ill-fitting or inappropriate shoes may affect their overall foot hygiene. Overly tight or non-sweat-permeable shoes can easily create a humid condition that will support fungal growth. For those at risk of foot complications more strongly, such as those with diabetes, there is a pressing need to choose shoes that are both correctly fitting and also supportive and well-ventilated. The new guidelines on diabetes-related foot ulceration in Australia emphasize appropriate footwear as essential to the prevention of conditions such as nail infection, in light of the importance of structured education on foot care and protective regimes within general health advice (Charles et al., 2022). Wearing appropriate footwear is both a requirement for everyday comfort and general well-being. Ergonomically designed shoes can help reduce the risk of mould infection through air circulation and minimizing moisture buildup in the region around the nails. This feature is particularly significant in warm weather or in persons who engage in work generating sweat and moisture around their feet. Moreover, orthotic therapy or medically engineered shoes can play a vital role for persons with a higher risk of developing foot disorders.

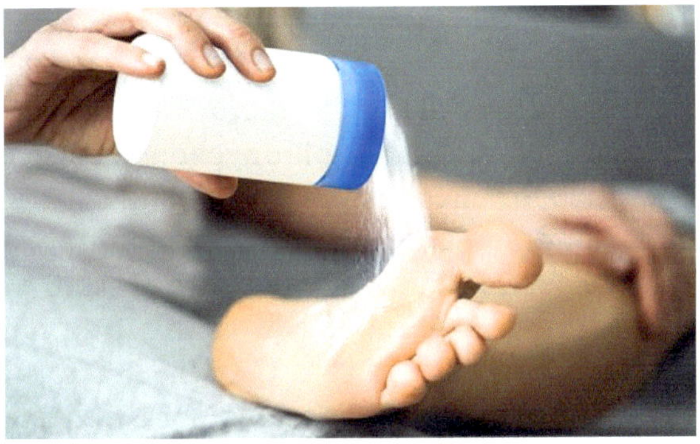

Figure 6.20. Regular cleaning and the use of antifungal powders can help minimize the growth of spores that can lead to nail infections.

Source: https://articles-1mg.gumlet.io/articles/wp-content/uploads/2022/06/Fungal-skin-infections.jpg?compress=true&quality=80&w=640&dpr=2.6.

The National Health and Medical Research Council has emphasized the critical role of organized education in promoting awareness about protection of the foot, inspection, and the right shoes as a preventive measure to nail mould infections, thereby maintaining enhanced health within the community (Charles et al., 2022). Footwear behavior extends beyond selection; maintenance and care contribute significantly towards foot health. Daily cleaning and application of antifungal powders can serve to reduce the development of spores that can cause nail infections. In addition, people should develop habits such as changing shoes every day and drying shoes properly before putting them on again so that they do not accumulate water. The cultural mindset toward footwear, as in the case of health talk, means that social norms will determine the selection of people, which can indirectly affect nail health. Optimal practice in footwear maintenance and selection is therefore important to reduce the incidence of nail mould infections. Such programs can give people the information they need to make informed decisions, leading to healthier feet in the long term (Figure 6.20).

6.5.3. Awareness of Risk Factors

Understanding the risk factors of mould infections of the nails, or onychomycosis, is imperative for effective prevention and control. Gender and age are some of the demographic characteristics that have a crucial role in determining the likelihood of contracting nail infections. Studies indicate that the 31 to 40 years age group is particularly vulnerable, perhaps due to occupational hazards with nails exposed to trauma and moisture (Kumar et al., 2018). Prevalence also increases by sex, where the female sex tends to be more vulnerable due to activities of prolonged wet exposure such as routine handwashing or doing wet work. These results are significant in raising awareness and leading in preventive measures among these risk groups. Environmental factors also play a decisive role in the causation of mould infections. For instance, moisture is at the center of the survival and development of fungi. People who live in humid climates or homes with poor ventilation can have increased cases of onychomycosis. Also, public gym and pool facilities have a shared risk factor in that these are fertile grounds for fungal spores to breed (Koticha et al., 2017). Awareness of the environmental conditions favorable to fungal growth can empower the individual to act proactively. Simple habits, for example, wearing suitable footwear in communal locker rooms or maintaining dry feet, might decrease exposure to these environmental risk factors and lower the chance of infection. Lastly, health factors, like medical conditions, contribute significantly to an individual's vulnerability to mould infections. These conditions like diabetes, circulatory disease, and compromised immunity heighten susceptibility to onychomycosis via compromised skin integrity and faulty healing. These susceptibilities emphasize the need for heightened vigilance and preventive measures in such cases. Regular medical check-ups and observation for nail deformities can ensure earlier detection and treatment, thus benefiting the high-risk group eventually. More public health education on these multifactorial risk factors needs to be available in order to reduce the frequency and severity of mould infections of the nails (Figure 6.21).

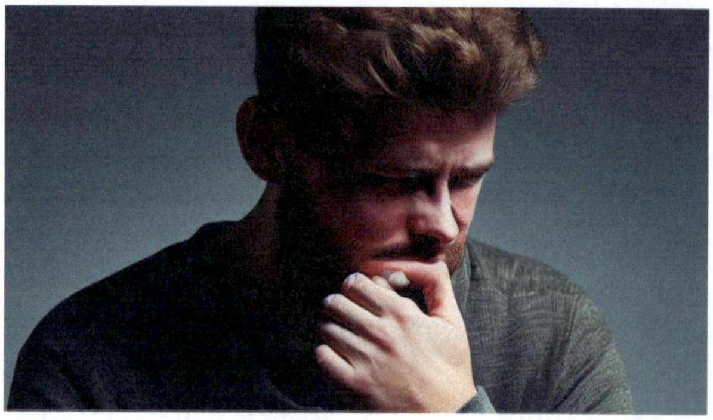

Figure 6.21. Recognizing the environmental variables that contribute to fungal growth can empower individuals to take proactive measures.

Source: https://sanixway.com/wp-content/uploads/0-28.jpeg.

SUMMARY

The prevalence of nail mould infections caused by fungal pathogens such as *Trichophyton* and *Aspergillus* is a causative public health issue. Scientifically, onychomycosis, the disease can lead to pain, discomfort, and severe psychosocial suffering. Moulds are happiest in warm and moist conditions, which is why the susceptibility of toenails, especially when proper hygiene and care protocols are neglected. Also, some underlying conditions, such as diabetes and immuno-deficiencies, can strengthen the severity of infection. An in-depth understanding of healthcare risks associated with mould infections is essential for prevention and treatment methods, which can be antifungal drugs and lifestyle modifications to avoid moisture accumulation and to enhance nail health. Antifungal susceptibility in mould species is a key concept employed in treating mould nail infections. High levels of resistance to common antifungal medications have been experienced, complicating treatment. As an example, research has reported that all *Fusarium* isolates tested were resistant to itraconazole, and high levels were also resistant to amphotericin B and voriconazole, which poses questions regarding the effectiveness of available medication (Restrepo et al., 2017). Such resistance points to the urgent necessity for ongoing research aimed at finding new antifungal drugs or other therapeutic strategies. Additionally, the risk of failure in treatment indicates how essential a proper diagnosis using mycological testing and sensitivity reporting is so that therapy can be appropriately adjusted for each patient. It is crucial to understand the complex interaction between health and environmental conditions in order to manage mould infections of nails. Climate change is a special challenge because it impacts the indoor prevalence of mould spores, particularly in regions where increased humidity and flooding are anticipated (Chalabi et al., 2015). This necessitates a multi-component approach to public health in the form of enhanced indoor air quality interventions and education aimed at preventing moulds. It is imperative to consider socio-economic inequalities since vulnerable populations may lack access to necessary sources for the sake of having healthy living conditions. Countermeasures to infections caused by mould have to therefore incorporate multi-strategic interventions that cover health promotion, environmental adaptation, and community-based efforts directed towards raising awareness and prevention of nail mould infections.

A CLOSER LOOK

VORICONAZOLE

Voriconazole belongs to the triazole class of broad-spectrum antifungal medication for the treatment of life-threatening and serious fungal infections, particularly in immunocompromised hosts. It suppresses the fungus's cytochrome P450 enzymes, hence impeding the production of ergosterol, a vital constituent of the fungal cell membrane.

Voriconazole is commonly used to treat infections such as:

- Invasive aspergillosis
- Candidemia (especially in non-neutropenic patients)
- Fusariosis
- Scedosporiosis

It comes in oral and intravenous preparations, depending on the severity of the infection.

Side effects include visual impairment (e.g., blurred vision, photophobia), increase in liver enzymes, rash, and hallucinations. Due to its low therapeutic ratio, therapeutic drug monitoring (TDM) is frequently recommended. Voriconazole also has extensive drug-drug interactions, particularly with liver metabolized drugs.

Because of its effectiveness and broad spectrum, it is a key drug in the treatment of life-threatening fungal infections, but it requires careful dosing and monitoring.

REFERENCES

1. Aleruchi, C., Emenike, A. O. I., James, D., Louisa, F., et al. (2012). Comparison of dermatophytes and other agents of human dermatitis between males and females in Jos, Plateau State, Nigeria. https://core.ac.uk/download/478291718.pdf (accessed on 27th June 2025).
2. Alessandrini, A., Apalla, Z., Bruni, F., Di Chiacchio, N., et al. (2025). Clinical and onychoscopy patterns in fingernail onychomycosis–A study by the International Dermoscopy Society "Tracheoscopy and Onychoscopy" Task Force. https://core.ac.uk/download/654521444.pdf (accessed on 27th June 2025).
3. Al-Hattab, K., Kadhum, M., Naher, O. H. S., Habeeb, H., et al. (2015). Clinical and histopathological study on dermatophytes infections caused by *Trichophyton mentagrophytes* using animal model. https://core.ac.uk/download/234656084.pdf (accessed on 27th June 2025).
4. Arabatzis, M., Emtestam, L., Faergemann, J., Hay, R. J., Lecerf, P., Nenoff, P., Nowicki, R. J., et al. (2019). A survey among dermatologists: Diagnostics of superficial fungal infections–What is used and what is needed to initiate therapy and assess efficacy? https://core.ac.uk/download/287184089.pdf (accessed on 27th June 2025).
5. Arendrup, M., Bruun, B., Gahrn-Hansen, B., Jensen, R. H., et al. (2004). *Fusarium* fungaemia in immunocompromised patients. https://core.ac.uk/download/pdf/82585933.pdf (accessed on 27th June 2025).
6. Arrese, M., Baran, R., Bruynzeel, D., De Doncker, P., De Hoog, G., English, M. P., Gianni, C., et al. (2012). Onychomycosis caused by *Scopulariopsis brevicaulis*: Report of two cases. https://core.ac.uk/download/pdf/8723791.pdf (accessed on 27th June 2025).
7. Bassett, A. (2013). Comparison test for infection control barriers for construction in healthcare. https://core.ac.uk/download/17050435.pdf (accessed on 27th June 2025).
8. Bii, C., Gitau, A. M., Mwangi, M., Ng'ang'a, Z., et al. (2012). Fungal infections among diabetic foot ulcer patients attending diabetic clinic in Kenyatta National Hospital, Kenya. https://core.ac.uk/download/478296609.pdf (accessed on 27th June 2025).
9. Borah, N., Hazarika, D., & Sharma, A. (2018). Clinic-mycological profile of onychomycosis in Assam, India. https://core.ac.uk/download/539912757.pdf (accessed on 27th June 2025).
10. Burak, I. I., Korikova, S. I., & Miklis, N. I. (2013). *Valeology*. https://core.ac.uk/download/53873566.pdf (accessed on 27th June 2025).
11. Cano Restrepo, L. E., Gaviria-Rivera, A. M., & Giraldo-López, A. D. (2017). *In vitro* antifungal susceptibility of clinical isolates of *Fusarium* from Colombia. https://core.ac.uk/download/427688208.pdf (accessed on 27th June 2025).
12. Chalabi, Z., Davies, M., Dimitroulopoulou, C., Heaviside, C., et al. (2015). Impact of climate change on the domestic indoor environment and associated health risks in the UK. https://core.ac.uk/download/42634309.pdf (accessed on 27th June 2025).
13. Charles, J., Cheney, J., Golledge, J., Kaminski, M. R., et al. (2022). Australian guideline on prevention of foot ulceration: Part of the 2021 Australian evidence-based guidelines for diabetes-related foot disease. https://core.ac.uk/download/559466781.pdf (accessed on 27th June 2025).

14. Conrado, P. C. V. (2019). Effect of photodynamic therapy with hypericin nano encapsulated in P123 on *Fusarium* spp. https://core.ac.uk/download/655371505.pdf (accessed on 27th June 2025).

15. Di Pietro, A., Reuben, A., Martinez-Rocha, A. L., Di Pietro, A., Musher, B., de Pauw, B. E., Foster, C. S., et al. (2014). Murine model for *Fusarium oxysporum* invasive fusariosis reveals organ-specific structures for dissemination and long-term persistence. https://core.ac.uk/download/20115566.pdf (accessed on 27th June 2025).

16. Fang, C. X., Lau, T. W., Leung, F. K. L., To, M. K. T., et al. (2017). Infection after fracture osteosynthesis–Part II: Treatment. https://core.ac.uk/download/95556650.pdf (accessed on 27th June 2025).

17. Fraser, S. (2013). The missing mass of morality: A new fit pack design for hepatitis C prevention in sexual partnerships. https://core.ac.uk/download/195674929.pdf (accessed on 27th June 2025).

18. Gierek, B. (2022). Nonverbal communication in rituals on Irish pilgrimage routes. https://core.ac.uk/download/552402549.pdf (accessed on 27th June 2025).

19. Gomathi Chitra, A. (2015). A study on mycological profile of onychomycosis in diabetic patients in a tertiary care hospital and their antifungal susceptibility pattern. https://core.ac.uk/download/235667628.pdf (accessed on 27th June 2025).

20. Koticha, A. H., Mehta, P. R., Suryawanshi, R. S., Wanjare, A., et al. (2017). Onychomycosis: Dermatophytes to yeasts–An experience in and around Mumbai, Maharashtra, India. https://core.ac.uk/download/539912865.pdf (accessed on 27th June 2025).

21. Kraft, W. K., Mantravadi, S., & Ogdie, A. (2017). Tumor necrosis factor inhibitors in psoriatic arthritis. https://core.ac.uk/download/83049994.pdf (accessed on 27th June 2025).

22. Kumar, M., Yadav, O. P., Kumar, R., & Pannu, S. (2018). The prevalence of onychomycosis in north western region of Rajasthan. https://core.ac.uk/download/233903002.pdf (accessed on 27th June 2025).

23. Macura, A., & Skóra, M. (2015). 21-year retrospective study of the prevalence of *Scopulariopsis brevicaulis* in patients suspected of superficial mycoses. https://core.ac.uk/download/286324201.pdf (accessed on 27th June 2025).

24. Mohideen Abdul Kadar, A. (2007). A study of otomycosis. https://core.ac.uk/download/235654258.pdf (accessed on 27th June 2025).

25. Nabulime, L. M. (2007). The role of sculptural forms as a communication tool in lives and experiences of women with HIV/AIDS in Uganda. https://core.ac.uk/download/40070140.pdf (accessed on 27th June 2025).

26. Nhlapo, N. (2013). Hygiene and nutritional content of the National School Nutrition Programmed in Bloemfontein, South Africa. https://core.ac.uk/download/222966369.pdf (accessed on 27th June 2025).

27. Pal, G. S., Kumar, R., Kumar, S., Ujjwal, R., & Pandey, V. S. (2024). Importance of *Achara Rasayana* in present era. https://core.ac.uk/download/617189883.pdf (accessed on 27th June 2025).

28. Palmqvist, C. (2020). Hygiene at CT and MRI. https://core.ac.uk/download/323274872.pdf (accessed on 27th June 2025).

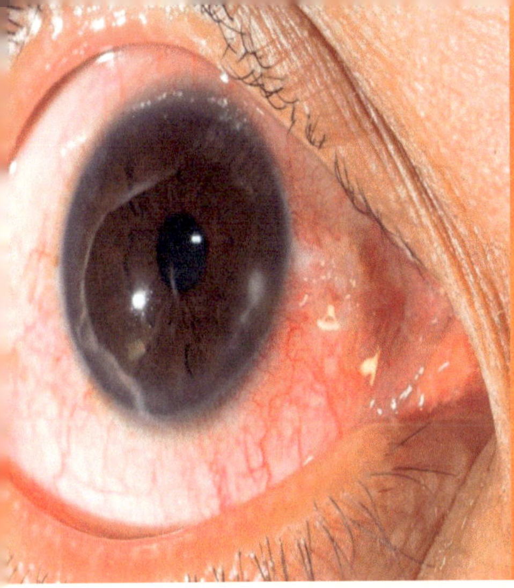

Chapter 7
KERATOMYCOSIS

Contents

Introduction

Fungal corneal infection of the eye, known as keratomycosis, is a particularly challenging issue in ophthalmology due to its capability to lead to extreme visual loss or even blindness if left untreated. Filamentous fungi, particularly *Fusarium* and *Aspergillus* species, are most prone to cause infection under certain environmental conditions and can easily infect the cornea through abrasions or underlying ocular surface disease. The first clinical presentation can be pain, redness, and blurring of vision, leading to delayed or misdiagnosis. Early diagnosis and prompt management are critical in keratomycosis because the course of the disease might lead to scarring of the cornea and perforation, which might necessitate surgery in the form of corneal transplant or even lead to blindness. Treatment of keratomycosis has evolved over time, with significant focus on antifungal therapy. Topical antifungal eye drops are conventionally employed, with Amphotericin B being a highly sought agent. However, effectiveness of such a treatment is generally hindered by two key points: compromised ocular bioavailability and the issue of the corneal barrier. The conventional drug delivery pathways cannot provide sustained release and good drug penetration of the drug in intraocular tissues, leading to therapeutic ineffectiveness. Based on research, new drug delivery systems such as microemulsions can enhance the bioavailability of Amphotericin B and their therapeutic action in treating keratomycosis (Chaudhari et al., 2016).

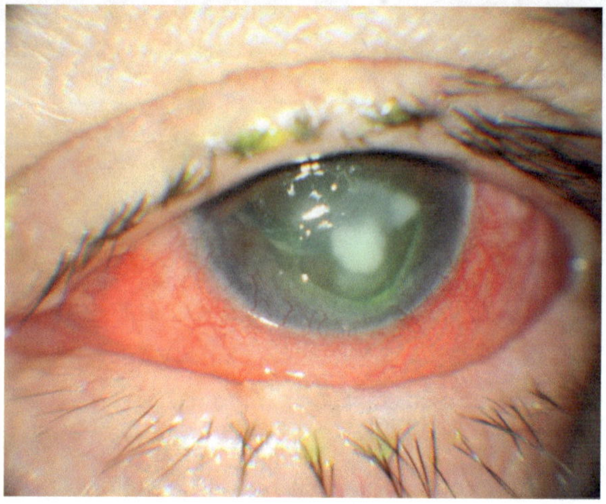

Figure 7.1. Keratomycosis.

Source: https://eyewiki.org/w/images/8/85/Fungal_ulcer.jpeg.

Thus, the development of novel delivery vehicles represents a viable solution for optimizing treatment regimens in these patients. The developments in pharmaceutical technologies over the past few years have made it possible to explore new drug delivery systems, especially ocular. A few examples of such innovations include the development of in situ gelling systems, which have been proven to increase the ocular residence time of topical ophthalmic medications. For instance, nanofibers electrospun, made up of Gellan Gum and Amphotericin B, provide the ability to gelate upon contact with the tear film, therefore promoting prolonged drug retention on the corneal surface and enhanced therapeutic efficacy (Göttel et al., 2022). Such an approach eliminates the defects in traditional drop formulations through the prevention of instantaneous clearance and promotion of controlled drug release. As the ophthalmology specialty continues to evolve, utilization of such advanced delivery systems would also revolutionize the dynamics of keratomycosis treatment, providing patients with more effective and longer-lasting therapeutic regimens (Figure 7.1).

7.1. Causes of Keratomycosis

The pathogenesis of keratomycosis is multi-factorial, with both host environment and susceptibility contributing. One of the significant factors in the causation of the ocular fungal infection is that the environment is inhabited by fungal organisms. Fungi inhabit all parts of the world and can be part of the commensal microflora present on mucosal surfaces like the eye. For instance, in the hot, humid environment of North Queensland in tropical regions, such organisms thrive. Corneal damage—either as a result of environmental exposure, trauma, or contact lens use—can upset the ocular surface, allowing the fungi to penetrate the corneal stroma and causing keratomycosis. These physical conditions combined with careless eye health practices maximize the risk and therefore the importance of investigating the role of outside conditions to this disorder (Gummow et al., 2023). Besides, host individual factors combined with the pathogenicity of specific fungal agents are important in the cause of keratomycosis. The variability in the immune response can affect vulnerability to fungal infections such that immunocompromised patients are at a higher risk. The prevalence of some fungal genera, such as *Aspergillus* and *Curvularia,* being present generally mirrors how the knowledge of certain strains is important in the prediction of the fate of an infection. Such fungi are capable of entering corneal tissue with ease, supported by the ability to adjust in different environments.

Intrinsic factors such as genetics and initial ocular disorders and extrinsic factors such as trauma or surface contact with contaminated materials combine and create a condition that makes keratomycosis more likely. Information regarding such interactions is important in preparing prevention measures (Lues et al., 2013). Preventive measures, therefore, must consider environmental cleanliness and personal hygiene to prevent the occurrence of keratomycosis. Studies indicate that fungi can live on contaminated surfaces, and this raises risks of transmission, especially in healthcare settings, where chances of exposure are increased. The detection of fungal organisms within kitchen areas, for instance, is a sign of a broader interest in environmental reservoirs as a factor in the spread of infection, such as keratomycosis. Promoting rigorous sanitation protocols in areas where eye care is provided has the possibility of reducing the amount of existing fungal load. Furthermore, public health interventions aimed at educating people on the safety of the eyes and adhering to compliance with appropriate treatment are significant factors in averting the causes of keratomycosis. Through proper comprehension of the reasons behind the disease, interventions could effectively be designed to negate this often-neglected ocular threat (Gummow et al., 2023; Lues et al., 2013) (Figure 7.2).

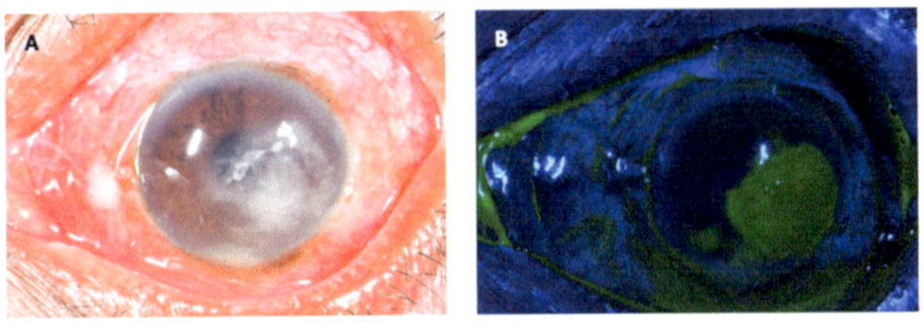

Figure 7.2. Fungi are ubiquitous and can be part of the commensal microflora residing on mucosal surfaces, including the eyes.

Source: https://pub.mdpi-res.com/jof/jof-07-00273/article_deploy/html/images/jof-07-00273-g001.png?1628048510.

7.1.1. Common Fungal Pathogens Involved

Within the context of keratomycosis, there are many fungal pathogens identified as key perpetrators behind this eye disease. Among these, *Aspergillus* species are notable in being one of the most frequent agents responsible, particularly within tropical regions where disease prevalence is quite high. According to epidemiological records, *Aspergillus* is seen to account for approximately 36% of occurrences of keratomycosis in South India, revealing its significant contribution toward infection of the cornea. The omnipresence of fungal spores, their ability to proliferate on organic media, and the opportunistic nature of these fungi make them formidable pathogens in the event of corneal compromise. Identification of the specific species and their niche in the environment is of extreme importance for the administration of targeted therapy and improving patient outcomes in managing keratomycosis. In addition to *Aspergillus*, several other fungal pathogens too carry the responsibility of keratomycosis. *Fusarium* species, though less frequently referenced in literature, are major pathogens for causing widespread corneal injury. While a few reports assert that *Fusarium* keratomycosis is less common than before estimated, its evolution as an opportunistic pathogen should be taken into account. Moreover, Dematiaceae fungi such as *Alternaria* and *Curvularia* are darker-colored fungi linked with corneal infection. The classification of such fungi into families, e.g., Moniliaceae and Dematiaceae, emphasizes the range of fungal pathogens having the potential to exploit compromised corneal surfaces to produce varying clinical presentations and complications related to keratomycosis (Fea et al., 2020). Management of keratomycosis is largely based on the identification of such opportunistic fungal pathogens and effective control of the infection through pharmacological interventions. Antifungal medications such as natamycin and azoles are frequently used to manage the infection. Current literature highlights the effectiveness of adjunctive treatments, such as 10% sodium chloride solution, in complementing the management of fungal keratitis. In addition to hastening healing, this combination treatment reduces the need for more aggressive surgical interventions, such as therapeutic keratoplasty. Since organisms like fungi are found in mycotic endophthalmitis after cataract surgeries, practitioners must remain vigilant about various pathogens involved in keratomycosis and modify treatment regimens accordingly to achieve the optimal patient outcomes (Fea et al., 2020) (Figure 7.3).

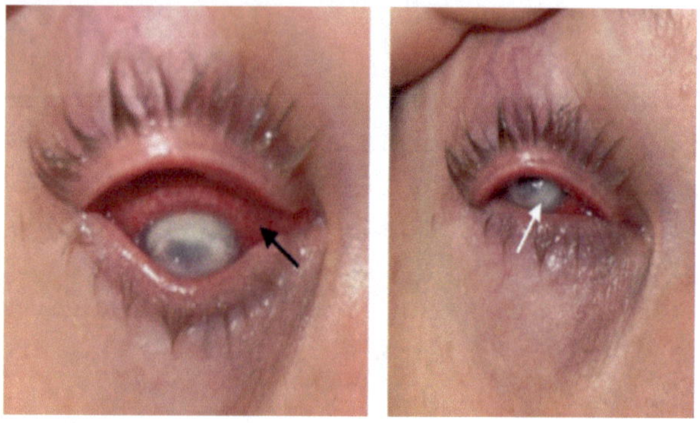

Figure 7.3. *Fusarium* keratomycosis.

Source: https://www.jem-journal.com/cms/asset/bca7b4ac-e1bd-416e-8444-fe9ef3084fe7/gr1.jpg.

7.1.2. Risk Factors for Infection

Risk factors for infection with keratomycosis are multifaceted, with a tendency to overlap environmental, physiologic, and behavioral variables. Environmental conditions conducive to the growth of fungi, such as tropical environments, highly predispose to infection of the cornea. An ideal region where there are favorable climatic conditions for fungal growth, including high temperatures and humidity, is North Queensland. Individuals, particularly outdoor workers or those with a history of ocular trauma, are thus at risk for keratomycosis. The presence of pathogenic fungi, which are capable of invading corneal tissue once corneal integrity is compromised, is the basis of the infection. Hence, an understanding of the environmental factors is the most important in the identification of risk groups and in devising prevention strategies that aim to minimize exposure and resulting infection rates. Physiological factors are a major contributor to the risk profile of keratomycosis. Individuals with compromised immune systems, e.g., diabetic patients with mellitus or patients undergoing immunosuppressive treatment, are at risk because they have diminished ability to resist opportunistic infections. Further, individuals with conditions leading to corneal destruction, e.g., prolonged use of contact lenses or underlying ocular surface disease, risk keratomycosis. In such instances, the corneal protective barriers are breached, so there is increased permeability to causative agents such as fungi. Considering such physiological risk factors not only places significant emphasis on patient-specific education but also reiterates the need for conscientious monitoring of those at risk in order to anticipate any emerging infections. Host lifestyle also represents a significant keratomycosis risk factor, particularly those activities that include ocular hygiene practices. For instance, improper contact lens management, i.e., under-disinfection or nighttime wear, facilitates fungal colonization of the cornea and subsequent infection. Furthermore, recreational water contact, e.g., in swimming pools or bodies of water, delivers pathogens directly into the eye, especially if it involves corneal abrasions. The occurrence of certain fungi in the environment, particularly in the tropics, highlights this fact, as is attested by the isolation of certain fungal strains from equine conjunctival swabs in North Queensland (Gummow et al., 2023). Knowledge of these behavioral risk factors in general is important in designing effective preventive interventions and educating patients on how to maintain proper ocular hygiene to prevent the incidence of keratomycosis (Figure 7.4).

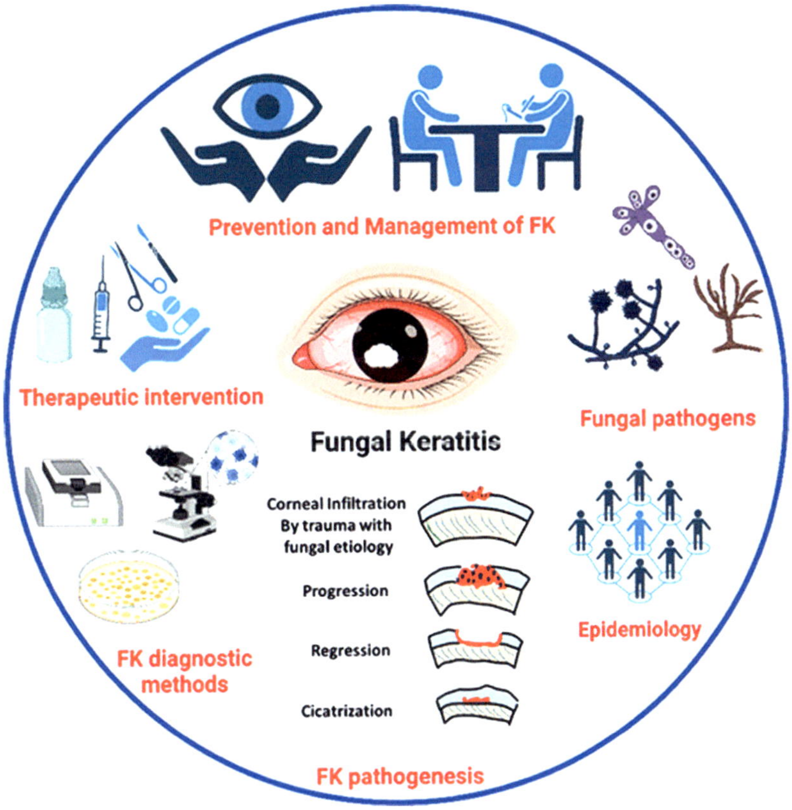

Figure 7.4. Personal behaviors also represent a significant risk factor for keratomycosis, particularly those associated with ocular hygiene practices.

Source: https://pubs.acs.org/cms/10.1021/acsinfecdis.4c00203/asset/images/medium/id4c00203_0009.gif.

7.1.3. Environmental Conditions Promoting Fungal Growth

Environmental conditions favoring the existence of fungi are paramount in the comprehension of keratomycosis, especially in the tropics such as North Queensland, Australia. Increased humidity and warm temperatures provide a favorable environment for fungal proliferation, triggering increased levels of keratinophilic fungi. Such organisms tend to thrive within moist conditions where organic matter contains the nutrients necessary for survival and reproduction. These conditions are especially pertinent following corneal trauma, which can compromise the eyes protective layers to facilitate entry by fungi into the corneal stroma. The prevalence of fungal species in the ocular microflora of horses, as evidenced in studies within North Queensland, corroborates the correlation between environmental factors and vulnerability to keratomycosis, as fungi can readily infiltrate damaged tissues to infect (Gummow et al., 2023). Moreover, the geographical location of the area affects the diversity of fungal pathogens that produce keratomycosis. In a Finnish retrospective review of infectious keratitis, *Aspergillus* sp. was identified as being among the invasive organisms prevalent with other organisms like *Cylindrocarpon* sp. (Aho et al., 2020). This variability emphasizes the significance of immediate environmental factors, such as seasonal variations and water content, in regulating the population of fungi within a region. Understanding the relative susceptibility of these microorganisms to antifungal treatment also relies upon an appreciation of their environmental proclivities. In tropical regions where humidity levels are consistently high, veterinary clinics must be careful for the likelihood of fungal keratitis, particularly during periods where there is heightened fungal activity owing to climatic factors. The findings suggest that veterinary treatments need to be adaptable to suit local environmental conditions supporting fungal growth.

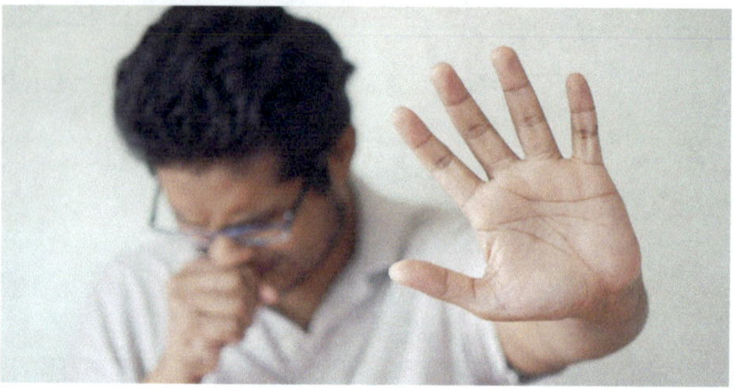

Figure 7.5. In tropical climates, where humidity remains consistently high, veterinary practices must remain vigilant regarding the potential for fungal keratitis, particularly during periods of heightened fungal activity due to climatic conditions.

Source: https://images.moneycontrol.com/static-mcnews/2023/07/Monsoon-fungal-infections.jpg?impolicy=website&width=1280&height=720.

For instance, the identification of various fungal genera like *Penicillium* and *Aspergillus* reveals the importance of selective antifungal therapies, particularly due to the varying sensitivities of these species to routine drugs (Gummow et al., 2023). Environmental factors, thus, cannot be left out during diagnosis and antifungal treatment of keratomycosis. Continuous surveillance and investigation are important in developing empirical guidelines that not only account for the biological characteristics of such pathogens but also for the environmental niches in which they live and thrive. A multi-component strategy therefore enables clinicians to appropriate treatment and employ effective preventive interventions into specific ecological contexts relative to fungal development (Figure 7.5).

7.2. Symptoms and Diagnosis

The symptoms of keratomycosis vary and can potentially have a significant impact on the patient's comfort and vision. The patient will typically present with a range of ocular discomforts in the form of pain, redness, and foreign body sensation. Keratomycosis involvement can also lead to visual disturbances in the form of blurring of vision or photophobia. As the disease progresses, patients also notice discharge, which is often of a purulent nature, causing further irritation of the corneal surface. The aforementioned clinical presentations highlight the importance of early recognition and diagnosis, since prompt management is crucial to prevent potential complications such as corneal scarring or perforation that may result in permanent loss of vision. Diagnosis of keratomycosis is made by detailed clinical evaluation aided by advanced laboratory techniques,. Initial assessment typically involves a thorough examination of the eye, during which the practitioner looks for common findings such as corneal opacity and infiltrates. Collection of a sample of the discharge or corneal tissue for microbiological culturing is essential in determining the presence of fungal pathogens. It is through this process that a number of isolates may be obtained, such as fungi such as *Aspergillus* species and *Cylindrocarpon* sp. being common culprits in keratomycosis cases, as supported by findings from the study that outlines the prevalence of such pathogens in clinical settings (Pietro et al., 2014). Proper diagnosis relies on the employment of clinical signs and laboratory results to diagnose accordingly, hence guiding proper modes of treatment. Further, the successful treatment of keratomycosis hinges on differentiation of other forms of keratitis, including bacterial infections. Differential diagnosis is necessary since identification of the type of keratitis wrongly can lead to improper therapies and poorer results. Laboratory findings, including culture and sensitivity, play a critical role in the differentiation process. To illustrate, studies indicate that while foscular agents like voriconazole are active against certain fungal organisms, others are resistant, and thus targeted therapy is crucial (Pietro et al., 2014). Duration of treatment in medicine also varies significantly in fungal and bacterial keratitis, as evidenced by research with the average duration of treatment being 38 days for fungal and just 25 days for bacterial infection (Aho et al., 2020). Through meticulous diagnostic processes, the outcomes of treatment can be maximized by establishing treatment plans based on the specific etiology of keratitis (Figure 7.6).

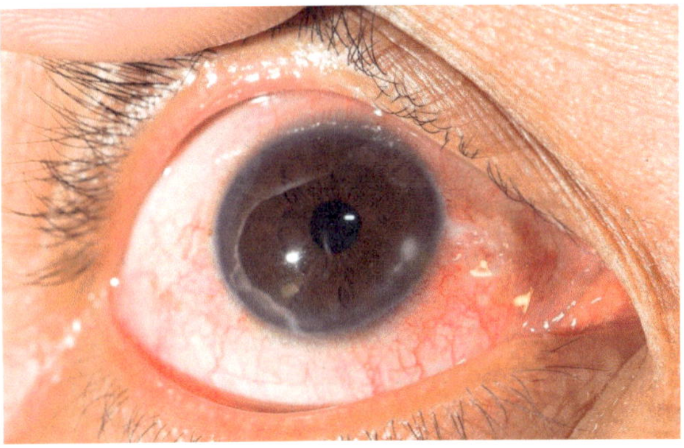

Figure 7.6. Collecting a sample of the corneal tissue or the discharge for microbiological culturing is vital in confirming the presence of fungal pathogens.

Source: https://media.allaboutvision.com/cms/caas/v1/media/571784/data/picture/b56756d9261adbd851e144f26934a78a.jpg.

7.2.1. Clinical Manifestations of Keratomycosis

The clinical manifestations of keratomycosis, or fungal keratitis, are diverse and may be quite distinct depending on the causative form of fungal organism and the extent of the disease. Symptoms in the patients are usually ocular pain, redness, and lacrimation, which may further exacerbate as the infection progresses. Visual symptoms, including blurred vision, are frequently encountered, reflecting an impairment of visual acuity due to corneal involvement. In more advanced stages, the cornea may present with opacity, which can lead to severe loss of vision if not attended to early. Additionally, the presence of corneal infiltrates or abscesses, commonly seen in microscopy in the process of diagnostic evaluation, further confirms the fungal etiology of the keratitis and necessitates immediate medical intervention to prevent potential complications. In animal medicine, particularly in the livestock, keratomycosis also poses significant health consequences, particularly in animals like buffaloes which are prevalent in agricultural lands. As revealed in a research conducted in the Thi-Qar province of Iraq, mycotic eye infection was prevalent among buffaloes with clinical presentations being the same as in humans. The infected animals also showed similar signs such as ocular inflammation, lacrimation, and corneal opacity—precisely the same as in human keratomycosis. The research indicated high correlation of early ages and male buffaloes' genders in susceptibility to such infections. The research also underscores the significance of keratomycosis not only in human subjects but also in veterinary medicine, towards a better understanding of its clinical presentations in different species (Salihi et al., 2021). Moreover, if left untreated, keratomycosis can lead to serious complications like the onset of endophthalmitis, a debilitating intraocular inflammation that will result in permanent loss of vision. The progression of a superficial keratomycosis to an invasive infection is typically a turning point when intensive treatment must be employed. Treatment typically consists of antifungal medication, which can be topical or intravitreal depending on the severity of the infections. Proper and early identification of clinical presentation is critical to avoid the progression of the infection and preservation of visual function. For this purpose, an overall understanding of clinical presentations that are seen with keratomycosis is crucial for effective diagnosis and treatment, particularly in the prevention of severe complications like endophthalmitis, which significantly complicates the course of the infection and therapeutic interventions (Durand et al., 2013) (Figure 7.7).

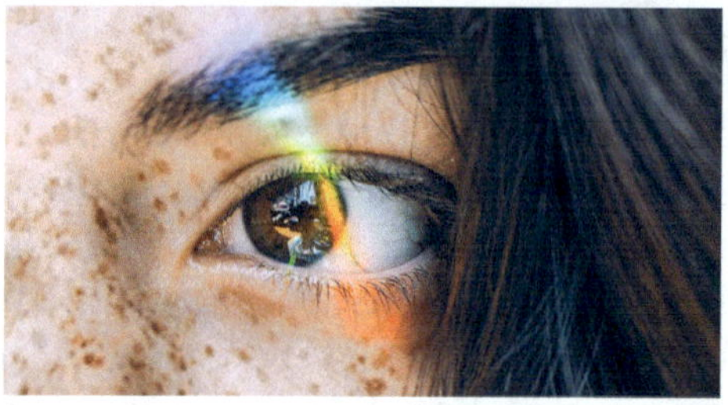

Figure 7.7. Visual disturbances, including blurred vision, are frequently reported, signaling an impact on visual acuity due to corneal involvement.

Source: https://media.post.rvohealth.io/wp-content/uploads/2020/08/Cropped-Image-Of-Young-Woman-Eye-1200x628-facebook-1200x628.jpg.

7.2.2. Diagnostic Methods Used in Identification

Diagnosis of keratomycosis, which is a fungal infection of the eye, is largely based on a correlation between clinical presentation and sophisticated diagnostic methods. Initial assessment typically involves intensive questioning of the patient's symptom and eye history, along with extensive slit-lamp examination to search for fungal infection lesions on the corneal surface. However, clinical presentations may not be adequate by themselves; hence, laboratory techniques are required for diagnosis confirmation. Laboratory diagnosis of these is most crucial with potentially catastrophic consequences of misdiagnosis, leading to appropriate antifungal treatment and early intervention to avert vision and ocular loss. Among the various diagnostic tests employed, culture and microscopy are significant in identification of the etiological fungal pathogens. Different media are used to isolate fungal cultures, and the resulting colonies are then inspected morphologically. Modern techniques like the polymerase chain reaction (PCR) are now being widely followed for their high sensitivity and specificity. PCR makes it possible to amplify the DNA of fungi, so that even minute traces of fungal components can be identified in ocular samples.

The technique, when used alongside traditional culture, boosts the accuracy in diagnosis, particularly where standard procedures may yield confusing results due to prior antifungal treatment or the fastidious nature of some microbes. The molecular techniques also supplement the diagnostic armamentarium with added depth in the form of species identification accuracy. For instance, sequencing analysis of specific genetic regions, such as the ITS 2 region, can yield comprehensive taxonomic information critical to the individualized approach for treatment. PCR-RFLP analysis is another new technique that enables differentiation of fungal species that induce keratomycosis. Such sophisticated diagnostic tools are priceless in a clinical setting where time matters because early detection can lead to immediate intervention and improved outcomes for the patient. Together, these diagnostic tests indicate the synthesis of traditional and modern methods in treating keratomycosis successfully and highlight the need to adopt a holistic approach in order to make accurate identification and treatment of this eye infection (Fea et al., 2020; Liu et al., 2011) (Figure 7.8).

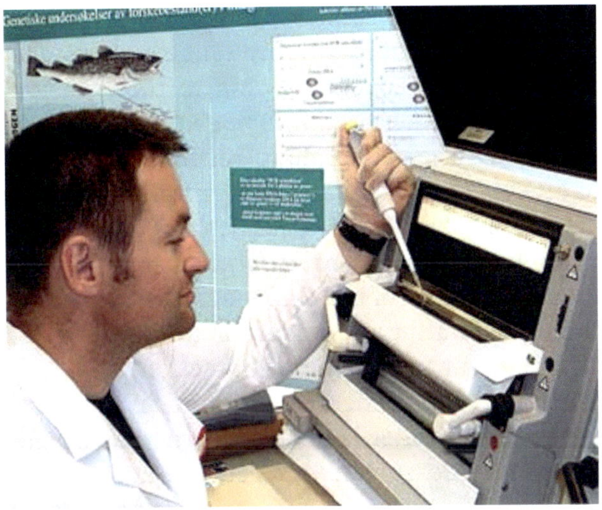

Figure 7.8. Molecular techniques further enrich the diagnostic arsenal, offering precision in species identification.

Source: https://lh3.googleusercontent.com/proxy/AyvcCxAyc6BVBAWhd2R1pnJ2twd-FiXJY5mfsU3ZtTEeAOMWbt8HDAFpAoCgW-11v5YBpJYAXsC488ZkTUou1hG6P43Bj7uTkcmzUp57ZA.

7.2.3. Differential Diagnosis with Other Ocular Conditions

Differential diagnosis of keratomycosis is relevant since it shares very similar symptomatology with other ocular infections. Corneal ulcers, for instance, also have similar presentation with clinical findings of redness, tear, and photophobia. These need careful clinical examination and workup to exclude keratomycosis from bacterial or viral infection, like herpes simplex keratitis, which also demonstrates epithelial defects and associated symptoms. Misdiagnosis would lead to unnecessary treatments, which would further exacerbate the condition and even lead to severe visual impairment. In endemic areas of fungal infection like in tropical areas, awareness of keratomycosis as a top cause of corneal disease becomes even more important because prevalence of the diseases makes the clinical presentation complicated (Gummow et al., 2023). The microbiologic analysis of corneal specimens plays an important part in differentiating keratomycosis from other infectious types of keratitis. In bacterial keratitis, ocular cultures often confirm characteristic bacterial isolates, but keratomycosis can sometimes require specific mycological cultures to confirm accurately.

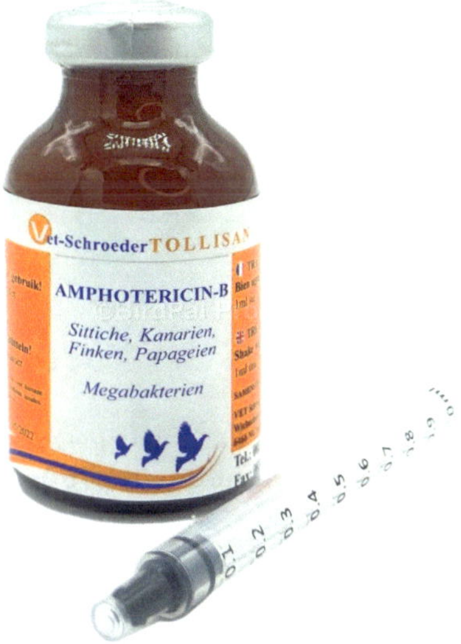

Figure 7.9. Amphotericin B.

Source: https://birdpalproducts.com/cdn/shop/products/Amphotethrin-3.jpg?v=1620863231.

A study presented results of abnormalities of ocular flora, including a number of fungal genera, which must be distinguished from normal commensal flora (Gummow et al., 2023). In addition, the clinic can apply imaging modalities that emphasize corneal lesion morphology. These imaging technologies are capable of providing information about corneal invasion depth and associated inflammatory reactions, which are critical factors in determining the disease pathology of an ocular process, for instance, hypopyon or massive corneal opacification. Newer therapies also provide insight into differential diagnoses of keratomycosis. Rising advancement involves the development of new drug delivery systems, such as nanofibers that enhance ocular bioavailability of antifungals like Amphotericin B. The systems enhance treatment effectiveness and create opportunities for distinguishing keratomycosis from less responsive diseases. Increased ocular surface retention can assist clinicians in being able to effectively treat fungal keratitis while ruling out bacterial or viral etiologies that could necessitate entirely different therapeutic regimens. The addition of novel therapeutic modalities emphasizes the need for accurate diagnosis, as proper treatment regimens hinge on distinguishing keratomycosis from the variegated spectrum of ocular disease (Figure 7.9).

7.3. Pathophysiology

Understanding the pathophysiology of keratomycosis is paramount in proper diagnosis and management of the condition, which is most frequently due to fungal infections, but more precisely those of the *Acanthamoeba* genus. Infection occurs when the corneal epithelium is compromised, allowing the deeper corneal structures to come into contact with the invading organisms.

Established risk factors include contact lens use, ocular trauma, and pre-existing ocular surface disorders. The corneal epithelium is a vital protective barrier against invading foreign pathogens; once broken, *Acanthamoeba* is able to grow, leading to inflammation and tissue destruction. This is facilitated by the recruitment of immune cells, which, in attempting to combat the infection, are also involved in continued damage to the cornea by the release of inflammatory mediators. The derangement of corneal homeostasis later aggravates the condition, making it very important to understand these mechanisms in formulating effective treatment modalities. The clinical presentation of keratomycosis is influenced by a range of pathophysiologic events and immune responses. The presentation usually consists of severe eye pain, redness, and blurred vision, manifestations basically brought about by the inflammatory response owing to the invasion of the fungus. The *Acanthamoeba* trophozoites initiate a series of immune responses, leading to corneal epithelial cell apoptosis and resultant ulceration. Microbial dysbiosis is also implicated, whereby the growth of *Acanthamoeba* disrupts the normal flora of the ocular surface, impairing the eyes native defenses and creating an environment for secondary infection. It is here crucial to comprehend the interaction of the pathogen's virulence factors with that of the host immune system to treat keratomycosis in a holistic manner. It aids in bringing into focus potential therapeutic choices centered on healing of the epithelial barrier and immune modulation to minimize tissue damage and yet achieve effective treatment of the infection.

Current advances in research aimed at the pathophysiology of keratomycosis hold promise for new therapeutic strategies, especially in the light of the inadequacies of existing antifungal treatments. The advent of novel anti-acanthamoebic drugs provides an exciting prospect, eliminating the issues of recurrent infection and suboptimal result with current therapies. Research emphasizes a demand for drugs with improved efficacy and safety profiles to target both the direct effects of *Acanthamoeba* and the secondary complications of inflammation and tissue damage. Emerging strategies such as drug repurposing, small interfering RNA (siRNA)-targeted therapy, and examination of derivatives of natural products mirror the current trend in this direction. With knowledge of the intricate pathophysiological mechanisms underlying keratomycosis, scientists are now in a position to continue to identify additional pharmacological targets, eventually maximizing treatment and enhancing quality of life for sufferers, as cited in the study of these parameters in recent literature (Elsheikha et al., 2020; Agache et al., 2024) (Figure 7.10).

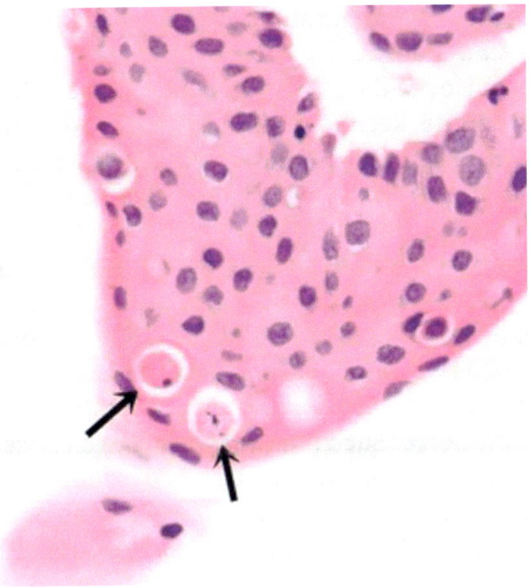

Figure 7.10. The *Acanthamoeba* trophozoites induce a cascade of immune responses, leading to corneal epithelial cell apoptosis and subsequent ulceration.

Source: https://www.researchgate.net/profile/Chien-Chin-Chen-2/publication/221740037/figure/fig1/AS:546934035148800@1507410643091/Photomicrographs-of-portions-of-full-thickness-corneal-epithelium-removed-by-peeling_Q320.jpg.

7.3.1. Mechanism of Fungal Invasion in the Cornea

The pathogenesis of fungal corneal invasion is a multifactorial interaction among the host factors and the biology of the fungus. Fungi, particularly those belonging to the *Aspergillus* and *Fusarium* genera, are opportunistic pathogens that invade pathologically altered corneal tissue unlike normal corneas. The presence of predisposing factors like trauma, intraocular surgery on the cornea, or ocular surface disease significantly raises the risk of corneal susceptibility to fungal invasion (Ravikumar et al., 2006). Once deposited onto the corneal surface, environmental spores germinate and penetrate the epithelial barrier, effectively utilizing the corneal stroma as a nutrient source. Spread from one corneal layer to another can lead to localized inflammatory reactions, which increase tissue damage and facilitate further colonization by fungi, thus laying the groundwork for more widespread keratomycosis. Apart from corneal tissue invasion, processes on how fungi injure tissues and evade immune detection are also crucial to the comprehension of keratomycosis. Fungal pathogens have evolved some methods to evade host defense mechanisms, including the production of mycotoxins and the formation of biofilms. These biofilms form an enclosed niche for the fungi, which can survive not only immune invasion but even topical antifungal therapy (Al-Otaibi et al., 2012). The inflammation resulting from such invasion exacerbates the disease, typically manifesting as corneal ulceration. The clinical presentation observed in patients suffering from keratomycosis is therefore determined by the interaction between the virulence of the fungal pathogen and hosts' immune response. Understandings of the mechanisms of fungal corneal invasion also have significant clinical relevance for diagnosis and treatment. Early diagnosis of fungal keratitis is critical, especially in hyperendemic regions where mycotic disease is the most frequent cause of keratitis due to environmental factors, such as agricultural practice (Al-Otaibi et al., 2012). Treatment typically consists of aggressive antifungal therapy, often with agents such as natamycin. Recent studies show that adjunctive therapies, such as the application of hypertonic sodium chloride, can enhance healing by reducing corneal edema and promoting ulcer regression (Ravikumar et al., 2006). These advances highlight the importance of a multi-disciplinary approach to keratomycosis management, with emphasis placed on tailored treatment protocols that consider both the pathogenic processes of the fungi and the hosts defense mechanisms (Figure 7.11).

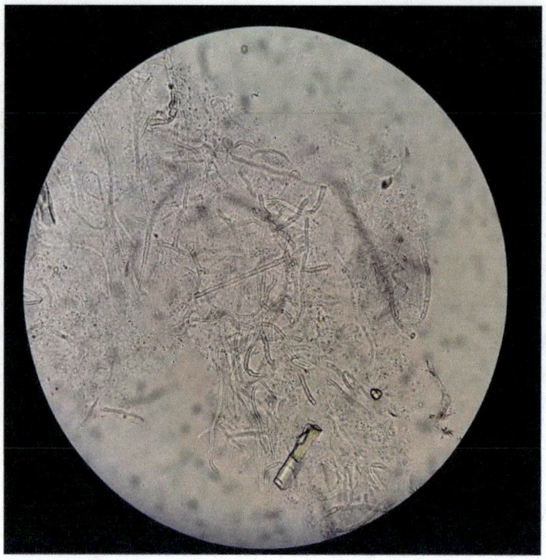

Figure 7.11. Prompt recognition of fungal keratitis is essential, especially in endemic regions where mycotic infections predominate due to environmental factors, such as agricultural practices.

Source: https://www.mdpi.com/jof/jof-07-00907/article_deploy/html/images/jof-07-00907-g002.png.

7.3.2. Immune Response to Fungal Infection

The immune response to fungus infection, particularly of keratomycosis, is complex involving both innate and adaptive immunity. Immune cells such as neutrophils and macrophages are the initial of several lines of defenses following the invasion of the cornea by fungi. The cells recognize fungal antigens such as polysaccharides and proteins that initiate multiple pathways of signaling that result in the production of pro-inflammatory cytokines. This initial inflammatory response is crucial since it attempts to wall off the infection and prevent additional fungal colonization. Furthermore, it also serves to bring additional immune cells to the site of infection and thereby enhance overall immunity against the pathogenic organisms. The efficacy of such immune activation is significant, as can be vouched for by the vast array of fungal organisms, for instance, those outlined in equine keratomycosis literature (Gummow et al., 2023) and (Aho et al., 2020), that take different measures to evade immune detection. While the innate immune response plays a key role in the initial defense, the adaptive immune response plays a key role in long-term immunity and control of fungal infections. T lymphocytes, i.e., CD4+ T helper cells, are activated by antigen-presenting cells presenting fungal antigens. Activation of such immunity leads to a concerted immune response through the production of antibodies as well as the differentiation of CD8+ cytotoxic T cells, which have the potential to play a crucial role in clearing infected cells. In keratomycosis, the net response of such adaptive mechanisms will determine clinical outcomes, particularly against different pathogens. The isolation of organisms such as *Aspergillus*, which is known to be prevalent in the instances of equine keratomycosis, is a test for host adaptive response since these can produce immunomodulatory substances, thereby determining the efficacy of treatment and healing (Gummow et al., 2023). Moreover, varied immunity to different fungal infections means that there must be a personalized therapeutic strategy. Studies of susceptibility of various fungal species to antifungal agents illustrate the importance of immune response as well as efficacy of the treatment in terms of available choices. Susceptibility findings for common fungi of keratomycosis, such as those under *Aspergillus*, for instance, imply that the immune response not only ought to respond effectively but also modify its strategy based on the particular needs of the pathogen (Aho et al., 2020). This equilibrium of immune response and antifungal treatment emphasizes the necessity of a multifaceted approach to treating keratomycosis in which understanding of the hosts immune mechanisms can lead to enhanced outcomes and guide the direction of future research in fungal infection (Figure 7.12).

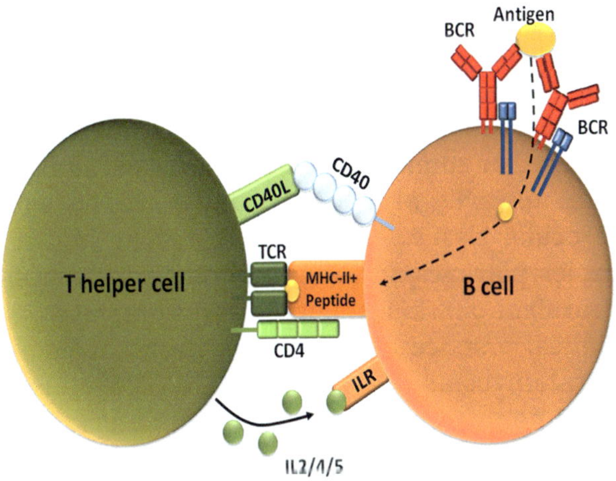

Figure 7.12. T lymphocytes, particularly CD4+ T helper cells, are activated by antigen-presenting cells presenting fungal antigens.

Source: https://upload.wikimedia.org/wikipedia/commons/thumb/d/df/T-dependent_B_cell_activation.png/500px-T-dependent_B_cell_activation.png.

7.3.3. Impact on Corneal Structure and Function

The impact of keratomycosis on corneal structure and function is widespread and multifaceted, primarily as a result of the invasion of fungal pathogens, which breaks the corneal integrity. The cornea is an important barrier that protects the internal ocular organs and allows for the transmission of light. Fungal invasion leads to thinning of the cornea, opacification, and perforation, which impair visual acuity and the eyes refractive potential. The inflammatory response elicited by fungal penetration also enhances tissue damage to the stroma of the cornea, in which collagen fibers are found, leading to a change in the curvature of the cornea and the development of astigmatism. This structural compromise has resultant effects on eye health, hence necessitating the importance of efficient therapeutic interventions to stem fungal infections (Göttel et al., 2022). Beyond mere erosion of structures is the functional implication of keratomycosis. The cornea is essential in maintaining the optical clarity required for vision; infection can therefore cause severe visual impairment. Photophobia and pain are caused by inflammatory mediators released during the immune response, making it even harder for normal corneal function. The tear film, which is needed to nourish and protect the cornea, can also be disturbed as a result of fungal activity, causing dry eye symptoms and secondary infections. Since the corneal surface is compromised, secondary bacterial infections are more probable, and treatment becomes more difficult and vision loss irreparable.

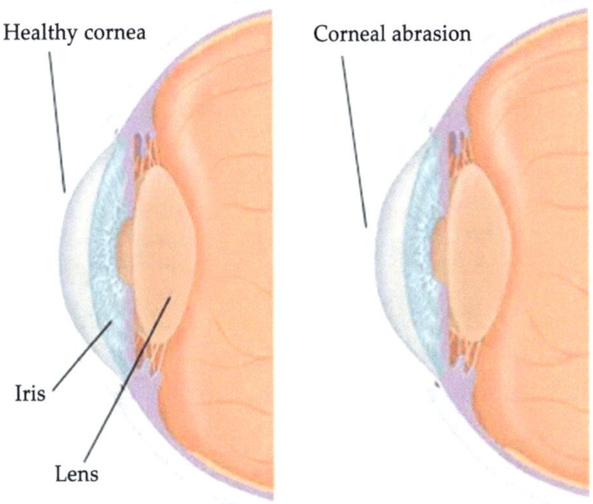

Figure 7.13. The cornea is critical for maintaining the optical clarity necessary for vision; thus, infections can lead to significant visual impairment.

Source: https://asiaretina.com/wp-content/uploads/2024/09/corneal-infections.jpg.

Proper understanding of the interplay of these variables is thus important for creating effective treatment protocols and sustaining corneal health (Abarca et al., 2017). New advances in therapeutic approaches, such as novel drug delivery systems, highlight the need for targeted therapy in order to combat the consequences of keratomycosis on corneal health. Illustrative examples include approaches using in situ gelling systems in order to enhance drug bioavailability and residence time on the ocular surface, one of the primary determinants of success in the battle against fungal infections such as keratomycosis. These systems are also able to provide prolonged antifungal activity and minimal systemic exposure and toxicity (Göttel et al., 2022). In addition, the thermogel delivery of therapeutic agents is also seen to be promising, as it is able to provide prolonged release of antifungal drugs like voriconazole and greater therapeutic effects in infected corneal tissue. These innovations must be assessed since their effectiveness can radically alter the clinical progression of keratomycosis and, in the long term, contribute to improved visual prognosis among infected patients (Abarca et al., 2017) (Figure 7.13).

7.4. Treatment Options

Management of keratomycosis, fungal corneal infection, is largely aimed at the eradication of infectious organisms with the preservation of ocular function and integrity. Antifungal treatment is the cornerstone of treatment of the infection, with the choice hinging on the causative fungal organism involved and their drug sensitivity pattern. As per research, fungal species most commonly involved in equine keratomycosis, including *Aspergillus* and *Curvularia*, vary in antifungal sensitivity. The treatment in practice is usually commenced using topical antifungals such as voriconazole and ketoconazole, which have proved highly effective against the majority of isolated fungal species while being resistant to fluconazole and amphotericin B, as reported in the research involving the tropical ecosystems that allow for fungal growth (Gummow et al., 2023). Earlier initiation of therapy is important, as delaying it leads to ulceration and loss of vision, and hence early clinical assessment is important. Topical treatment alone might not be enough in some cases, where systemic antifungal treatment would be required. Intravitreal injection, particularly in severe and complicated cases, allows direct intraocular administration of antifungals into the vitreous cavity with greater drug concentrations in ocular tissues. According to recent studies, azoles, polyenes, and echinocandins are the most prevalent pharmacological classes employed in clinical practice for ocular infection, including keratomycosis (Fea et al., 2020). Systemic treatment selection should be determined by the rate of fungal growth and the degree of penetration of the cornea, which needs to be aggressively controlled without causing complications such as endophthalmitis.

Ultimately, an integrated therapeutic regimen, in certain instances blending systemic and topical antifungals, has a comprehensive approach to its treatment of this ocular threat. Beyond medication therapy, correction of risk factors is essential to an optimal outcome in keratomycosis. Underlying conditions such as ocular surface disease, prior trauma, or prolonged wear contact lenses can predispose to fungal infection.

Clinical management, therefore, has to include extensive patient education about proper eye care, heightened awareness of hygiene to mitigate the risk of damage, and regular follow-up to evaluate the effectiveness of treatment. Furthermore, studies in horse populations have attributed environmental factors to play a significant role in the endemicity of keratomycosis in the tropics, so prevention strategies have to incorporate both clinical and environmental conditions (Gummow et al., 2023). Following an overall approach that integrates sound pharmacotherapy with prevention measures, prevalence and severity of keratomycosis can significantly be reduced to preserve long-term ocular well-being (Figure 7.14).

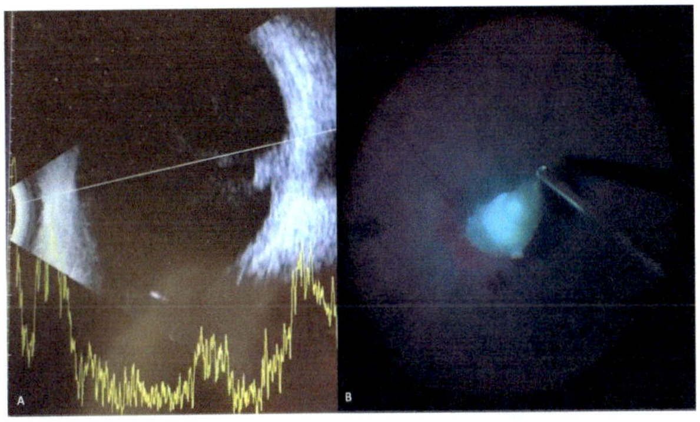

Figure 7.14. The choice of systemic therapy must consider the rapidity of the fungal spread and the degree of corneal involvement, which necessitates a controlled, aggressive approach to prevent complications such as endophthalmitis.

Source: https://pub.mdpi-res.com/jof/jof-07-00996/article_deploy/html/images/jof-07-00996-g005.png?1637652296.

7.4.1. Antifungal Medications and Their Effectiveness

Among the antifungals employed for keratomycosis treatment, drug choice has a big bearing on patient outcomes. Natamycin, voriconazole, and amphotericin B are most commonly employed as antifungals, each with mixed efficacy against various fungal pathogens. Of particular interest, natamycin has shown itself to be highly effective against filamentous fungi such as *Fusarium* and *Aspergillus*, with which keratomycosis infections are most often associated. Studies have shown that patients treated with natamycin tend to have better clinical outcomes when compared to patients treated with voriconazole, especially if the microbiological cure rates and visual acuity are taken into consideration. This revelation is highlighted by research implying that natamycin reduces the risk of complications like corneal perforation by a considerable margin, highlighting its importance in the clinical treatment of fungal keratitis. Voriconazole is yet another option, most especially in cases where fungi are resistant to the traditional treatments. Its broad spectrum of action against a variety of fungal pathogens makes it a desirable option in some clinical situations. Response variability may be experienced because all the fungal pathogens do not respond uniformly to voriconazole. It has been indicated through research that while voriconazole might be effective, natamycin is often more effective in the management of keratomycosis, particularly for the *Fusarium* species (Gummow et al., 2023). Hence, the use of an antifungal should be done with great caution and taking into consideration the causative fungal strain and its pattern of susceptibility.

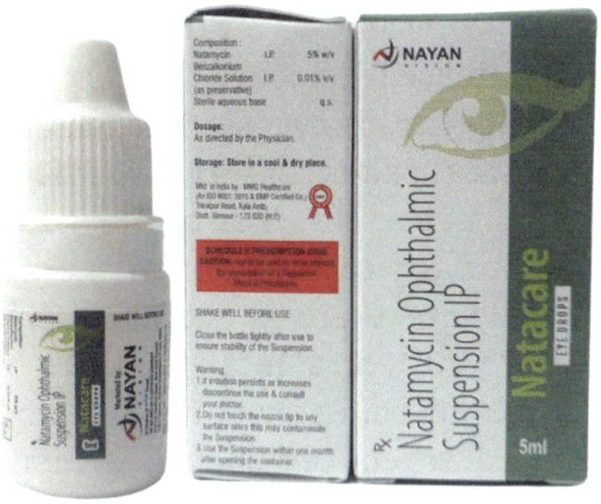

Figure 7.15. Natamycin.

Source: https://ww w.nayanvision. com/public/images/product/ Rf7J7DQ PqylvNhjlcDJhaW5odwwo2m7ptHcMIOhD.jpg.

In treating keratomycosis, clinicians must be aware of resistance and modify the treatment strategy accordingly to optimize patient outcomes. At the end of the day, success of antifungal therapy involves more than basic clinical cure rates; it involves issues of patient compliance and quality of life. Because keratomycosis is a chronic disease process, long-term compliance with therapy can become a problem with some antifungals' side effects.

Effective communication between health care professionals and patients can counteract such issues by producing a better understanding of the treatment regime and its importance. Also, studies on other formulations and delivery systems like combination therapy or adjunct therapy can create easier efficacy and less side effect. This dynamic setting of antifungal therapy highlights the need for continuing research into optimal therapeutic strategies, whereby efficacy is optimized in tolerable treatment regimens (Gummow et al., 2023). With the establishment of an integrated strategy, health professionals can actually improve patient outcomes in this challenging condition (Figure 7.15).

7.4.2. Surgical Interventions for Severe Cases

Surgical intervention comes to the forefront in managing keratomycosis, particularly in its advanced stages after conservative management has been unsuccessful. The traditional therapy begins with topical antifungal medications; however, where there is extensive or central corneal ulceration, a more invasive method must be employed. Referral to a tertiary center is indicated whenever clinical evidence that indicates involvement of the anterior chamber becomes apparent. These procedures may include ulcer debridement, which facilitates proper penetration of topical medications, bolstering the overall outcome of treatment. The success of such surgeries emphasizes the importance of early and appropriate management in patients with serious keratomycosis because prolonged therapy, extending to four weeks or more, becomes pivotal in clearing infection (Tuli et al., 2011). Compounding the complexity of treating keratomycosis is the mixed group of fungal pathogens responsible for causing advanced stages of the condition. To illustrate, deep keratomycosis may be caused by pathogens *Scopulariopsis brevicaulis* and *Fusarium verticillioides*, which are not amenable to traditional therapies. In cases where initial antifungal therapy is unsuccessful, surgical options become a central issue. A case in recent years was successful in management through a combination of surgery and topical treatment, again asserting that surgical debridement of infected tissue can be highly effective in enhancing the effectiveness of subsequent medical interventions.

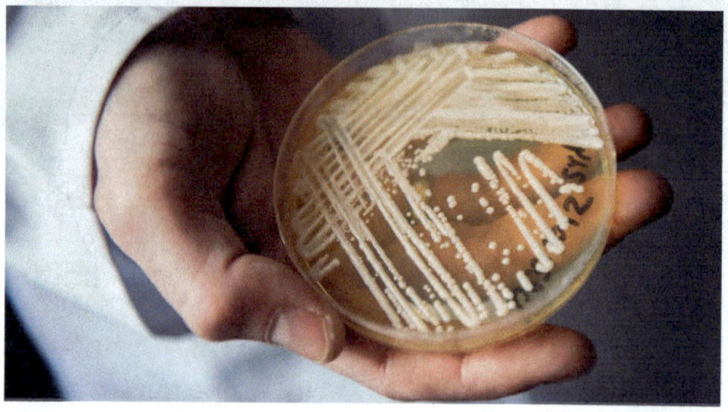

Figure 7.16. Combination therapy, involving the use of multiple antifungal agents, has shown promise in synergistically combating resilient fungal organisms.

Source: https://medicalrealities.com/wp-content/uploads/2025/05/image-131.png.

This approach not only cures the chronic infection but also enables the penetration of antifungal medications deeper, resulting in improved patient outcomes when treating recalcitrant fungal strains (Allbaugh et al., 2021). The addition of surgery in the management of advanced keratomycosis not only provides prompt relief from the infection but is also parallel to advancements in antifungal treatment. Combination therapy involving the use of two or more antifungal drugs has been promising in synergizing the treatment of recalcitrant fungal pathogens. For instance, combined use of caspofungin and terbinafine along with surgical debridement has been said to have promising results. This serves to illustrate the necessity of a multidisciplinary approach, both surgical and pharmacologic, in treating severe instances of keratomycosis appropriately. As more research continues to evolve, such approaches will play an increasingly prominent role in simplifying treatment protocols, thus enhancing the prognosis for individuals afflicted with this potentially vision-destroying disease (Allbaugh et al., 2021) (Figure 7.16).

7.4.3. Role of Supportive Care in Recovery

Support care plays a crucial role in the management of keratomycosis, as it assists antifungal medication and addresses patients' general physical and psychological needs. Support care is a holistic approach, involving not only direct medical interventions but also support intended to enable individuals to cope with the impact of the disease. Since the severe challenges associated with keratomycosis, including potential vision loss or blindness, pose a big risk to patients, working towards a robust supportive care program can enhance patient outcomes. Proper communication between healthcare providers, patients, and relatives is crucial in this situation. By offering a supporting platform, patients are also likely to adhere to treatment plans, receive proper medical assistance in due time, and cooperate fully with the healing process. Thus, supportive care comes forth as a determinant role in the management of keratomycosis, and it has direct effects on recovery pathways and overall quality of life. Integration of supportive care interventions into the treatment of keratomycosis allows for the integrative healing process, reaching out to physical and psychological elements of recovery. Education emerges as a fundamental component among supportive care interventions, which equips patients with necessary knowledge pertaining to the disease and its treatment. Providing patients with information on the nature of keratomycosis, potential complications, and why adhering to antifungal drops is important enables them to be active partners in their care. It is important to avoid misbeliefs regarding the disease, especially in resource-limited settings, where such knowledge may be further tainted by the existence of inappropriate interventions, like corticosteroid eye drops or delayed diagnoses that become driver factors for unfavorable ocular outcomes (Brown et al., 2022).

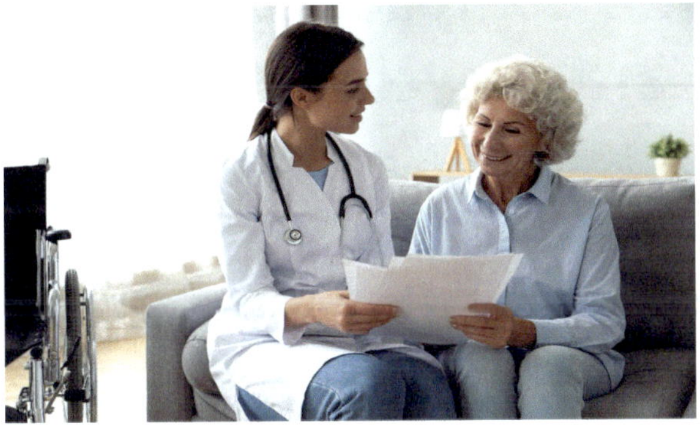

Figure 7.17. Effective communication among healthcare providers, patients, and their families is critical in this context.

Source: https://www.oneeducation.org.uk/wp-content/uploads/2021/09/communication-skills-in-healthcare.jpeg.

Efforts in education can also make clinicians and patients collaborate more efficiently, generating well-trained individuals who are empowered to take an active role in their conditions. Lastly, supportive care has an additional role in the context of trends in antifungal treatment that have been witnessed with novel breakthroughs in ocular formulations like PEG-NLC-AmB to enhance drug delivery as well as efficacy (Lakhani et al., 2019). Such formulations have increased residence time and tissue penetration, which are necessary for successful therapy. The benefit of such advancements is that the patient is able to receive supportive care in the form of constant supervision and advice throughout the course of treatment. Supportive care is able to ensure patients can remain in their normal setting for as long as possible with minimal interference, hence enhanced overall compliance of patients to treatment protocols. Merging therapeutic breakthroughs with care support mechanisms can lead to enhanced clinical results and therefore proves that an integrative approach is central to successful recovery from keratomycosis (Figure 7.17).

7.5. Complications of Keratomycosis

The keratomycosis complications can cause extensive morbidity and permanent vision loss unless they are promptly and effectively treated. One of the significant complications occurs in the form of an atypical occurrence following ocular surgery, e.g., pterygium removal. A case study explains that a patient contracted keratomycosis caused by *Fusarium dimerum* just one month after surgery with the manifestation of a corneal abscess. This identifies the potential for fungal infection to make healing processes more complex, particularly where surgical trauma has opened the corneal epithelium to invasion by pathogens into lower layers of the eye. Although more common following such procedures are bacterial infections, the example shows that fungi can represent a risky but occasional outcome that practitioners must be vigilant against, particularly in patients with additional risk factors or those undergoing similar procedures (Desbois et al.). Further complications may arise as exogenous fungal endophthalmitis (EXFE), an fulminant infection normally reserved for penetrating eye trauma or unmanaged keratitis. Complication often happens a few weeks to months after an inciting incident and may lead to the development of fungi in intraocular structures. The most frequent pathogens in such a situation are molds, with *Aspergillus* species being the most probable culprits. Prompt identification and intervention are crucial, as delay in treatment can lead to permanent ocular damage and loss of vision. Topical, intravitreal, and systemic antifungal treatment are some of the methods adopted to treat this condition, pointing towards cautious clinical management in the event of fungal complications that comprise a small, yet important, part of keratomycosis (Fea et al., 2020). In addition to surgical complications and infections secondary to trauma, keratomycosis can lead to long-standing corneal issues, including scarring and chronic corneal ulcers. These can be due to delayed diagnosis or improper management. Keratomycosis can make patients very uncomfortable with pain, photophobia, and visual loss, hence making their daily lives more difficult. It results in extensive scarring of the corneal stroma, which can make corneal transplantation a last resort to regain the vision. So, an early diagnosis of the symptoms and immediate therapeutic measures are essential to avoid such complications. Education about the risk factors and presentation of keratomycosis is essential for both patients and healthcare providers in order to improve outcomes and minimize the burden of this eye condition (Desbois et al.; Fea et al., 2020).

7.5.1. Potential for Vision Loss

Vision loss risk is a significant concern in keratomycosis, and this serves to emphasize the need for early detection and effective therapeutic intervention. Keratomycosis, or fungal keratitis, typically occurs with redness, pain, and reduced visual acuity that, if left unattended, can lead to severe complications such as corneal scarring or perforation. The disease process associated with keratomycosis is most frequently the result of invasion of the eye by fungal organisms and can be initiated by environmental exposures, contact lens abuse, or ocular trauma. It has been shown that the longer the symptom duration prior to intervention, the greater the risk for permanent ocular tissue damage, ultimately resulting in a heightened risk of visual loss. Vigilance and awareness are thus necessary in reducing the long-term impact of the ocular disease, particularly in immunocompromised patients or with existing ocular surface pathology. Prevention or management of vision impairment requires immediate treatment from a health professional. The treatment used are primarily antifungal medications administered topically, systemically, or through intravitreal injection. Efficiency of these therapies, to a large degree, is dependent on early detection of the etiological organism, which is crucial in directing appropriate therapy. Studies have established that polyenes and azoles are among the classes of antifungal medications commonly used to achieve optimal drug concentration in the vitreous as well as ocular tissues, effectively combating the infection as well as restoring ocular health. Despite such advancements, though, there still remains a window of risk, since a late intervention can rapidly accelerate the condition to lead to complications such as exogenous fungal endophthalmitis, which in turn can aggravate the vision loss possibility (Fea et al., 2020). Doctors must be very vigilant about such matters and prioritize early assessment and management on a high scale in such patients. Surgical interventions may also play a definitive role in the avoidance of vision impairment in keratomycosis. When medical treatment is not effective, other reconstructive procedures like corneal transplantation may be necessary to rehabilitate vision. Amniotic membrane transplantation (AMT) has been a promising adjunct treatment which, if used, may enhance healing and stimulate tissue regeneration on the corneal surface following extensive fungal destruction. AMT has proved to be significantly successful in a number of ocular surface disorders, including keratomycosis, in performing as a biological dressing that aids in epithelial repair and reduces inflammation. Its potential in restoring the corneal anatomy and function emphasizes the status of a multidisciplinary treatment modality in preserving sight, particularly in patients with serious keratitis (Barachetti, 2010). Finally, early diagnosis combined with proper medical and surgical management protocols is essential to reduce the risk of vision loss due to keratomycosis (Figure 7.18).

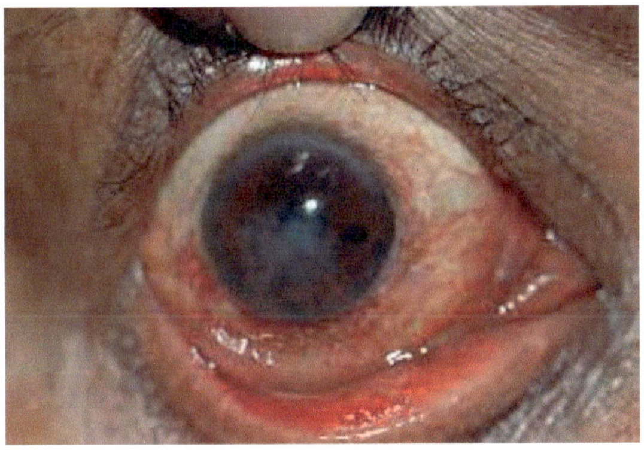

Figure 7.18. The threat of vision loss is a significant concern in cases of keratomycosis, highlighting the need for prompt diagnosis and effective therapeutic interventions.

Source: https://encrypted-tbn0.gstatic.com/images?q=tbn:ANd9GcQ_JmzJ0D9qXY_KdSu4BzX-AeJtCoMZalcPWbffxyAcY88Gy1LWb_Codkeyc_DhvycrViw&usqp=CAU.

7.5.2. Risk of Corneal Scarring

Scarring of the cornea is a significant problem in a patient diagnosed with keratomycosis, an infection caused by fungi that live in the cornea. Scarring generally occurs due to trauma or with contact with organic material, which can infect the eye using the causative organisms including *Candida albicans* and *Fusarium* spp., which are found commonly in fungal keratitis patients. The prevalence of corneal scarring is particularly high in regions that lack easy access to medical treatment, such as developing nations where predisposing factors like trauma and immunocompromised states are prevalent. By the time patients present symptoms of infection, immediate intervention is necessary to save the disease from progression and further damage to the corneal tissue, leading to irreparable scarring and even blindness. Hence, an understanding of keratomycosis causes of corneal scarring is vital in ensuring effective management and prevention (Alli et al., 2013). The interaction of infection and inflammation in keratomycosis significantly contributes to the potential for corneal scarring. Infective keratitis first produces very severe inflammation which, despite being part of the body's immune response, results in widespread corneal tissue damage. This inflammatory process, as a pathological one, can result in scarring that is observable by the eye even after the infection is successfully eradicated. Further, the application of corticosteroids, which are used to abate inflammation, is two-edged; while they can alleviate pain and reduce scarring, they also concurrently suppress the immunity needed to eliminate fungal infection. Consequently, the balance between balancing antifungal therapy and inflammation control is tenuous, particularly considering that the use of steroids in fungal keratitis is not widely established (Keenan et al., 2023). Knowledge of these mechanisms is critical for the best possible design of treatment approaches to keratomycosis. Furthermore, management of corneal scarring in keratomycosis calls for robust clinical acumen and preemptive action.

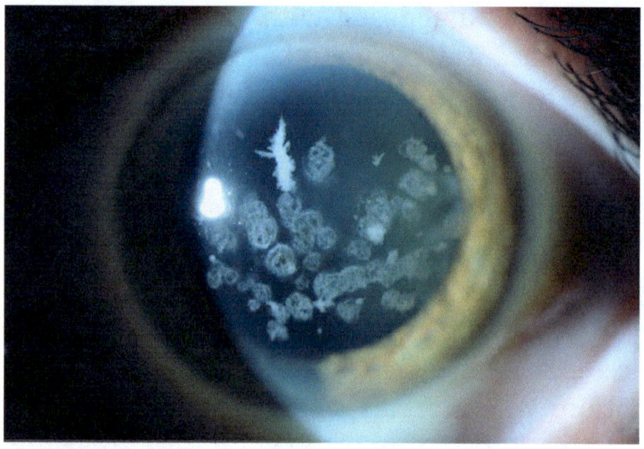

Figure 7.19. Corneal scarring.

Source: https://www.willseye.org/wp-content/uploads/2020/07/Corneal-dystrophy-scaled.jpg.

The clinicians should be cautious about fungal infection in those with history of corneal trauma, particularly vegetable material, to prevent worsening to severe keratitis and its consequences. Existing evidence indicates that corneal scarring ranks among the top causes of monocular blindness and thus deserves regular monitoring and follow-up of vulnerable groups. With increased knowledge of the immunocompromised state and therapeutic intervention impact, prevention mechanisms for incidence and severity of scarring of the cornea will be increasingly significant. Enhanced understanding of the etiologic agents and their treatment can translate into improved outcomes for patients, and additional studies should target developing guidelines for the use of corticosteroids in such infections (Alli et al., 2013) (Figure 7.19).

7.5.3. Systemic Implications of Untreated Infections

The progression of keratomycosis, an infection of the eye caused by fungi, can have significant systemic effects if not managed. Fungal infections, like that of keratomycosis, can penetrate local tissue and even reach the blood, resulting in disseminated infections. As the body attempts to combat the initial infection of the eye, inflammatory mediators and immune responses can result in a generalized response that affects other organs. This systemic inflammatory response syndrome can lead to such complications as organ dysfunction or sepsis, underlining the extremely critical importance of earlier diagnosis and treatment in keratomycosis cases. Additionally, if not treated, keratomycosis can compromise the integrity of the eye, leading to loss of vision and additional complications that can have systemic consequences. Compromise to ocular health might compromise the general health of an individual, resulting in compromised quality of life as well as vulnerability to further infections. The eye is a critical part of the sensory system, and compromised vision might lead to accidents or injury, thereby affecting systemic health. Ocular health being related to general health, ignoring the treatment of keratomycosis complements not only visual impairments but also puts patients at disadvantage in terms of systemic health. Recent advances in drug technology highlight the necessity of creating new efficient ocular drug delivery systems for keratomycosis treatment. For instance, proof has established that the production of electrospun fibers from gellan gum can be used to increase ocular bioavailability of antifungal medication and maximize therapeutic effect while concurrently minimize systemic consequences of treatment deficiency (Göttel et al., 2022). Further, antifungal drug development using cyclodextrins has emerged as a viable route to designing new topical ophthalmic drugs that ensure sustained ocular surface contact while minimizing systemic infection risk (Díaz Tomé et al., 2023). These advances may not only optimize therapeutic outcomes but also highlight the key role for effective treatment of keratomycosis in averting systemic complications from untreated infection (Figure 7.20).

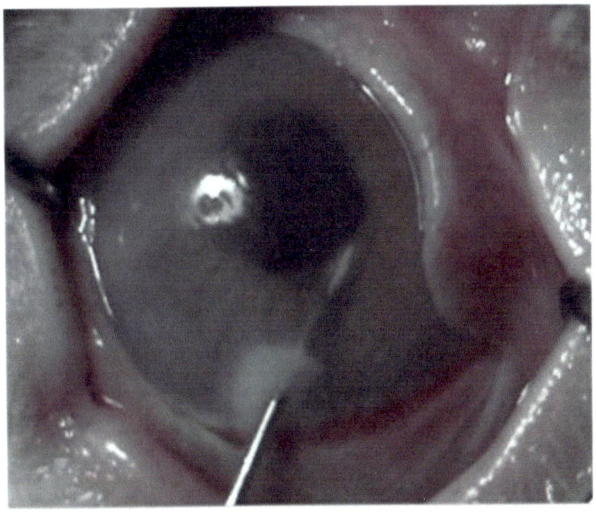

Figure 7.20. Untreated keratomycosis can compromise the integrity of the eye, leading to vision loss and further complications that may have systemic ramifications.

Source: https://ars.els-cdn.com/content/image/1-s2.0-S2214250919302288-gr3.jpg.

7.6. Prevention Strategies

Prevention of keratomycosis, a major cause of corneal blindness, is of significant concern since it is on the increase more than ever before, particularly in tropical and subtropical regions. One of the strategies involves educating communities on the ways of taking care of their eyes, e.g., refraining from unhygienic activities that expose the eyes to environmental pathogens. Public health campaigns may emphasize the risk of bathing or washing the eyes with contaminated water, which can directly deposit fungal spores onto the cornea. Furthermore, health education in the community can highlight the need for prompt visitation to a physician for eye injury or evidence of infection and hence check the onset of blinding diseases like fungal keratitis. By establishing a culture of vigilance with regard to eye care, these prevention mechanisms can reduce the incidence of keratomycosis by a significant amount. In addition to community-level education, designing and implementing creative pharmacy solutions are also critical in preventing the development of keratomycosis. The development of novel antifungal medications that can be delivered topically, such as those in which cyclodextrins play a key role, has emerged as a promising avenue for further enhancing ocular treatments. (Díaz Tomé et al., 2023) presents some topical-ophthalmic formulations focused on maximizing the delivery and efficiency of drugs in treating fungal infection. The innovation ensures that antifungal products become even more efficient in being absorbed by ocular tissues, thus reducing risks of infections. Making such efficient medication available to rural and urban healthcare facilities could bridge the gap in treatment accessibility, leading to reduced cases of keratomycosis ultimately. Such programs not only cure infection better but also develop a robust health infrastructure that can counter the strength of this preventable disease. Lastly, healthcare industries must accord highest priority to implementing guidelines for keratomycosis diagnosis and treatment so that prevention measures are further streamlined. Lack of established protocols can lead to treatment delays, deteriorating conditions of the affected individuals. (Brown et al., 2022) emphasizes the lack of existing guidelines and the urgent need for an integrated framework to guide practitioners in both high- and low-resource settings. Establishing clear diagnostic criteria and treatment protocols will enable healthcare workers to respond more effectively to putative presentations of fungal keratitis. Consequently, increased diagnostic capability can ensure early intervention, averting long-term visual complications. Through joint efforts on both the educational and clinical sides of keratomycosis prevention, stakeholders are able to come together in mitigating this public health hazard to the vision of at-risk populations.

7.6.1. Importance of Proper Eye Hygiene

Proper eye hygiene is relevant in the prevention of a chain of ocular conditions, among them keratomycosis, which may lead to serious visual disability or blindness if not treated promptly. Mycotic keratitis, which is a frequent form of keratomycosis, according to research, has a tendency to be precipitated by factors like vegetable matter trauma or unsanitary practices on the part of agricultural laborers, particularly in the tropics (Premalatha et al., 2017). Precautions to ensure that individuals practice good eye care, including washing hands frequently before accessing the face and avoiding the use of contaminated water for the eyes, can reduce chances of infection. Public education campaigns targeting eye cleanliness could teach vulnerable groups on the need for having clean environments and proper care methods to prevent ocular complications. In addition to overall hygiene protocols, proper use of contact lenses is also a significant aspect of eye care. Many individuals, particularly in situations where keratomycosis is endemic, actually wear contact lenses with insufficient consideration of the risks involved. Improper cleaning and manipulation of contact lenses can transfer microorganisms to the eye, which augments the chance of fungal infections (Ramasundar et al., 2009). In addition, environmental factors like dust or organic contaminants common in farm environments can exacerbate this risk. Therefore, subjects would be taught safe lens wear, i.e., regular replacement schedules and disinfection practices to limit the risk of fungal colonization and associated ocular injury.

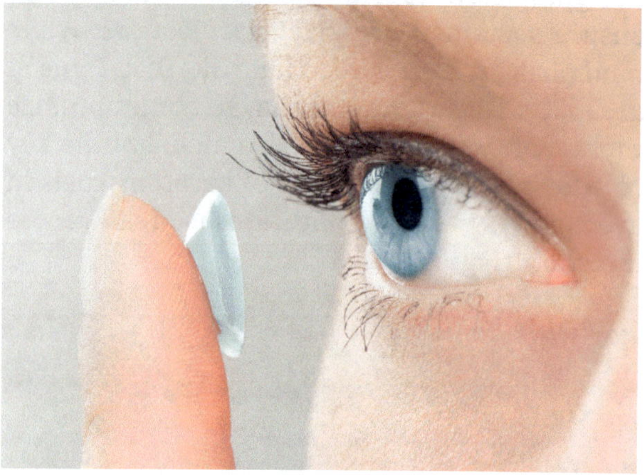

Figure 7.21. Proper eye hygiene is essential in preventing a range of ocular conditions, including keratomycosis, which can lead to significant visual impairment or blindness if left untreated.

Source: https://cdn.sanity.io/images/0vv8moc6/optometrytimes/c97595494e609c814262d8c5961872d28a990b1d-1478x792.png?fit=crop&auto=format.

Also, the promotion of educational programs to focus on the relationship between ocular hygiene and overall eye health is essential in the prevention of keratomycosis spread. Medical professionals need to engage in interaction with communities, especially those highly engaged in agricultural work, to highlight the importance of treating eye injury early since an untreated injury is an entry point for fungal infection

(Premalatha et al., 2017). Regular eye checkup can also enable early detection of abnormalities to enable early intervention after symptoms of keratomycosis start. Through incorporation of teaching on eye hygiene in public health interventions, society can effectively prevent on-the-rise cases of mycotic keratitis and protect people from avoidable vision loss (Figure 7.21).

7.6.2. Protective Measures for at-Risk Populations

The prevalence of keratomycosis in risk groups, particularly vulnerable groups, necessitates the mobilization of special preventive strategies. Individuals at high risk, including those with weakened immunity and pre-existing ocular disorders, require vigilant preventative strategies to avoid maximum exposure to fungal infections. Personal hygiene, cleanliness in the environment, and the necessity for early medical intervention through awareness programs can effectively promote readiness and vigilance among such risk groups. Accessibility of information that describes the signs and risk indicators of keratomycosis can make such a population self-motivated to seek medical care in time, hence reducing the chances of late complications. Additionally, it can be an important platform for community outreach programs to spread information on prevention strategies, resulting in overall resilience against the challenging ocular fungal infection. Prevention of the risk of keratomycosis is crucial, and environmental control plays an essential part, especially where vulnerable populations reside. Increasing air cleanliness and eliminating contact with airborne fungal spores is crucial, especially in hospitals and residential areas where compromised-immunity patients are accommodated. Keeping strict hygiene and sanitation measures in place, particularly in common areas, will serve a long way in prevention of fungal transmission. The use of air filtration equipment, coupled with educating caregivers about the correct procedures for cleaning, can offer a safer space for at-risk patients. These measures, combined with implementation of strict standards for going outside in areas very well known for high fungal spore content, will further enhance security and reduce keratomycosis incidence. Lastly, nutritional interventions also enhance the immune system of susceptible groups to avoid keratomycosis. Clearly established diets with high vitamin and mineral intake can enhance ocular as well as general immune function. Some nutrients have been observed to influence susceptibility to eye infections, thereby even pointing to the role played by personalized dietary counseling in individuals at risk of fungal infection. For instance, promoting the consumption of antioxidant-rich foods has the potential to enhance the body's immunity against fungal infections. As suggested by research correlating diet and ocular illnesses, nutritional enhancement can lead to positive outcomes on conjunctivitis as well as potentially keratomycosis, and thus, the continued study into food recommendations for prevention of such eye ailments is pertinent, including references to seminal research on dietary research on populations (Martins et al., 2022) (Figure 7.22).

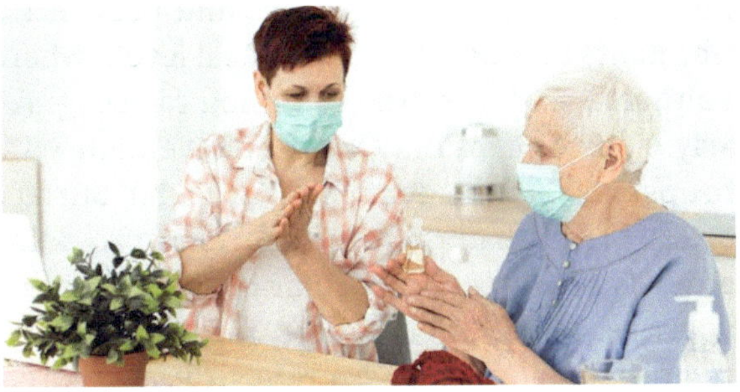

Figure 7.22. The use of air filtration systems, alongside educating caregivers on proper cleaning practices, can create a safer surrounding for susceptible individuals.

Source: https://cdn.growtha.dev/658e94199b4bd43921c76b20/670c9c434ff15097ec9f6f9a_HomeTeam%20(3).jpg.

7.6.3. Public Health Initiatives to Raise Awareness

Public health programs play a key role in educating communities about keratomycosis, which is a severe fungal eye infection that overwhelms communities in tropical regions beyond measure. Communication strategies must be developed and used in an effort to educate communities about the risk factors of keratomycosis, such as poor hygiene, environmental exposure, and utilization of traditional medicines for eye trauma. By using various mediums, including social media, grass roots mobilization, and educational workshops, health organizations can disseminate crucial information. Such initiatives not only inform the public but also create a sense of urgency for preventive measures. Collaboration with local leaders and respected community icons can make messages more credible, thereby increasing outreach and participation. This multi-faceted approach is meant to reach a broader population and potentially reduces keratomycosis incidence via increased public education. Another key strategy involves integrating keratomycosis awareness programs into existing public health infrastructure. This might entail regular screenings and preventive treatments at health centers at local levels where healthcare workers can be trained to recognize early signs of keratomycosis. Involvement with groups such as the Tear Film & Ocular Surface Society (TFOS) can aid these efforts by providing access to resources and ocular health education expertise. TFOS Ambassadors, for instance, can provide sessions to at-risk groups, disseminating the findings and recommendations of current research useful to keratomycosis prevention and management. In addition, data from local research can be used to guide these campaigns so that messaging would ring true with the specific challenges people would face within communities, as would be indicated by continuing research on the etiology and prevalence of keratomycosis among at-risk populations. Public health action against keratomycosis is heavily reliant on community engagement and input. Engaging local communities in the development and evaluation of awareness strategies can lead to more effective programs. For instance, qualitative research, such as research conducted in Sub-Saharan Africa, has established that misconceptions about traditional medicine are significant determinants in the context of keratomycosis. Through communication between healthcare providers and the community, programs can dispel these misconceptions, ensure timely treatment, and establish trust in the healthcare system. Moreover, routine evaluation should be conducted to assess the impact of such interventions on health outcomes. Through the recognition of the community's perspective, public health interventions can further be enhanced to address the needs of the vulnerable population and ultimately reduce the burden of keratomycosis and promote eye health among the population (Figure 7.23).

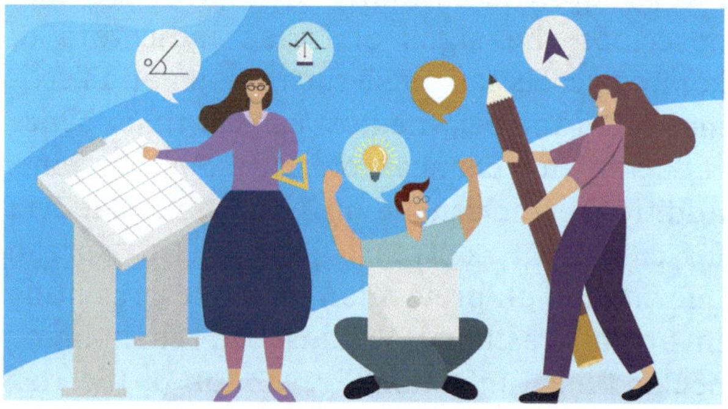

Figure 7.23. Collaborations with local leaders and trusted figures in communities can enhance message credibility, facilitating better outreach and engagement.

Source: https://cdn-cchkmpj.nitrocdn.com/CJXGnJvCvbQYOSNVvxpLvOYcHhpJDKbH/assets/images/optimized/rev-f91b43e/ossisto.com/wp-content/uploads/2024/04/What-is-a-community-engagement-manager.webp.

SUMMARY

When looking at keratomycosis, or fungal keratitis, one of the most important points is the pathology and incidence of the condition in question. Fungal keratitis occurs largely as a result of filamentous fungi and yeasts, with the greatest incidence being described in agricultural areas, especially in poorer nations. This is related to a higher exposure to pathogens as a result of farming-type activities, which adds to the general worldwide burden of the infection. The disease, although relatively uncommon in economically developed nations, is a significant issue on the basis of the differing levels of access to proper healthcare and antifungal treatments. An understanding of the demographic parameters and environmental conditions causing keratomycosis is important in the context of assessing epidemiological trends and establishing effective prophylactic measures. Keratomycosis is difficult to treat, primarily due to the variety of pathogenic fungal species involved and the corresponding efficacy of treatment. Topical Natamycin has been the drug of choice for filamentous fungal infections traditionally, while Amphotericin B is favored in the case of yeast infections. However, Voriconazole is now increasingly becoming a drug of choice due to its broad activity and better penetration in the cornea, as highlighted in recent literature (Tuli et al., 2011). Management of it also entails appropriate clinical assessment to distinguish between local and more complex cases, the former of which may need referral to specialized centers for intensive treatment. This multi-pronged approach emphasizes the need for specific therapy depending on fungal species and clinical presentation to improve outcome and prevent complications, such as corneal perforation. Literature review of existing studies indicates that comparative effectiveness research in antifungal therapy yields inconsistent results, complicating clinical decision-making (Evans et al., 2015). While Natamycin presents superior results in some studies, Voriconazole remains a viable option, particularly for some strains of fungi. Yet, the quality of the existing studies is also heterogeneous with the majority having high risk for bias. The majority of trials focus on short-term clinical outcomes such as cure and visual acuity but refuse to address longer-term effects on compliance with treatment and quality of life. Subsequent research, therefore, should not only aim to account for these discrepancies but also to explore longer-term outcomes and patient-centered measures, ultimately driving technological development in the keratomycosis treatment process and enhancing the quality of patient care.

A CLOSER LOOK

NATAMYCIN

Natamycin is a polyene antifungal medication utilized primarily to treat fungal eye infection, such as keratitis and conjunctivitis. It inhibits by chelating ergosterol within fungal cell membranes, leading to cell lysis. Natamycin most commonly comes as a 5% ophthalmic suspension and is active against fungi like *Fusarium*, *Aspergillus*, and *Cand*ida spp. It has minimal systemic absorption, so it is safe for local use with very few side effects. Besides, it is also employed as a food preservative to retard the development of mold on milk products.

REFERENCES

1. Abarca, E. M., Babu, R. J., Cuming, R. S., Duran, S. H., et al. (2017). Development of a sustained-release voriconazole-containing thermogel for subconjunctival injection in horses. https://core.ac.uk/download/83988258.pdf (accessed on 27th June 2025).
2. Agache, I., Akdis, C. A., Akdis, D., Akdis, M., et al. (2024). The epithelial barrier theory and its associated diseases. https://core.ac.uk/download/636779829.pdf (accessed on 27th June 2025).
3. Aho, R., Brooks, D. E., Brooks, D. E., CLSI, Davis, J. L., European Committee on Antimicrobial Susceptibility Testing, Finnish Meteorological Institute (FMI), et al. (2020). Equine infectious keratitis in Finland: Associated microbial isolates and susceptibility profiles. https://core.ac.uk/download/286810615.pdf (accessed on 27th June 2025).
4. Al Salihi, K. A., Karim, A. J., & Khalaf, J. M. (2021). Buffaloes (*Bubalus bubalis*) mycotic eye infection: Reported herd cases in Thi-Qar province, Iraq. https://core.ac.uk/download/478746551.pdf (accessed on 27th June 2025).
5. Allbaugh, R. A., Bowden, A. C., Foote, B. C., Sebbag, L., et al. (2021). Case report: Successful management of refractory keratomycotic in an alpaca using penetrating keratoplasty and combination antifungal therapy (Caspofungin 0.5% and Terbinafine 1%). https://core.ac.uk/download/478577945.pdf (accessed on 27th June 2025).
6. Alli, A. J., Ashaye, A. O., Bakare, R. A., Fayemiwo, A. S., et al. (2013). Causative agents of keratomycosis in Ibadan: Review of laboratory reports. https://core.ac.uk/download/478291750.pdf (accessed on 27th June 2025).
7. Al-Otaibi, A. G. (2012). Non-viral microbial keratitis in children. https://core.ac.uk/download/pdf/82636611.pdf (accessed on 27th June 2025).
8. Arunga, S. (2025). The epidemiology of microbial keratitis in South Western Uganda. https://core.ac.uk/download/287606692.pdf (accessed on 27th June 2025).
9. Barabino, S., Begovic, E., Benitez-del-Castillo, J. M., Bonini, S., et al. (2020). TFOS European Ambassador meeting: Unmet needs and future scientific and clinical solutions for ocular surface diseases. https://unsworks.unsw.edu.au/bitstreams/237e1df5-4727-410e-b42d-2501bfaae03e/download (accessed on 27th June 2025).
10. Barachetti, L. (2010). Amniotic membrane transplantation for ocular surface reconstruction in veterinary medicine. https://core.ac.uk/download/187845811.pdf (accessed on 27th June 2025).
11. Brown, L., Burton, M. J., Denning, D. W., Kamwiziku, S., et al. (2022). The case for fungal keratitis to be accepted as a neglected tropical disease. https://core.ac.uk/download/571216905.pdf (accessed on 27th June 2025).
12. Chaudhari, D. R., & Chirlekar, R. (2016). Fundamental aspects in the development of microemulsion systems containing amphotericin B for ophthalmic use. https://core.ac.uk/download/230735554.pdf (accessed on 27th June 2025).
13. Desbois, N., Donnio, A., Dueymes, M., Guyomarch, S., et al. (2025). Keratomycotic complicating pterygium excision. https://core.ac.uk/download/pdf/8631833.pdf (accessed on 27th June 2025).

14. Di Pietro, A., Reuben, A., Martinez-Rocha, A. L., Di Pietro, A., Musher, B., de Pauw, B. E., Foster, C. S., et al. (2014). Murine model for *Fusarium oxysporum* invasive fusariosis reveals organ-specific structures for dissemination and long-term persistence. https://core.ac.uk/download/20115566.pdf (accessed on 27th June 2025).

15. Díaz Tomé, V. (2023). Development of topical ophthalmic formulations for fungal keratitis treatment. https://core.ac.uk/download/570984894.pdf (accessed on 27th June 2025).

16. Durand, M. L. (2013). Endophthalmitis. https://core.ac.uk/download/28943507.pdf (accessed on 27th June 2025).

17. Elsheikha, H. M., Khan, N. A., & Siddiqui, R. (2020). Drug discovery against *Acanthamoeba* infections: Present knowledge and unmet needs. https://core.ac.uk/download/323358175.pdf (accessed on 27th June 2025).

18. Evans, J. R., & FlorCruz, N. V. (2015). Medical interventions for fungal keratitis. https://core.ac.uk/download/84659989.pdf (accessed on 27th June 2025).

19. Fea, A. M., De Rosa, F. G., Petrillo, F., Polito, M. S., Galdiero, M., Fallico, M., Reibaldi, M., et al. (2020). Exogenous fungal endophthalmitis: Clues to *Aspergillus* etiology with a pharmacological perspective. https://core.ac.uk/download/534959248.pdf (accessed on 27th June 2025).

20. Göttel, B. N. (2022). *In situ* gelling nanofibers: An innovative strategy for the treatment of keratomycotic. https://core.ac.uk/download/619989577.pdf (accessed on 27th June 2025).

21. Gummow, B., Mo, P. M., & Picard, J. (2023). The conjunctival fungal microflora of horses in a North Queensland tropical environment and their *in vitro* susceptibilities to antifungal agents. https://core.ac.uk/download/577868489.pdf (accessed on 27th June 2025).

22. Kayalvizhi, E. (2009). Isolation and identification of bacterial and fungal agents in patients with corneal ulcer in a tertiary care ophthalmic hospital. https://core.ac.uk/download/235655415.pdf (accessed on 27th June 2025).

23. Keenan, J. (2023). Steroids in the management of infectious keratitis. https://core.ac.uk/download/622529291.pdf (accessed on 27th June 2025).

24. Lakhani, P. M. (2019). PEGylated nanostructured lipid carriers for amphotericin B ocular delivery. https://core.ac.uk/download/288062984.pdf (accessed on 27th June 2025).

25. Liu, D., & Paterson, R. R. M. (2011). *Coprinopsis/Hormographiella*. https://core.ac.uk/download/55633726.pdf (accessed on 27th June 2025).

26. Lues, J. F. R., Malebo, N. J., Setlhare, G. G., Shale, K., et al. (2013). Microbial levels on the food preparation areas of a typical district hospital in South Africa. https://core.ac.uk/download/222967670.pdf (accessed on 27th June 2025).

27. Martins, L. (2022). Allergy to fungi in veterinary medicine: *Alternaria*, dermatophytes and *Malassezia* pay the bill. https://core.ac.uk/download/491624501.pdf (accessed on 27th June 2025).

28. Premalatha, S. (2017). Spectrum of mycotic keratitis and their antifungal susceptibility pattern in a tertiary care hospital, Chennai. https://core.ac.uk/download/327695868.pdf (accessed on 27th June 2025).

29. Ramasundar, P. (2009). A study of fungal diseases of nose and paranasal sinuses. https://core.ac.uk/download/235654338.pdf (accessed on 27th June 2025).

30. Ravikumar, K. (2006). A study on 100 cases of keratomycoses to compare the efficacy of topical 10% sodium chloride with 5% natamycin versus 5% natamycin alone as a treatment strategy. https://core.ac.uk/download/235656733.pdf (accessed on 27th June 2025).
31. Tuli, S. S. (2011). Fungal keratitis. https://core.ac.uk/download/pdf/8545706.pdf (accessed on 27th June 2025).
32. Vasanthapriyan, M. R. (2011). Study on isolation and identification of fungal agents in patients with corneal ulcer in tertiary care ophthalmic hospital. https://core.ac.uk/download/235654820.pdf (accessed on 27th June 2025).

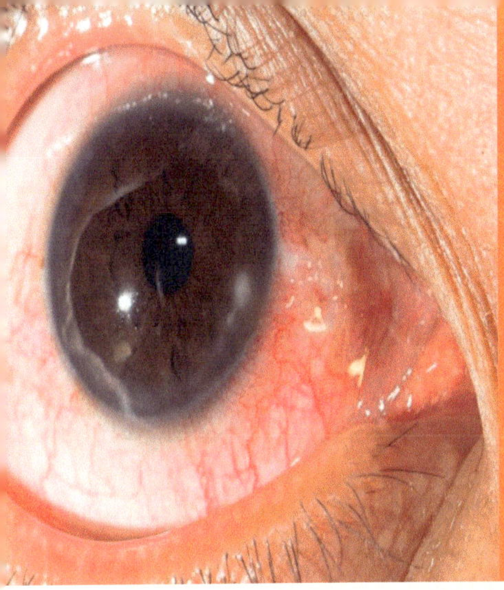

Chapter 8
OTOMYCOSIS

Contents

Introduction

Otomycosis, which is a frequent fungal infection of the outer ear, is largely coupled with severe pain and discomfort for those afflicted by it. It is seen to contribute to more than 9% of the cases of external otitis, with some 80% of its cases being due to the *Aspergillus* genus (Ali et al., 2024). The condition is predominantly seen in individuals who are constantly exposed to humidity or users of hearing aids, thus being extremely susceptible to fungal colonization within the external auditory canal. Understanding otomycosis dynamics would be essential for both clinical practice and public health because proper diagnosis and treatment at an early stage would significantly reduce the symptoms as well as the quality of life among sufferers. The therapy of otomycosis, in the majority of instances, employs antifungal agents, whose success is most commonly ascribed to the combination treatment. A systematic review of the condition has mentioned the therapeutic effect of patients' reactions to both Betadine and Clotrimazole, testifying to their high therapeutic effectiveness (Ali et al., 2024). In particular, symptom severity before and after treatment are analyzed with harsh contrasts for example, the patients had a significantly reduced symptom score after the intervention. This indicates that it is imperative to employ a customized approach towards treatment because response varies so widely based on several factors, including age, overall health, and individual clinical presentations specific to the infection.

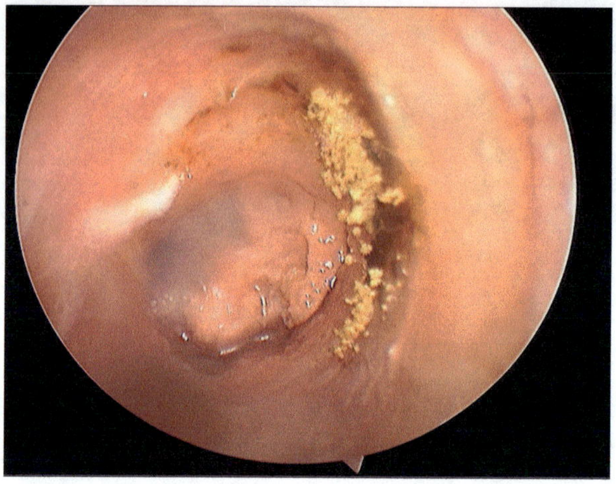

Figure 8.1. Otomycosis.

Source: https://img1.wsimg.com/isteam/ip/6f769e17-ab0a-4d5f-9481-df0b962b6689/IMG_20240720_185009.jpg.

Moreover, patient profiles for otomycosis have marked trends that may be employed to inform prevention. Research establishes a peak incidence rate of the infection among individuals 40 to 49 years of age, suggesting an association between work or lifestyle factors and increased exposure to risk (Ali et al., 2024). Symptoms are usually itching, which is present in a high percentage of patients, and pain that disrupts daily activity. Identification of such populations enables healthcare providers to better serve vulnerable populations by educating them on prevention strategies, including proper ear hygiene and prudent protection of the ears from water exposure. Addressing treatment and prevention in a comprehensive manner, the treatment of otomycosis can be significantly enhanced, eventually resulting in improved patient outcomes (Figure 8.1).

8.1. Causes of Otomycosis

Otomycosis etiology is varied, and the pathology tends to lie on environmental factors that create an optimum breeding ground for fungi. The outer canal of the ear, characterized by a warm and humid environment, is most susceptible to a fungal infection. This optimum environment offers the ideal situation for the growth of fungi, and this leads to an infection with symptoms such as itching and pain. The most common causative agent is *Aspergillus* species and is accountable for most of the reported cases. Recent studies have shown that individuals in the age group of 40-49 years had the highest infection rates, which can be suggestive of either pre-existing susceptibility or yet to be understood exposure patterns (Ali et al., 2024). This susceptibility of the population can be attributed to lifestyle choices or wear of such devices as hearing aids that can allow water to pool inside the ear canal unintentionally. Apart from external risk factors, individual risk factors also contribute significantly towards the development of otomycosis. Individuals who are immunocompromised, for example, diabetics or individuals suffering from chronic illnesses, are highly susceptible to fungal infection since their immune reactions are less effective (Naseeruddin et al., 2011). Moreover, behavior such as prolonged water immersion or behavior that causes irritation of the ear canal can predispose one to otomycosis occurrence. For instance, taking a shower or swim without thoroughly drying the ears can lay down moisture conducive to fungal growth. Furthermore, the improper use of cotton swabs disrupts the ears natural protection, leading to damage that creates a window for entry by fungi. The treatment not only involves curing the fungal infection but also removing these risk factors to keep recurrence rates in check. Treatment of otomycosis is antifungal-based, involving clotrimazole and betadine, which have been found effective in curing the disease (Ali et al., 2024). However, the underlying reasons for the fungal infection must be treated in order to treat the condition in the long run. Treatment can be successful and may differ based on the overall health of the patient because those who are immunocompromised will require more aggressive and longer treatment and higher recurrence rates (Naseeruddin et al., 2011). The intricacy of treating otomycosis highlights the value of an integrated approach with educating the patient on prevention of moisture buildup and minimizing irritants to the ear. Through treating the acute fungal infection and the causative factors, medical practitioners are then better positioned to help patients control and even prevent recurrent instances of otomycosis (Figure 8.2).

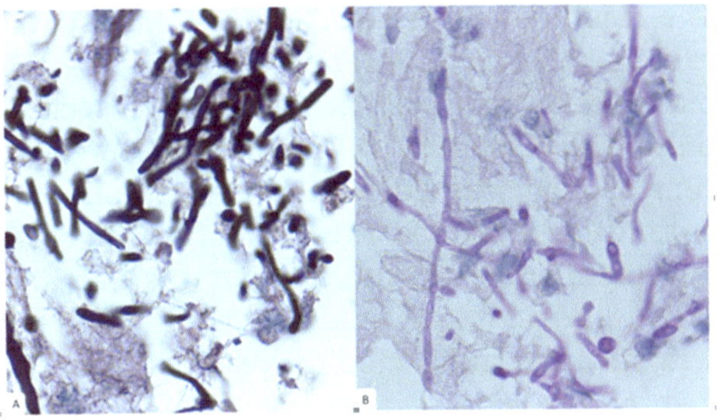

Figure 8.2. The most common causative agent is *Aspergillus* species, which accounts for a majority of recorded cases.

Source: https://clinicsearchonline.org/uploads/articles/external/0-49440900-1685450171.png.

8.1.1. Fungal Pathogens Involved

Of the numerous fungal pathogens that have been reported to cause otomycosis, the most prevalent ones are *Aspergillus* species and *Candida* species. *Aspergillus niger* is the most prevalent isolate, which accounts for a high percentage of cases. *Aspergillus niger* is a filamentous fungus that proliferates best under warm and humid temperatures and therefore is a very significant pathogen where otomycosis is most prevalent, i.e., in tropical and subtropical parts of the world. *Aspergillus* spp. grow and survive. within the external ear canal can lead to inflammation, discomfort, and itchiness, therefore great discomfort for infected patients. The understanding of their own role in the disease is crucial for accurate diagnosis and effective treatment, since studies have indicated increased prevalence of *Aspergillus niger* in combined infections complicating the treatment process and implying the necessity for evidence-based therapeutic approaches (Ajay et al., 2012). Aside from *Aspergillus* species and *Candida* species, and most notably *Candida auris*, have emerged as serious health issues in recent years. *C. auris* is unique in that it is able to form biofilms, which by their very nature enhance the resistance of the organism to antifungal treatment and create difficulties within clinical settings. The increasing incidence of *C. auris* infections, with the added feature of multidrug resistance, complicates the treatment of otomycosis, when this pathogen is responsible. In addition, misidentification of *C. auris* can further hinder ideal treatment interventions, with precise diagnostic methods being a priority. The progression of *C. auris* and mechanisms of resistance necessitate further research on effective treatments in overcoming the barrier, emphasizing the importance of determination of the exact fungal pathogens involved in each case for ideal planning of management interventions (Brás et al., 2021). The higher otomycosis rates mean that there is an even greater necessity for more information regarding the characteristics of the involved fungal pathogens. The host factor interaction, such as anatomical variation, levels of humidity, and immune status, is crucial for the onset of disease. A patient history of ear canal self-cleaning can predispose them to fungus infections since such an action might rupture the natural barrier provided by the cerumen (earwax). Furthermore, predisposing factors such as humidity and skin integrity play an important role in favoring the growth of fungi. This synergy indicates the necessity of integrated management procedures that target not only the pathogens but also the predisposing factors and overall well-being of the ear canal environment. Robust clinical interventions with intensive diagnostics and advanced therapy will ultimately improve results for all who suffer from otomycosis (Ajay et al., 2012) (Figure 8.3).

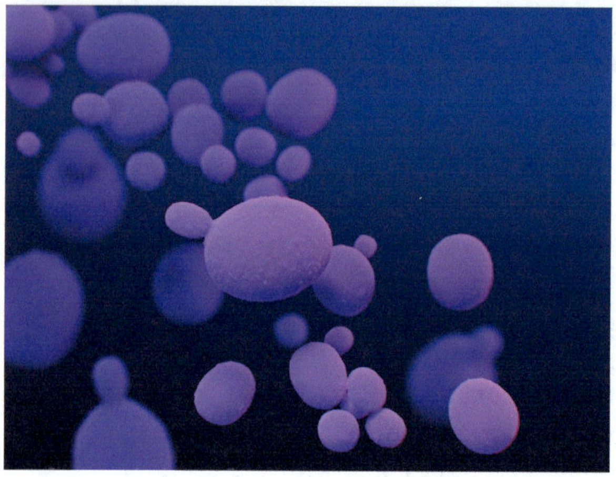

Figure 8.3. The increasing incidence of *C. auris* infections, characterized by multidrug resistance, complicates the management of otomycosis when this pathogen is involved.

Source: https://www.mdpi.com/jof/jof-09-00913/article_deploy/html/images/jof-09-00913-g001.png.

8.1.2. Risk Factors for Developing Otomycosis

Development of otomycosis, a fungal infection of the external auditory meatus, is made possible by various risk factors that predispose a person to the condition. Among these is ear moisture, most often due to excess swimming or bathing. Warm and humid environments present an ideal habitat for fungi that thrive in such environments. Therefore, individuals who expose their ears to water regularly without protection or drying them are prone to developing otomycosis. This is particularly the case in communities that practice water sports or humid climates. Utmost awareness of such environmental and behavioral nuances is crucial in an effort to minimize the vulnerability of fungal ear infections among susceptible persons. Additionally, anatomical factors also play a key role in the causation of otomycosis. Individuals with anatomical abnormalities, i.e., narrow ear canal or excessive earwax hypersecretion, may be more prone to fungal infections. These anatomical predispositions lead to the entrapment of moisture and dirt in the ear, which increases the chance of infection. Moreover, certain chronic medical illnesses, such as diabetes or immunocompromised conditions, weaken the body's resistance to fungal infection. The concomitance of these health conditions with risk of otomycosis underscores the value of targeted prevention in high-risk populations. The resolution of these anatomical and health-related factors is essential in reducing the incidence of otomycosis in individuals, especially those with confirmed predispositions. Moreover, some otologic practice and interventions can potentially enhance the risk of otomycosis development. Over-cleansing of the ear and the use of topical medications in the ear without consulting medical practitioners can disturb the ear's natural flora. Uncontrolled use of ear drops, particularly those containing antifungals, might be the cause of disorder in the ears microbial balance with a bias towards opportunistic development of fungi. To address these concerns, studies confirm that healthcare experts need to embrace practices for safer ear care interventions, particularly among patients with current infection or disorders of the ears. This entails careful use of topical substances and educating the patients on the importance of seeking professional medical experts' advice on issues concerning the ears' health in order to prevent otomycosis and maintain overall hearing wellness (M et al., 2017; Aziz et al., 2020) (Figure 8.4).

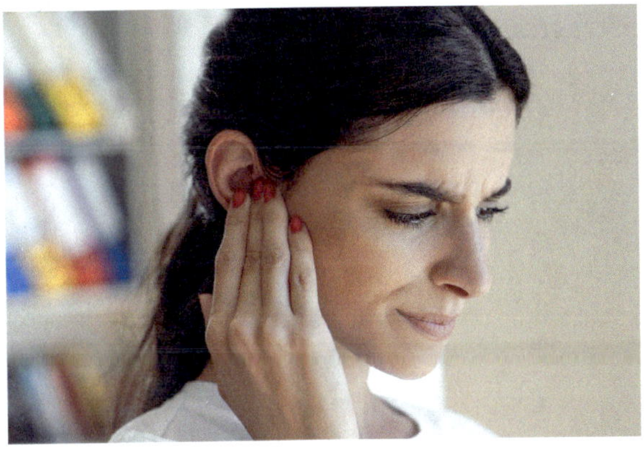

Figure 8.4. One significant factor is the presence of moisture in the ear, often resulting from excessive swimming or bathing.

Source: https://assets.clevelandclinic.org/m/63172d6aabadfaa1/webimage-ear-1731055025.png.

8.1.3. Environmental Conditions Contributing to Infection

The widespread nature of otomycosis, particularly in warm climatic zones and in individuals presenting certain risk factors, underlines the importance of environmental factors in the etiology of fungal infection of the ear. Warm temperature and high humidity are conducive to the growth of fungi, particularly of *Aspergillus* and *Candida* species. Evidence shows that such conditions significantly increase the risk of infection since high levels of moisture make it easy for fungi to thrive (Karami et al., 2019). In addition, behaviors that destroy the pH balance in the ear canal, such as swimming or excessive cleaning, can further expose individuals to otomycosis in such vulnerable surroundings. Greater understanding of how such conditions predispose the patient towards fungal colonization can also serve to enhance prevention and therapy measures to combat the incidence of otomycosis in various groups that are at risk. Geographic and socio-economic factors also play tremendous roles in the incidence of otomycosis, particularly in developing nations. Scarce healthcare centers are usually the culmination of issues in the diagnosis and treatment of ear infections. Where preventive practices, such as education concerning ear cleanliness and early intervention, are weak, the likelihood of otomycosis is very high.

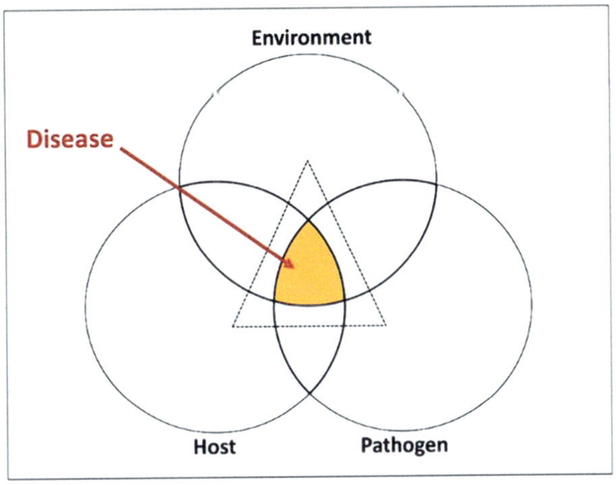

Figure 8.5. As fungi often infect patients already colonized by resistant bacterial strains, the environmental dynamics influencing such resistances may contribute to an increase in the severity and duration of otomycosis.

Source: https://www.mdpi.com/pathogens/pathogens-13-00426/article_deploy/html/images/pathogens-13-00426-g001-550.jpg.

Fungal infection can dominate where the subjects continually come into contact with water, accompanied by poor practice in ear drying and cleanliness. Thus, these socio-cultural aspects highlight the interconnection between environmental causes and health outcomes. Therefore, therapy for such imbalances can lead to a reduction in otomycosis cases in vulnerable populations (Angelis et al., 2023). Care should also be taken against the establishment of resistance to antibiotics by bacterial pathogens, complicating clinical management of otomycosis. Because fungi preferentially infect already colonized patients by strains of resistant bacteria, environmental situations influencing such resistances can lead to the exacerbation and prolongation of otomycosis. Misuse of antibiotics in human treatment and agriculture has the ability to disrupt the microbial balance and create situations favorable to fungal growth (Angelis et al., 2023). Additionally, the application of certain agricultural produce and their environmental by-products inherently enhances fungal virulence. This requires comprehensive environmental assessments in infection dynamics research, as such conditions not only account for traditional risk indicators but also the emerging issues presented by resistant pathogens in otomycosis research (Figure 8.5).

8.2. Symptoms of Otomycosis

Otomycosis, or fungal infection of the external auditory canal, is marked by a host of signs and symptoms that significantly contribute to the morbidity of the patient. The most striking symptom is pruritus, reported by approximately 70% to 80% of patients, which leads to discomfort and increased vulnerability to further inflammation. Irritation due to mechanical scratching-induced inflammation can compromise the cover of the skin, further increasing the infective potential. In addition, patients normally experience ear pain that varies in severity and may develop into a chronic condition if not treated. Pain is accompanied by ear fullness and will impact daily activities, further demystifying the impact of otomycosis on the health and day-to-day life of the patients (Ali et al., 2024). Appreciation of these symptoms is important for early diagnosis and treatment, and symptom awareness is an important element of successful management. In a few instances, otomycosis patients can present with changes in hearing as well, like muffled hearing or even transient loss of hearing. The symptoms are due to the collection of fungal debris and inflammation within the ear canal, resulting in obstruction.

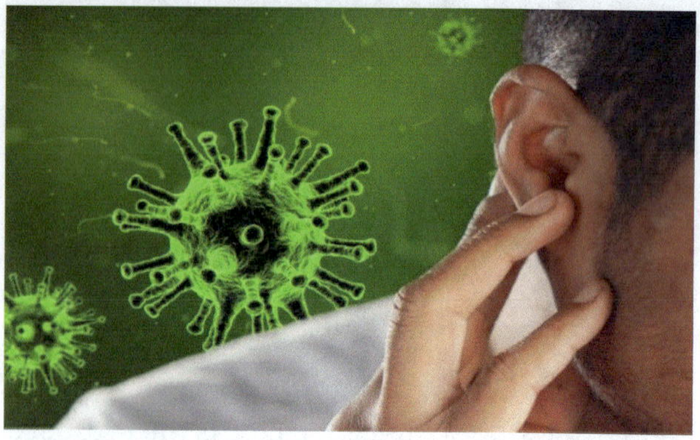

Figure 8.6. Mechanical irritation from excessive scratching can compromise the skin barrier, potentially exacerbating the infection.

Source: https://drdarakshanent.com/wp-content/uploads/2025/02/Fungal-Infections.jpg.

These hearing disturbances also cause worry and loneliness in the patients who depend on unobstructed hearing for communication and interaction. Notably, discharge (which can be preceded by an offensive smell) could also occur, which further contributes to the clinical presentation. Observations of these signs in a holistic way are important for healthcare workers so that appropriate assessment is conducted leading to treatment and care interventions (Akram et al., 2023). As the infection progresses, chronic illness might result, causing long-term discomfort and other effects on the patient's wellbeing, thus the need for prompt medical treatment. The success of treatments for otomycosis depends to a great extent on early recognition of its symptoms and resultant therapy. Clinical findings indicate that clotrimazole and isoconazole nitrate have yielded variable success in alleviation of symptoms, radically improving the patient's quality of life following treatment. For instance, one study identified that the majority of patients reported notable relief from symptom severity upon receiving isoconazole nitrate treatment, which shows its potential as an ideal treatment. Alternatively, other interventions such as Nystatin were less effective, illustrating the importance of making evidence-based choices for managing otomycosis (Akram et al., 2023). Considering the impact of the symptoms on daily functioning and potential chronicity, the availability of a timely and effective treatment plan is imperative to the alleviation of the discomfort endured by the patient with this disorder (Figure 8.6).

8.2.1. Common Signs and Symptoms

Otomycosis, a disease of the outer ear canal in the majority of cases, is characterized by a series of common signs and symptoms that will significantly impact a patient's quality of life. The most common reported symptom is the intense itching, affecting virtually 80.43% of patients suffering from this disease. This sensation may prompt individuals to play with their ears in an attempt to alleviate the discomfort, further complicating the condition. In addition, hearing loss is also frequently encountered in around 78.26% of patients, with debris and fungus accumulation in the ear canal. Blockage sensation is also frequently felt by the majority of patients to the extent of around 73.91% of cases, which might increase the pain and nourish frustration and anxiety regarding their capacity to hear, hence emphasizing the importance of detecting these signs in an effort to intervene in time (Darmawan et al., 2024). The clinical presentation of patients of otomycosis is characterized by a variety of findings that further confirm the conditions effect. A typical finding is the presence of a fungal mass in 100% of cases studied. The fungal mass is normally represented as a white, grayish material with a mixed texture and density according to the causative fungal agent. This is accompanied by the occurrence of discharge from the ear in approximately 64.04% of patients, ranging from serous to purulent consistency. Tympanic membrane perforation occurs in approximately 60.87% of patients, which accounts for more severe cases of otomycosis that require urgent treatment.

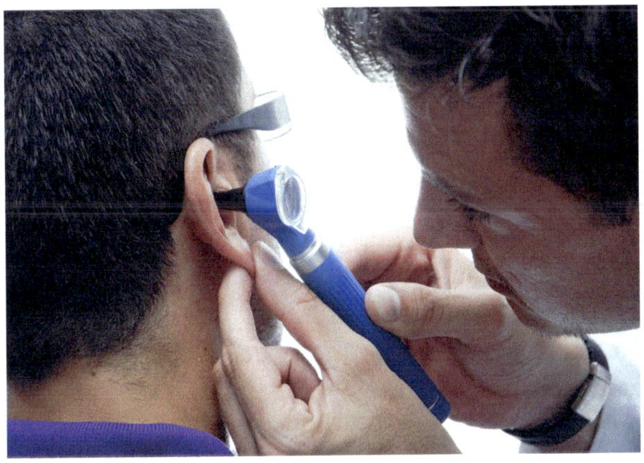

Figure 8.7. Delaying diagnosis and treatment of otomycosis can lead to complications and prolonged suffering due to its uncomfortable symptoms.

Source: https://cdn-prod.medicalnewstoday.com/content/images/articles/321/321910/doctor-examining-otomycosis.jpg.

These symptoms coupled with the attendant signs are crucial to clinical diagnosis and management of the condition, necessitating higher patient and health worker awareness (Aziz et al., 2020). Otomycosis delayed treatment and diagnosis can lead to complications and prolonged misery due to its painful nature. Widespread sign and symptom reporting requires those experiencing ear pain to seek medical attention promptly. Particularly, the apparent relationship between signs and symptoms can be instructive to clinicians in creating effective treatment regimens. For instance, a comparative study established that some antifungal treatments have been equivocal in efficacy, with 7.5% Povidone-iodine being more efficacious at clearing both symptoms and signs compared to

1% Clotrimazole ear drops and lignocaine (Aziz et al., 2020). This comprehension of successful treatment supports the importance of ongoing research and education about otomycosis because familiarity with typical symptoms and signs can lead to quicker solutions and better patient outcomes (Figure 8.7).

8.2.2. Variability in Symptoms Based on the Causative Fungus

The variability of the symptom in otomycosis is also significantly influenced by the causative organism of the fungus. The most common implicated samples are *Aspergillus* and *Candida* species. The outcomes in *Aspergillus* species infections tend to be more acute and typically lead to intense itching, pain, and black discharge typical of the disease, which may be indicative of the virulence pattern of the organisms. The presence of these clinical manifestations concurs with the findings that emphasize the fungus capacity to produce virulence factors such as biofilms and mycotoxins, especially aflatoxins, which further exacerbate tissue inflammation and irritation. In addition, the symptoms may also be accompanied by fullness or pain in the ear, impacting the quality of life of the patient.

This calls attention to the remarkable ability of different fungal pathogens to adjust and to their modalities of interacting with the host immune apparatus, and provides a clue that the therapy for otomycosis must be choreographed in accordance with the particular fungi responsible for a case. *Candida* organisms, particularly *Candida albicans*, have been implicated in otomycosis with comparatively milder symptomatology than *Aspergillus*. *Candida* patients may present with less severe itching and white discharge, which is of creamy description. The relatively benign presentation of symptoms of *Candida* infections can be attributed to the organisms unique interaction with the immune defense of the host, which in certain instances may limit the extent of mucosal damage. Notably, studies have indicated that *Candida* infection has the ability to induce biofilm formation in the ear canal, which needs long courses of treatment to efficiently clear fungi. Thus, the clinical presentation depends not only on the etiologic pathogen but also on the patient factors like immune status, so a wide variety of potential symptoms related to otomycosis (Jayachitra et al., 2018).

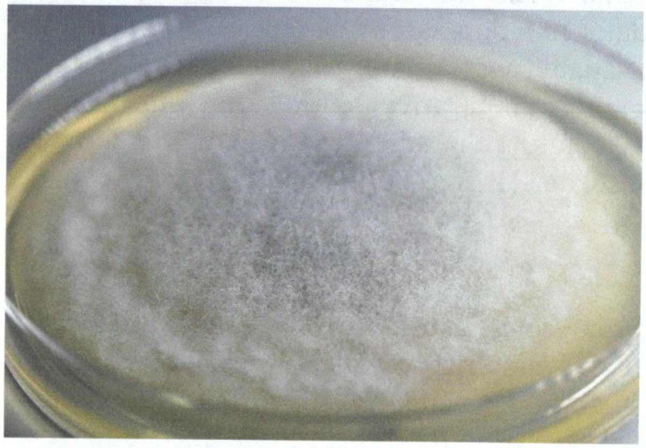

Figure 8.8. *Rhizomucor.*

Source: https://i.redd.it/70ucw0vf2aq21.jpg.

8.2.3. Impact of Symptoms on Daily Life

Less commonly, other fungal genera such as *Cladosporium* and *Rhizomucor* produce otomycosis with varying symptoms. Incidence of these less common pathogens also bears secondary symptoms such as chronic irritation and long-term sensation of fullness in the ear in comparison to the more typical presentations with *Candida* or *Aspergillus*. These fungi are more likely to have less typical symptoms, typically rendering exact diagnosis impossible and necessitating more extensive clinical evaluations. Moreover, the identification highlights the importance of knowledge regarding the diverse nature of fungi found in the external auditory canal because environmental factors and personal habits, such as ear cleansing habits, may lead to outbreaks among different species of fungi. Thus, this signifies the necessity of the patient receiving a tailored diagnosis and treatment approach, as the efficacy of the treatment can hugely vary from one causative agent to the other (Resca et al., 1948) (Figure 8.8).

The presence of otomycosis seriously disrupts the daily life of an individual due to its predisposed nature, which in most instances manifests as ear ache. Most of the patients complain of persistent itching and discomfort in the ear canal, which may divert their attention from normal behaviors such as work, school, or recreational activities. Moreover, this discomfort can lead to a higher degree of irritability and anxiety since the lack of control over the symptoms can provide room for repetitive thinking or worrying regarding the condition. Because otomycosis is usually symptomatic of hearing impairment and aural fullness, people would find it challenging to engage in conversations or activities that involve auditory attention, thus leading to isolation and compromised quality of life. Such implications are meant to highlight the overwhelming emotional and psychological load that otomycosis symptoms can put on a person, the need for proper management and treatment in consequence.

Besides pain, otomycosis has massive social implications due to its symptoms, which typically involve ear discharge. This release can be an acute cause of embarrassment for the affected individuals, leading to avoidance of public and social activities. Fear of judgment or stigma, especially from colleagues or peers, can further enhance feelings of self-consciousness and apprehension, restricting social interactions further. Furthermore, when signs such as hearing impairment develop, individuals may withdraw from social interactions entirely or rely on others to assist them, which suggests a likely change in interpersonal relationships. These alterations can enhance increased feelings of loneliness and alienation, implying that the impact of otomycosis extends from mere physical manifestations to have far-reaching effects on interpersonal relationships and social well-being, which are essential for good mental health and general satisfaction with life. The chronic nature of otomycosis, particularly in immunocompromised individuals, can render it difficult for the impact of symptoms on daily life. The severity of the symptoms necessitates prolonged treatment cycles, leading to frequent hospital visits and possible work or academic interference. As (Arijit et al., 2017) describes, a patient whose immune system has been weakened suffers greater complications, which further make their state of health worse, hence leaving them trapped in a vicious cycle of sickness and increased symptom burden. This can turn into a time-consuming situation spent managing symptoms rather than doing enjoyable activities or work. To boot, frequent symptoms like tinnitus can lead to sleep disruptions, causing fatigue and impaired cognitive function during the day. These effects not just drain one's ability to perform daily tasks effectively but also contribute to the decline of physical and emotional well-being, thus the need for complete care and management of otomycosis (Figure 8.9).

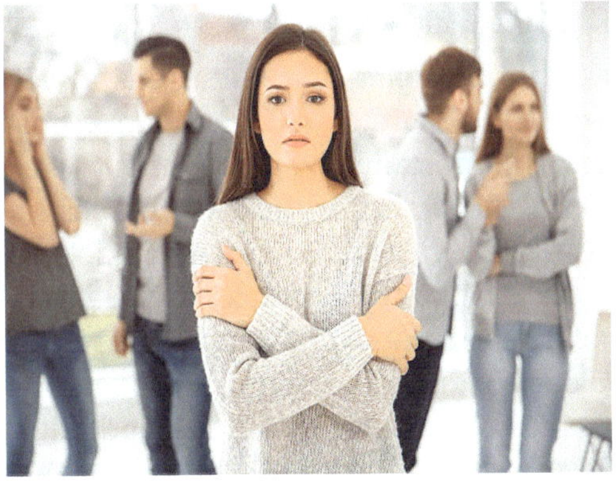

Figure 8.9. Fear of judgment or stigma, particularly from peers or colleagues, can exacerbate feelings of self-consciousness and anxiety, further limiting social interactions.

Source: https://patnaneuroandchildpsychiatry.in/wp-content/uploads/2025/01/Why-Social-Anxiety-Disorder-Happens.jpg.

8.3. Diagnosis of Otomycosis

The diagnosis of otomycosis is mostly dependent on a thorough clinical examination and taking of history to search for characteristic signs. The patients typically present with a complaint of pruritus, otalgia, ear fullness, and occasionally hearing impairment. Indeed, literature indicates that pruritus is seen in up to 88.73% of the cases, pain and discomfort in 72.09% of the patients with this condition. The environmental factor consideration by the clinician, such as humidity and swimming habits, is most important in detecting risk factors that predispose an individual to fungal infection. Diagnostic procedures can also incorporate otoscopy to look at purulent discharge, debris, or mycelium growth within the external ear canal, thus being part of making a definite diagnosis of otomycosis. The laboratory tests are also important in the confirmation of the diagnosis of otomycosis, particularly through microbiological culture. Fungal specimens are aspirated with ear canal swabbing and cultured to identify the-species of infection. *Aspergillus* species, particularly *Aspergillus niger* and *Aspergillus flavus,* have been reported to be significant pathogens in various studies and, therefore, identification of the species is important in the treatment planning (Ali et al., 2024). In addition, the association of the fungal species with patient demographics and corresponding systemic diseases will supplement the clinical strategy. For instance, the prevalence of diabetes mellitus or chemotherapy may indicate enhanced susceptibility to otomycosis, necessitating intervention strategies according to the patients' individual health status. Treatment of otomycosis relies on accurate diagnosis and determination of the etiologic agent, with antifungal therapy serving as the cornerstone of treatment. Such successful treatments as betadine and clotrimazole have seen good success with studies showing significant relief in patients' symptoms after treatment (Ali et al., 2024). Follow-up evaluation again supports the need for monitoring treatment efficacy, as symptom severity scores have been demonstrated to significantly improve, indicative of a favorable response to antifungal treatment. In the case of complications arising or the patient returning with recurrent infection, further investigation may be necessary to address underlying conditions. Ultimately, successful diagnosis and treatment of otomycosis requires a recognition and multidisciplinary approach incorporating both clinical acumen and evidence-based treatment protocol (Figure 8.10).

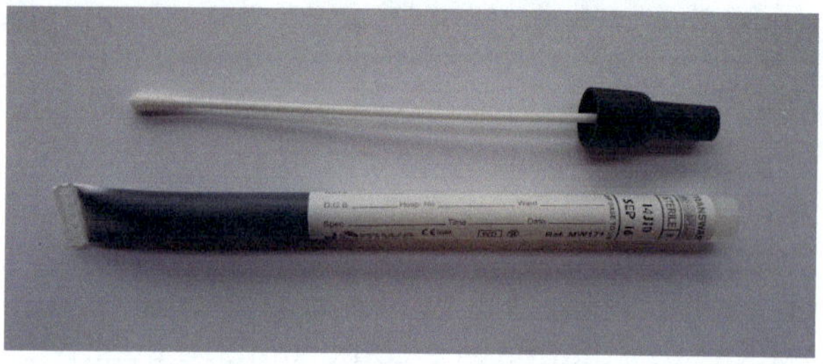

Figure 8.10. Fungal specimens are obtained via swabs of the ear canal and cultured to identify the-species responsible for the infection.

Source: https://www.exeterlaboratory.com/wp-content/uploads/charcoal-swab.jpg.

8.3.1. Clinical Examination Techniques

Clinical examination techniques are important in the diagnosis of otomycosis, a prevalent fungal infection of the external ear. The assessment begins with thorough patient history, beginning with the onset history of symptoms such as itchiness, pain, and discharge. Patients context, including hearing aid use or water exposure, gives clues about the potential risk factors. This is accompanied by a physical examination where an otoscope is used to inspect the ear canal and tympanic membrane. During the inspection, the clinicians can view common evidence of otomycosis such as inflammatory and fungal debris that have the capability of directing treatment selection. The clinical processes used during evaluation in addition to confirming diagnosis support determination of the severity of infection, which ultimately results in effective curative intervention. Following the examination, the process involves the use of the respective clinical methods for assessment of treatment outcomes. In a recent study of 110 patients with otomycosis, researchers quantitatively documented symptom severity before and after treatment with pain and discomfort scales. This uniform procedure facilitated an appropriate evaluation of the efficacy of antifungals such as betadine and clotrimazole. The results showed a substantial reduction in symptom scores from a mean of 89.10 ± 4.25 during the initial visit to 11.79 ± 2.58 following treatment. These clinical practices are part of the foundation of an evidence-based practice, as they not only represent an indicator of the success of treatment but also allow for greater patient outcomes and quality of life, as seen in the recorded outcomes of decrease in both pain and symptoms. Furthermore, the utilization of follow-up visits cannot be overemphasized in clinical management of otomycosis. Follow-up clinic visits are crucial to ascertain that healing is on course and to manage complications when they arise. During these visits, clinicians can adapt exam techniques to incorporate assessments for residual fungal infection in the ear canal. In the aforementioned study, an impressive 87 patients responded favorably to betadine treatment by the second visit and 97 patients to clotrimazole. Such details emphasize the need for constant monitoring and modification of treatment regimens based on unique patient reactions. Ultimately, clinical examination techniques not only facilitate early detection but also promote a more participatory approach to managing otomycosis, so that treatment protocols remain effective and tailored to the unique demands of each patient and thereby optimize the overall process of therapy(Ali et al., 2024; Ali et al., 2024) (Figure 8.11).

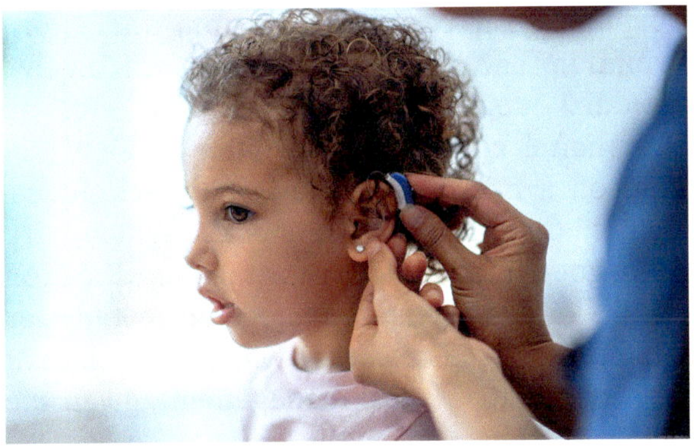

Figure 8.11. Understanding the patients context, including the use of hearing aids or exposure to water, offers insights into potential risk factors.

Source: https://assets.clevelandclinic.org/m/51c2aa14bbe541fa/webimage-child-hearing-aid-2160289598-r.png.

8.3.2. Laboratory Tests for Fungal Identification

The diagnosis of etiological fungi of otomycosis is dependent to a large extent on laboratory examinations using diversified microbiological methods. Samples of the ear canal are initially taken because the specimen is the immediate source of fungal infections. Following sample collection, numerous culture media are utilized in an attempt to stimulate fungal growth. Potato Dextrose Agar (PDA) is one of the most universally used culture media for fungi because of its high carbohydrate content and support for a broad spectrum of fungal growth. Alternative culture media have also been tested for their effectiveness in isolating fungi in some studies, showing large differences in growth among the different types of media. In particular, semi-synthetic media like PDA have documented very prominent results in culturing organisms like *Candida albicans*, which is normally suspected in otomycosis infections (Nurdin et al., 2020). Once fungi are cultured, microscopic and morphological examination is significant in species determination. Characterization techniques include the assessment of colony morphology, hyphal organization, and spore formation. Laboratory techniques can involve standard identification techniques, such as lactophenol cotton blue staining to view the fungi on a microscope. Molecular techniques, such as PCR followed by Sanger sequencing, are also a good line of inquiry for the identification of rare fungal isolates. Molecular techniques enhance diagnostic accuracy, which is paramount for appropriate clinical management, given the nuance between fungal species.

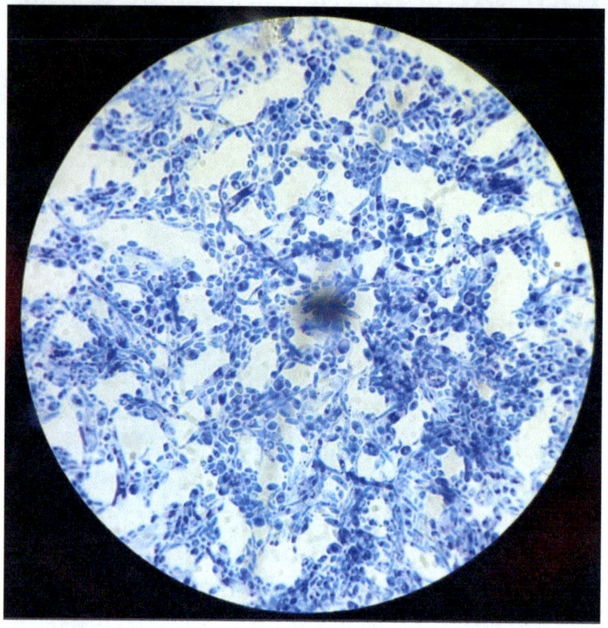

Figure 8.12. Laboratory protocols can incorporate standard identification techniques, such as the use of lactophenol cotton blue staining to visualize the fungi under a microscope.

Source: https://media.licdn.com/dms/image/v2/D5622AQE5x9xZ1C9SMg/feedshare-shrink_800/feedshare-shrink_800/0/1723040588149?e=2147483647&v=beta&t=UIxgrj3GzJ-8iuvem658NX7jj2b55rxZLtIM0ZUZKxo.

As the figures highlighted show, *Aspergillus* and *Candida* are most commonly isolated from individuals with otomycosis and need precise identification to guide treatment (Jayachitra et al., 2018). Antifungal susceptibility testing is also an extremely critical laboratory test that guides therapeutic regimens for treating otomycosis. Identification of resistance patterns is critical, especially during a period when increasing antifungal resistance is an issue. Microbroth dilution and disc diffusion are commonly employed to determine the susceptibility of fungal isolates to a number of antifungal agents. Most filamentous fungi were found susceptible to common antifungals, but certain species of *Candida* are resistant to some of the prominent drugs such as Fluconazole and Itraconazole. It has serious clinical implications as identification of resistance patterns enables the healthcare workers to tailor the antifungal treatment accordingly, improving the outcome of patients. This overall quality method of fungal identification and susceptibility testing emphasizes the role of rigorous laboratory protocols in otomycosis treatment (Jayachitra et al., 2018) (Figure 8.12).

8.3.3. Differential Diagnosis Considerations

In clinical diagnosis of otomycosis, thorough differential diagnosis should be performed to properly diagnose the condition and rule out other otologic conditions having a similar presentation. Clinicians should first think of bacterial infections, particularly those caused by *Pseudomonas aeruginosa*, which are similarly presenting as itching and discharge of otomycosis. A complete history and physical examination are most important, often identifying various attributes of the discharge color and odor that help distinguish between fungal and bacterial etiology. Furthermore, the presence of pain, fever, and systemic signs may be suggestive of a bacterial etiology, in which case further laboratory investigation is undertaken to allow for definitive diagnosis. These early evaluations form the foundation for proper diagnosis and tailored treatment, essential to prevent complications from misdiagnosed conditions (University, 2014). In addition to bacterial pathogens, differential diagnosis should also account for strict attention to other fungal infections, such as aspergillosis and candidiasis. While otomycosis is most frequently due to superficial fungal infection of the external ear canal, it should be remembered that *Aspergillus* organisms can penetrate deep structures, with more severe clinical manifestations. Such differentiation between such fungal infections can typically be achieved with biopsies or fine needle aspirates, which provide direct evidence of fungal spores or hyphae within the infected tissue.

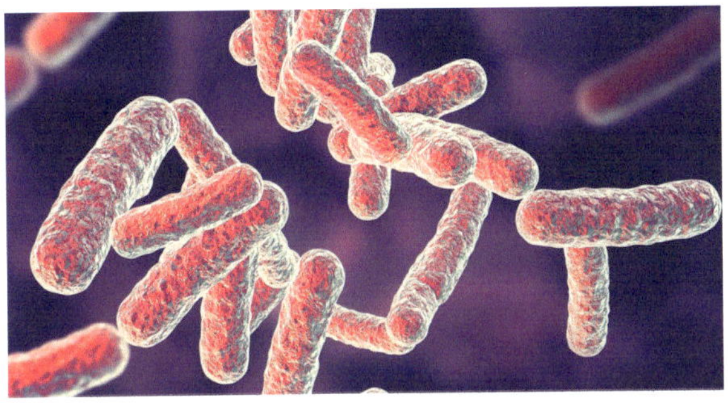

Figure 8.13. Clinicians must first consider bacterial infections, particularly those caused by *Pseudomonas aeruginosa*, which can mimic the itching and discharge associated with otomycosis.

Source: https://media.post.rvohealth.io/wp-content/uploads/sites/3/2020/02/322386_2200-1200x628.jpg.

Further, the recognition of specific risk factors, such as immunocompromised states that put one at risk of infection by these pathogens, is mandatory. Diagnosis is not only dependent on clinical acumen but also on reflective ordering of diagnostic examinations (Akinbobola et al., 2024). Finally, clinicians must remain always wary of maintaining a long list of conditions that can confound the diagnosis of otomycosis. Conditions such as eczema or psoriasis may have a presentation that is the same but necessitates entirely different treatment plans. Additionally, history-taking should also encompass recent antibiotic use, which makes patients susceptible to excessive fungal growth. An effective treatment regimen demands proper knowledge of the patient's complete medical history, which may hold significant clues to their predisposition to otologic disease. Thus, the intricate process of differential diagnosis becomes an important aspect of appropriate treatment and management, resulting in improved patient outcomes and avoiding the likelihood of chronicity of otomycosis (University, 2014) (Figure 8.13).

8.4. Treatment Options for Otomycosis

Treatment of otomycosis has also diversified to encompass various methods, depending on the severity of infection and overall health of the patients. Traditional treatment of this fungal infection has been through the use of topical antifungal drugs such as nystatin and clotrimazole. The treatments are not sufficient for chronic cases, as evident in a case of a 45-year-old woman who failed to respond to multiple topical treatments. Cultures of fungi revealed *Aspergillus niger* as the causative agent, and this motivated investigating more advanced treatments. The application of a 1% solution of voriconazole revealed an effective alternative solution, illustrating the importance of innovative approaches in managing refractory otomycosis that is resistant to traditional methods (Lagarce et al., 2018). If the patients present a perforated tympanic membrane, their treatment scenario is more complex. Topical therapy with conventional drugs can be risky, for example, ototoxic. Systemic therapy with oral itraconazole has been found to be safe and effective in such patients. In a study of 34 patients, patients on oral itraconazole, along with conventional antibiotic ear drops, achieved an excellent response. Within a week, 25 patients were completely cured, showing the possible effectiveness of the treatment even with complex otomycosis (M et al., 2017). This is a hint towards why parameters specific to each patient need to be considered while determining the most effective treatment. A holistic approach to treating otomycosis isn't just about using effective medicine, but also about understanding the causative factors of the infection. Patient education is also an important element in prevention of recurrence because control of moisture and proper ear hygiene can contribute significantly to the success of the treatment. Moreover, awareness about indwelling risk factors such as diabetes or prolonged hearing loss caused by hearing aid use can lead the clinician to customize their therapeutic protocol. A combination of pharmacotherapy such as voriconazole or itraconazole with life-style changes provides a balanced approach to the management of otomycosis. Eventually, ongoing research into the pathophysiology and efficacy treatment of the conditions will enhance clinical success for affected individuals, paving the way toward more targeted therapeutic regimens (Figure 8.14).

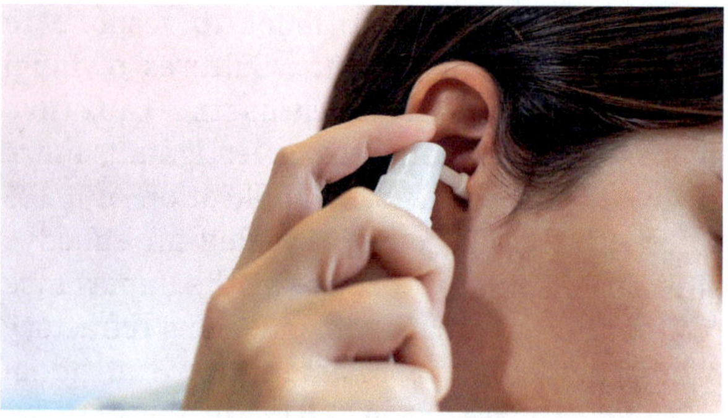

Figure 8.14. Patient education plays an essential role in preventing recurrence, as moisture control and proper ear hygiene can significantly impact the success of treatment.

Source: https://earwaxmove.com/wp-content/uploads/2024/06/girl-using-a-spray-to-clean-the-ears-clogged-by-t-2023-11-27-05-34-55-utc-scaled.jpg.

8.4.1. Antifungal Medications

Treatment of otomycosis, an outer ear fungal infection, significantly depends on the application of antifungal drugs to treat the symptoms as well as destroy the causative agents. Of the different treatment options that exist, the antifungal to be used can make a difference in the success of the therapy. For example, it was the effectiveness of isoconazole nitrate over nystatin in the treatment of otomycosis that was revealed by a recent study. Patients treated with isoconazole showed notable relief in their symptoms within two weeks, which confirms the superiority of some antifungal drugs over others in treating this prevalent disorder. This suggests that clinical efficacy must be utilized when selecting antifungal therapy to enhance patient success and enhance their way of life (Akram et al., 2023). In addition to isoconazole and nystatin, other medications such as clotrimazole and betadine were also used to test their efficacy against otomycosis. A general assessment of the patients' reactions showed that both clotrimazole and betadine showed significant therapeutic benefits, particularly if used within a predetermined regimen of treatment. These medications not only reduce the severity of symptoms like itching and pain but also improve the overall quality of life of patients. The trials illustrate that the regular application of effective antifungal therapy can lead to dramatic clinical improvements following a course of one month of treatment.

Such findings accentuate the importance of proper selection of the antifungal treatment in order to enable effective management of otomycosis (Ali et al., 2024). Despite the efficacy of antifungal therapy, possible factors causing vulnerability of patients to otomycosis need to be determined. Detection of common risk factors, such as hearing aid use or water exposure in the ear, can assist in reinforcement of preventive measures and planning for treatment. Awareness of the attendant symptoms also allows providers to anticipate complications and individualize therapeutic measures. Therefore, the integration of comprehensive patient assessments with their respective antifungal therapies is key in achieving the optimal treatment results in treating otomycosis. As a testament of clinical evidence, managing both risk factors and the regimen of medications can significantly reduce recurrence rates as well as improve patient satisfaction (Akram et al., 2023; Ali et al., 2024) (Figure 8.15).

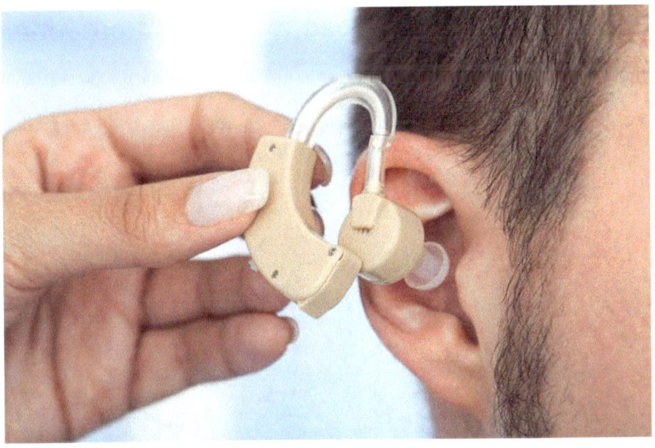

Figure 8.15. Awareness of common risk factors, such as the use of hearing aids or exposure to water in the ear, can enhance preventive measures and guide treatment decisions.

Source: https://lirp.cdn-website.com/6cabce8a/dms3rep/multi/opt/latest-2-404204b4-640w.jpg.

8.4.2. Surgical Interventions if Necessary

Surgical intervention may become unavoidable in the treatment of chronic cases of otomycosis, particularly if the conservative treatment is not effective. Otomycosis or fungal infection of the outer ear canal can in some instances lead to sequelae such as chronic inflammation or formation of granulation tissue. These are sequelae that arise due to the virulence of certain fungi that will not be treated by standard antifungal agents and proceed to exacerbate the disease. In such instances, surgery is employed for the reasons of removal of infected tissue and alleviation of symptoms to enable healing. Whether or not to have surgery is generally based on the duration of infection and patients' general health, with the importance of early diagnosis and treatment emphasized in the avoidance of advanced states of disease. The most common surgery for severe otomycosis is myringotomy, in which incisions are made to relieve pressure and drain infected secretions out of the middle ear. Not only is it useful as a relief from symptoms, but also as an opportunity to have samples for further microbiological evaluation. Early myringotomy can reduce the risk of more serious complications like tympanic membrane perforation or spread of infection to adjacent structures. Surgery also provides a platform for the use of adjuvant therapies, such as the application of medical-grade honey, which has proved useful for the prevention of fungal infection due to its antimicrobial properties. This new approach has the potential to supplement unsuccessful conventional antifungal treatment regimens, and better patient outcomes will be realized in otomycosis therapy (Dahiya et al., 2024). Postoperative care is equally important to get the desired results and prevent otomycosis recurrence. Patients after surgery must adhere to strict aftercare, encompassing medical interventions and lifestyle modifications. Topical antifungal therapy and regular cleaning of the ears may also reduce the risk of reinfection significantly. Even patient education regarding measures of prevention, i.e., avoiding damp environments, can minimize recurrences. As outlined in more recent literature, proper management protocols involving all of the above elements have been effective in reducing the occurrence of recurring cases of fungal infection within the ear canal (University, 2014). Therefore, integration of surgical treatments with comprehensive aftercare can optimize treatment interventions for otomycosis, optimizing quality of life for patients and minimizing complications (Figure 8.16).

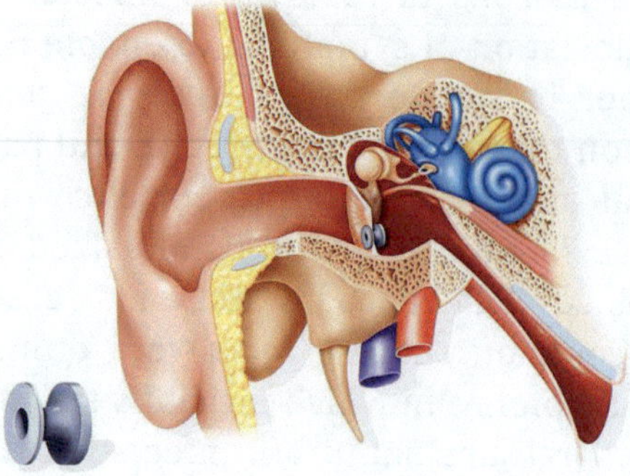

Figure 8.16. Timely myringotomy can reduce the risk of more serious complications like tympanic membrane perforation or the spread of infection to adjacent structures.

Source: https://healzone.co.in/storage/app/public/directories/June2023/Myringotomyy.jpg.

8.4.3. Home Remedies and Preventive Measures

In the management of otomycosis condition, home treatment and prevention play an important role in managing and minimizing the risk of fungal ear infections. One of them is having good ear hygiene involving cleaning the outer ear canal with a moist cloth without using cotton swabs. These habits all serve to help prevent the accumulation of moisture and debris that would result in fungal development. Symptomatic relief has also been found by others by applying natural products such as apple cider vinegar or tea tree oil, which are antifungal. These remedies not only provide symptomatic relief but are also part of a healthier general ear environment more likely to prevent recurrent infections. By adopting daily hygiene practices and learning about natural antifungals, one can minimize significantly the possibility of contracting otomycosis. Preventive practice extends beyond the individual method and may involve lifestyle changes that are advantageous to the ear. For instance, being cautious about drying the ears—particularly for swimmers or those who engage in water sports—is important. The application of earplugs or a swim cap will keep the ears away from water, thus reducing the risk of otomycosis. The individuals who sweat should also apply drying agents such as isopropyl alcohol to remove moisture within the ear when swimming or bathing. According to studies, drying the environment within the ear is critical in resisting fungal pathogens (Gill et al., 2024). Therefore, including these preventive aspects not only guarantees ear well-being but also ensures quality of life through prevention of infections that could lead to pain and potential complications.

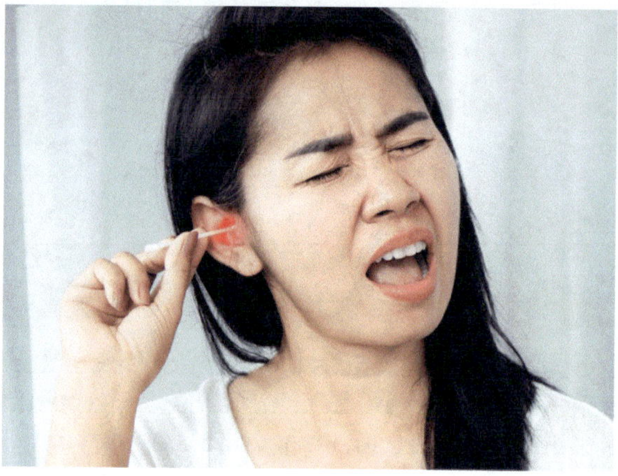

Figure 8.17. One effective method is maintaining proper ear hygiene, which includes cleaning the external ear canal with a damp cloth while avoiding the insertion of cotton swabs.

Source: https://www.allswabs.com/product_images/uploaded_images/how-to-get-cotton-out-of-your-ear.png.

Moreover, familiarity with how diet prevents otomycosis is one feature of ear health that is oftentimes overlooked. A balanced diet with probiotics and antioxidants can help to boost the immune system, thereby stimulating the body to effectively fight off infections such as ear infections. Yogurt, garlic, and green leafy vegetables have been shown to possess antifungal activity that may help protect against fungal infection (Gall et al.). As individuals are keeping a close eye on their total health, adding these food components to the diet can assist in constructing a robust defense against otomycosis. Through the application of a combination of effective home remedies, prevention methods, and dietary adjustments, individuals can utilize a complete system of ear care that reduces the danger of this prevalent fungal infection and supports long-term health (Figure 8.17).

8.5. Prevention of Otomycosis

Prevention of otomycosis is crucial due to the rise in the infection of the ear by fungal organisms, especially in tropical and subtropical regions. One of the primary causes of the development of otomycosis is the accumulation of moisture in the ear canal, which can facilitate the development of fungi. Therefore, it is important to develop dry conditions in the ear for prevention. Individuals are recommended to avoid excessive exposure to water, particularly swimming or bathing. This can be supported through the use of earplugs or earmolds which are specifically tailored to deflect water. According to recent literature, exposure to the environment is an important factor in the development of otomycosis, which requires preventive action against vulnerable populations (University, 2014). Better individual hygiene is also accountable for the prevention of otomycosis. Their ears must be instructed on how to clean them, emphasizing the avoidance of cotton swabs that can push dirt further into the ear canal and lead to infection. Instead, a gentle cleansing technique is recommended, using a soft tissue to wipe the outer ear. Regular checks for moisture accumulation or fungal infection in high-risk individuals, such as those with compromised immune systems, can assist in early recognition. Moreover, the population must be informed about the dangers of using over-the-counter ear cleaners, where some will disrupt the ears natural flora and cause growth of fungi (Gill et al., 2024). The presence of fungal spores in the entire environment means that preventive measures must be taken strongly against otomycosis. Healthcare providers should promote appropriate interventions in high-risk populations, such as those with a history of recurrent ear infections or pre-existing skin disease. Consideration should also be given in the management of underlying diseases like eczema or diabetes because they predispose individuals to fungal infections. Community ear cleanliness awareness campaigns to establish the importance of ear cleanliness and the danger of moisture build-up will also be helpful in prevention. Education, personal responsibility, and professional recommendations coming together can form a comprehensive approach, ultimately reducing the incidence of otomycosis and overall ear health (University, 2014) (Figure 8.18).

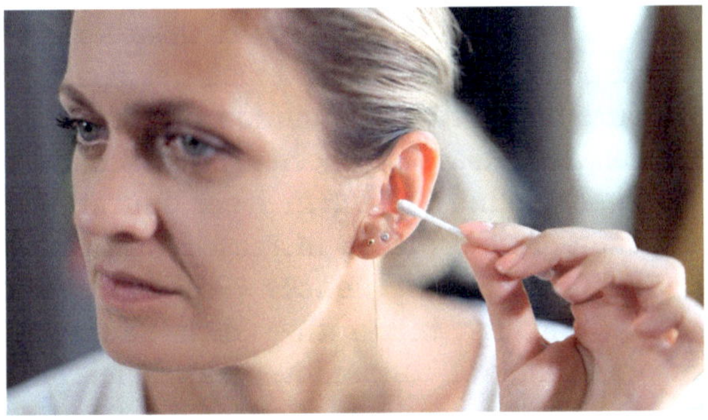

Figure 8.18. Patients should be educated on proper ear cleaning techniques, emphasizing the avoidance of cotton swabs that can push debris further into the ear canal and potentially lead to infection.

Source: https://www.touchwoodpharmacy.com/wp-content/uploads/2023/12/Expert-tips-for-avoiding-ear-wax-blockages-and-infections.jpg.

8.5.1. Personal Hygiene Practices

Personal cleanliness practices play a crucial role in prevention and control of otomycosis, an infection of the ear caused by fungus.

Maintenance of routine cleanliness practices, such as daily cleaning of the outer ear using damp cotton, will ensure that the possibility of fungal growth is reduced to a minimum. Dirt and moisture in the ear canal create a good place for fungi to grow, and this leads to infection. Therefore, individuals prone to ear issues should be more cautious to have clean and dry ears as a part of their routine daily hygiene. By adopting these practices, not just the incidence of otomycosis can be reduced, but even overall ear health can be improved, which is crucial in maintaining auditory function and preventing other related complications. Moreover, personal hygiene entails attention to the environment and cleanliness of shared facilities. Research has indicated that bacterial and fungal microorganisms can thrive on surfaces, including treatment beds within the healthcare setting, where patients are exposed to risk of infection by infective agents (Edwards et al., 2020). This, in turn, identifies the necessity for ensuring that any shared facilities used for the purpose of ear examination or treatment are well cleaned and disinfected. School children have been found to benefit from educational programs that promote increased awareness of proper hygiene practices (Prakash et al., 2014). Through integrating such education into programs of community health, personal hygiene's role in preventing otomycosis can be effectively disseminated and foster a culture of health consciousness. Outside cleansing aside, individual habits regarding moisture control are responsible for the central role in preventing otomycosis. People who engage in water sports or live in hot and humid climates must be especially careful. The use of earplugs and ear drying following swimming or showering can be helpful preventive measures. Furthermore, patients who have a history of infections in the ears should be careful not to overuse cotton swabs, as this will push debris down into the ear canal and continue to foster moisture retention. Overall, a comprehensive plan for personal hygiene with education on environmental and behavioral factors can effectively minimize the risks of otomycosis, obtaining an environmentally sound ear that deters excess growth of fungi (Figure 8.19).

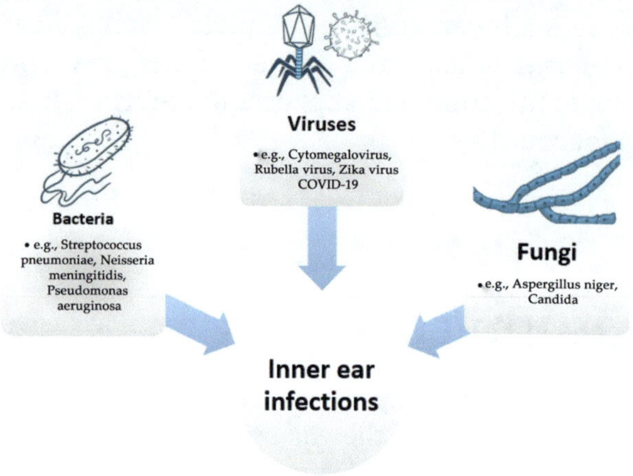

Figure 8.19. The presence of moisture and debris in the ear canal creates an ideal environment for fungi to proliferate, leading to potential infections.

Source: https://www.mdpi.com/nanomaterials/nanomaterials-11-01311/article_deploy/html/images/nanomaterials-11-01311-g001-550.jpg.

8.5.2. Environmental Control Measures

The case of otomycosis emphasizes the role of control measures of the environment in the prevention of the risk of fungal ear infection. Preceding the latter are typically numerous environmental conditions such as temperature and humidity, which provide a favorable setting for fungi growth. Therefore, reduced contact with these factors is critical in preventing otomycosis, especially in tropical regions or rainy weather patterns. Additionally, poor ear care behavior that leads to moisture retention adds to susceptibility. Good ear hygiene education is an important aspect of a broader effort to minimize risks associated with fungal infection. Public health announcements can focus on keeping ears dry and avoiding the use of cotton swabs, which push dirt further into the ear canal, creating conditions for easier growth of fungi. Another area of control measures of the environment takes into consideration the identification and modification of potential reservoirs for potential fungi in domestic situations. Fungi develop in wet conditions, and therefore new solutions to domestic environments are essential to aid in prevention. Eliminating contact with standing water and the application of sufficient ventilation can significantly decrease the possibility of fungal spores settling and propagating within domestic spaces. Additionally, attention should be drawn to public swimming areas, such as pools or lakes, where water environments pose greater risks for fungal exposure. As reported in research, fungal infections can result from exposure to freshwater sources, relating group habits to individuals' genetic effects. Consequently, establishing protocols for frequent cleaning and monitoring of such settings can become an essential part of public health programs aimed at reducing the incidence of otomycosis (Dennis, 2017). Introducing environmental control measures goes beyond individual means to encompass mass measures for the community and healthcare policies for maintaining public health. Monitoring and observation of onsite environmental conditions may guide targeted interventions to reduce rates of otomycosis among high-risk populations. For instance, in areas of flooding or high humidity, doctors may collaborate with municipal health authorities to introduce fungal screening and ear hygiene education specifically for adaptation to such special risks. Furthermore, clinics and hospitals can institute practices that guide patients with repeated bouts of otomycosis to evaluate their homes proactively. Therefore, comprehensive approaches that integrate education, environmental management, and health policy may not only promote better individual-level health results but also strengthen community resilience to fungal infection such as otomycosis (University, 2014) (Figure 8.20).

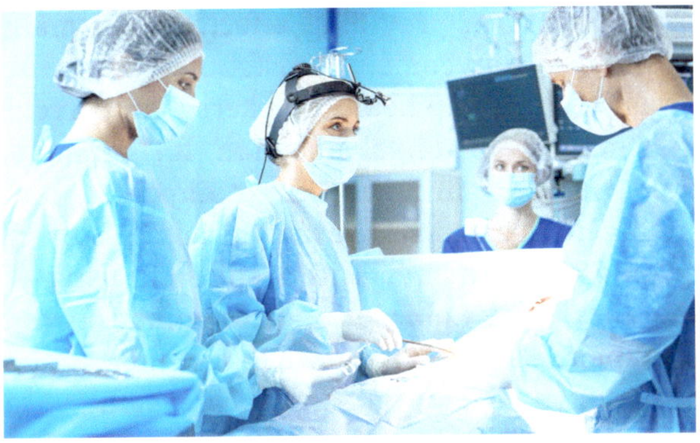

Figure 8.20. Hospitals and clinics can adopt guidelines that encourage patients with recurrent otomycosis to evaluate their living environments proactively.

Source: https://advantumhealth.com/wp-content/uploads/2020/03/dreamstime_m_99735813-optimize-rcm-surgeon-1500x956-1-1080x675.jpg.

8.5.3. Education and Awareness Initiatives

There is a critical role for education and awareness campaigns in breaking the challenges posed by otomycosis, especially in regions where the condition is most widespread. With greater knowledge of the major causes, symptoms, and treatment, these campaigns can significantly reduce the incidence of the condition. Educational campaigns can be carried out in any one of a number of formats such as community workshops, printed information pamphlets, and health care provider and population social media outreach. In addition to educating individuals about the importance of early detection, these campaigns emphasize ear hygiene practices and dangers of self-medication. Through targeted messaging, individuals can be enabled to recognize early signs and the appropriate type of medical intervention, thereby eliminating the risk of complications due to untreated otomycosis. Yet another extremely crucial aspect of education and awareness programs is that they can enhance the competence of healthcare practitioners in providing effective treatment against otomycosis. Workshops may be organized to equip health workers with current information on fungal infection, for example, the etiologic pathogens in otomycosis, and treatment protocols, for example, administering antifungal medicines and aseptic cleaning of the ears. This information dissemination not only benefits the patients but also builds the confidence level of health professionals to render timely and effective services. Besides, continuous professional education schemes have the ability to ensure an environment in which health practitioners are updated with current research and developments in the management of otomycosis to allow them to deliver quality service to their communities. Through bridging gaps in knowledge, such programs will go a great distance in ensuring quality healthcare provision for otomycosis. In addition, collaboration among stakeholders can advance the effectiveness of education and awareness programs for otomycosis. Alliances among government health authorities, non-governmental organizations, and schools can increase reach and impact. Such collaborations can facilitate cross-sharing of resources and encompassing strategies towards not only otomycosis but also co-morbidities. For instance, coordinating educational activity on otomycosis with broader public health campaigns can promote a greater profile for this illness as well as address relevant underlying risk determinants such as hygiene practices and environmental health. Broadening the focus of awareness programs will more probably lead communities to have increased health literacy regarding otomycosis, which in turn will result in improved prevention and treatment. Collaborative approaches are important in formulating a sustainable framework for ongoing education of the general public and healthcare providers in the effective management of otomycosis (Figure 8.21).

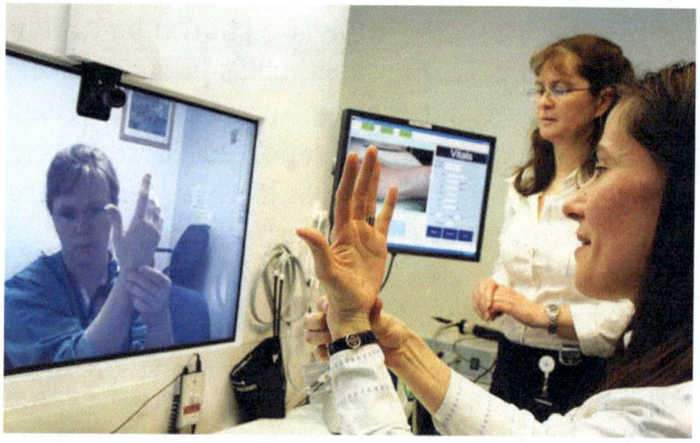

Figure 8.21. By bridging knowledge gaps, these initiatives can significantly advance the overall quality of healthcare delivery related to otomycosis.

Source: https://ehealth.eletsonline.com/wp-content/uploads/2011/04/Telemedicine.jpg.

SUMMARY

Otomycosis, the most prevalent fungal infection of the ear canal, is usually due to the proliferation of non-pathogenic fungi that belong to the normal flora. These belong to the genus *Aspergillus* and occur when the environmental conditions favor their growth at the expense of the ear's health, e.g., excessive humidity or damage to the ear canal skin. The predisposing factors for otomycosis are humid weather, chronic otitis externa, and incorrect ear hygiene habits. This infection, although widely misunderstood, is a significant matter of public health, particularly for tropical and subtropical regions where the prevalence is even greater. Understanding the balance of the ears microflora ecologic is crucial to identifying the reasons behind the occurrence of fungal overgrowth and its subsequent infection, as is represented by various studies on fungal pathogens and how they influence the external auditory canal (University, 2014). The symptoms of otomycosis most commonly include itching, discharge, and a fullness of the ear. Diagnosis is largely clinical, with evidence of fungal structures on microscopic examination. The etiology can vary, but *Aspergillus* species are still the most commonly diagnosed culprits. While the infection is not usually life-threatening in and of itself, it can lead to chronic otitis if left untreated. Effective management methods will involve antifungal therapy and copious cleaning of the outer auditory canal, being careful to put emphasis on correct medical treatment. Improper or nontreatment of earwax by self or untrained attempts will aggravate the situation, leading to further damage and susceptibility to infection (Resca et al., 1948). Prophylaxis plays an important role in the management of otomycosis, particularly for those who are more susceptible. Education on proper ear cleanliness, for example, the prevention of insertion of foreign bodies into the ear canal and minimizing exposure to dampness, may significantly influence occurrence rates. Public health campaign messages explaining the possible danger of certain behaviors, for instance, the use of cotton swabs, can encourage better habits of ear care. Moreover, alleviation of infection in the high-risk populations, via accessible medical infrastructures and early means of treatment, can minimize the incidence of such fungal infections. Ultimately, familiarity with this salient information that guides otomycosis—from cause and sign to practical means of prevention and management—provides better health outcomes and enhances public awareness for this often-overlooked disease (University, 2014).

A CLOSER LOOK

EAR CANAL

The ear canal, or external auditory canal, is a narrow tube that connects the outer ear to the eardrum. It facilitates the passage of sound waves to the middle ear as well as protects the ear by trapping dust and microbes with earwax (cerumen). The canal is lined with cartilage and bone, and its smoothly curved configuration protects against damage to the eardrum. Shared conditions that impact the ear canal are infections such as otitis externa and obstruction due to earwax blockage.

REFERENCES

1. Afolabi, S. O., Fansula, A. J., & Ogunkeyede, S. A. (2019). Hearing loss among adolescents on antiretroviral therapy: A need for periodic hearing assessment. https://core.ac.uk/download/478397490.pdf (accessed on 27th June 2025).
2. Ajay, P. (2012). Effectiveness of 7.5 percent povidone iodine in comparison to 1 percent clotrimazole in the treatment of otomycosis. https://core.ac.uk/download/235654978.pdf (accessed on 27th June 2025).
3. Akinbobola, A., Kean, R., & Quilliam, R. S. (2024). Plastic pollution as a novel reservoir for the environmental survival of the drug-resistant fungal pathogen *Candida auris*. https://core.ac.uk/download/595730342.pdf (accessed on 27th June 2025).
4. Akram, A. U., Alamgir, A., Chaudhry, S., Hussain, S., et al. (2023). Comparison of isoconazole nitrate versus nystatin for the treatment of otomycosis. https://core.ac.uk/download/587960476.pdf (accessed on 27th June 2025).
5. Ali, A. K., & Altimimi, M. L. M. (2024). Evaluation and treatment of the incidence of otomycosis in patients visiting the ENT clinic. https://core.ac.uk/download/612988619.pdf (accessed on 27th June 2025).
6. Arijit, D. (2017). A study on incidence and types of otomycosis in patients diagnosed with chronic suppurative otitis media. https://core.ac.uk/download/235661341.pdf (accessed on 27th June 2025).
7. Aziz, T., Qureshi, N., Khawaja, M., Ulfat, R., Muhammad, T., Malik, A., Aziz, T., et al. (2020). Comparison of effectiveness of 7.5% povidone-iodine with 1% clotrimazole ear drops and lignocaine in otomycosis. https://core.ac.uk/download/555274568.pdf (accessed on 27th June 2025).
8. Bajpai, N., & Wadhwa, M. (2019). Health and wellness centers: Expanding access to comprehensive primary health care in India. https://core.ac.uk/download/226761821.pdf (accessed on 27th June 2025).
9. Baumgardner, D. J. (2017). Freshwater fungal infections. https://digitalrepository.aurorahealthcare.org/cgi/viewcontent.cgi?article=1262&context=jpcrr (accessed on 27th June 2025).
10. Brás, S. M. P., Cernáková, L., Rodrigues, C. F., Roudbary, M., et al. (2021). *Candida auris*: A quick review on identification, current treatments, and challenges. https://core.ac.uk/download/428286057.pdf (accessed on 27th June 2025).
11. Dahiya, D., Mackin, C., & Singh-Nee Nigam, P. (2024). Studies on bioactivities of Manuka and regional varieties of honey for their potential use as natural antibiotic agents for infection control related to wound healing and in pharmaceutical formulations. https://core.ac.uk/download/613688097.pdf (accessed on 27th June 2025).
12. Darmawan, A. B., Kinanthi, R., Krisniawati, N., Kusdaryanto, A., et al. (2024). Gambaran klinis otomycosis di RS Margono Soekarjo. https://core.ac.uk/download/622344384.pdf (accessed on 27th June 2025).
13. De Angelis, G. (2023). Internalization mechanisms of biopolymeric nanoparticles in plants and fungi and application in integrated pest management. https://core.ac.uk/download/599513660.pdf (accessed on 27th June 2025).

14. Dekhil, K. R. (2018). Presentation pattern and fungal agent's spectrum causing otomycosis. https://core.ac.uk/download/477854097.pdf (accessed on 27th June 2025).
15. Edwards, A. G. (2020). Cross sectional analysis of the presence of airborne bacteria and fungi within the UJ Chiropractic Clinic. https://core.ac.uk/download/479290330.pdf (accessed on 27th June 2025).
16. Farooqi, J., Jabeen, K., & Zafar, A. (2017). Practical guide and atlas for the diagnosis of fungal infections. https://core.ac.uk/download/212878268.pdf (accessed on 27th June 2025).
17. Gall, L. S., & Riely, P. E. (2025). Effect of diet and atmosphere on intestinal and skin flora. *Volume II – Literature survey*. https://core.ac.uk/download/pdf/85249155.pdf (accessed on 27th June 2025).
18. Giannotti, G. (2022). Modelling of the antifungal activity of propionic and sorbic acid against spoilage molds and validation in bread and cake. https://core.ac.uk/download/570944655.pdf (accessed on 27th June 2025).
19. Gill, E. G. (2024). Consideration for expanding the audiology scope of practice to include prescription medication authority. https://core.ac.uk/download/616442610.pdf (accessed on 27th June 2025).
20. Jayachitra, J. (2018). Isolation, characterization and antifungal sensitivity pattern of fungi causing otomycosis in patients reporting in a tertiary care hospital. https://core.ac.uk/download/235668323.pdf (accessed on 27th June 2025).
21. Karami, M., Khademian, A., Kiakojuri, K., Omran, M., et al. (2019). Outer ear infections in Iran: A review. https://core.ac.uk/download/196239682.pdf (accessed on 27th June 2025).
22. Kasimjanovna, D. O. (2024). Foreign body in the respiratory tract. https://core.ac.uk/download/612989432.pdf (accessed on 27th June 2025).
23. Lagarce, F., Legrand, G., de Gentile, L., Chappe, M., Vrignaud, S., & Le Govic, Y. (2018). Successful treatment of a recurrent *Aspergillus niger* otomycosis with local application of voriconazole. https://core.ac.uk/download/156875504.pdf (accessed on 27th June 2025).
24. Naseeruddin, K., & Viswanatha, B. (2011). Fungal infections of the ear in immunocompromised host: A review. https://core.ac.uk/download/pdf/8571099.pdf (accessed on 27th June 2025).
25. Nurdin, E. (2020). Comparison growth of *Candida albicans* in alternative media and semi-synthetic on fisheries cerumen in Bastion Karaca, Ternate City. https://core.ac.uk/download/328104115.pdf (accessed on 27th June 2025).
26. Raja, K. (2024). The current state of digital health access for patients with chronic diseases in rural India: A scoping review. https://core.ac.uk/download/628714907.pdf (accessed on 27th June 2025).
27. Resca, H. G. (1948). The occurrence of pathogenic fungi in the normal human body. https://open.bu.edu/bitstream/2144/6263/1/Resca_Helen_1948_web.pdf (accessed on 27th June 2025).
28. Sagesh, M., & Ravindran, A. (2017). Effectiveness of oral itraconazole in the management of otomycosis with tympanic membrane perforation. https://core.ac.uk/download/544391331.pdf (accessed on 27th June 2025).

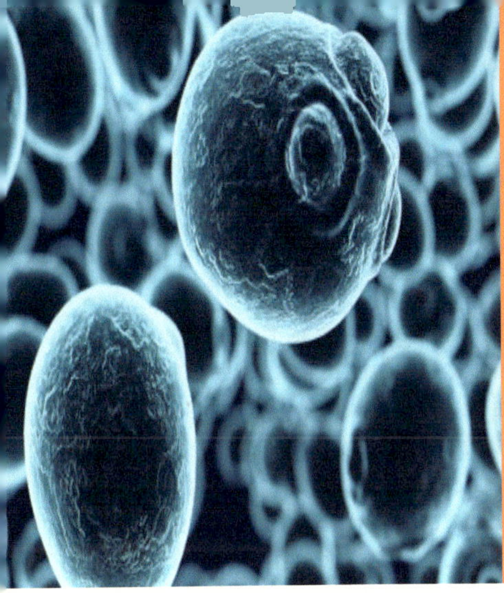

Chapter 9
ASPERGILLOSIS

Contents

Introduction

Aspergillosis is a serious infection that is caused by *Aspergillus* species members, which are ubiquitous molds found in various environments. The molds inhabit rotting organic matter, and their spores tend to be inhaled by humans. Under healthy conditions, the immune system is able to suppress the dangers posed by the spores. In immunocompromised individuals or people with predisposing respiratory diseases, *Aspergillus*, however, leads to severe health complications, i.e., invasive aspergillosis. New insight into the mechanisms of the immune response to such mold exposure indicates that while the interaction between mold species and human disease is complex, it is important in successful diagnosis and therapy, especially in risk groups. The expanded knowledge of the immune response to *Aspergillus* exposure has been upheld by recent studies on the impact of various fungal species on human health. Studies have shown that allergic responses may happen when exposed to molds, discussing in detail how particular molds can trigger strong immunological reactions. New developments in immunology indicate that the identification of these reactions is vital in developing effective treatments against mold diseases. Most notably, the relationship between mold spore exposure and human disease continues to be a concern, bringing attention to one area of future research into effective prevention and treatment for diseases like aspergillosis (Gorham et al., 2010). Further, as knowledge of the medical implications of mold exposure increases, the need for careful investigation into diagnostic and therapeutic modalities grows more evident. Human variability in response to different species of mold requires a nuanced understanding of individuals' immune profiles. Such variability underscores the necessity of targeted interventions aimed at ensuring specific vulnerabilities in patients. By determining associations between environmental factors and therapeutic outcomes, researchers seek to chart the interactions between exposure to molds, allergic responses, and the development of diseases such as aspergillosis (Baldin et al., 2014). In so doing, they leave room for valuable innovations in public health guidance and clinical interventions, ultimately a step towards minimizing the dangers of this widespread fungal disease (Figure 9.1).

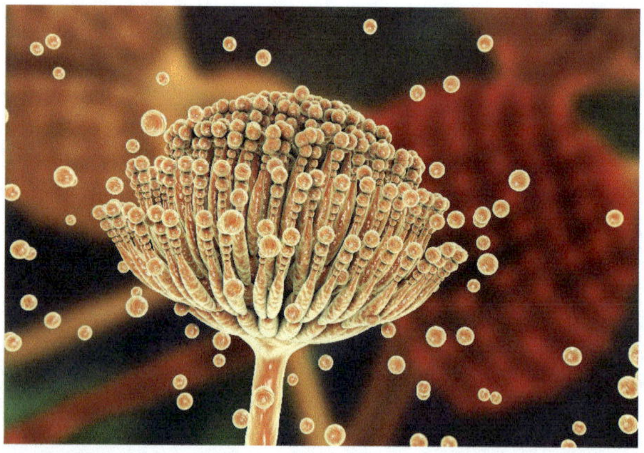

Figure 9.1. Aspergillosis.

Source: https://medlineplus.gov/images/Aspergillosis_share.jpg.

9.1. Causes of Aspergillosis

The etiology of Aspergillosis is most frequently due to environmental factors and the immune status of the patient. *Aspergillus* fungi, particularly *Aspergillus fumigatus*, thrive on decaying organic matter, like soil and plant detritus, and thus are ubiquitous in nature. When spores are inhaled, individuals with compromised immunity—e.g., organ transplant recipients or patients who are on immunosuppressive therapy—are at high risk. A sample case of this risk includes that of a 2-month-old child following liver transplantation who developed an unusual central nervous system infection by *Aspergillus fumigatus*. Management involved a combination of antifungal treatment and cessation of immunosuppression, highlighting the way in which these immunocompromised periods increase the invasive potential of the pathogen (Green et al., 1991). Thus, individuals with pre-existing conditions must also be vigilant about their environments to reduce exposure to probable *Aspergillus* sources. In addition to environmental exposure, there are also predisposing medical conditions that lead to Aspergillosis. Allergic bronchopulmonary aspergillosis (ABPA) is a case in point, occurring nearly exclusively in patients with asthma and cystic fibrosis due to an unusual immune response to antigens of *Aspergillus fumigatus*. In these patients, augmented IgE and allergic inflammation can exacerbate respiratory manifestations, ultimately leading to severe bronchiectasis, a permanent ABPA complication (Cinicola et al., 2016). Furthermore, difficulty in early ABPA diagnosis can hinder the application of effective treatment, with secondary damage to the lungs. It is essential to make recognized the complicated interaction among such predisposing health conditions and *Aspergillus* infection to install adequate preventative measures as well as therapeutic interventions. Apart from the above causes, occupational factors such as exposure to work in agriculture and construction increase the susceptibility to Aspergillosis, particularly in individuals who work in these sectors. Such occupations involve working with organic materials, and this increases susceptibility to the inhalation of *Aspergillus* spores. Individuals with existing chronic respiratory conditions are especially vulnerable, as their pre-existing respiratory conditions make it highly challenging for the body to fight fungal infection. Higher incidence among at-risk groups is a call for greater vigilance and preventative action within the workplace. Continued research into the cause of Aspergillosis, inherently multifaceted in nature, ensures that these risk factors are dealt with by education and rigorous safety protocols. Appreciation of the confluence of environmental, medical, and lifestyle factors ultimately provides a comprehensive strategy for avoiding the impact of this highly invasive fungal infection (Figure 9.2).

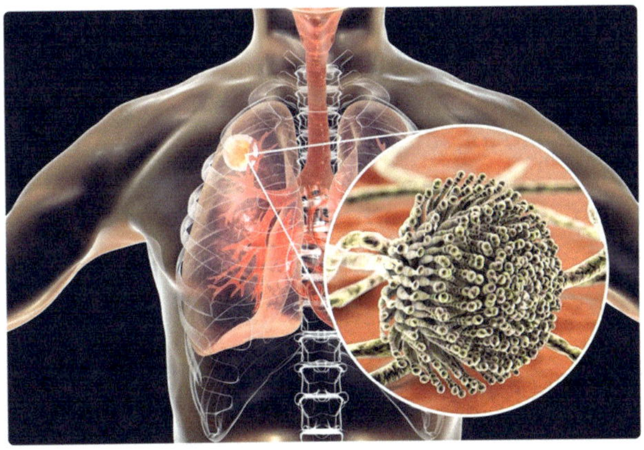

Figure 9.2. *Aspergillus fumigatus.*

Source: https://www.news-medical.net/image-handler/picture/2020/11/shutterstock_1107032042.jpg.

9.1.1. Aspergillus Species and Their Characteristics

Aspergillus consist of a large class of filamentous fungi with an enormous number of species that play important roles in various ecological systems, especially nutrient cycling and decomposition. *Aspergillus* are characterized by their septate, branched hyphae and the production of asexual spores, or conidia, which are key to their success at reproduction. Among the more than 180 described species, *Aspergillus fumigatus* stands out because of its clinical importance as a well-known pathogen in immunocompromised patients. Some other species, including *Aspergillus flavus* and *Aspergillus niger*, are similarly known to cause opportunistic infections. Understanding the morphological and genetic characteristics of these fungi not only facilitates their identification in clinical settings but also contributes to understanding their pathogenic mechanisms, which are crucial for the creation of effective therapeutic strategies against aspergillosis. Pathogenicity in *Aspergillus* species is established by their capacity for adaptation to various environments and endurance under various conditions, particularly in decaying organic substrates, in soil, and even indoors. Omnipresence like this allows for regular exposure, particularly in immunocompromised patients. Environmental conditions, such as temperature and humidity, are mostly responsible for spore germination and development, and therefore affect *Aspergillus*-associated infection rates. As discussed in the literature review, some populations, such as solid organ transplant recipients or those with hematological malignancies, are susceptible to invasive aspergillosis due to their compromised immune status. Epidemiology of infections like these highlights the need for detailed information regarding the nature of *Aspergillus* species, since considerable information is beneficial in applying preventive measures and performing effective outbreak control. New advances in diagnostic methods for invasive fungal disease have been a paradigm shift for the management of aspergillosis. Development of some imaging techniques, molecular tests, and serologic tests facilitates timely and precise identification of *Aspergillus* species from the infected patient, which is important for timely intervention. Based on various studies such as aspergillosis case review among transplant patients, the role of determination of clinical presentation, diagnosis, and treatment outcome has become increasingly significant, especially among high-risk populations. Through advancing the understanding of the behavior and characteristics of *Aspergillus* species, medicine is able to customize therapeutic approaches, including judicious use of antifungal drugs. This is in accordance with new invasive fungal diseases definitions that are intended to expand the representativeness of diagnostic criteria to include a broad patient population and thereby advance the clinical mycology science and improve patient outcomes, as necessary because of evolving healthcare needs (Green et al., 1991; Akan et al., 2019) (Figure 9.3).

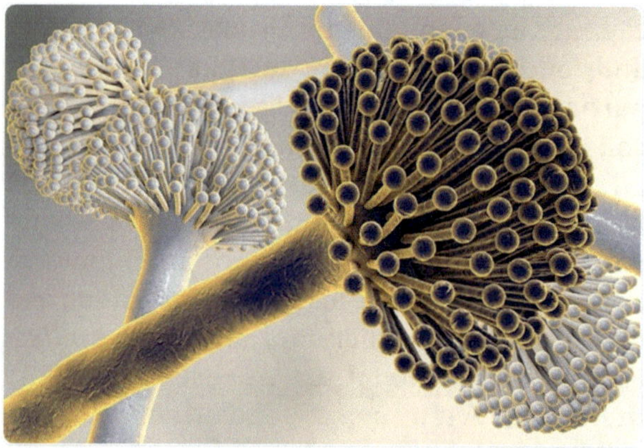

Figure 9.3. *Aspergillus niger.*

Source: https://www.news-medical.net/image-handler/picture/2018/9/shutterstock_308094836.jpg.

9.1.2. Environmental Factors Contributing to Infection

Environmental conditions play a central role in the development and incidence of infectious disease, particularly invasive aspergillosis. *Aspergillus* spp. is an environment fungus which may thrive in any environment, and hence exposure is continuous, particularly in immunocompromised individuals. The fungi are widespread on soil, decaying plant matter, and even within homes, with severe implications on health. The abundant sporulation capacity of *Aspergillus* renders it a widespread organism that can easily disseminate by air. Studies have demonstrated that inadequate environmental control techniques, such as ineffective ventilation systems or dirty cleaning practices, increase the risk of exposure to infection, particularly in hospitals where vulnerable people reside. Therefore, detection and prevention of such environmental factors are essential to the efficient implementation of prevention modalities for invasive aspergillosis (Puglia et al., 2024). Environmental contamination is also a significant risk factor for aspergillosis, especially among patients with cancer undergoing treatment for hematologic malignancies. Neutropenia, perhaps the most common side effect of chemotherapy, severely compromises a patient's ability to defend against fungal infections. Air-borne fungal spores in hospital settings are responsible for high incidence rates of invasive aspergillosis, which are the reasons behind stringent environmental control being unavoidable. HEPA (particulate air) filters and laminar airflow units have been proven to substantially reduce air-borne fungal spores.

This protects immunocompromised patients. Incorporation of regular environmental surveillance is unavoidable in order to guarantee the implementation of the set guidelines. By modifying the infection prevention practices based on individual environmental risk factors, hospitals can more effectively reduce the incidence of invasive aspergillosis (Puglia et al., 2024). The interaction between viral infections and fungal susceptibility adds another angle to the environmental risk factors in aspergillosis. The ongoing research has unveiled that acute viral infections such as influenza and COVID-19 significantly enhance the risk for developing invasive pulmonary aspergillosis. This condition, known as influenza-associated pulmonary aspergillosis (IAPA) and COVID-19-associated pulmonary aspergillosis (CAPA), is a testament of how environmental stressors can feed into risk factors for infection. Such patients with the said viral infections have compromised immunity, and this is a predisposing condition for opportunistic pathogens like *Aspergillus* to thrive in. The advancement of animal models has provided new insight into the pathogenesis of such co-infections and emphasized the need for further research to reveal the synergism between environmental exposures and host genetics. Ultimately, it is crucial to remain cognizant of these multifactorial factors in making effective strategies for minimizing the risks of aspergillosis (Figure 9.4).

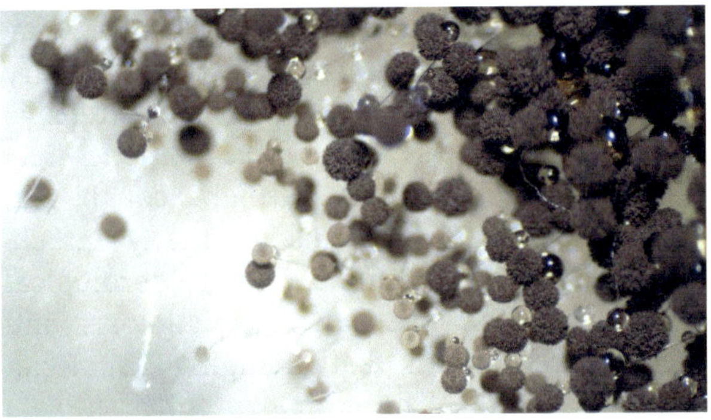

Figure 9.4. *Aspergillus* spp. is an environmental mold that thrives in various settings, making exposure an ever-present risk, particularly for immunocompromised individuals.

Source: https://www.intertek.com/siteassets/blogs/mold-blog.jpg.

9.1.3. Risk Factors for Developing Aspergillosis

The development of Aspergillosis, particularly in invasive cases, is governed by several significant risk factors that further enhance the vulnerability of an individual to *Aspergillus* species infections. Individuals with prior respiratory infections, such as asthma and cystic fibrosis, are especially more susceptible. These states are likely to weaken the integrity of the airway and predispose the patient to easy colonization by *Aspergillus* species with resultant Allergic Bronchopulmonary Aspergillosis (ABPA) or more serious forms of disease. For instance, the derangement of an immune response characterized as a T-helper 2 lymphocyte response has been linked with ABPA in asthma and implies a profound interdependency between respiratory function and susceptibility to fungi (CInicola et al., 2016). Also, the subtle nature of accurate diagnosis and management of ABPA underscores the importance of preventive screening in such high-risk groups. Beyond respiratory illness, immunocompromised states also have a primary role in the development of invasive Aspergillosis. Patients undergoing immunosuppressive treatment, as well as those who are post-organ transplant, are particularly at risk due to compromised immune status. Studies conducted on liver transplant recipients revealed that the presence of increased levels of creatinine and the use of OKT3, an intense immunosuppression agent, were associated with higher numbers of invasive *Aspergillus* lung infection (Fung et al., 1992). This indicates that both the constitution of the underlying condition and the treatment regimen can increase susceptibility to fungal infections, with a particular emphasis placed on surveillance in subjects receiving immunosuppressive treatment. Environmental factors such as the ability to develop Aspergillosis are also dependent on the susceptibility factors, particularly in subjects who have pre-existing medical conditions. Protracted exposure to environments rich in *Aspergillus* spores, such as building environments or environments of rotting organic material, is a prominent risk factor, especially for individuals with weakened respiratory defenses. In addition, the presence of fungal spores indoors—often combined with dampness or poor ventilation—can be an indicator for repeated exposure. These environmental determinants are particularly relevant to patients who are already predisposed due to conditions like asthma or cystic fibrosis, additionally putting them at risk of developing ABPA. As epidemiologic understanding progresses about risk factors, there remains a very compelling necessity for risk-adjusted preventive strategies and guidelines that protect susceptible groups from the risk of Aspergillosis (Figure 9.5).

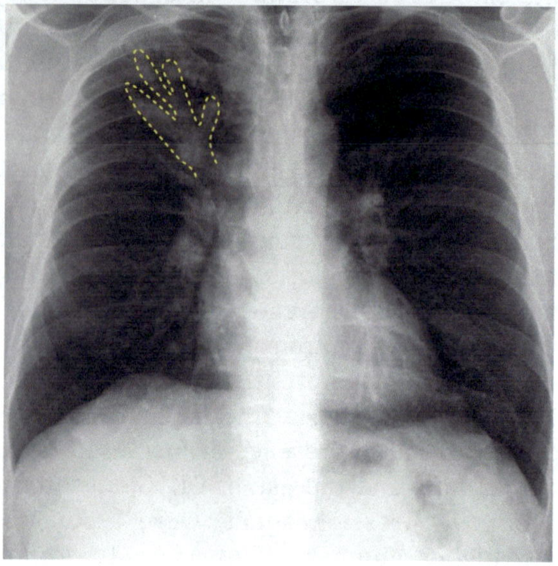

Figure 9.5. Allergic bronchopulmonary aspergillosis (ABPA).

Source: https://prod-images-static.radiopaedia.org/images/3001319/b21053fa9f9dcfc867600adf0886b3_big_gallery.jpeg.

9.2. Types of Aspergillosis

A variety of *Aspergillus* species can produce a spectrum of aspergillosis, which is classified in general into four forms: allergic bronchopulmonary aspergillosis (ABPA), invasive aspergillosis (IA), chronic pulmonary aspergillosis (CPA), and aspergilloma. ABPA usually occurs in individuals with asthma or cystic fibrosis and is caused by a hypersensitivity response to the fungal antigens. Symptoms are typically wheezing, coughing, and respiratory distress, which are like asthmatic symptoms but aggravated by hyperresponsiveness of the immune system. Diagnosis is typically through serum IgE levels, and treatment can involve corticosteroids to block inflammation and antifungal treatment to cure infection. The importance of accurate diagnostics comes to the forefront with novel molecular techniques that improve sensitivity in the identification of such types of aspergillosis, particularly pronounced with the addition of RT-qPCR technology, emphasized in findings presented by Gibert et al., (2024). Chronic pulmonary aspergillosis (CPA) is another common type that attacks patients who have pre-existing lung infections such as tuberculosis. It is a disease with chronic respiratory presentation and may present in various forms, such as simple cavitary disease and complicated disease with extensive lung damage. The symptoms that patients may experience include loss of weight, cough, and hemoptysis as the fungus gradually infects the lung tissue. Imaging tests with serological markers are the most used for diagnosis, and the galactomannan test is highly beneficial in identification. The management of CPA is typically long-term antifungal therapy but with the complicating factor of the relapsing nature of the disease. Clinical presentation heterogeneity corroborates the necessity of clinician close monitoring of patients along with individualized treatment modalities for the management of this disorder, as indicated by results of Badillo-Almaraz et al., (2022) on CAPA. The most severe form is invasive aspergillosis (IA), and it is most frequently seen in immunocompromised hosts. The fulminant nature of IA can lead to significant morbidity and mortality since the fungus becomes invasive of vascular structures and leads to necrotizing pneumonia and disseminated complications. Diagnosis is normally challenging due to the non-specific nature of clinical signs and necessitates the use of advanced diagnostic modalities such as imaging and galactomannan assays to determine the presence of *Aspergillus*. The addition of RT-qPCR techniques has shown promising improvements in the early diagnosis, particularly in patients with low fungal burdens, enhancing the prognosis in high-risk patients. Along with the advance of knowledge about aspergillosis pathogenetic mechanisms and classification, additional research is still required to improve diagnostic sensitivity and therapeutic efficacy for affected patients, especially in the case of the new cases emerged in the context of events like the COVID-19 pandemic, such as discussed in Badillo-Almaraz et al., (2022) (Figure 9.6).

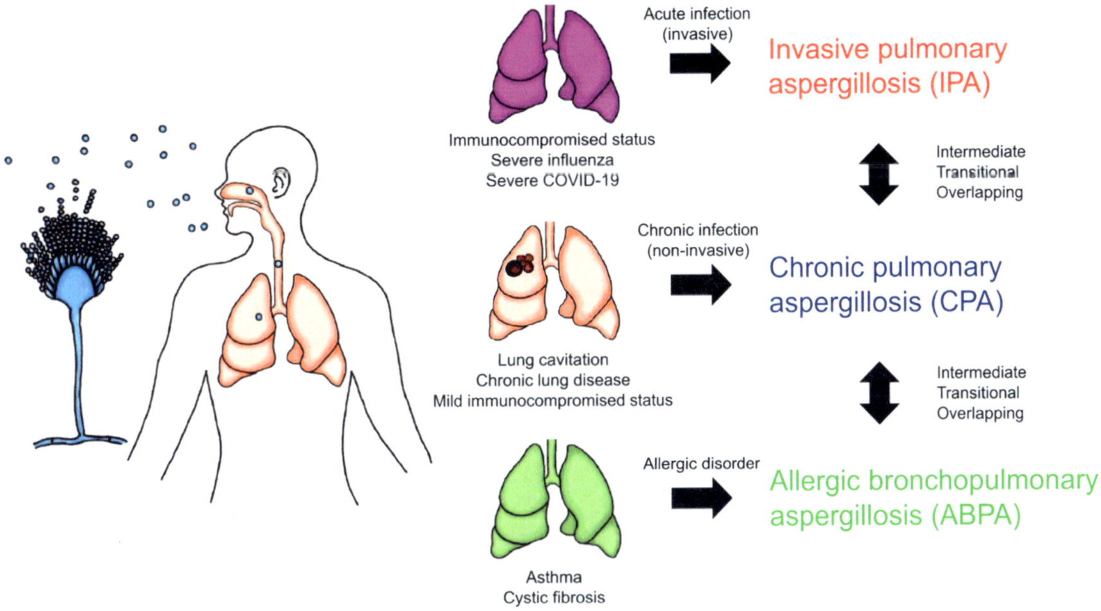

Figure 9.6. The management of CPA typically involves long-term antifungal therapy, but this can present challenges due to the recurring nature of the disease.

Source: https://journals.sagepub.com/cms/10.1177/20499361241253751/asset/3f2cf483-d22d-4e5f-85ba-72304458d9ea/assets/images/large/10.1177_20499361241253751-fig2.jpg.

9.2.1. Allergic Aspergillosis

Allergic Aspergillosis, primarily in the guise of Allergic Bronchopulmonary Aspergillosis (ABPA), is a serious pulmonary disease that needs attention from clinicians and researchers alike. It predominantly affects individuals with underlying respiratory diseases, such as asthma and cystic fibrosis, and is an abnormal immune response to *Aspergillus fumigatus* antigens. The diagnosis of ABPA involves a clinical history of symptomatic asthma, cutaneous reactivity to A. fumigatus antigens, elevated total serum IgE concentration above 1000 IU/mL, and prominent radiological findings like transient pulmonary opacities and central bronchiectasis. Central bronchiectasis, described as a distinctive finding of ABPA, is difficult to diagnose in its initial phase and treat because the majority of clinicians miss potential cases in patients with uncontrolled asthma, thereby creating delays in treatment that may result in irreparable lung damage (Cinicola et al., 2016). The complex pathogenesis of Allergic Aspergillosis, even with the advancements in realizing its place in respiratory illnesses, remains much to be unraveled. The treatment regimens adopted are largely based on clinical evidence and not on rigid protocol, resulting in varied practices among caregivers. However, appropriate management of ABPA is necessary, given that it can lead to chronic pulmonary sequelae in case of neglect. Long-term treatment typically involves the use of corticosteroids to regulate acute inflammatory responses; however, the role of azoles and anti-IgE antibodies is increasingly valued. The latter drugs are employed as steroid-sparing agents, thereby prolonging remission periods and minimizing the cumulative toxicity of side effects of corticosteroids.

The inability to come to an agreement on therapeutic and diagnostic procedures once more stresses that the investigation of new immunomodulatory treatment and early screening in high-risk populations continues (Cinicola et al., 2016). Of main significance when treating Allergic Aspergillosis is an awareness of its association with bronchiectasis, a condition where the permanent widening of the bronchi by inflammation and damage takes place. Diagnosis of bronchiectasis is often multidimensional, including thorough examinations like clinical history, HRCT scan, and certain laboratory investigations.

The European Respiratory Society suggests extensive evaluation for identification of treatable conditions underlying the disease, and allergic bronchopulmonary aspergillosis is a primary consideration. The understanding of the interaction between bronchiectasis and Allergic Aspergillosis is imperative to facilitate early diagnosis and effective management, as a number of patients presenting with respiratory symptoms are not provided with appropriate management due to a lack of specificity in their symptoms. There is a necessity for enhanced awareness and education of practitioners on the clinical phenotypes of bronchiectasis to facilitate effective identification and management of the complex interaction (Figure 9.7).

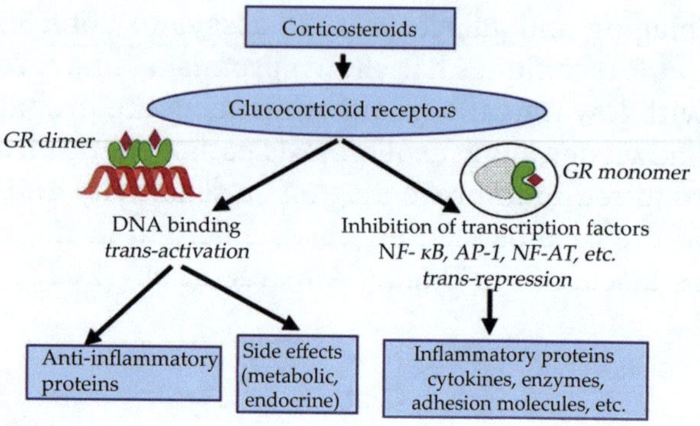

Figure 9.7. Long-term management often involves corticosteroids to mitigate acute inflammatory responses; however, the role of azoles and anti-IgE antibodies is increasingly recognized.

Source: https://media.springernature.com/full/springer-static/image/art%3A10.1038%2F35037026/MediaObjects/41586_1999_Article_BF35037026_Fig1_HTML.gif.

9.2.2. Invasive Aspergillosis

Invasive Aspergillosis (IA) is a significant clinical issue, particularly in immunocompromised patients, such as recipients of chemotherapy or bone marrow. The organism, primarily the species *Aspergillus fumigatus*, is extremely common within the environment, and contact is effectively unavoidable. Pathogenesis of IA is characterized by extreme preference for lung tissue and adjacent structures with associated lethal respiratory impairments. The illness is characterized by the invasion of blood vessels, resulting in acute pulmonary hemorrhage and secondary respiratory failure. These extreme consequences show the importance of early diagnosis and effective therapeutic management in patients infected with it. Recent work highlights the correlation of early antifungal therapy and improved survival rates, highlighting the importance of early clinical evaluation in treating this otherwise fatal condition. The diagnosis of Invasive Aspergillosis requires a multi-dimensional approach, with clinical, radiological, and mycological assessment. Diagnostic criteria have been modified to include varied non-culture-based diagnostics such as PCR and galactomannan testing that enhance detection rates. In spite of this, challenges remain—diagnostic failure can lead to delayed treatment and increased mortality. According to recent data, patients with hematological malignancies who experience acute respiratory failure often have undetermined etiologies despite extensive diagnostic regimens of which IA is responsible for a considerable proportion (Azoulay et al., 2016).

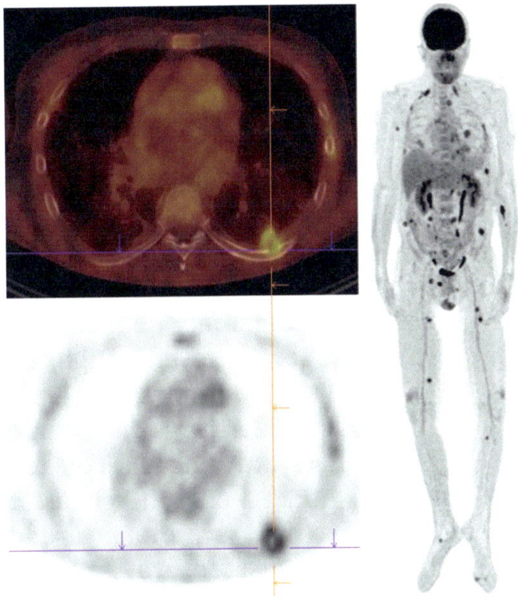

Figure 9.8. Invasive Aspergillosis (IA) represents a significant clinical challenge, particularly among immunocompromised patients, such as those undergoing chemotherapy or bone marrow transplantation.

Source: https://pub.mdpi-res.com/jof/jof-09-00131/article_deploy/html/images/jof-09-00131-g003.png?1675150835.

Moreover, invasive pulmonary aspergillosis has also been linked to high hospital mortality rates, and therefore it is an important determinant that requires immediate clinical intervention. These complexities necessitate profound understanding of IA to improve diagnostic sensitivity and patient management. In spite of a rise in the availability of treatment options for Invasive Aspergillosis, antifungal resistance is becoming a growing issue. Voriconazole remains a first-line therapy; however, resistant organisms complicate therapeutic strategies and adversely affect the prognosis. The increasing incidence of IA makes more effective antifungal treatments such as combination therapy or newer drugs targeting resistant infections important. Prevention, in the form of antifungal prophylaxis in high-risk patient populations, is also crucial in minimizing the occurrence of IA. Additionally, research activities supported by agencies with the vision to drive medical mycology are vital in widening the frame of knowledge and control over this invasive infection (King et al., 2017). Overall, an integrated approach consisting of rapid diagnosis, customized therapies, and efficient preventive strategies is vital in combating the rising threat of Invasive Aspergillosis in medical settings (Figure 9.8).

9.2.3. Chronic Aspergillosis

Chronic Aspergillosis, or chronic pulmonary aspergillosis (CPA), is a chronic infection of the lung by the species *Aspergillus*, primarily *Aspergillus fumigatus*. It typically arises in the presence of underlying lung disease, such as tuberculosis or chronic obstructive pulmonary disease (COPD), where the lung tissue is compromised. The clinical presentation of CPA can include weight loss, chronic cough, and hemoptysis, and hence it is essential that the clinicians detect the symptoms early. Delayed diagnosis and inappropriate treatment of CPA can lead to progressive lung damage, and hence right knowledge of its pathophysiology is significant. Notably, the patients typically exhibit an aberrant immune reaction to the antigens of fungi that results in heightened inflammation and tissue destruction, which complicates the whole clinical presentation and management strategy. The challenge in the diagnosis of this CPA is also added to by the overlap of symptoms with other pulmonary conditions and the lack of uniform diagnostic criteria. The clinicians should make use of findings obtained from combined clinical assessment, radiographic imaging, and mycological analysis, to make an accurate diagnosis. Nonetheless, existing mycological tests are not very sensitive, and this can lead to delayed or incorrect diagnosis with consequent effect on the outcome of treatment in patients. Consequently, according to existing literature, it is necessary for patients to receive prompt and targeted systemic antifungal therapy, and antifungal drug selection, e.g., itraconazole or voriconazole, is patient-reliant.

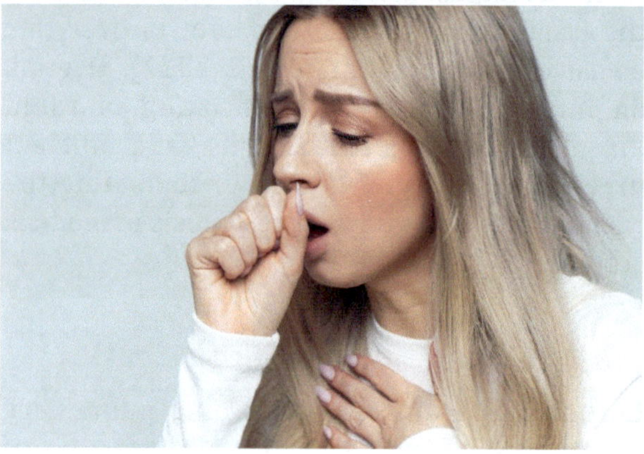

Figure 9.9. Chronic cough.

Source: https://familypracticecenterpc.com/wp-content/uploads/2018/12/4-Potential-Causes-of-Your-Chronic-Cough.jpg.

Given the high morbidity of CPA, vigilant follow-up care and watch for arising complications are crucial components of effective management protocols. Moreover, new therapy approaches for CPA have been established, yet significant effort still remains to be undertaken in standardization and chronic management protocols. Initial treatments currently employed also rely mostly on antifungal medications to control the infection and alleviate symptoms, but they may not be successful in resolving the root immune response. New therapies, including immunomodulatory treatments, are promising but require further research to establish their role in clinical practice. As per latest research, urgent research is necessary to establish improved diagnostic criteria and treatment regimens incorporating novel therapies. By solving these determinants, health workers can enhance the life quality of patients with Chronic Aspergillosis, reducing the chance of irreversible lung damage and associated complications (Cinicola et al., 2016; Hoenigl et al., 2018) (Figure 9.9).

9.3. Symptoms of Aspergillosis

The presentation of aspergillosis can be quite diverse based on the nature of the disease and the status of health in the infected person. In immunocompromised patients, invasive aspergillosis (IA) commonly presents with acute symptoms such as fever, cough, chest pain, and dyspnea. These symptoms are often overwhelmed by an underlying condition, thus becoming difficult to attribute directly to the fungal infection. Additionally, the clandestine character of IA so that symptoms are only manifest late in the disease process, making clinical presentation more complex. That late presentation of symptoms makes it imperative to detect and treat early, which, based on current guidelines, plays a vital role in improving patient outcomes. Thus, detection of the urgency of such symptoms is thus imperative in managing and treating effectively at-risk populations (King et al., 2017). On the other hand, chronic manifestations of aspergillosis, like chronic pulmonary aspergillosis (CPA), usually manifest with more subtle symptoms. The patients usually present with a chronic cough, intermittent hemoptysis (coughing up blood), tiredness, and weight loss over several years. CPA is often underdiagnosed since the non-specificity of such symptoms may overlap with other respiratory conditions. Chronic hemoptysis and coughing can be a source of significant distress for patients and compromise their quality of life. The resulting pulmonary changes, which manifest as cavitary lesions on imaging examinations, can eventually lead clinicians to diagnose CPA.

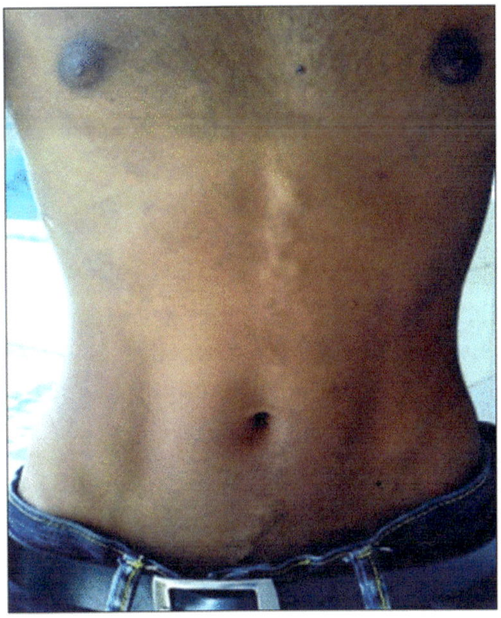

Figure 9.10. In immunocompromised patients, invasive aspergillosis (IA) often presents with acute symptoms such as high fever, cough, chest pain, and difficulty breathing.

Source: https://www.annsaudimed.net/cms/asset/35a554bc-6ab9-4fbb-94ba-17cf8f9dd12a/asm-5-409f1.gif.

It is important to recognize such chronic symptoms as they underpin early interventions that will alleviate suffering and improve health outcomes in affected individuals (Hoenigl et al., 2018). Furthermore, the allergic forms of aspergillosis, such as ABPA, present particular challenges in symptom identification and management. The symptoms of asthma, including wheezing, shortness of breath, and persistent cough, may occur in these patients, and management of such symptoms may prove unfruitful. *Aspergillus* species-induced allergic reaction precipitates worsening of asthma symptoms and makes underlying pulmonary conditions challenging by allowing chronic inflammation. Diagnosis can also include serological examinations for the detection of specific IgE antibodies to *Aspergillus*, as well as imaging investigations to picture typical bronchial hyperinflation and plugging of mucus. Early detection of ABPA manifestations is also of particular importance to initiate appropriate antifungal treatment and control the asthma-like exacerbations and so better manage patients affected by this allergic condition to aspergilli (King et al., 2017) (Figure 9.10).

9.3.1. Respiratory Symptoms

The respiratory manifestations of aspergillosis are the greatest concern due to their potential severity and the involved mechanisms. Ingestion by inhalation or aspiration of *Aspergillus* spores may generate a spectrum of respiratory illnesses, including cough, wheezing, and dyspnea. They usually mimic the symptoms of other pulmonary diseases, hence the potential risk of misdiagnosis and delayed treatment. The clinical presentation of invasive pulmonary aspergillosis (IPA) is very threatening in immunocompromised individuals, where the disease can progress rapidly. Evidence shows that IPA can unexpectedly arise in individuals who do not display conventional risk factors, proving the opportunism of the pathogens. For instance, patients who are seriously ill with COVID-19 have been observed to develop IPA even when there is no classic predisposition that has usually been associated with fungal infections, as they can acquire respiratory symptoms that will become advanced within a very short time and require urgent medical attention (Eller et al., 2021). Aspergillosis diagnosis complicates the management of respiratory symptoms, for which the total clinical examination and diagnostic workup are mandatory. Clinicians traditionally rely on a combination of imaging studies, such as chest CT scans, and laboratory studies to diagnose the presence of *Aspergillus* species in respiratory secretions. The challenge is due to the variability of symptoms and clinical presentations among patients, particularly in patient populations with underlying respiratory disease such as pneumonia or COPD. During acute exacerbation, corticosteroids can suppress airway inflammation, thereby making it more challenging to diagnose and less likely to recognize aspergillosis in a timely manner. Additionally, research sponsored by premier grants highlights the importance of understanding interactions between respiratory status and fungal infection, a variable that can realign diagnostic strategies and treatment algorithms for individuals with early respiratory symptoms (King et al., 2017).

Management of respiratory symptoms secondary to aspergillosis must be intensive and tailor-made to the specific needs of the patient and also taking into consideration the potential for rapid deterioration. Antifungal treatment in the form of voriconazole or amphotericin B is essential in treating *Aspergillus* and alleviating respiratory distress.

In addition to pharmacotherapy, supplemental oxygenation and bronchodilator therapy may be used to alleviate evidence of hypoxemia and bronchospasm. Diligent monitoring of respiratory performance on an ongoing basis should identify a priority, especially among patients with pre-existing lung disease or immunocompromised status. Lastly, management of aspergillosis respiratory symptoms involves not only the healing of fungal infection but also an interdisciplinary measure to arrange for the comprehensive respiratory health of individuals who might be at risk. Also, an understanding of these complexities will enhance patient outcomes against this opportunistic pathogen (Eller et al., 2021) (Figure 9.11).

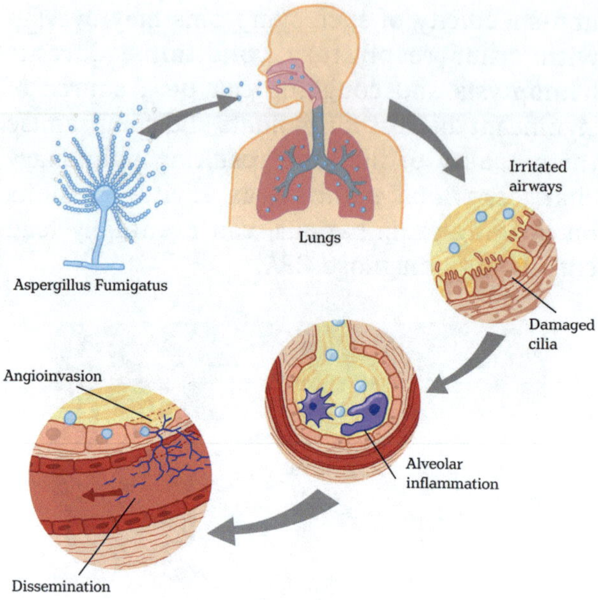

Figure 9.11. The clinical manifestation of invasive pulmonary aspergillosis (IPA) is particularly alarming in immunocompromised patients, where rapid progression can occur.

Source: https://onlinelibrary.wiley.com/cms/asset/006a646b-868a-44b5-b881-11c19a88dca5/apm13316-fig-0001-m.png.

9.3.2. Systemic Symptoms

Systemic manifestations of aspergillosis represent a prominent indicator of disease progression, often occurring when the infection has spread past the localized stages. Systemic manifestations involve fever, malaise, and weight loss, and may be accounted for by the inflammatory response of the body against the *Aspergillus* species. Patients, especially those immunocompromised, may manifest with an exaggerated host response that renders their clinical presentation more complicated. The presence of systemic symptoms is generally a sign of a more severe expression of the disease, such as invasive aspergillosis, where fungal spores penetrate into body systems and lead to complications such as pneumonia or disseminated infection. Early detection of these systemic symptoms plays a significant influence on patient management and outcome through early intervention and potential improved prognosis. The challenge in making a diagnosis of systemic aspergillosis is that its symptoms are nonspecific. Fever and malaise, while common in the majority of infectious diseases, are not pathognomonic for fungal infection and therefore present a diagnostic challenge. Furthermore, as suggested by recent reports, invasive aspergillosis mycological examinations are of low sensitivity, and diagnoses in high-risk patients are often delayed. If the patients are not neutropenic, manifestations of systemic symptoms may be atypical, posing another degree of difficulty in the clinical assessment. Therefore, clinicians should be vigilant and keep an open differential diagnosis in mind while seeing systemic symptoms in aspergillosis patients. In the absence of pathognomonic diagnostic procedures, familiarity with the context of these symptoms allows for better clinical decision-making. Treatment of systemic symptoms in aspergillosis patients is significantly linked to the early initiation of antifungal therapy. New recommendations emphasize that early and targeted systemic antifungal treatment is the most important prognostic factor for a favorable outcome, especially in immunocompromised patients. As per recommendations described in the recent standards, drugs such as voriconazole and isavuconazole are recommended for primary treatment of invasive aspergillosis, and liposomal amphotericin B remains the first alternative. This tailored therapy plays a critical role in managing the systemic manifestation of the disease, such that early action will be able to avoid further complications. As antifungal therapy and knowledge of the disease process advance with ongoing innovations, opportunities for improved management regimes that take into account both the complexities of systemic signs and overall patient health in victims of aspergillosis are enhanced (King et al., 2017; Hoenigl et al., 2018) (Figure 9.12).

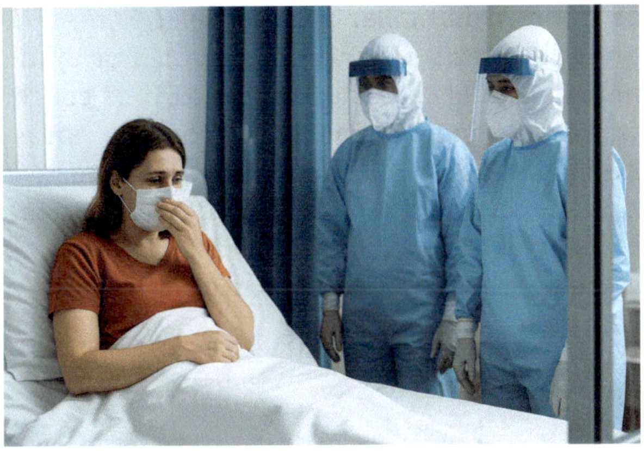

Figure 9.12. Patients, especially those who are immunocompromised, may experience an overwhelming host response that complicates their clinical picture.

Source: https://skycare.uk/wp-content/uploads/2025/05/air-travel-immunocompromised-patient-1024x683.png.

9.3.3. Symptoms Specific to Different Types of Aspergillosis

Aspergillosis is defined by a widespread spectrum of clinical features based on the specific type of infection as well as the overall state of health in the infected individual. In its most severe form, invasive aspergillosis (IA) presents with an acute onset of symptoms, particularly in immunocompromised persons, such as those undergoing cancer therapy or stem cell transplant. Symptoms are typically fever, cough, and chest pain with the frequent accompanying hemoptysis or sputum expectoration with blood. The diagnosis of IA is still problematic with presenting patients having non-specific radiological findings that pose difficulties in effective treatment protocols. Since the risk of unfavorable outcomes is present, particularly in the intensive care unit (ICU) setting, early detection is critical as delay in diagnosis can cause significantly higher mortality rates (Bassetti et al., 2017). Non-invasive aspergillosis presentation, such as allergic bronchopulmonary aspergillosis (ABPA), follows an entirely dissimilar symptom pattern. ABPA typically affects patients with asthma or cystic fibrosis and is characterized by chronic cough, wheezing, and intermittent chest tightness. ABPA pathophysiology involves an overactive immune response to *Aspergillus* species. Patients present with recurrent respiratory infections and may develop bronchiectasis due to lung damage if left untreated.

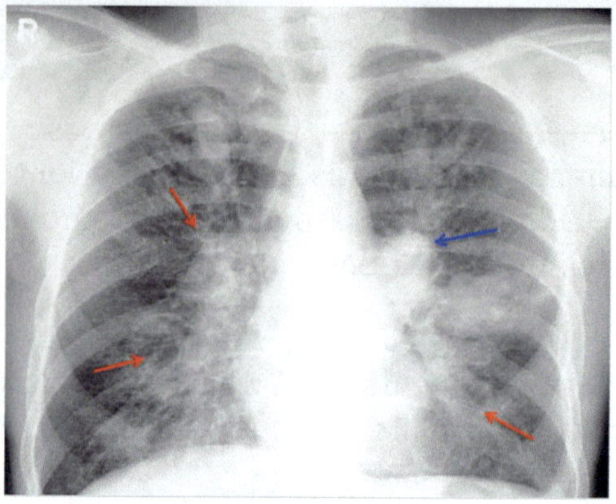

Figure 9.13. Non-invasive forms of aspergillosis, such as allergic bronchopulmonary aspergillosis (ABPA), exhibit a markedly different symptom profile.

Source: https://upload.wikimedia.org/wikipedia/commons/d/da/Article_river_5800d6205cfa11e99c51c512b70b63f3-Fig-1.png.

Another typical presentation, aspergilloma, is responsible for a ball of fungus most commonly within a pre-existing pulmonary cavity, producing such findings as chronic cough and frequent hemoptysis. This symptom dichotomy highlights the necessity to individualize diagnostic plans and treatment modalities to the specific form of aspergillosis being presented by the patient (Bassetti et al., 2017). Chronic pulmonary aspergillosis (CPA) is characterized by another spectrum of symptoms, months to years after the onset in people with previous lung disease, such as COPD or tuberculosis. Patients have chronic cough, weight loss, fever, and nocturnal sweats, which can be mistaken for chronic respiratory disease. If left untreated, CPA can cause severe lung damage and respiratory failure. CPA diagnostic workup usually involves imaging and serology testing for fungal biomarkers such as galactomannan and beta-D-glucan, which are useful but not specific. A consideration of the nuances of presentation of different aspergillosis forms should be maintained to facilitate early detection and proper management, particularly in individuals at risk who might present with similar overlapping symptoms (Lamoth et al., 2016) (Figure 9.13).

9.4. Diagnosis of Aspergillosis

The diagnosis of aspergillosis is mostly a combination of clinical tests, imaging studies, and microbiological studies. The physicians typically begin with the assessment of the patients symptoms and clinical history that may include respiratory disease, fever, and chest pain. These clinical presentations are significant as they guide further investigations for diagnosis. High-resolution computed tomography (HRCT) scanning is crucial in the identification of particular pulmonary features of the disease, including the distinctive air crescent sign. This radiological feature is indicative of invasive pulmonary aspergillosis and is critical evidence that guides the clinical strategy toward treatment. While imaging findings are informative, they are most useful in combination with the patient's symptomatology and overall state of health to create a complete diagnostic template required for effective management. Microbiological techniques are equally important in establishing the diagnosis of aspergillosis. Bronchoalveolar lavage (BAL) is a procedure frequently employed to yield respiratory secretions, which may be directly visualized. The isolation of *Aspergillus* species from BAL fluid can provide definite evidence of infection, particularly when complemented with tissue histopathology. Serum markers such as galactomannan can also be measured, offering a non-invasive means of detecting invasive aspergillosis in immunocompromised patients. The sensitivity and specificity of these tests vary; hence, a multi-dimensional approach that incorporates both clinical and microbiologic data has to be employed. The ability to balance these investigative tools helps establish an appropriate diagnosis, having a significant effect on the treatment to be undertaken and the outcome of the patient afterwards.

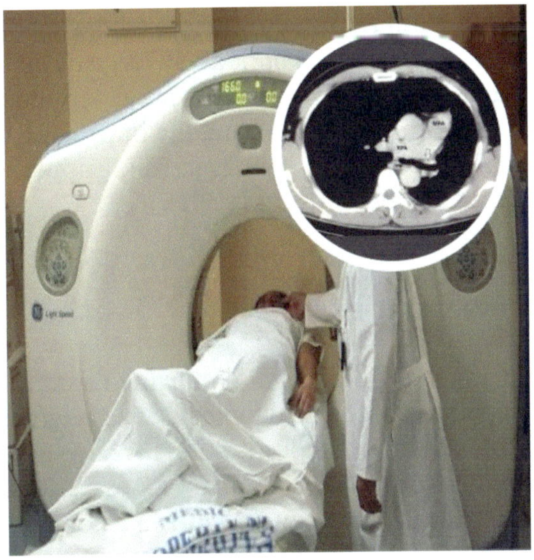

Figure 9.14. High-resolution computed tomography (HRCT) scans play a significant role in identifying specific pulmonary manifestations of the disease, such as the characteristic air crescent sign.

Source: https://www.ganeshdiagnostic.com/admin/public/assets/images/product/1663661991-HRCT%20Thorax.webp.

In case the initial conservative treatment proves to fail, radical surgical treatment may be necessary, particularly in patients with localized invasive pulmonary aspergillosis. Lobectomy or pneumonectomy can be contemplated when no improvement is seen after antifungal treatment, as shown through clinical and radiological assessments. In a clinical trial with 18 patients, surgical treatment led to the prognosis for such patients being greatly improved, demonstrating the effectiveness of such treatment in managing the disease (Baron et al., 1998). Additionally, such a surgical intervention tends to distinguish aspergillosis from non-fungal infections, thereby reducing the clinical diagnosis. As patients are still suffering from underlying immunocompromised conditions, ongoing monitoring and more robust treatments are required (Groll et al., 2012). The depth of diagnosis and treatment indicates the thorough processes involved in effective perhaps calving of aspergillosis (Figure 9.14).

9.4.1. Clinical Evaluation and Patient History

A clinical examination and full patient history are important in aspergillosis diagnosis and treatment. *Aspergillus* species can cause a range of diseases from allergic reaction to invasive disease, particularly in immunocompromised patients such as transplant recipients. Comprehensive patient history should involve details about past medical conditions, recent surgeries, and immunosuppressive therapy, all contributing significantly to determining risk for fungal infection. Furthermore, information regarding the patients exposures to the environment—e.g., exposure to wet or moldy settings—can provide invaluable clues in identifying the source of the infection. Clinicians can pay attention to symptoms such as chronic cough, hemoptysis, or fever because these may align with the variable presentations of aspergillosis. The association of clinical presentation and patient history ultimately guides subsequent diagnostic testing and therapeutic intervention, acknowledging the sophistication in the treatment of this fungal infection. Invasive fungal diseases, including aspergillosis, have become leading causes of illness within susceptible populations. Based on revised guidelines, the definition of invasive fungal infections demands a complex understanding that transcends traditional paradigms of immunocompromised individuals.

Clinical diagnosis must therefore entail thorough examination of imaging and laboratory results alongside patient history. Computed tomography and bronchoscopy, among other advanced methods, may be utilized for more accurate detection and identification of aspergillosis. The dynamic and progressively broadening categorizations also highlight that current diagnostic criteria can be applied to more patient populations, invalidating the idea that only immunocompromised patients are at risk. This evolution identifies the necessity to include patient-specific variables like their psychosocial background and symptomatology, which may influence clinical presentation and management, necessitating therapeutic individualization. Finally, aspergillosis treatment is based on its clinical evaluation and patient history complexity. Each case presents a unique challenge, so it requires a multidisciplinary strategy from medical practitioners in order to be able to make decisions regarding appropriate antifungal treatment.

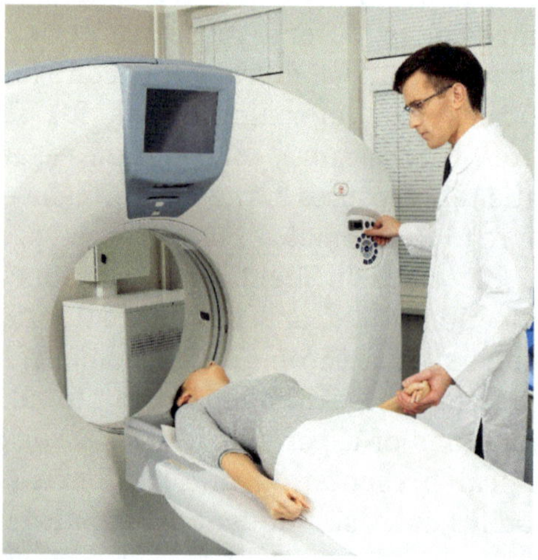

Figure 9.15. Clinicians must be vigilant in recognizing symptoms such as chronic cough, hemoptysis, or fever, as these can align with the diverse presentations of aspergillosis.

Source: https://helma.healthians.com/stationery/mailer-assets/6332d70084714.jpg.

Such complexity occurs particularly in the patient with comorbid disease or recent surgery, as reflected by clinical experience among transplant recipients. For instance, in a noted case, effective treatment of an aspergillosis central nervous system infection in a young patient was through careful evaluation and tailored treatment with the use of a regimen of multiple antifungals and surgery (Green et al., 1991). Furthermore, the new definitions of invasive aspergillosis emphasize the use of multidisciplinary teams to formulate targeted approaches that are appropriate to the specific circumstances of each patient. Synergistic action is vital to reduce the risk of severe aspergillosis-related complications, ultimately improving the clinical outcomes in this high-risk population (Akan et al., 2019) (Figure 9.15).

9.4.2. Laboratory Tests and Imaging Techniques

Both laboratory testing and imaging techniques are reliant on accurate diagnosis of aspergillosis and are pivotal in differentiating invasive fungal infections from other pulmonary illnesses. Serum beta-D-glucan assays and serum galactomannan are significant serological tests that provide feedback on *Aspergillus* species presence within the bloodstream. Galactomannan detection, in particular, is a helpful invasive aspergillosis marker offering great sensitivity in immunocompromised patients, as suggested by current research guidelines. Furthermore, the addition of newer molecular techniques, such as polymerase chain reaction (PCR), helps to further improve diagnostic accuracy through rapid detection of fungal DNA. New laboratory methods not only provide prompt results but also enable early interventions, which are critical in reducing morbidity and mortality of such life-threatening infection. Imaging is also a central feature of the diagnostic process of aspergillosis, particularly in assessing disease extent and complications. Computed tomography of the chest at high resolution (HRCT) is currently the gold standard for imaging pulmonary aspergillosis, and it shows characteristic imaging findings in the form of air crescent signs or halo signs consistent with necrotizing lesions. Imaging signs are particularly important in coming to a probable diagnosis with clinical presentations and laboratory findings. The correlation of imaging findings with established criteria for classification—proved, probable, and possible invasive fungal diseases—is a testament to the effectiveness of rigorous evaluation in the process of diagnosis. Moreover, the ability of imaging evaluations to demonstrate change over time is crucial in tracking therapeutic response and directing further management plans. Recent criticisms and advancements in invasive fungal infection diagnostic criteria, as observed in current literature, reflect a need for continued refinement in diagnosis. Collaboration among disparate specialists has led to new definitions and classifications better capturing the current diagnostic capabilities. (Akan et al., 2019) states the necessity to narrow down invasive fungal infection classification categories to cover a greater number of high-risk patients, indicative of a shift towards expanding the categories. Moreover, findings from (Blasco-Navalpotro et al., 2015) show the clinician's immediate need to make correct diagnoses of invasive aspergillosis among critically ill patients, with a need for collaboration across disciplines to improve patient outcomes. As the latest diagnostic equipment is developed, the specialty will be enriched by the incorporation of advances in laboratory technology and imaging modalities, further increasing the prognostic utility of these tests in clinical practice (Figure 9.16).

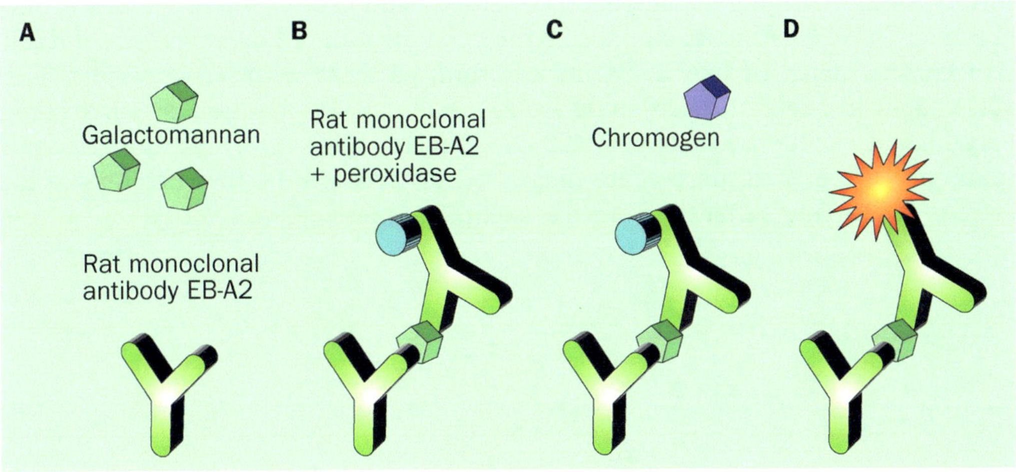

Figure 9.16. Galactomannan detection, in particular, is a valuable marker for invasive aspergillosis, yielding high sensitivity among immunocompromised populations, as noted in contemporary research practices.

Source: https://microbeonline.com/wp-content/uploads/2022/05/Platelia-*Aspergillus*-Galactomannan-Enzyme-Immunoassay.jpg.

9.4.3. Differential Diagnosis

Differential diagnosis plays a critical role in the diagnosis of allergic bronchopulmonary aspergillosis (ABPA) and differentiation from other respiratory diseases, particularly in individuals with cystic fibrosis and asthma. The reason for the difficulty in diagnosing ABPA is the overlapping clinical manifestation with asthma exacerbation and cystic fibrosis pulmonary infections. Definitive diagnostic criteria are clinical history, serologic testing for evidence of the presence of specific IgE responses to *Aspergillus fumigatus* antigens, and imaging studies that may demonstrate central bronchiectasis or fleeting opacities. As the literature explains, the challenge is distinguishing cystic fibrosis patients with ABPA from those without, since many common tests lack sensitivity in distinguishing between these subgroups (Bansal et al., 2006). There is thus a call for a sensitive approach to avoid misdiagnosis and avoid unnecessary management with a lot of morbidity. The detection of ABPA requires careful evaluation of immunological response and clinical presentation. It can be presented by patients with an elevated total serum IgE level of over 1000 IU/mL, a common diagnostic marker of ABPA indicating a chronic allergic process (Cinicola et al., 2016). Nonetheless, because asthma and cystic fibrosis are heterogeneously presented, the clinicians must use a predetermined set of diagnostic criteria encompassing both clinical and laboratory findings. The absence of consensus on diagnostic thresholds would render the evaluation process complicated, so that repeat testing and careful clinical assessment might need to be considered. Thus, early diagnosis is limited, and this is extremely crucial in the early treatment initiation as well as preventing irreversible lung injury. Therefore, the development of standardized diagnosis guidelines is imperative to improve patient outcomes in ABPA. Current approaches to the differential diagnosis of ABPA also indicate a requirement for chronic management regimens based on patient individual profiles. While corticosteroids remain the primary treatment, awareness of the requirement for adjunct therapies such as azoles and anti-IgE antibodies in managing uncontrolled conditions and prolonging remission (Cinicola et al., 2016) is growing. These treatments emphasize the need for tailored management of the individual patient with chronic diseases like ABPA. In addition, patients with hard-to-control asthma or cystic fibrosis ought to qualify for screening for A. fumigatus sensitization, as early recognition of ABPA is very likely to influence management. Last but not least, improved understanding of the disease's pathophysiology and more acute diagnostic criteria will be instrumental to the success of interventions in patients suffering from this complex illness (Figure 9.17).

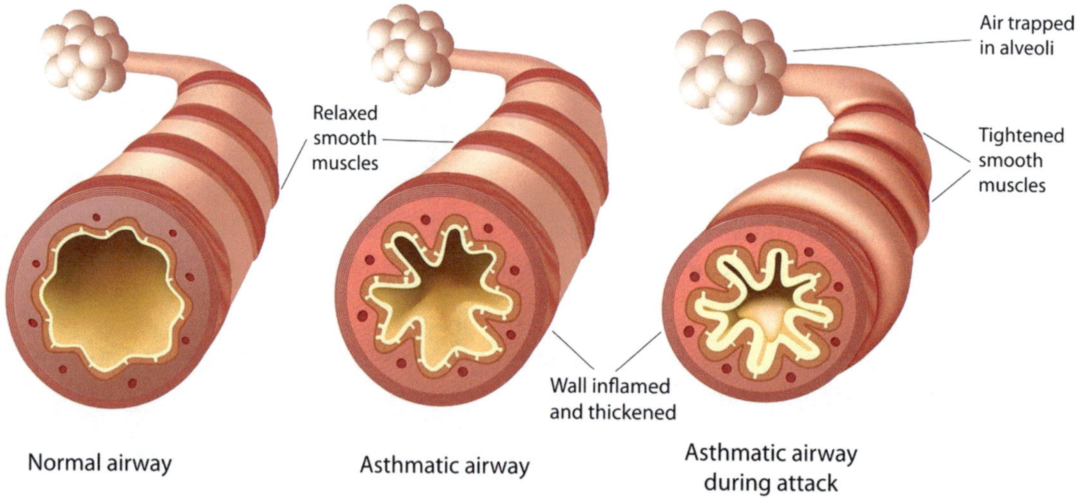

Figure 9.17. Asthma exacerbations.

Source: https://canadiem.org/wp-content/uploads/2017/07/asthmatic-airway-Shutterstock.jpg.

9.5. Treatment Options

The treatment of Aspergillosis, particularly in immunocompromised individuals, warrants a careful and specific approach to attain the best treatment and improved outcomes for the patient. Voriconazole is currently the first-line treatment of choice for invasive aspergillosis (IA) and has been shown to be active against most *Aspergillus* species. As IA carries a high morbidity and mortality rate, immediate initiation of appropriate systemic antifungal therapy is necessary. Guidelines of current clinical practice have recommended voriconazole and/or isavuconazole as first-line treatments, with liposomal amphotericin B being a good alternative. It is very important to treat these antifungals at an early stage in the case of clinical suspicion of IA to ensure the highest success of treatment and possibly balance the serious consequences that the disease bears (Hoenigl et al., 2018). Treatment of chronic pulmonary aspergillosis (CPA) is very different. Prolonged oral therapies, including itraconazole and voriconazole, are the current gold standard for CPA treatment. Unlike IA in its acute form, CPA has chronic treatment challenges where patients must be put on long-term antifungal therapy as a result of the chronic infection and primary underlying lung disease. CPA care not only demands cautious application of antifungal therapy but also vigilant surveillance for side effects and drug-drug interactions, especially in patients with complex comorbidities. Moreover, individualized treatment regimens based on the individual patient's unique clinical scenario, including the degree of immunosuppression, are pivotal to long-term care (Stewart et al., 2016). Salvage therapy is also important in the management of aspergillosis when initial options are not successful or in breakthrough infections among patients. Polyenes, new triazole compounds, or echinocandins combined with voriconazole can be employed in patients with poor response to initial treatments. These approaches emphasize the importance of formulating a high level of clinical suspicion and establishing proper diagnostic maneuvers at the time of infection. Since resistance patterns towards antifungal drugs continue to evolve, the potential for combination therapy can become an increasingly important consideration for effective treatment of aspergillosis. Developing an integrative treatment plan with multidisciplinary teams of infectious disease physicians and pulmonologists will enhance outcomes for patients faced with the challenge of this complex fungal infection (Hoenigl et al., 2018) (Figure 9.18).

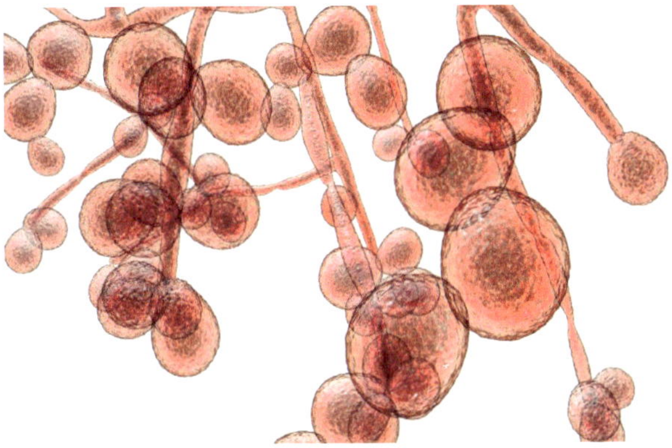

Figure 9.18. Echinocandins.

Source: https://prdmspst.blob.core.windows.net/images/articles/invasive-candidiasis-2f08666c-949d-436c-8062-f8381dc25134-thumbnail.jpg.

9.5.1. Antifungal Medications

The treatment of aspergillosis, which is primarily due to the *Aspergillus* species, has evolved with the use of various antifungal medications. Traditional antifungal medications such as azoles, polyenes, and echinocandins have played a key role in the treatment of invasive aspergillosis. Azoles such as voriconazole and itraconazole are typically the initial line in treatment due to their efficacy against *Aspergillus* species and favorable pharmacokinetics. Nevertheless, the resultant issue of drug resistance calls for continuous evaluation of treatment regimens.

The use of combination therapies would enhance the efficiency of antifungal therapy and decrease the chance for the emergence of resistance, thus demanding continuous studies to investigate these mechanisms under clinical conditions. Recent studies have shown novel ways to enhance antifungal delivery, such as curcumin-loaded lipid nanoparticles (CLNs). This new formulation is prepared to increase the bioavailability and therapeutic activity of curcumin, a bioactive compound with known antifungal action. Traditional treatment with curcumin is typically hampered by its low solubility; however, its encapsulation within lipid nanoparticles can considerably enhance its pharmacological profile. CLN formulation has appeared not only higher antifungal activity against pathogens *Aspergillus niger* and *Candida albicans* but also lower systemic toxicity. Moreover, this method is promising to overcome existing antifungal resistance, which remains a major challenge to treating aspergillosis (TM et al., 2025). On comparative analysis of monotherapy versus combination antifungal therapy, new meta-analyses offer a large amount of information regarding their clinical relevance. The combination of echinocandins with SOC antifungal therapy indicated no detectable differences in clinical cure rates or mortality rates compared to SOC monotherapy. However, an emergent clinical advantage with combination of echinocandins and SOC therapies is indicated, and it is stated that further studies may elucidate more clearly the advantage of combination therapy (Alsowaida et al., 2024). These emerging data justify our efforts in modifying our treatment paradigms and emphasize the need for further research toward optimizing antifungal regimens against aspergillosis and improving patient outcomes (Figure 9.19).

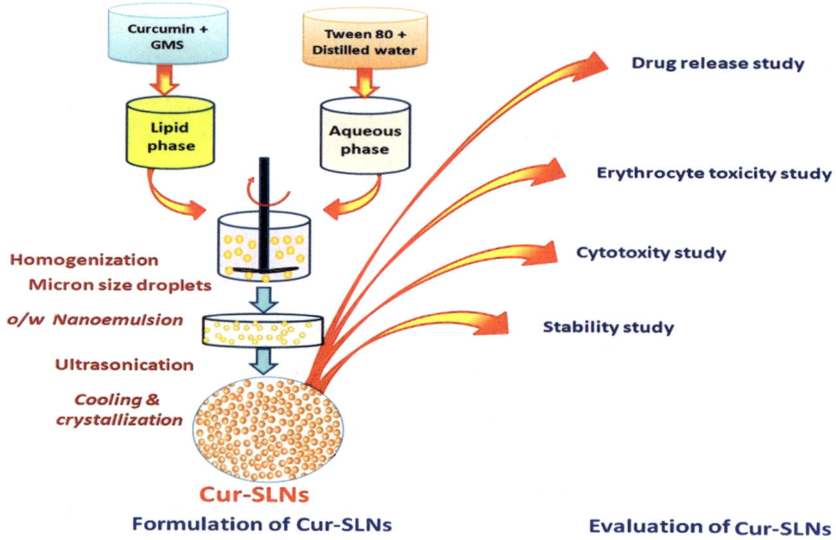

Figure 9.19. Curcumin-loaded lipid nanoparticles (CLNs).

Source: https://www.pharmaexcipients.com/wp-content/uploads/2023/02/Fabrication-of-Sustained-Release-Curcumin-Loaded-Solid-Lipid-Nanoparticles-Cur-SLNs-as-a-Potential-Drug-Delivery-System-for-the-Treatment-of-Lung-Cancer.png.

9.5.2. Surgical Interventions

Surgical procedures come into play to treat aspergillosis, especially when standard medical treatments no longer work or when the disease has become complicated. Invasive pulmonary aspergillosis with its rapidly advancing nature and mortality rate tends to require a multi-faceted strategy that incorporates surgical intervention. Applying surgical techniques such as lobectomy or decortication can be of benefit in isolating and excising the infected lung parenchyma, thereby alleviating the local disease burden and hopefully improving patient outcomes. For instance, when a patient with chronic necrotizing pulmonary aspergillosis was managed using surgical procedures in combination with antifungal therapy, the outcome showed the potential efficacy of integrating surgery and medicine in complex situations (Cho et al.). Surgical methods should be chosen with careful regard to the patient variables and the severity of the illness. Research shows that early surgical resection of the disease can improve survival, particularly for those models of local invasive aspergillosis. In a study involving rats with neutropenia, those who were subjected to early lobectomy demonstrated markedly enhanced survival rates in relation to their non-operated controls, which shows the possible advantages of early surgical resections in inhibiting local dissemination of disease (Adler et al., 2017). These findings highlight the importance of patient-specific treatment regimens that include surgical intervention as an adjunct to medical therapy, particularly in the immunocompromised host who is most likely to develop severe infection. While signs for surgical intervention in the management of aspergillosis are present, they are not without risk and limitation. The surgical interventions themselves carry risk of complications like infection, hemorrhage, and extended hospital stay. Therefore, proper patient evaluation is required prior to choosing surgical methods, weighing the potential benefits against inherent risks. The type of surgical intervention also must be appropriate to the individual case, considering severity of fungal infection, patients overall health, and severity of symptoms. Therefore, while surgical procedures might be a necessary component of aspergillosis treatment, particularly in complicated or refractory disease, they must be utilized as part of a broader, overall treatment regimen with close observation and proper medical treatment (Figure 9.20).

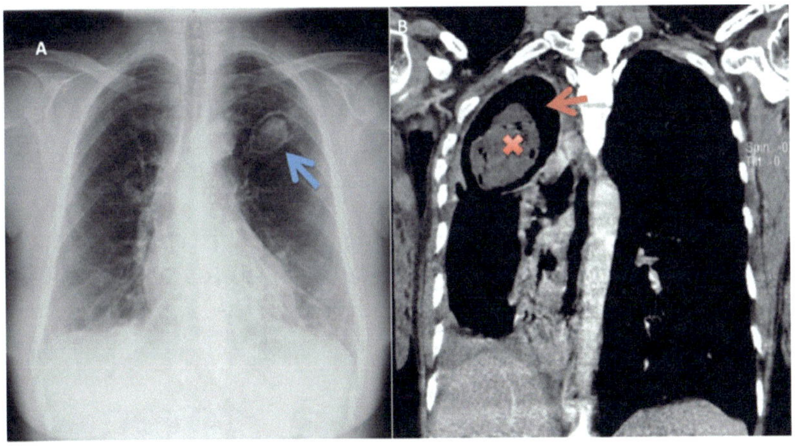

Figure 9.20. When a patient diagnosed with chronic necrotizing pulmonary aspergillosis underwent surgical treatments alongside antifungal therapy.

Source: https://pub.mdpi-res.com/jof/jof-06-00075/article_deploy/html/images/jof-06-00075-g003.png?1591931469.

9.5.3. Management of Underlying Conditions

Good control of baseline conditions is paramount in the setting of aspergillosis, a fungal infection that largely involves immunocompromised hosts. Diabetes mellitus, chronic lung disorders, and immunosuppressive conditions have a high predisposing potential for more debilitating manifestations of aspergillosis. Treatment of these underlying conditions involves a multi-pronged strategy that includes normalizing diabetic patients' glycemic levels and treating chronic pulmonary disorders to improve overall lung function. Effective management of these comorbidities has the potential to cancel out aspergillosis progression risk, thereby improving patient outcomes. Furthermore, regular health assessment for the purpose of diagnosing the incidence and severity of underlying disorders of health is important in prescribing treatment guidelines that prevent further complications of *Aspergillus* infection. Moreover, recognition of interconnected states of underlying disorders of health and aspergillosis is essential for patient treatment in its totality. A study pointed out that fatigue is an often neglected factor in the treatment of chronic disease; therefore, clinicians need to take precedence in addressing such symptoms in addition to the main treatment for aspergillosis (Mulligan et al., 2024). Fatigue-slowing interventions such as supporting physical activity can significantly enhance quality of life in already disease-burdened patients. It accentuates the need to integrate the management of fatigue into the treatment regimens of patients suffering from chronic diseases, such as those who are predisposed to aspergillosis. This helps to enhance the overall success of the treatment and the satisfaction level of the patient. Apart from directly treating the underlying diseases, education as well as preventive care is also helpful in diminishing the risks associated with aspergillosis. Healthcare practitioners should promote patients' active participation in symptom recognition of their underlying disease and informing them on *Aspergillus* exposure and its risks, particularly in immunocompromised individuals. Empowering patients through education programs on the importance of living a healthy lifestyle and developing knowledge regarding environmental determinants leading to fungal infections is possible. Moreover, as pointed out in the lower urinary tract disease guidelines, routine diagnostic evaluation is instrumental to the diagnosis of complicating conditions that could exacerbate aspergillosis symptoms (Samantha et al., 2025). Such a comprehensive approach ensures the disease and its risk factors are handled accordingly, ultimately leading to better health outcomes for the patient (Figure 9.21).

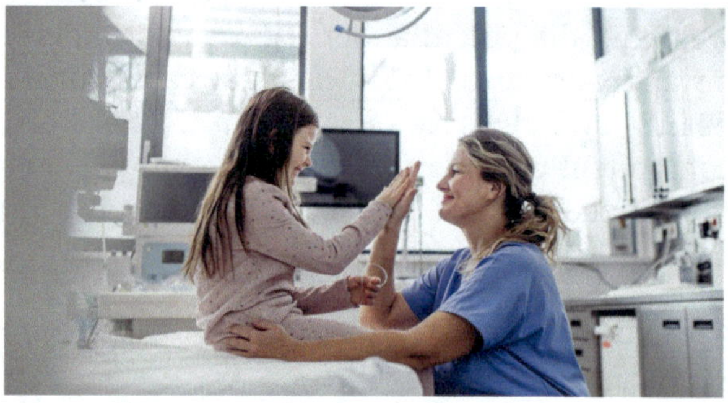

Figure 9.21. Healthcare providers can enhance the overall treatment efficacy and patient satisfaction.

Source: https://www.sermo.com/wp-content/uploads/2025/04/improve-patient-satisfaction-01.jpg.

9.6. Prevention Strategies

Preventive interventions against aspergillosis are generally effective in limiting exposure to *Aspergillus* species in vulnerable populations such as immunocompromised hosts. Management of environmental fungal contamination by rigorous air quality control is one of the main approaches.

High-efficiency particulate air (HEPA) filters in healthcare facilities and maintenance of cleanliness and dryness of environments to prevent spore growth are components of this. Regular monitoring of infected areas and decontamination can contribute substantially to the avoidance of infection. For instance, scientific studies have shown that detection of fungal spores is possible to enhance by utilizing specific methods of sampling, thereby allowing the application of certain cleaning and prevention measures. Research indicates that cotton pads and DC pads are far more effective at gathering fungal spores than traditional Rodac contact plates, enabling improved monitoring and environmental control (D'Alessandro et al., 2008). In addition to environmental monitoring and control, preventive action on the basis of the patient is of absolute significance. In the case of patients undergoing treatments such as allogeneic hematopoietic stem cell transplantation (HSCT), dysfunction of the immune system renders the patient more susceptible to infections, including aspergillosis. Immunotherapeutic interventions thus take center stage. Such treatments could entail the infusion of granulocytes or donor-derived antifungal T cells to boost the patient's immune system against fungal infections. There is evidence that such treatments could drastically lower the rates of invasive fungal infections among recipients of HSCT and consequently enhance overall survival. Further research on the use of natural killer cells to fight such infections also presents promising new paths for prevention and treatment. These immunologic treatments combined show a multi-component approach to lowering the burden of aspergillosis in vulnerable populations (Klingebiel et al., 2013). Finally, public health interventions through education and awareness can have a direct impact on the prevention of aspergillosis. Physicians should go out of their way to inform susceptible patients about the dangers of mold exposure, especially in environments like home repair or when switching from warm to cold weather when spores in the air may be able to proliferate. Providing advice on reducing indoor humidity, using mold-resistant materials in building construction, and appropriate ventilation are easy practices that can be adopted by individuals. Community monitoring systems are also effective in finding and mitigating sources of fungal spores in public spaces. Healthcare providers and public health agencies can collaborate to create a comprehensive prevention plan based on individual practices and community-wide efforts. This holistic strategy is an indication of appreciation for the complex interplay between environmental and health status to ensure effective control of aspergillosis.

9.6.1. Environmental Control Measures

Environmental management plays a crucial role in a vertibility of the risk of aspergillosis, particularly where vulnerable populations exist, such as health care units and hospitals. Air quality control plays a central role among these interventions because spores of *Aspergillus* organisms suspended in the air are ubiquitous in the environment and can pose serious infections, particularly in immunocompromised persons. HEPA filtered ventilation systems are to be installed to reduce airborne fungal contamination. Low humidity conditions in controlled environments are also required because high moisture content leads to spore germination and colonization. Adherence to stringent cleaning routines that include regular disinfection of surfaces and the removal of biological material is equally vital in minimizing spore deposition and the related inhalation exposure. Further, strict compliance with the use of personal protective equipment (PPE) among patients' visitors and medical personnel will greatly influence the transmission dynamics of aspergillosis. Simple interventions involving the use of masks and gloves when coming into contact with patients or contaminated areas represent an initial barrier to airborne particulate matter and direct contact with contaminated surfaces. As also suggested by prior research, prevention of transmission controls, treatment controls, and environmental disinfection controls remain the major strategies proven through various numerical experiments, which corroborate their effect in curbing disease spread prior to individual interventions. Given that healthcare facilities continue to struggle with outbreaks, integrated strategies stress the importance of integrated measures for infection prevention, hence safeguarding vulnerable groups while tackling aspergillosis effectively.

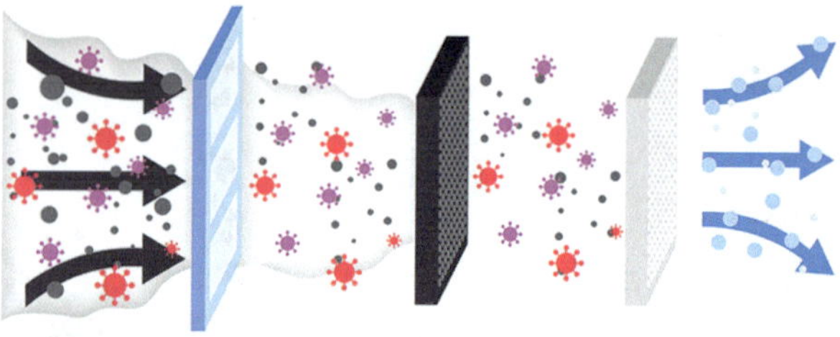

Figure 9.22. Ventilation systems should be equipped with high-efficiency particulate air (HEPA) filters to reduce airborne fungal contamination.

Source: https://sites.manchester.ac.uk/covid19-national-project/wp-content/uploads/sites/276/2022/09/air-filtration.jpg.

Lastly, the role played by training and education towards environmental control measures cannot be overestimated. Provision for health-care staff to be properly sensitized on the environmental risks of *Aspergillus* exposure and being properly trained in the correct use of control measures is likely to create a more responsive and proactive health-care setting. This is aligned with the present health policy of encouraging whole infection prevention policies that are crucial in evading the emergence of aspergillosis among vulnerable populations. Greater awareness will mean actual compliance with infection control measures, resulting in decreased rates of transmission. The blend of environmental controls and education gives rise to a foundation for a heightened sustainable approach toward the management of aspergillosis, thereby improving patient outcomes in addition to protecting healthcare environments from outbreak risks (Kuehn et al., 2024; Mohankumar et al., 2023) (Figure 9.22).

9.6.2. Personal Protective Equipment

The use of personal protective equipment (PPE) in aspergillosis exposure prevention cannot be overestimated. Aspergillosis, a serious health risk that is caused primarily by the fungus *Aspergillus*, poses a significant threat to immunocompromised individuals. Adequate-fitting PPE creates a necessary barrier against airborne spores potentially created in environments where *Aspergillus* dominates, e.g., construction sites or hospitals. There is evidence that unclean environments, especially where the construction work takes place, serve as reservoirs for spores, which further lead to more infections of surgical sites and the respiratory system in patients and healthcare workers. Strategic management of PPE, including gloves, gowns, and masks, is therefore paramount in averting such risks and creating a safe environment for vulnerable groups (Sexton et al., 2005). Moreover, effective PPE procedures are developed and implemented based on awareness of bioaerosol risks, as defined by emerging studies. These studies have shown that specific working environments, e.g., composting plants, host elevated levels of bioaerosols, which are prone to create issues in human health, such as respiratory diseases linked with *Aspergillus*. In such working environments, increased monitoring and use of high-quality PPE become the requirement to minimize risks. For instance, workers in areas with known high bioaerosol concentrations must be equipped with the appropriate respiratory protection to reduce inhalation exposure to the fungus spores. The study shows that areas like pre-treatment and screening processes are very hazardous, and better PPE standards are necessary to protect the employees from airborne contaminants (Anedda et al., 2020). Training and education on the proper use of PPE are important aspects of infection control practices, especially in preventing the risk of aspergillosis. It is not sufficient to provide protective equipment at hand; health workers and other personnel must be equipped with the knowledge on how to use it to maximize protective advantages. Standard training drills can help to enforce adherence to PPE protocols and educate individuals on the exact dangers of *Aspergillus* exposure. Coupling environmental surveillance, such as in the surgical environment and bioaerosol investigations, with these training drills can provide an additional level of these training drills with actual data regarding potential threats. Finally, holistic education with keen attention and strict PPE measures can prevent the occurrence of aspergillosis and general well-being in susceptible populations (Sexton et al., 2005) (Figure 9.23).

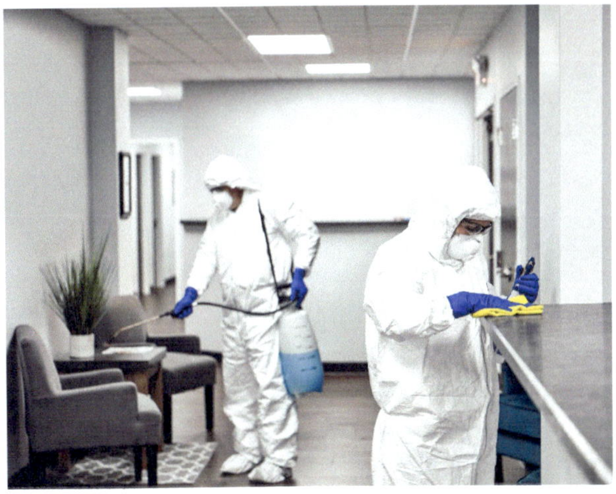

Figure 9.23. Effective PPE serves as a critical barrier, mitigating exposure to airborne spores that may arise in environments where *Aspergillus* is prevalent, such as in construction areas or healthcare facilities.

Source: https://ncceh.ca/sites/default/files/GettyImages-1215724939.jpg.

9.6.3. Education and Awareness Programs

Awareness and education programs are equally important in defeating the limitations of aspergillosis, which is a severe invasive fungal infection. With the increasing burden of invasive fungal infections (IFIs) globally, there is a pressing need for systematic awareness among the healthcare providers and the general population alike. Effective programs must address a wide array of educational elements, including being aware of the symptoms, risk factors, and the importance of early diagnosis and treatment. With greater knowledge of aspergillosis, these programs can realistically reduce misdiagnosis and create improved patient outcomes, subsequently alleviating the healthcare burden placed by this disease. As pointed out, there are broad gaps in the education of healthcare workers in the management of IFIs, and therefore the incorporation of educational models into the health system to bridge the gaps (Haderi et al., 2025). The Mycoses Study Group Education and Research Consortium is a new paradigm for improving the perception of invasive fungal diseases, including aspergillosis. This consortium promotes discussion of timely topics of the day, keeping educators, researchers, and clinicians abreast of the evolving landscape of clinical mycology. By providing initiatives such as the Clinical Mycology Today biennial meeting, the Consortium promotes networking and research synergy required to overcome upcoming fungal challenges. Such sessions not only enable the sharing of treatment and diagnostic innovation but also create avenues through which future mycologists can be mentored, thus ensuring an educated workforce that will be able to deal with the complexity of fungal infections (Little et al., 2024). Moreover, to ensure maximum return on education and awareness efforts, it is imperative to include a variety of lively teaching methods so that these can be offered before many different audiences. Online courses, workshops, and community outreach can each play a role in spreading information regarding aspergillosis to high-risk groups. Interactive visual aids, patient narratives, and simple educational terminology can each enhance understanding and render information more susceptible to learning. By employing technology and interactive systems, the programs can enhance comprehension and retention of critical information regarding aspergillosis, resulting in an educated populace. Last but not least, integrated education and targeted awareness programs play an important role in the battle against invasive fungal infection spread, enabling both patients and healthcare workers to overcome the complexities of diseases like aspergillosis successfully.

SUMMARY

Aspergillosis, which is largely due to the air-borne fungus *Aspergillus fumigatus*, primarily affects immunocompromised hosts. The mold is present throughout the environment and occurs in soil and compost organic matter, and its conidia are daily inhaled by humans without harming them in normal individuals. But in the case of compromised natural immunity by disorders such as long-term corticosteroid therapy, cancer treatment, or chronic infections in the lungs, these conidia will germinate within lung tissue and establish severe infection. This highlights the importance of understanding host immunity in the combating of this fungal infection, as the immune system has a crucial role in suppressing the progression of aspergillosis, especially among immunocompromised populations whose defenses are already weakened (McCormick et al., 2012). Research into the pathogenesis of aspergillosis has shown the role of immune mechanisms, specifically neutrophil extracellular traps (NETs) and natural killer (NK) cells, in controlling the growth of fungi. NETs are networks of structural proteins derived from neutrophils that are employed to entrap and destroy pathogens but are insufficient to eliminate A. fumigatus by themselves. They are able to inhibit hyphal growth by mechanisms that presumably include starvation for nutrients, e.g., zinc deprivation by the NET-associated protein calprotectin. NK cells, in contrast, release interferon-gamma (IFN-γ), which also inhibits hyphal elongation by as-yet-undefined mechanisms. The interaction of these immune components reveals the complexity of the host immune response to *Aspergillus* and the challenge of initiating effective therapeutic interventions that can restore immunity functions and combat infection effectively (McCormick et al., 2012). The study of health-related quality of life (HRQoL) among patients with chronic disease such as cystic fibrosis can generate useful information on the disease burden of diseases like aspergillosis. Longitudinal studies have also shown that many demographic and clinical factors—e.g., age, sex, nutritional status, and other comorbidities—have significant impacts on HRQoL in the long term. These factors are particularly relevant to the context of aspergillosis, since the opportunistic fungal infections are highly capable of impairing lung function and thereby further impairing quality of life. By not only focusing on clinical outcomes but also on the psychosocial elements of patients' existence, researchers are capable of acquiring a better understanding of how aspergillosis affects individuals in the long term. Thus, including the measurement of HRQoL can enhance the treatment of aspergillosis-at-risk patients and inform healthcare policies aimed at improving the overall well-being of such groups.

A CLOSER LOOK

NEUTROPHIL EXTRACELLULAR TRAPS (NETS)

Neutrophil extracellular traps (NETs) are networks of DNA, histones, and antimicrobial proteins formed by neutrophils upon exposure to infection or inflammation. NETosis, the process by which they form, captures and kills microorganisms outside cells, restricting their dissemination. Although NETs serve an important function in innate immunity, abnormal or excessive NET formation is associated with tissue injury and a variety of diseases, including autoimmune conditions, thrombosis, and sepsis.

REFERENCES

1. Adler, H., Dalquen, P., Frei, R., Habicht, M., et al. (2017). Invasive pulmonary aspergillosis: Effects of early resection in a neutropenic rat model. https://core.ac.uk/download/85219980.pdf (accessed on 27th June 2025).
2. Agarwal, R., Agarwal, A., Bonaiti, G., Cartier, Y., Chu, J., Cole, B., Erasmus, J., et al. (2018). Bronchiectasis: A case-based approach to investigation and management. https://core.ac.uk/download/195289411.pdf (accessed on 27th June 2025).
3. Akan, H., Alexander, B. D., Andes, D., Azoulay, E., et al. (2019). Revision and update of the consensus definitions of invasive fungal disease from the European Organization for Research and Treatment of Cancer and the Mycoses Study Group Education and Research Consortium. https://core.ac.uk/download/287649722.pdf (accessed on 27th June 2025).
4. Alsowaida, Y., Alshoumr, B., Alowais, S. A., Bin Saleh, K., Alshammari, A., Alshurtan, K., & Wali, H. A. (2024). Effectiveness and safety of echinocandins combination therapy with the standard of care compared to the standard of care monotherapy for the treatment of invasive aspergillosis infection: A meta-analysis. *Frontiers in Pharmacology, 15*. https://www.semanticscholar.org/paper/4eba1694399643f2b0a602b7ded7d5579e772cfe (accessed on 27th June 2025).
5. Anedda, E., & Traversi, D. (2020). Bioaerosol in composting facilities: A survey on full-scale plants in Italy. https://core.ac.uk/download/326908486.pdf (accessed on 27th June 2025).
6. A-Rahman, M., Abbott, J., Abbott, L., Arrington-Sanders, R., Bradley, J., Bradley, S., et al. (2015). Longitudinal impact of demographic and clinical variables on health-related quality of life in cystic fibrosis. https://core.ac.uk/download/42137142.pdf (accessed on 27th June 2025).
7. Audebert, C., Delhaes, L., Deschaght, P., Loywick, D., et al. (2016). Effects of propidium monoazido (PMA) treatment on mycobiome and bacteriome analysis of cystic fibrosis airways during exacerbation. https://core.ac.uk/download/84596094.pdf (accessed on 27th June 2025).
8. Azoulay, E., Benoit, D., Bruneel, F., Contejean, A., et al. (2016). Increased mortality in hematological malignancy patients with acute respiratory failure from undetermined etiology: A Groupe de Recherche en Réanimation Respiratoire en Onco-Hématologique (Grrr-OH) study. https://core.ac.uk/download/84044246.pdf (accessed on 27th June 2025).
9. Badillo-Almaraz, J. I., Cardenas-Cadena, S. A., Gutierrez-Avella, F. D., Villegas-Medina, P. J., Garza-Veloz, I., Badillo Almaraz, V., & Martinez-Fierro, M. (2022). COVID-19 syndetic: Convergence of COVID-19, pulmonary aspergillosis (CAPA), pulmonary tuberculosis, type 2 diabetes mellitus, and arterial hypertension. *Diagnostics, 12*. https://www.semanticscholar.org/paper/7bbaa739eabcccc80aa9be8fb8e4a1527f7b295e (accessed on 27th June 2025).
10. Baldin, C., Brakhage, A. A., Castanheira, S., Di Pietro, A., et al. (2014). Fungal model systems and the elucidation of pathogenicity determinants. https://core.ac.uk/download/25497497.pdf (accessed on 27th June 2025).
11. Bansal, N. K., Knutsen, A. P., Kurup, V. P., Moss, R. B., et al. (2006). Specific antibodies to recombinant allergens of *Aspergillus fumigatus* in cystic fibrosis patients with ABPA. https://core.ac.uk/download/213082106.pdf (accessed on 27th June 2025).

12. Baron, O., De Lajartre, A. Y., Despins, P., Germaud, P., et al. (1998). Aggressive surgical management in localized pulmonary mycotic and nonmycotic infections for neutropenic patients with acute leukemia: Report of eighteen cases. https://core.ac.uk/download/pdf/82703914.pdf (accessed on 27th June 2025).
13. Bassetti, M., & Bouza, E. (2017). Invasive mold infections in the ICU setting: Complexities and solutions. https://core.ac.uk/download/80137827.pdf (accessed on 27th June 2025).
14. Blasco-Navalpotro, M., Blot, S. I., Bulpa, P., Cardoso, T., et al. (2015). Epidemiology of invasive aspergillosis in critically ill patients: Clinical presentation, underlying conditions, and outcome. https://core.ac.uk/download/55762158.pdf (accessed on 27th June 2025).
15. Cho, S. J., Lee, K. H., Lee, K. H., Park, S., et al. (2025). A surgically treated case of chronic necrotizing aspergillosis with pleural invasion. https://core.ac.uk/download/pdf/8685202.pdf (accessed on 27th June 2025).
16. Cinicola, B. L., Duse, M., Laitano, R., Leonardi, L., et al. (2016). Allergic bronchopulmonary aspergillosis: Diagnostic and treatment challenges. https://core.ac.uk/download/54537073.pdf (accessed on 27th June 2025).
17. D'Alessandro, D., Vescia, N., Osborn, J. F., & Grillot, R. (2008). Development of an innovative method for the evaluation of fungal contamination of surfaces. https://core.ac.uk/download/54352187.pdf (accessed on 27th June 2025).
18. Eigl, S., Flick, H., Heldt, S., Hoenigl, M., et al. (2019). Using interleukin 6 and 8 in blood and bronchoalveolar lavage fluid to predict survival in hematological malignancy patients with suspected pulmonary mold infection. https://core.ac.uk/download/323066120.pdf (accessed on 27th June 2025).
19. Eller, P., Hoenigl, M., Prattes, J., Reisinger, A. C., et al. (2021). Invasive pulmonary aspergillosis complicating COVID-19 in the ICU–A case report. https://core.ac.uk/download/323311046.pdf (accessed on 27th June 2025).
20. Fang, W., Wu, J., Cheng, M., Zhu, X., Du, M., Chang, C., Liao, W., et al. (2023). Diagnosis of invasive fungal infections: Challenges and recent developments. *Journal of Biomedical Science, 30*. https://doi.org/10.1186/s12929-023-00926-2 (accessed on 27th June 2025).
21. Fung, J., Irish, W., Kusne, S., Martin, M., et al. (1992). Factors associated with invasive lung aspergillosis and the significance of positive *Aspergillus* culture after liver transplantation. https://core.ac.uk/download/12204865.pdf (accessed on 27th June 2025).
22. Gibert, C., Tirard-Collet, P., Miossec, C., Dupont, D., Persat, F., Wallon, M., Ader, F., et al. (2024). Reverse-transcriptase real-time PCR in the diagnostic strategy for invasive infections caused by *Aspergillus fumigatus*. *Journal of Clinical Microbiology, 62*. https://www.semanticscholar.org/paper/d94825ae4bef55200ec1f977ed3cb8c35940c6c9 (accessed on 27th June 2025).
23. Gonçalves, S., Pereira, I., Feys, S., Cunha, C., Chamilos, G., Hoenigl, M., Wauters, J., et al. (2024). Integrating genetic and immune factors to uncover pathogenetic mechanisms of viral-associated pulmonary aspergillosis. *mBio, 15*. https://www.semanticscholar.org/paper/68eb04d54f3564c05e0ec2ce4c298b83a06645ce (accessed on 27th June 2025).
24. Gorham, K. (2010). Effects of mold exposure on immune cells. https://core.ac.uk/download/56727991.pdf (accessed on 27th June 2025).

25. Green, M., Starzl, T. E., Todo, S., Tzakis, A., et al. (1991). Aspergillosis of the CNS in a pediatric liver transplant recipient: Case report and review. https://core.ac.uk/download/12204611.pdf (accessed on 27th June 2025).

26. Groll, A. H., Pham, A. S., De Pauw, B., Costa, C., Girmenia, C., Halliday, C., Mengoli, C., et al. (2012). A MIQE-compliant real-time PCR assay for *Aspergillus* detection. https://core.ac.uk/download/30696634.pdf (accessed on 27th June 2025).

27. Haderi, A., Altevogt, B., Denning, D. W., Chavez, E., Armstrong, H., Aram, J. A., Perfect, J. R., et al. (2025). Antifungal policy and practice across five countries: A qualitative review. https://core.ac.uk/download/644552488.pdf (accessed on 27th June 2025).

28. Heldt, S., & Hoenigl, M. (2017). Lateral flow assays for the diagnosis of invasive aspergillosis: Current status. https://core.ac.uk/download/323065685.pdf (accessed on 27th June 2025).

29. Hoenigl, M., & Jenks, J. D. (2018). Treatment of aspergillosis. https://core.ac.uk/download/323064842.pdf (accessed on 27th June 2025).

30. King, J., Lehrnbecher, T., Pana, Z. D., Steinbach, W. J., et al. (2017). Recognition and clinical presentation of invasive fungal disease in neonates and children. https://core.ac.uk/download/131024549.pdf (accessed on 27th June 2025).

31. Klingebiel, T., Lehrnbecher, T., Schmidt, S., Tramsen, L., et al. (2013). Immunotherapy of invasive fungal infection in hematopoietic stem cell transplant recipients. https://core.ac.uk/download/14528617.pdf (accessed on 27th June 2025).

32. Kuehn, R., Fox, T., Guyatt, G., Lutje, V., & Gould, S. (2024). Infection prevention and control measures to reduce the transmission of mpox: A systematic review. *PLOS Global Public Health, 4*. https://www.semanticscholar.org/paper/3ffaab650f148c81270d3fa8f0c09f41f71f7c11 (accessed on 27th June 2025).

33. Lamoth, F. (2016). Galactomannan and 1,3-β-d-glucan testing for the diagnosis of invasive aspergillosis. https://core.ac.uk/download/84059936.pdf (accessed on 27th June 2025).

34. Little, J., McCarthy, T., Pappas, P., Perfect, J., et al. (2024). Clinical mycology today: Emerging challenges and opportunities. https://core.ac.uk/download/619402138.pdf (accessed on 27th June 2025).

35. McCormick, A. (2012). Studies on the release of neutrophil extracellular traps and IFN-γ as part of the innate immune response to *Aspergillus fumigatus* and on the fungal stress response via the hybrid sensor kinase TcsC. https://core.ac.uk/download/11033812.pdf (accessed on 27th June 2025).

36. Mohankumar, N., Rajagopal, L., & Nieto, J. (2023). Optimal control for co-infection with COVID-19-associated pulmonary aspergillosis in ICU patients with environmental contamination. *Mathematical Biosciences and Engineering: MBE, 20*(6), 9861–9875. https://www.semanticscholar.org/paper/ffbb9cd48d824b41ff3ed50ca40e57570a4ebada (accessed on 27th June 2025).

37. Mulligan, K., Harris, K., Rixon, L., & Burls, A. (2024). A systematic mapping review of clinical guidelines for the management of fatigue in long-term physical health conditions. *Disability and Rehabilitation, 47*, 531–548. https://www.semanticscholar.org/paper/9309c2ce9ca7707b3b6568cbd6bdeab13ed240d9 (accessed on 27th June 2025).

38. Nast, A., Smith, C., Spuls, P. I., Avila Valle, G., Bata-Csörgő, Z., Boonen, H., de Jong, E. M. G. J., et al. (2020). EuroGuiDerm guideline on the systemic treatment of *Psoriasis vulgaris*–Part 1: Treatment and monitoring recommendations. *Journal of the European Academy of Dermatology and Venereology, 34*, 2461–2498. https://doi.org/10.1111/jdv.16915 (accessed on 27th June 2025).

39. Puglia, D. R., Puglia, J. Á. R., García-Cabrera, E., Morales, F., Camacho-Vega, J. C., & Vilches-Arenas, Á. (2024). Risk factors and environmental preventive actions for aspergillosis in patients with hematological malignancies. *Clinics and Practice, 14*, 280–292. https://www.semanticscholar.org/paper/4f894b2ad522a9e2539751780ad467ad51cfb818 (accessed on 27th June 2025).

40. Sexton, S. (2005). Hospital epidemiological surveillance during a major construction project. https://core.ac.uk/download/232787829.pdf (accessed on 27th June 2025).

41. Stewart, E. R., & Thompson, G. R. (2016). Treatment of primary pulmonary aspergillosis: An assessment of the evidence. https://core.ac.uk/download/323070109.pdf (accessed on 27th June 2025).

42. Taylor, S. S., Boysen, S., Buffington, T., Chalhoub, S., Defauw, P., Delgado, M. M., Gunn-Moore, D. A., et al. (2025). 2025 iCatCare consensus guidelines on the diagnosis and management of lower urinary tract diseases in cats. *Journal of Feline Medicine and Surgery, 27*. https://www.semanticscholar.org/paper/18bc9e6b3ad8829ccdb3aebc32cfe38af39cf874 (accessed on 27th June 2025).

43. Venugopal, T. M., Yadav, S., Patil, M. B., Sindhu, Y. R., Patel, J., Uttekar, P. S., Aranha, I., et al. (2025). Nano formulation of phytochemicals to increase antifungal effectiveness against pathogens resistant to drugs. *Journal of Neonatal Surgery*. https://www.semanticscholar.org/paper/7c5417093fda3948934d99d4989eb88422f963bf (accessed on 27th June 2025).

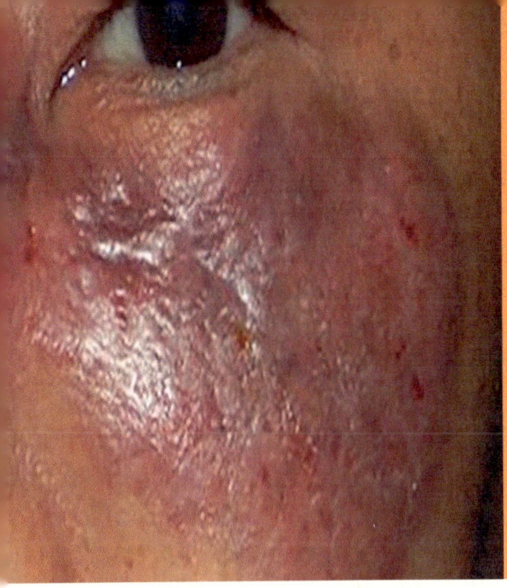

Chapter 10
MUCORMYCOSIS

Contents

Introduction

The development of mucormycosis, or black fungus, has gained much focus in recent public health debate, particularly in the context of the COVID-19 pandemic. In most countries, such as India, an increasing number of mucormycosis cases have been observed, which occurred at times when waves of COVID-19 infections were reported. The fungal infection, predominantly seen in immunocompromised patients, has remained a persistent problem in medical mycology. When populations experience vulnerabilities with severe health conditions, the prevalence of consequences of mucomycosis grows, and a more thorough examination of its epidemiology, symptomatic presentation, and prevention is necessary. A lot of research has emerged that associates the growth in mucormycosis with the immunosuppressive nature of COVID-19, and underlying factors warrant skeptical analysis (Naeini et al., 2022). Understanding the pathogenesis of mucormycosis is also going along with an understanding of its underlying biological mechanism and advances in medical science. Advances made in diagnostics and treatment over the last few years have transformed the approach to this invasive fungal infection. Advances in molecular biology have upgraded diagnostic equipment so that cases of mucormycosis can be detected earlier and with greater accuracy compared to conventional methods. For instance, rapid antigen detection systems have been at the forefront in the identification of invasive pulmonary fungal infections, thus allowing timely interventions. The introduction of new antifungal agents has also complemented therapeutic strategies, deviating from traditional modes, e.g., amphotericin B, which pose heightened risks of toxicity. Such advancements in clinical practice merely serve to amplify a broader trend in the continued fight against fungal disease, emphasizing the need for continued research and innovation (Ampel et al., 2012). As the world continues to evolve in the context of global health, there must be heightened awareness and education about mucormycosis and further advancements in treatment and diagnostic methods. Public health initiatives in terms of revealing the prevalence of the disease, especially in times of peak susceptibility, are essential to prevent its impact on susceptible populations. Furthermore, when clinicians address the complexities involved in managing immunocompromised patients, it becomes imperative to develop certain measures of prevention and treatment of mucormycosis effectively. To this end, collaboration among clinicians, researchers, and public health officials becomes important in addressing the challenges related to this opportunistic infection. Lastly, better knowledge of mucormycosis, risk factors, and association with broader health conditions like diabetes mellitus/COVID-19 would pave the way for improved management protocols and better patient outcomes, greatly helping the field of infectious disease (Naeini et al., 2022) (Figure 10.1).

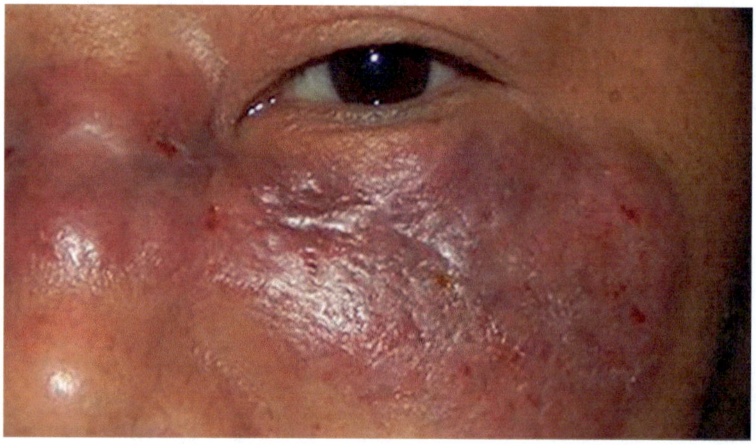

Figure 10.1. Mucormycosis.

Source: https://images-prod.healthline.com/hlcmsresource/images/Image-Galleries/mucormycosis/1220-Mucormycosis-642x361-slide2.jpg.

10.1. Causes of Mucormycosis

Mucormycosis, a fulminant and frequently fatal fungal infection, predominantly affects immunocompromised patients. The opportunistic fungus *Lichtheimia corymbifera* is one of the prime culprits of this infection, which has been shown to infect the body predominantly in immunocompromised hosts, such as diabetic, cancer, or immunosuppressed therapy patients.

Infection is caused when the spores of the fungus are inhaled or touch damaged skin, and the disease progresses very rapidly. The death rate for Mucormycosis is characteristically high based on reasons like the paucity of antifungal drugs available and also because the infection is usually diagnosed very late. This emphasizes infection mechanisms and the immune response to Mucorales as central factors to the critical outcome observed among infected patients (Montaño et al., 2024).

The second reason why Mucormycosis develops is the presence of certain environmental conditions for fungal development. Hot and humid environments, particularly those with organic disintegration, are significant reservoirs for spores of Mucorales. These are compounded within clinical settings, where the control of ventilation and cleanliness may be lost. In addition, factors such as the extended hospital stay, surgery, or the wear of medical devices implanted inside the body can predispose the patient to infection. Immunocompromised individuals are particularly at risk because they already have existing illness and compromised defense against opportunistic pathogens. A well-informed understanding of the environmental risks is crucial to implement effective preventive measures in the risk groups, thus reducing the incidence of Mucormycosis in high-risk patients (Hamilos et al., 2012). The interaction between host immunity and Mucormycosis also plays a significant role in the severity of infections. *Lichtheimia corymbifera* recognition by human monocytes is an essential element of the immune response since these cells are responsible for recognizing and reacting to fungal pathogens. In the event of infection, the monocytes release cytokines like Interleukin 1 beta (IL-1β) and Tumor Necrosis Factor-alpha (TNF-α), which play a fundamental role in the development of an early inflammatory response. However, *Lichtheimia corymbifera* is intracellularly resistant and can potentially survive inside monocytes, hindering the hosts from combating the infection. The intracellular resistance disregards the effective immunity, thus leading to a faster development of disease and ultimately high mortality due to Mucormycosis. Thus, host-pathogen interactions are significant to recognize as well as to have a chance of discovering novel therapeutic methods (Montaño et al., 2024) (Figure 10.2).

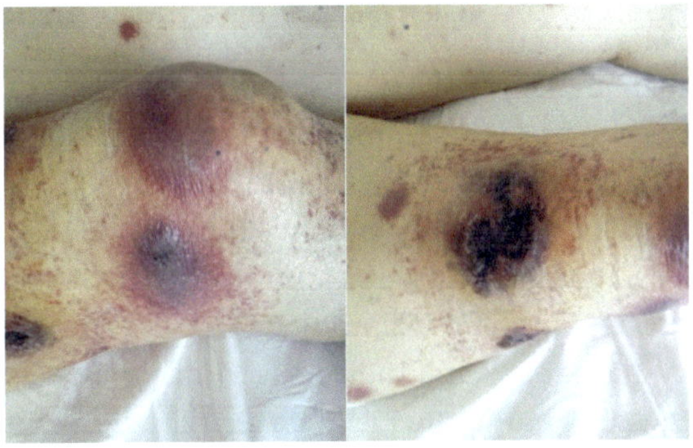

Figure 10.2. Mucormycosis, a critical and often fatal fungal infection, primarily afflicts individuals with compromised immune systems.

Source: https://www.mdpi.com/curroncol/curroncol-30-00599/article_deploy/html/images/curroncol-30-00599-g001.png.

10.1.1. Fungal Pathogens Responsible

Mucormycosis pathogenesis is attributed primarily to fungal pathogens within the class Zygomycetes, specifically to the genera *Mucor, Rhizopus,* and *Lichtheimia*. They are omnipresent in the environment and are found ubiquitously in soil, decaying organic matter, as well as in hospitals. They are saprophytes by nature, which under normal circumstances would not infect immunocompetent hosts. Mucormycosis has become much more prevalent in immunocompromised patients. Risk factors such as uncontrolled diabetes, malignancy in the blood, and organ transplant have rendered these patients vulnerable to these opportunistic pathogens. Part of the rising prevalence can be explained by the increasing application of antifungal treatment, selectively targeting familiar pathogens and indirectly paving the way for the emergence of uncommon fungi such as *Mucor* species (Alcazar-Fuoli et al., 2009). Under recent worldwide health emergencies, such as the COVID-19 pandemic, mucormycosis has seen a record increase. Fungal infections following viral diseases in patients suffering from COVID-19 show varying correlations with the reactivation of opportunistic agents such as *Mucor*. The immunocompromised status caused by the viral infection, combined with the glucocorticoid therapies often used to treat the more severe cases, provides the ideal setting for the growth of fungi. Cautious research has identified *Mucor* species as the most prevalent pathogen in COVID-19 patients, where it manifests as a prime secondary infection in recovering patients. Detection of such fungal pathogens in clinical settings underscores the need for clinicians to remain vigilant of the risks created by opportunistic infections (Agarwal et al., 2021).

In order to effectively combat the menace of mucormycosis, early diagnosis and targeted therapeutic management are required. The intricacies involved in the diagnosis of mucormycosis extend beyond routine laboratory tests; early identification of the specific causative fungal pathogens is mandatory for timely effective therapy. Secondly, the common occurrence of predisposing risk factors necessitates a multimodality approach to patient management consisting of aggressive screening for fungal infections among high-risk groups. An understanding of the dynamic interaction between such pathogens and their host could give clues towards antifungal prophylaxis recommendations and treatment modalities. Ultimately, the determinants responsible for the emergence of opportunistic fungal pathogens must be dealt with to reduce the morbidity and mortality caused by mucormycosis and other infections in susceptible groups of patients (Alcazar-Fuoli et al., 2009) (Figure 10.3).

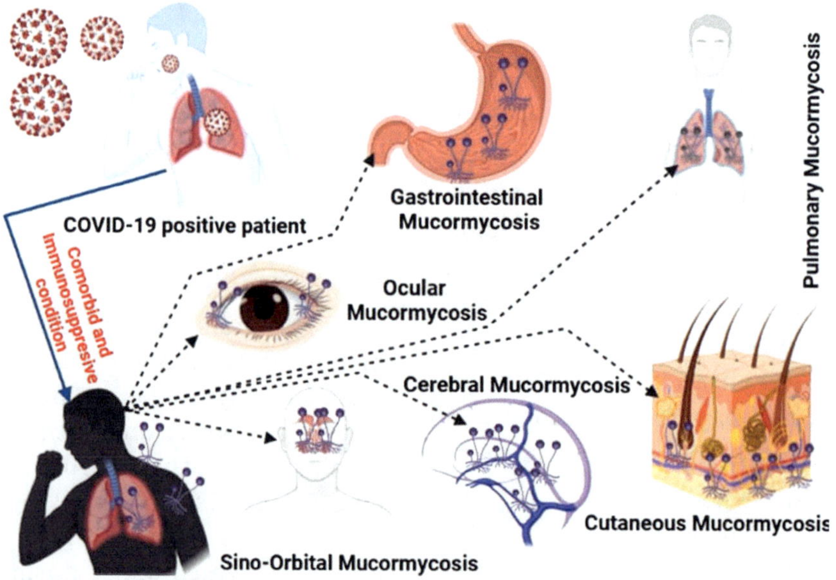

Figure 10.3. Post-viral fungal infections among COVID-19 patients reveal a correlation with the reactivation of opportunistic pathogens like *Mucor*.

Source: https://media.springernature.com/lw685/springer-static/image/art%3A10.1007%2Fs11356-022-22204-8/MediaObjects/11356_2022_22204_Fig3_HTML.png.

10.1.2. Environmental Factors Contributing to Infection

The environmental factors of the development of mucormycosis are of paramount significance to an understanding of the epidemiology of this opportunistic infection. Of the most important of these factors is the presence of specific molds, such as *Rhizopus oryzae*, within the environment. Such molds have a tendency to infest decaying organic matter and reproduce in warm, moist environments, thus creating an optimal setting for infection, especially among compromised individuals. Places with poor hygiene or high organic wastes are especially susceptible, as they can harbor fungal spores which can be breathed in or which may become introduced into open wounds. Furthermore, certain agricultural methods, particularly those involving composting, do the opposite – they increase exposure to these pathogens – and need targeted public health measures and environmental regulations to curb these threats, particularly where there are both environmental degradation and health crises such as pandemics. The nexus between environmental exposure and health consequence is further brought out by surges in mucormycosis cases during the COVID-19 pandemic's aftermath. As outlined in recent studies, individuals recovering from COVID-19 exhibit a heightened susceptibility to opportunistic infections, including mucormycosis, largely due to weakened immune systems and the potential effects of steroid treatments. The interplay between high levels of iron, diminished immunity, and environmental molds presents a critical nexus of factors that exacerbate infection rates in post-COVID patients. In nations like India, where the second wave of COVID-19 witnessed an abnormal predominance of cases involving mucormycosis, these environmental connections must be known to effectively manage public health threats. Hence, more studies and health awareness programs must be oriented towards informing healthcare workers as well as the masses about the environmental vectors that promote this fatal disease (Rauf et al., 2022). In addition, socioeconomic status convergence with environmental elements is also at the heart of mucormycosis epidemiology. Such people at risk of the infection are usually located in disadvantaged environments where diabetes and other comorbidities are prevalent, coupled with poor access to quality healthcare and hygiene facilities. Malnutrition, driven by inadequate medical care, can weaken immunity and make populations susceptible to infections from environmental reservoirs. In these contexts, the symbiotic environment of fungal molds, coupled with the immunocompromised state created by these social determinants, creates a staggering susceptibility to mucormycosis. To mitigate these risks, there needs to be an interdisciplinary understanding of both the biological subtleties of mucormycosis and the environmental contexts that foster these diseases. Interventions should not only address the medical care of current diseases but also implement broader environmental health interventions that reduce exposure to fungal spores in higher-risk settings (Kumar et al., 2022) (Figure 10.4).

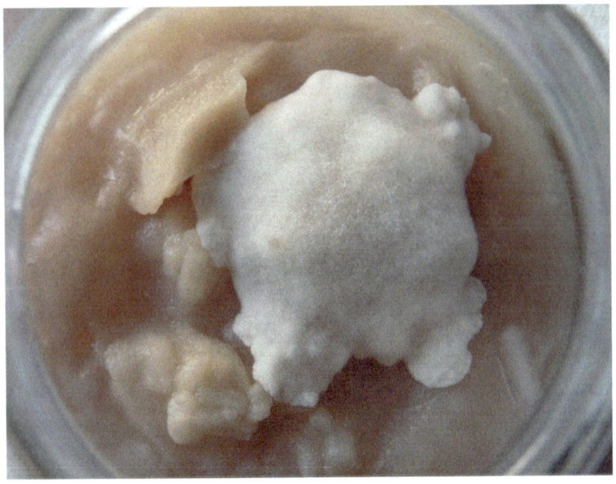

Figure 10.4. *Rhizopus oryzae.*

Source: https://upload.wikimedia.org/wikipedia/commons/d/df/*Rhizopus*_Oryzae.jpg.

10.1.3. Risk Factors Associated with Mucormycosis

The emergence of mucormycosis as an aggressive clinical syndrome has been closely linked with some predisposing factors that render a person vulnerable to the invasive fungal infection. The most salient risk factor is uncontrolled diabetes mellitus. Hyperglycemic patients often present with impaired immune response and vascular compromise, and this creates a ground for fungal infections. In addition, prolonged corticosteroid treatment, not uncommon in patients with chronic inflammatory diseases, once more weakens immune defenses so that the opportunistic character of Mucorales can manifest. Infections of mucormycosis have considerably increased in the times of critical illness such as COVID-19 infections, wherein diabetes, immunosuppression, and pulmonary disorders enhance the susceptibility for the infection. This growing comorbidity overlap demands an urgent appeal to healthcare providers to more accurately detect those at risk and implement early therapeutic interventions. Trauma, particularly with severe soft tissue damage, is also a significant risk factor in mucormycosis development. In post-traumatic infection, Mucorales can thrive in circumstances of open contaminated organic debris wounds, leading to the development of invasive fungal infections.

The military forces and non-combat populations typically encounter such circumstances, whereby severe injuries result in lengthy medical interventions, thus putting them at higher risk for post-traumatic mucormycosis. Additionally, other critically ill patients who are admitted to intensive care units and are already struggling with other life-threatening diseases are also at higher risk. The interaction of underlying medical conditions and traumatic injuries primes the pattern of development of mucormycosis, causing high mortality and morbidity in patients (Bochicchio et al., 2017).

Another challenge to meet is hospital-acquired infections, and these are most prevalent among immunocompromised individuals. Organ transplant, hematological malignancy, and prolonged neutropenia dramatically increase the risk of a variety of healthcare-associated infections, including mucormycosis. In these patients, any delay in recognizing the onset of infection may lead to rapid progression of the disease, with widespread tissue necrosis in the majority of cases.

The diagnostic challenge in mucormycosis renders it all the more challenging to treat, since clinicians must keep themselves alert to its non-specific presentation. Reliance on advanced diagnostic techniques, such as molecular techniques and tissue biopsy, becomes essential in confirming the diagnosis and initiating early treatment (Bassetti et al., 2017). As these risk factors get intertwined, it continues to remain essential to appreciate their role in mucormycosis development as a cornerstone to enhancing prevention and cure (Figure 10.5).

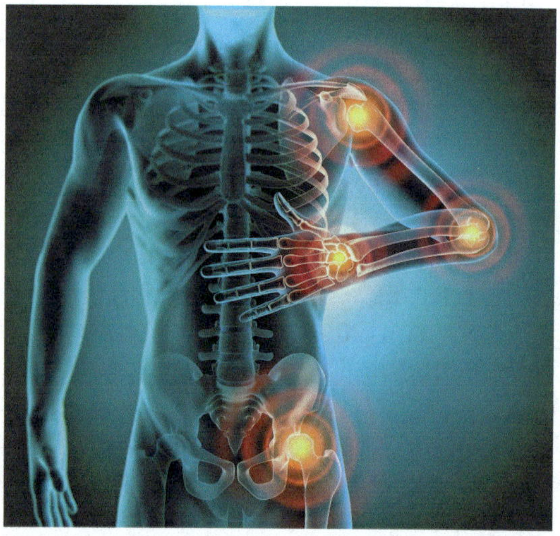

Figure 10.5. Chronic inflammatory conditions.

Source: https://domf5oio6qrcr.cloudfront.net/medialibrary/6202/a4886852-65ff-49e6-9d21-9a5d08b77dad.jpg.

10.2. Symptoms and Diagnosis

The clinical presentation of mucormycosis can vary greatly depending on the site of infection, but common presentations are facial pain or swelling, nasal discharge, and black necrotic skin lesions surrounding the eyes and nose. Pulmonary infection usually presents with cough, fever, and hemoptysis as evidence of the virulent capacity of the organism to invade adjacent tissue. In immunocompromised individuals, for instance, in those with diabetes or undergoing chemotherapy, the symptoms progress very rapidly, and hence awareness at the right time is critical. Notably, acute presentation and mortality related to these symptoms also underscore awareness among clinicians, as early intervention can limit life-threatening complications and improve outcomes in such patients. Diagnosis of mucormycosis is heavily reliant on a combination of imaging, clinical assessment, and laboratory tests. History and physical examination to identify risk factors and clinical findings present in disease cases are applied. Imaging tests, such as CT scans or MRIs, can illustrate tissue destruction and other classic findings of mucormycosis. However, diagnosis still depends on microbiologic proof, traditionally by histopathologic examination and biopsy material culture. This multi-pronged approach in diagnosis is well supported by the fact that a significant percentage of invasive fungal disease patients have atypical presentation, thereby requiring a high level of suspicion combined with alertness among clinicians to identify potential cases of mucormycosis (Bochicchio et al., 2017). In clinical practice, the diagnostic dilemma presented by mucormycosis highlights the significance of standardized methods and recognition of its insidious onset. As research evolves, it becomes clear that risk factors and presentation patterns may differ across populations, and therefore, the requirement for the establishment of specific diagnostic protocols. Familiarity with the epidemiological background of mucormycosis can also enhance diagnostic skill and treatment outcomes (King et al., 2017). This underscores the necessity of an interdisciplinary strategy, blending information from infectious disease specialists, pathologists, and radiologists so that effective diagnosis is possible. Identification of signs and systemic diagnostic methodology are imperative in improving patient outcomes because timely and effective interventions can significantly enhance the morbidity and mortality of this pathogenic fungal infection (Figure 10.6).

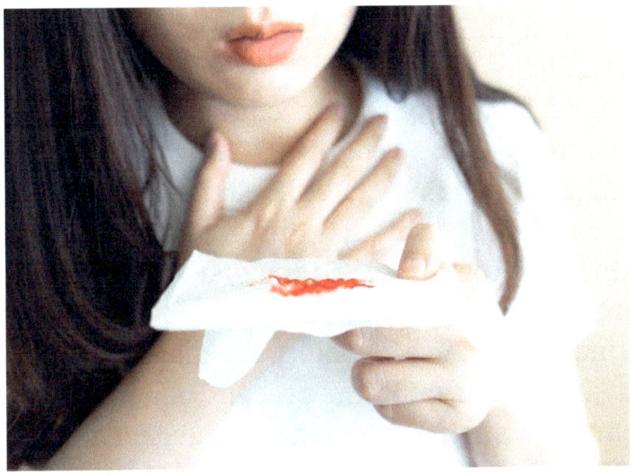

Figure 10.6. Hemoptysis.

Source: https://cdn.apollohospitals.com/health-library-prod/2021/08/shutterstock_1660999831-scaled.jpg.

10.2.1. Common Symptoms of Mucormycosis

Mucormycosis is an opportunistic fungal infection that typically occurs in individuals with compromised immune systems. The initial symptoms of this disease may vary widely and, most frequently, depend on the site of infection. Initial presentation usually includes facial swelling of the face, the eyes, or other facial structures, accompanied by nasal congestion and black or discolored nasal discharge. Patients will present with severe facial pain or headache depending on the course of the infections.

Symptoms are highly likely to be mimicked by other upper respiratory tract infections, and therefore, medical practitioners will not easily suspect a mucormycosis infection. Recognition of these symptoms is, therefore, highly critical to enable early treatment as well as institute effective treatment procedures against possible mucormycosis-related complications, thus improving patient outcomes and survival rates in general. As the infection progresses, mucormycosis may have more solidified signs, particularly with its invasive nature penetrating the sinuses, brain, and lungs. Pulmonary mucormycosis patients may present with cough, dyspnea, and chest pain, which can quickly deteriorate. Presentation can also include hemoptysis, or coughing up blood, indicating severe lung involvement. While that is happening, the systemic signs of fever and malaise are generally present as well, along with the pulmonary findings, so it makes the clinical picture a rather formidable diagnosis to make. Because of the great disparity in the way in which symptoms present, clinicians need to have a high suspicion of mucormycosis in the face of risk factors. Early detection and aggressive treatment of such symptoms can do much towards limiting morbidity and mortality from this fulfilment infection. In some situations, mucormycosis can result in ocular manifestations, further complicating the clinical presentation. Visual disturbances, swelling of the eyes, and even proptosis can occur, highlighting the need for prompt management of ocular manifestations. A study highlighted that although ocular presentations resulting from mucormycosis are not very frequent, their implications on disease progression can be devastating, leading to possible functional deficits and even blindness if left untreated at an early stage (Haseli-Mofrad et al., 2023). The association of systemic diseases like COVID-19 with mucormycosis is particularly significant, where patients run the risk of further deteriorating symptoms or even new ophthalmic complications emerging during their time under hospitalization (King et al., 2017). The identification of the entire spectrum of symptoms among the at-risk patients is therefore of utmost importance in planning effective management strategies for managing mucormycosis and its subsequent complications (Figure 10.7).

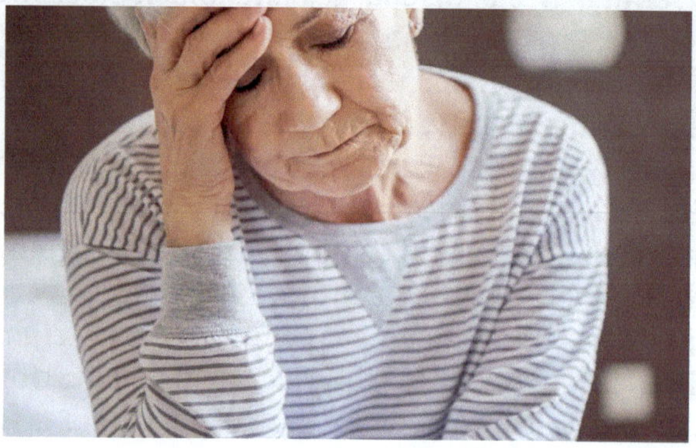

Figure 10.7. Patients might experience significant facial pain or headache due to the infections progression.

Source: https://images.ctfassets.net/222znibi5gto/ppm_ppm_article_fid8395_asset/3e65890ec974cb95d88a3abe97e242d6/42470759xl.jpg?fm=webp&q=50&w=1200&h=600&fit=thumb.

10.2.2. Diagnostic Methods Used

Correct diagnosis of mucormycosis is critical, given the fulminant course and severe morbidity of this invasive fungal infection. Diagnosis often begins with careful clinical examination and history taking of the patients, particularly for any pre-existing condition such as uncontrolled diabetes, immunosuppression, or recent trauma. The practitioners should be highly suspicious, as mucormycosis can have nonspecific clinical presentations mimicking other infections. Early diagnosis is imperative, especially in intensive care units since the margins are much bigger here because of the high likelihood of disastrous outcomes. Early identification of clinical signs such as facial swelling, nasal discharge, and necrotic lesions, therefore, warrants prompt diagnostic tests to confirm the presence of the etiological fungi in affected tissue. Laboratory tests are pivotal to the confirmation of mucormycosis diagnosis. The histopathological demonstration of invasion of tissue by non-septate hyphae in tissue biopsies is considered the gold standard to establish the diagnosis. It allows pathologists to see the characteristic morphology of Mucorales, thus enabling differentiation of mucormycosis from other fungal infections.

Use of ancillary diagnostic tests, such as serum testing for biomarkers, can enhance diagnostic sensitivity. For instance, serum β-D-glucan elevation, though not specific for Mucorales, can be helpful when taken together with clinical presentation. Additionally, newer molecular tools, such as PCR to detect the presence of fungal DNA, have proved useful adjuncts. These can accelerate diagnosis and thus potentially permit earlier therapeutic intervention, which is critical in maximizing outcomes in involved patients. Despite advancements in medical technology, mucormycosis remains a challenging diagnosis, particularly in the intensive care unit (ICU) setting. High rates of mortality and morbidity are involved, and as such empirical antifungal therapy has to be started on the basis of a high level of suspicion of the infection even prior to definitive diagnostic proof. (Bassetti et al., 2017) emphasizes that timely intervention can markedly improve survival rates, which puts focus on vigorous clinical decision-making. Reliance on non-culture-based diagnostic tests, coupled with clinical experience, can enable quicker management strategies. As mucormycosis epidemiology continues to evolve, additional work optimizing and validating new diagnostics needs to be done. This undertaking is critical not only to enhance diagnostic sensitivity but to ultimately reduce the severe burden this deadly fungal infection has on healthcare networks (Figure 10.8).

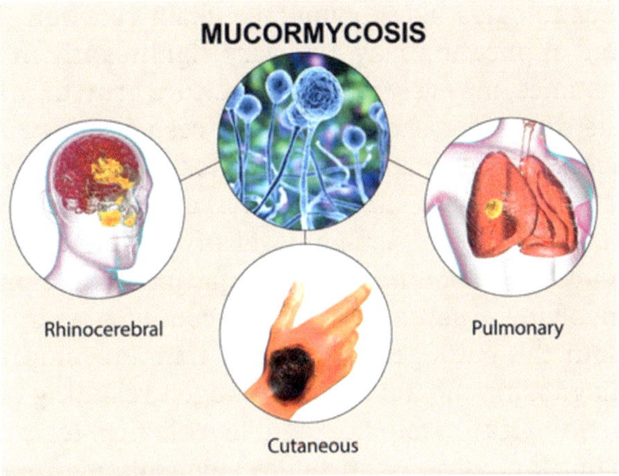

Figure 10.8. Effective diagnosis of mucormycosis is critical, given the rapid progression and severe morbidity associated with this invasive fungal infection.

Source: https://www.tandfonline.com/cms/asset/bd6651a1-a918-4498-9e22-29ca3990008f/iero_a_2233906_f0001_oc.jpg.

10.2.3. Challenges in Diagnosing Mucormycosis

Mucormycosis has serious diagnostic difficulties that usually make it difficult to treat in a timely and effective manner. One of the main challenges is the fact that its clinical symptoms are non-specific and may resemble other more prevalent conditions or infections. The patient may present with fever, cough, or pain localized to the affected area early on, prompting the clinician to overlook it as one of the more common diseases. This lack of a clear diagnosis results in low clinical suspicion, and thus health care providers postpone initiating significant diagnostic testing. Time is thus lost that could possibly have been used to initiate early antifungal treatment, a relevant consideration based on the aggressive nature of the disease (Bassetti et al., 2017). Compounded to these diagnostic difficulties is the challenge to obtain proper microbiological confirmation. Mucormycosis requires histopathological identification of non-septate hyphae and, while newer molecular technologies like polymerase chain reaction (PCR) offer promising alternatives, their availability and application may also vary significantly in diverse clinical settings. Diagnosis of Mucorales, for instance, may rely mostly on culture growth, which will take some weeks, thereby further extending the delay in treatment. Where resources are limited, such as in most intensive care units, timely access to these advanced diagnostic methods might not be feasible, and the patients are subjected to the invasive characteristics of the disease, ultimately affecting their mortality rates (Nosari et al., 2010). A further level of challenge arises when it is a matter of differentiating between mucormycosis and other fungal infections, particularly when co-infection exists. Mixed infection involving *Aspergillus* species is complicated by the diagnosis as also proved by case reports in which both the pathogens coexist in immunocompromised hosts. This ambiguity leads to confusion in diagnosing the dominant pathogen resulting in the worsening of the patients. Divergence between histological, cytological, and mycological tests is also likely to yield conflicting results, confusing the clinical picture. Accordingly, a consolidated model that includes clinical assessment and advanced molecular diagnosis is required to increase the precision and speed of mucormycosis diagnosis, which is crucial to achieve better outcomes of treatment (Nosari et al., 2010) (Figure 10.9).

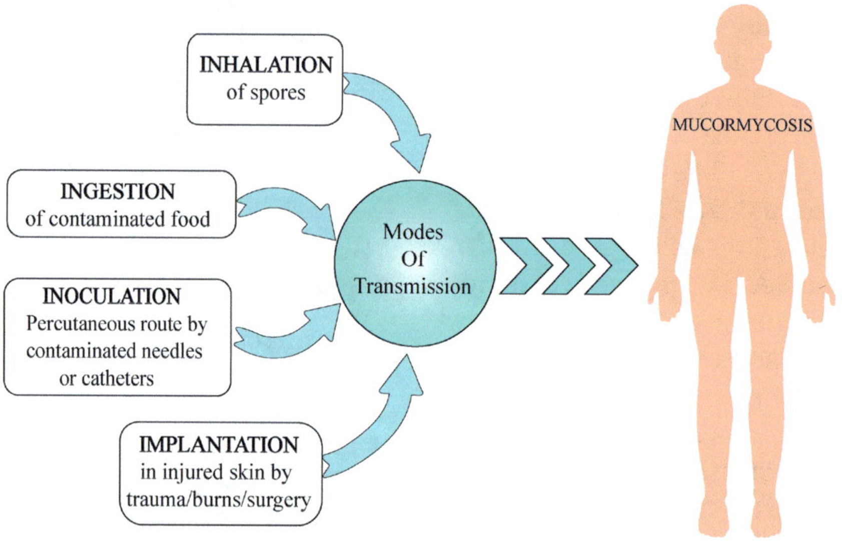

Figure 10.9. Mucormycosis presents significant diagnostic challenges that often hinder timely and effective treatment.

Source: https://www.frontiersin.org/files/Articles/794176/fmicb-12-794176-HTML/image_m/fmicb-12-794176-g003.jpg.

10.3. Pathophysiology

Mucormycosis opportunistic infection pathophysiology is largely dependent on the immune response of the hosts and the virulence of the etiologic fungi, primarily belonging to the Mucorales order. Infection is most devastating in immunocompromised hosts, such as patients with poorly controlled diabetes mellitus or undergoing extensive immunosuppressive therapy, such as organ transplantation. In these hosts, an impaired immune system cannot provide an adequate defense, and

Mucorales overgrow. The presence of ketoacidosis, a commonly-related condition for diabetics, also contributes to the risk, offering a rich growth medium for fungi. Furthermore, the recent increase in mucormycosis has generated questions about the association of fungal infection frequency with the use of voriconazole prophylaxis among high-risk patients, implying a potential link between evolving treatment trends and the incidence of this rare yet perilous infection (Kontoyiannis et al., 2009). The pathophysiologic mechanisms of mucormycosis also involve widespread inflammatory reactions, which can lead to tissue damage and disease worsening. Hyperinflammatory states are reported to complicate the immune response by enlisting the recruitment of neutrophils and macrophages to the infected site, thereby hastening tissue destruction. In COVID-19-associated rhino-orbital-cerebral mucormycosis infection, elevated levels of inflammatory biomarkers like serum ferritin and D-dimer have been correlated with the severity of the disease. These markers not only signify inflammation markers but also can potentially serve as triage agents for assessing the status of patients. The host-pathogen interaction between hosts inflammatory responses and the pathogens capacity to evade immune recognition is thus a key area of study in mucormycosis pathophysiology (Bhagat et al., 2023).

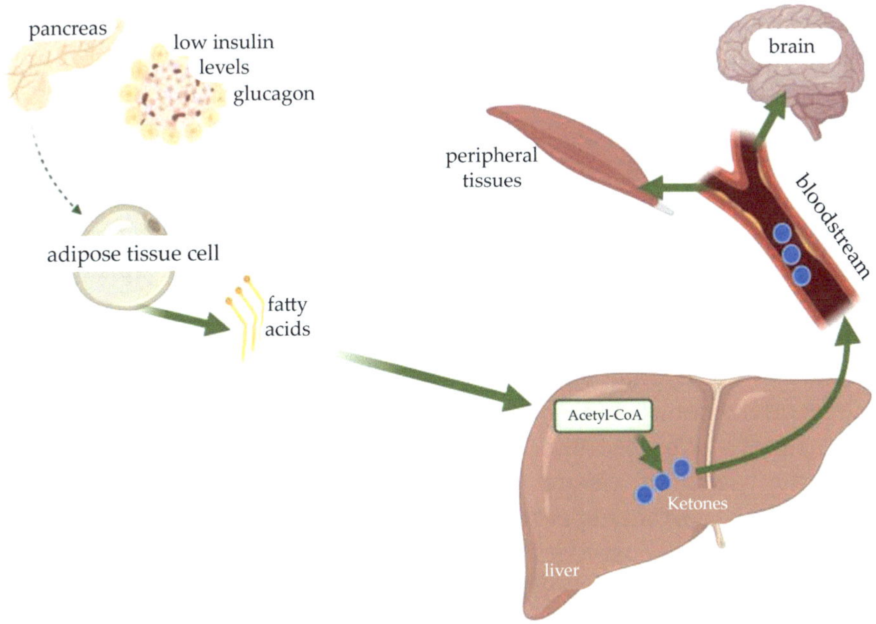

Figure 10.10. The presence of ketoacidosis, an often-associated state in diabetic patients, further exacerbates the risk, creating an environment conducive to fungal growth.

Source: https://pub.mdpi-res.com/nutrients/nutrients-15-04383/article_deploy/html/images/nutrients-15-04383-g001.png?1697448405.

Finally, obtaining an understanding of the pathophysiology of mucormycosis necessitates a detailed examination of host-pathogen interactions, particularly within vulnerable populations. Fungal potential to infect tissues over a background of dysregulated immunity marks out an urgent clinical issue, making preidentification and treatment urgently needed. More than that, insofar as increasing reports of mucormycosis cases keep step with shifts in clinical practice such as antifungal prophylaxis, healthcare providers must remain vigilant. This vigil is not only crucial to minimize the risk of mucormycosis but also to tailor treatment approaches considering the absolute immunocompromised status of the patients. Hence, ongoing research into the pathophysiologic mechanisms involved in this complex fungal infection is warranted for the optimization of preventive and therapeutic interventions (Figure 10.10).

10.3.1. Mechanism of Fungal Invasion

The mode of invasion of fungal in mucormycosis is largely attributed to the opportunistic fungus *Rhizopus oryzae*, which has an evident adaptation to environment. Spore germination is the initial invasion and can be rapid upon contact with host tissues under conditions of compromised immunity. Upon germination of the spores, *R. oryzae* results in dense growth of hyphae that invades the tissues and blood vessels and leads to necrosis of tissues as well as the interference with normal physiological processes. Invasion is facilitated by the organism's ability to manipulate the host's immunity, thereby allowing extensive dissemination within the body of the host. The process of interaction of the hyphae with host cells is also an important infection establishment factor because the fungus uses proteins and enzymes to degrade the host tissue and facilitate colonization. An important aspect of *R. oryzaes* ability to live within the host is its iron acquisition system. It has been established well that patients undergoing deferoxamine therapy represent a special risk group for mucormycosis development. Deferoxamine creates a condition under which free iron is not much, but *R. oryzae* has developed a successful mechanism to use iron from the chelator itself. The presence of some receptors, i.e., Fob1 and Fob2, on the yeast cell surface is required for the purpose. These receptors are induced under conditions of high concentrations of ferrioxamine so that *R. oryzae* is able to bind and use iron efficiently. Experiments have shown that mutants with decreased expression of these proteins have impaired virulence, suggesting that targeting the iron acquisition machinery could be a novel therapeutic target for managing the invasive capacity of this pathogen in immunocompromised patients (Chou et al., 2015). In addition to iron acquisition, invasive enzyme production by *Rhizopus oryzae* enhances its invasive capacity and contributes to tissue destruction. Enzymes such as proteases, lipases, and phospholipases facilitate the breakdown of extracellular matrix components that facilitate hyphal invasion in host tissues. The symbiotic interaction between these enzymes and the fungal hyphae not only facilitates further invasion but also enhances the inflammatory process, thus predisposing to increased growth of the fungus. Both invasion mechanisms of invasion and host degradation emphasize the necessity of investigating these mechanisms in the context of mucormycosis. Further research needs to be directed towards elucidating intricate pathways involved in host interaction and fungal pathogenicity, which could lead to improved treatment options (Leon et al., 2017) (Figure 10.11).

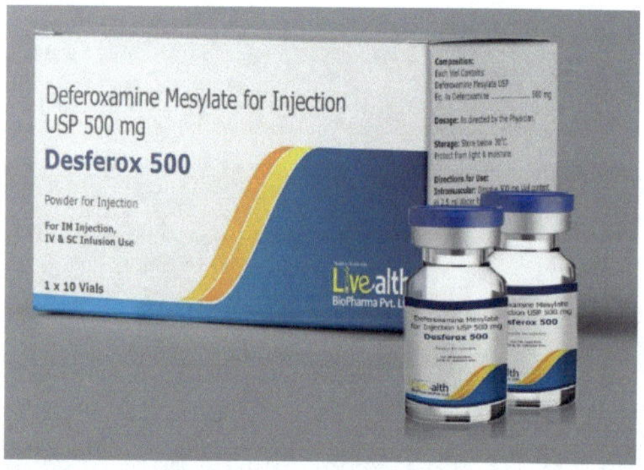

Figure 10.11. Deferoxamine.

Source: https://5.imimg.com/data5/ANDROID/Default/2024/8/445263099/IE/OY/WU/25156975/product-jpeg.jpg.

10.3.2. Immune Response to Mucormycosis

The immune response to mucormycosis is critically dependent upon the hosts overall health status and availability of immunosuppressive factors. Mucorales, particularly species like *Rhizopus oryzae*, employ iron acquisition mechanisms to live in host niches, and the immune systems involvement in combat against such infections is critical. Iron overload conditions, such as in patients receiving deferoxamine for chronic renal failure, significantly elevate the risk for mucormycosis. Specifically, the deferoxamine siderophore facilitates iron uptake in *Rhizopus* species as indicated by research demonstrating the cell surface expression of CBS domain proteins Fob1 and Fob2 in *R. oryzae* iron acquisition. Strains with reduced expression of these proteins have reduced virulence, highlighting the importance of iron in the pathogen's life cycle and the complexity of the immune system in preventing the pathogen from invading and replicating (Chou et al., 2015). The innate immunity is the first line of defense against mucormycosis and comprises phagocytic cells such as neutrophils and macrophages that attempt to clear the invading fungi. Nevertheless, Mucorales have also developed mechanisms to overcome these host defense mechanisms. Mucorales can germinate quickly and invade the vascular system of the blood vessels, causing thrombosis and necrosis of the tissues, a process fueled by their capacity to control the availability of iron in the host (Kousser et al., 2019).

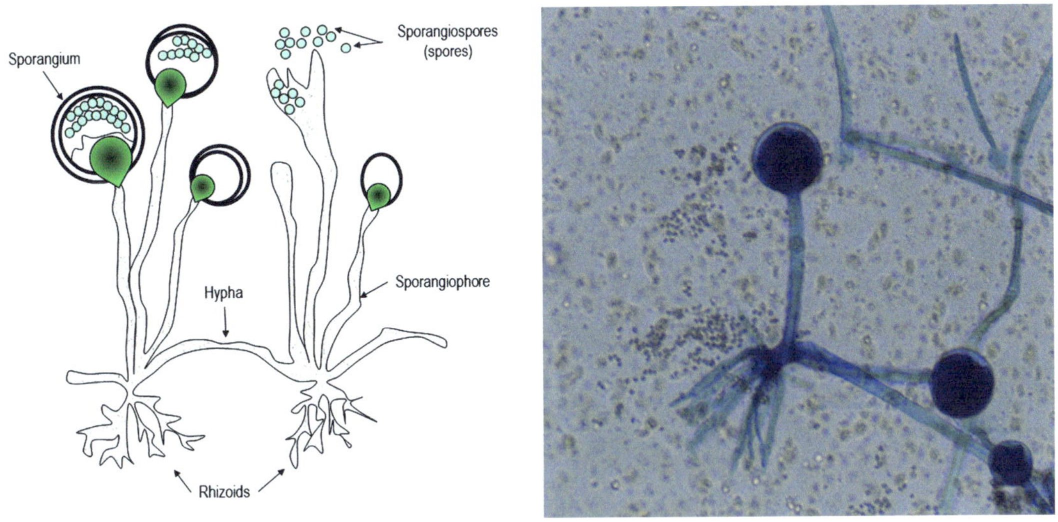

Figure 10.12. Mucorales, particularly species like *Rhizopus oryzae*, exploit iron acquisition mechanisms to thrive in host environments, making the immune systems role in combating such infections vital.

Source: https://www.id.theclinics.com/cms/10.1016/j.idc.2021.03.009/asset/6ce1c713-e7b7-4b66-babf-c561b4c1e964/main.assets/gr1_lrg.jpg.

This complicates the immune response further since factors resulting from competing pathogens, like *Pseudomonas aeruginosa*, may enhance susceptibility of tissue to infection by inhibiting germination of *Rhizopus microsporus*. Such intricate interaction not only displays how challenging it is to develop a proper immune response but also how significant it is to comprehend the full range of microbial interaction and how they affect mucormycosis pathogenesis. An understanding of the immune response to mucormycosis is required for devising effective therapeutic protocols. The available treatment modalities, typically antifungal agents such as amphotericin B, may not be sufficient in cases where the fungal invasion is further compounded by the hosts' immunocompromised status and dysregulation of iron. The dynamic equilibrium between the immune response and pathogens like Mucorales highlights the need for new therapies that could target the mechanisms through which such fungi obtain iron or escape the immune system. Moreover, information gathered from identifying inter-microbial relationships, such as between *Rhizopus* species and *Pseudomonas aeruginosa*, can yield new therapeutic models that enhance the host's immune response and reverse the current trend of mucormycosis infections among vulnerable groups (Kousser et al., 2019). Research advances notwithstanding, the goal remains the same: to improve patient outcomes overall through better understanding and management of mucormycosis and its immunological repercussions (Figure 10.12).

10.3.3. Impact on Human Health

Mucormycosis, an invasive fungal infection produced predominantly by fungi in the order Mucorales, is a severe medical hazard to human health, particularly to immunocompromised hosts. Infection is associated with high morbidity and mortality and is fueled with severe complications such as surgery debridement and prolonged hospitalization. The impact on the health system is considerable; mucormycosis patients usually have lengthy and expensive medical interventions since the infection is virulent and consequently difficult to cure, which makes its treatment complicated (Bochicchio et al., 2017). The spread of mucormycosis incidence, especially in patient populations with conditions such as diabetes or malignancies, illustrates the necessity of understanding the diseases' epidemiology and risk factors to facilitate better prevention and curative strategies (Bochicchio et al., 2017). The effect of mucormycosis extends beyond the immediate physical health of infected patients. Patients recuperating from the disease often experience long-term health conditions, including psychological trauma secondary to the disease process and treatment. The requirement for extensive surgical intervention, such as amputation or the removal of a large quantity of tissue by debridement, may lead to extremely low quality of life and therefore the specific focus on rehabilitation and psychiatric support. Moreover, the threat of secondary complications, including further invasive fungal infections, adds to the overall cost burden on the healthcare system. Patient analysis of those who already have existing invasive fungal infections reveals that the pre-and post-treatment setting for mucormycosis presents unique challenges that can further impact patient outcomes and survival rates (Aljurf et al., 2017).

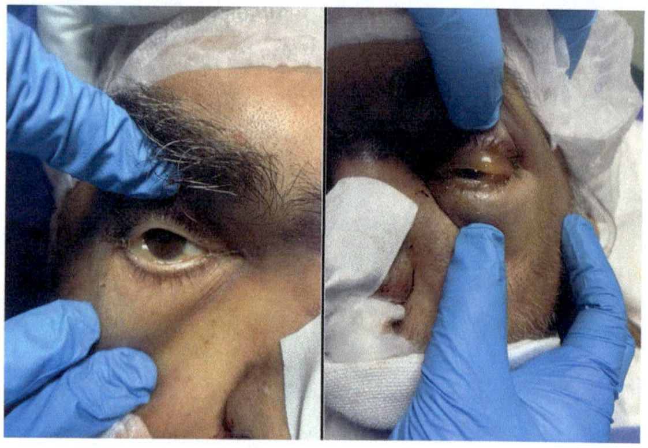

Figure 10.13. Analysis of patients with pre-existing invasive fungal infections indicates that the pre- and post-treatment landscape of mucormycosis presents unique challenges that can significantly affect patient outcomes and survival rates.

Source: https://images-provider.frontiersin.org/api/ipx/w=1200&f=png/https://www.frontiersin.org/files/Articles/645270/fmed-08-645270-HTML/image_m/fmed-08-645270-g001.jpg.

Overall, the social burden of mucormycosis cannot be overlooked. The financial burden on the patient and the healthcare system is staggering, particularly with the cost of extended hospital stays and costly therapies required for treatment. Public health initiatives that prevent mucormycosis infections, particularly among high-risk populations, need more awareness and education on the disease. With the worldwide rise in risk factor prevalence like diabetes, healthcare professionals need to remain alert and detect and manage these groups to prevent mucormycosis from causing potential harm to human health. Planning for prevention and early intervention would go a long way in cutting down the prevalence of the diseases and its harmful impact on people and society as a whole (Bochicchio et al., 2017) (Figure 10.13).

10.4. Treatment Options

Successful treatment of mucormycosis is multimodal and should include a complete attack with both pharmacologic and surgery aspects. The groundwork for drug therapy here is antifungal drug therapy, and liposomal amphotericin B is now employed as the drug of choice in serious infections. The drug has proved to penetrate the tissue and be effective against the Mucorales species responsible for the infection. In addition, newer agents such as isavuconazole are also proving to be effective alternatives with efficacy comparable to traditional treatments. Early detection and antifungal treatment are crucial, especially among critical patients or those presenting with initial symptoms characteristic of mucormycosis. The delayed intervention will lead to greater morbidity and mortality and highlights the necessity of early therapeutic interventions. Surgical debridement is also an essential part of the management of mucormycosis, particularly if necrotizing lesions are present. Removal of infected necrotic tissue through surgery has as its goal to avoid further progression of infection and maximize overall efficacy of antifungal therapy. Debridement success is largely based on the extent of tissue involvement and surgical response rate. Where the conditions causing causation, such as uncontrolled diabetes or immunocompromised status, cannot be reversed in the short term, effective surgical treatment becomes all the more important. As seen in intensive care units, combined management strategies with aggressive surgical debridement as well as systemic antifungal therapy can have a favorable outcome in involved patients, particularly when lesions rapidly progress in the rhino-sinusal cavity or lungs. Management of predisposing conditions remains central to avoiding the severity and frequency of mucormycosis. Individuals with comorbid conditions such as diabetes mellitus, chronic renal impairment, or those being treated with deferoxamine are at risk for the onset of mucormycosis due to the involvement of the disease with iron overload (Chou et al., 2015).

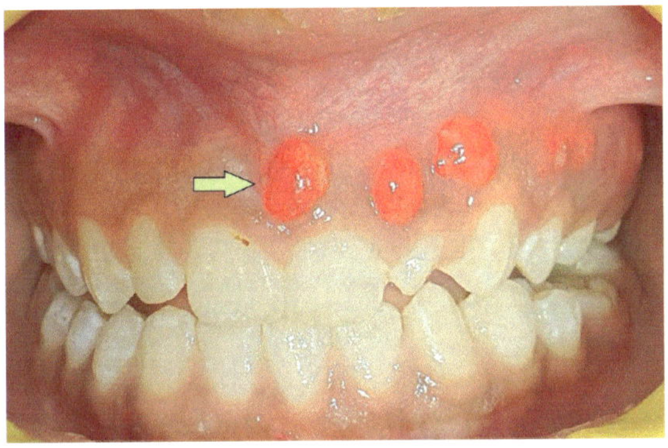

Figure 10.14. Rapid identification and initiation of antifungal therapy are critical, especially in patients who are critically ill or have presenting symptoms characteristic of mucormycosis.

Source: https://www.ccjm.org/content/ccjom/89/10/553/F1.large.jpg.

As the pathophysiology of infection by Mucorales is increasingly elucidated, focused therapy addressing these pathologic processes may enhance overall therapeutic result. Management of hyperglycemia and refined immunosuppression therapy might reduce the incidence of fungal infections among these high-risk groups. Further investigation into the mechanisms of iron uptake in R. might yield leads for therapy in the future. oryzae suggests promising avenues for new therapeutic approaches that would be able to maintain the use of current treatments without imposing associated risks (Chou et al., 2015) (Figure 10.14).

10.4.1. Antifungal Medications

Therapy of mucormycosis, a lethal and often fatal fungal infection, relies heavily on the strategic use of antifungal medications. The most widely known of these is amphotericin B, and it is drug of choice due to its efficacy against the broad range of fungi comprising the Mucorales order. Amphotericin B acts through chelation of ergosterol in the fungal cell membrane, causing cell death via increased permeability. This pharmacological effect is of significance in the treatment of mucormycosis and other fungal diseases, particularly in immunocompromised subjects. Amphotericin B's effectiveness is also demonstrated by in vitro studies, which attest to its superior antifungal efficacy against mucormycosis, and underscore its role in clinical practice where prompt action is required (Gopal et al., 2022). In addition to amphotericin B, other antifungals such as posaconazole and isavuconazole play a significant part in the treatment of mucormycosis. The triazole antifungal, posaconazole, represents a second-line agent for patients who may not tolerate side effects of amphotericin B or present with refractory disease. It inhibits the fungal lanosterol 14α-demethylase enzyme involved in ergosterol synthesis.

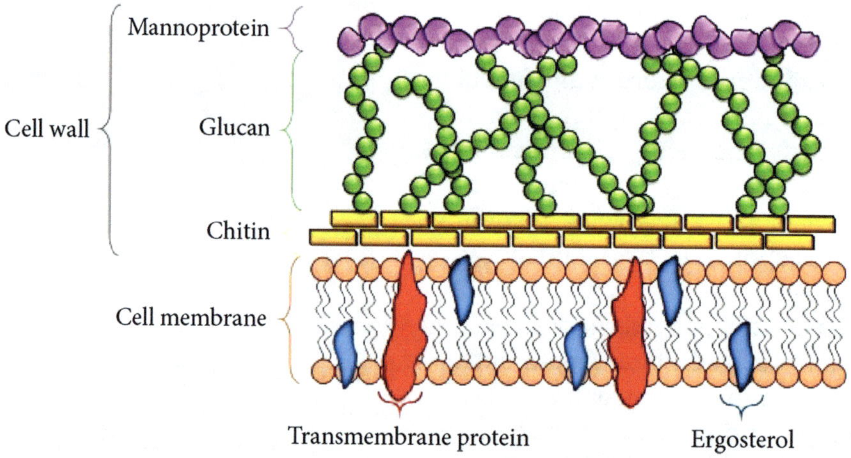

Figure 10.15. Amphotericin B acts by binding to ergosterol in the fungal cell membrane, leading to increased permeability and ultimately cell death.

Source: https://pub.mdpi-res.com/nanomaterials/nanomaterials-12-04470/article_deploy/html/images/nanomaterials-12-04470-g001.png?1671609941.

This disruption not only inhibits the development of fungi but is also utilized in the therapy of invasive mucormycosis. Isavuconazole is another newer triazole that has shown to be an option of interest due to its favorable pharmacokinetic properties and low toxicity over conventional antifungals. These advances in antifungal drugs emphasize the importance of individualized therapeutic approaches in combating the complexity of mucormycosis (Singh et al., 2021). The choice of antifungal medication in the treatment of mucormycosis must consider several factors, including the overall condition of the patients, the extent of fungal invasion, and some risk factors like diabetes or recent surgery. Early antifungal treatment is extremely crucial, particularly in immunocompromised hosts, who have a significant risk of aggressive disease progression. Physicians, thus, need to stay current and vigilant about the evolving profile of antifungal medications and mechanisms of resistance that may render them obsolete. While seeking to mitigate the impact of mucormycosis, medical professionals also emphasize early detection and aggressive surgical treatment, as the combination of antifungal medication and surgical debridement can significantly improve outcomes in patients. The convergence of these factors is a testament to the multi-faceted characteristics required in combating this deadly infection and proves the central position held by novel antifungal therapies in modern medicine (Gopal et al., 2022) (Figure 10.15).

10.4.2. Surgical Interventions

Surgery is an integral part of mucormycosis therapy, particularly where the infection is accompanied by aggressively progressing necrotizing lesions. The invasive fungal infection has a tendency to lead to widespread tissue loss among affected patients, and this renders prompt surgical debridement a necessary procedure for halting further proliferation of the fungus as well as in salvaging healthy tissue in the area. Surgical management is paired with systemic antifungal therapy, since the two-tiered approach can improve outcomes more optimally. Surgical treatment is not only to debride dead tissue but also to allow better penetration of antifungal medications into the affected tissues, thereby improving clinical success. Timing and the extent of surgical debridement are important because delays are related to increased mortality and complications, particularly in immunocompromised patients who are more prone to rapid disease progression and systemic extension. Apart from the acute requirement of surgical therapy, post-operative management of mucormycosis patients requires cautious observation. Following debridement, patients need to be closely monitored for clinical evidence of re-disease, as well as for re-disease-carrying complications like wound healing and requirement of additional surgery. It has been demonstrated in studies that treatment with state-of-the-art imaging techniques, supplemented with clinical evaluation, is essential in order to follow disease evolution and to assess response to therapy. Moreover, the association of antifungal medications, e.g., liposomal amphotericin B or the new molecules isavuconazole, again emphasizes the value of the multi-disciplinary treatment strategy. With improvements in surgery and a better realization of antifungal pharmacology, clinicians are optimistic to decrease the extremely high mortality from mucormycosis and enhance the quality of life for infected patients. The employment of surgical procedures to manage mucormycosis is also underscored by the epidemiology of the disease, which usually presents in individuals with underlying health disorders. Diabetics, immunocompromised individuals, and those with open wounds are most susceptible to this virulent infection. Surgical debridement thereby not just becomes a procedure of treatment but also prophylactic against further complications. As highlighted in current studies, prompt surgical management along with systemic antifungal treatment significantly reduces the incidence of amputations and improves overall results in patients who come with post-traumatic mucormycosis (Bochicchio et al., 2017; Bassetti et al., 2017). Synergy among early detection, aggressive surgical treatment, and targeted medical therapy is the cornerstone of an efficacious treatment program, ultimately striving to mitigate morbidity and mortality associated with this pathogenic fungal infection (Figure 10.16).

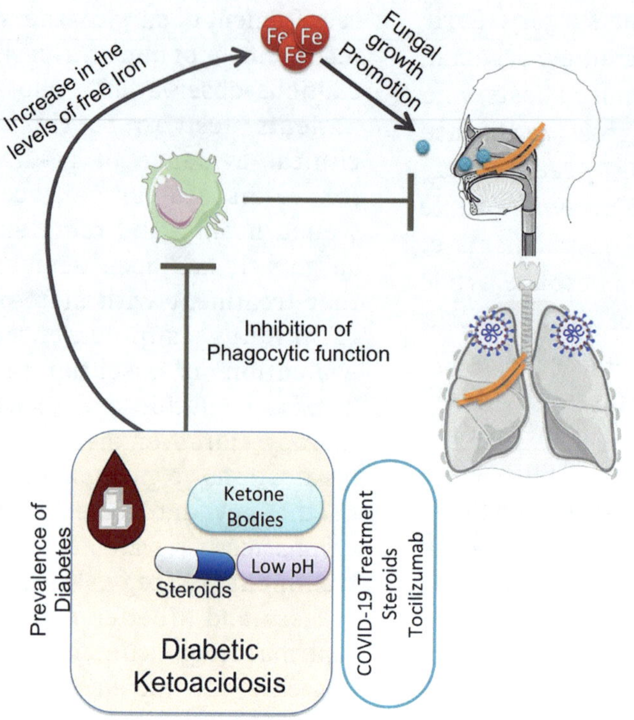

Figure 10.16. Surgical interventions play a crucial role in the management of mucormycosis, particularly when the infection is characterized by rapidly progressing necrotizing lesions.

Source: https://www.frontiersin.org/files/Articles/937481/fcimb-12-937481-HTML/image_m/fcimb-12-937481-g006.jpg.

10.4.3. Supportive Care and Management

In mucormycosis, supportive care and management play a key role in improving patient outcomes, particularly during the COVID-19 pandemic, which had boosted the incidence of this opportunistic fungal disease. There is ample evidence indicating that individuals suffering from predisposing conditions such as diabetes mellitus and those on high doses of corticosteroids are most vulnerable to mucormycosis. The Uttar Pradesh observational study identified that a great proportion of the afflicted were diabetic, unvaccinated, and steroid users, highlighting the need for careful surveillance and control of these risk factors. Institution of rigorous protocols for blood sugar control and tapering of immunosuppressive therapy can minimize risks and enhance responsiveness to treatment, reiterating the importance of specific supportive care interventions among these patients (Bansal et al., 2021). Therapy for mucormycosis not only involves immediate antifungal treatment but also supportive therapy targeted at the individualized needs of infected individuals. Clinical examination indicates that a prompt diagnosis is essential, as early intervention would decrease morbidity and mortality significantly. In particular, it is essential to assess and maintain the patients nutritional condition, hydration level, and overall physical status throughout treatment. This not only encompasses pharmacological treatment but also psychological intervention since the physical presentation of mucormycosis can be annoying and may coexist with mental illness. Besides, oral health and hygiene education is pivotal in preventing secondary infections and enhancing patient recovery, highlighting the complementary role of supportive care in managing this severe condition (Bhandari et al., 2022). Finally, harmony among an interdisciplinary healthcare team is paramount in optimizing supportive care for mucormycosis patients. This process needs to include infectious disease specialists, endocrinologists, and critical care clinicians in order to address all aspects of a patient's status. Regular monitoring for the efficacy of therapy and toxicities of antifungal medications is necessary in fine-tuning therapy appropriately. Also, educating patients and caregivers comprehensively about the disease process, treatment, and prevention maximizes their involvement and compliance with treatment protocols. As highlighted in more recent studies, the development of a positive culture through sound communication and shared decision-making not only improves results but also the patient experience navigating the intricacies of mucormycosis treatment (Bansal et al., 2021; Bhandari et al., 2022) (Figure 10.17).

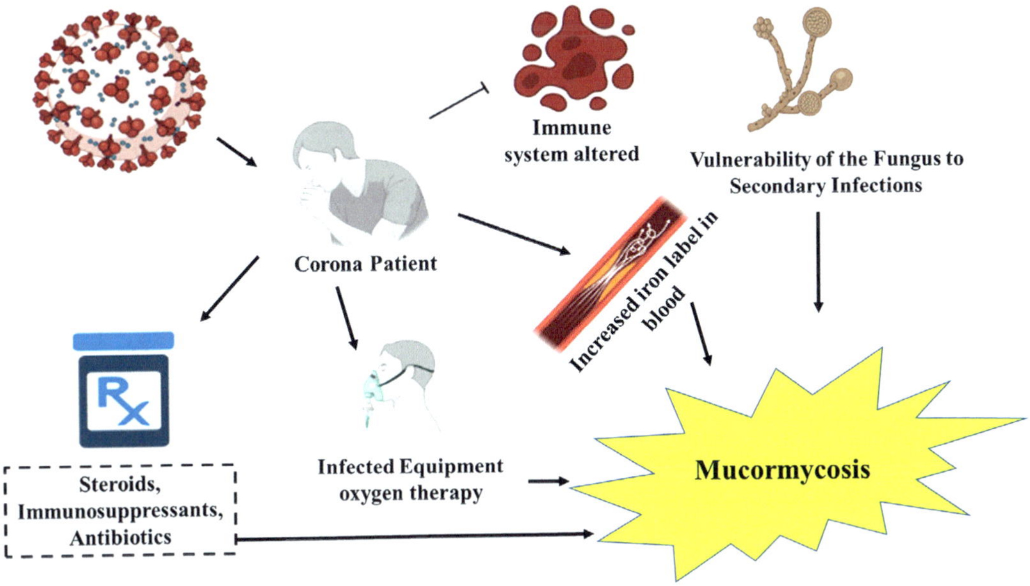

Figure 10.17. In the context of mucormycosis, supportive care and management play a crucial role in improving patient outcomes, particularly in the wake of the COVID-19 pandemic, which heightened the incidence of this opportunistic fungal infection.

Source: https://ars.els-cdn.com/content/image/1-s2.0-S2772431X24000261-gr1.jpg.

SUMMARY

Mucormycosis, an opportunistic fungal disease by the Mucorales order of fungi, is a serious threat to health, particularly for individuals who are immunocompromised. The most significant predisposing factors for the diseases' occurrence are diabetes mellitus, hematologic malignancies, and iron overload disorders. Of note is that deferoxamine-treated individuals are at risk, given the drug's function to assist iron acquisition for pathogens like *Rhizopus oryzae*, the most common species associated with mucormycosis. Experiments have shown that surface presentation of CBS domain proteins Fob1 and Fob2 on *R. oryzae* enhances acquisition of iron from ferrioxamine, enhancing the virulence and pathogenicity of the fungus. This partnership underscores the critical role iron metabolism plays in pathogenesis and severity of mucormycosis and underscores the need for vigilant monitoring within high-risk populations. Pathogenesis of mucormycosis is also directly linked to how *R. oryzae* accesses iron, presenting yet another complicating factor when it comes to treating those who are infected. Studies indicate that ferric receptor proteins Fob1 and Fob2 play a critical role in the acquisition of iron from ferrioxamine, essential for growth and virulence of the fungus. *R. oryzae* mutants with altered receptor expression in experiments resulted in a highly impaired ability to utilize ferrioxamine as the source of iron, along with reduced virulence in murine models. This discovery not only contributes to our understanding of Mucorales survival and iron homeostasis interaction but also offers avenues for novel therapeutic approaches toward the iron acquisition mechanism in Mucorales. The observations on iron uptake in R. are invaluable for treatment and prevention of mucormycosis in immunocompromised patients, particularly in deferoxamine-treated individuals. Beyond immediate implications for therapy, the iron uptake observations in *R. oryzae* also present more general concerns for the long-term management of patients with iron overload disease. As deferoxamine continues to be a significant therapeutic agent for conditions such as thalassemia and sideroblastic anemia, balancing its value against the risk of mucormycosis is necessary. Additional research is needed to explore possible therapeutic options that can minimize the danger of fungal infections while not compromising the efficacy of iron chelating treatment. The preservation of receptors like Fob1 and Fob2 across Mucorales suggests that targeting these pathways could offer a promising direction for the development of antifungal therapy. With the ongoing global increase in mucormycosis incidence, especially during the COVID-19 pandemic, targeting these areas becomes growing significance towards safeguarding public health as well as improving outcomes among high-risk populations (Chou et al., 2015; Adam et al., 2012).

A CLOSER LOOK

DEFEROXAMINE

Deferoxamine is a chelating agent used in the treatment of acute and chronic iron overload, most commonly found in states of thalassemia or following multiple transfusions of blood. It binds free iron within the bloodstream, which enters into a compound that is both excreted primarily through the urine and bile. Administered subcutaneously, intramuscularly, or intravenously, deferoxamine prohibits iron-related organ damage, particularly of the liver and heart. Though effective, use is strictly checked for side effects such as auditory or visual symptoms, allergy, and slowing of growth in children with long-term use.

REFERENCES

1. Abtahi Naeini, B., Abtahi, S. H., Ahmadikia, K., Alijani, R., et al. (2022). COVID-19 associated mucormycosis: A review of an emergent epidemic fungal infection in the era of COVID-19 pandemic. https://core.ac.uk/download/533464400.pdf (accessed on 27th June 2025).
2. Adam, A., Boelaert, M., Calfee, C., Douglas, C., Wallace, E., Kontoyiannis, D., et al. (2012). "Different strokes for different folks." https://deepblue.lib.umich.edu/bitstream/2027.42/90351/1/1924_ftp.pdf (accessed on 27th June 2025).
3. Agarwal, R., Asija, R., Sharma, A., Tanwar, P., et al. (2021). Fungal infections associated with COVID-19. https://core.ac.uk/download/482241778.pdf (accessed on 27th June 2025).
4. Alcazar-Fuoli, L., Bernal-Martinez, L., Buitrago, M. J., Cuenca-Estrella, M., et al. (2009). Incidence of zygomycosis in transplant recipients. https://core.ac.uk/download/pdf/82273109.pdf (accessed on 27th June 2025).
5. Aljurf, M., Auletta, J. J., Battiwalla, M., Boeckh, M., et al. (2017). Pre-existing invasive fungal infection is not a contraindication for allogeneic HSCT for patients with hematologic malignancies: A CIBMTR study. https://core.ac.uk/download/323072284.pdf (accessed on 27th June 2025).
6. Ampel, N. M., Anstead, G. M., Babady, N. E., Baddley, J. W., Bariola, J. R., Ben-Ami, R., Bialek, R., et al. (2012). Pulmonary fungal infections. https://deepblue.lib.umich.edu/bitstream/2027.42/92435/1/j.1440-1843.2012.02150.x.pdf (accessed on 27th June 2025).
7. Artes Haderi, A., Altevogt, B., Denning, D. W., Chavez, E., Armstrong, H., Aram, J. A., Perfect, J. R., et al. (2025). Antifungal policy and practice across five countries: A qualitative review. https://core.ac.uk/download/644552488.pdf (accessed on 27th June 2025).
8. Ascioglu, S., Chamilos, G., De Pauw, B., Duarte, R. F., Even, G., Girmenia, C., et al. (2016). Pulmonary fungal infections in patients with acute myeloid leukemia: Is it time to revise the radiological diagnostic criteria? https://core.ac.uk/download/54529664.pdf (accessed on 27th June 2025).
9. Bal, A. M., Brüggemann, R., Chowdhary, A., Ghafur, A., et al. (2023). The battle against fungi: Lessons in antifungal stewardship from COVID-19 times. https://core.ac.uk/download/591798215.pdf (accessed on 27th June 2025).
10. Bansal, M. K., Kumar, M., Kumar, V., Singh, R., et al. (2021). Mucormycosis during second wave of COVID-19 in India: Exploratory analysis from tertiary care center of Uttar Pradesh. https://core.ac.uk/download/586040549.pdf (accessed on 27th June 2025).
11. Bassetti, M., & Bouza, E. (2017). Invasive mold infections in the ICU setting: Complexities and solutions. https://core.ac.uk/download/80137827.pdf (accessed on 27th June 2025).
12. Bhagat, S., Chopra, S., Kaur, M., Yadav, R., et al. (2023). The role of inflammatory markers in COVID-19 associated rhino-orbital-cerebral mucormycosis patients. https://core.ac.uk/download/591405016.pdf (accessed on 27th June 2025).
13. Bhandari, S., Sharma, S., & Singhal, M. (2022). Clinical profile of recent progressive illnesses in patients with mucormycosis: A comprehensive analysis. https://core.ac.uk/download/539911999.pdf (accessed on 27th June 2025).
14. Bochicchio, G., Bochicchio, K., Kronen, R., Liang, T., et al. (2017). Invasive fungal infections

secondary to traumatic injury. https://core.ac.uk/download/129069519.pdf (accessed on 27th June 2025).

15. Bonifaz, A., Bonifaz, A., Bonifaz, A., Bruder-Nascimento, A., Lindenberg, A., Silva-Hernández, A. G., Tichellio, A. G., et al. (2012). Epidemiology of invasive fungal infections in Latin America. https://core.ac.uk/download/pdf/8681425.pdf (accessed on 27th June 2025).

16. Castro, G. K., Chiller, T. M., Davis, T., Ferretti, M., et al. (2024). Shared vision for improving outcomes for serious fungal diseases: Report of a patient, caregiver, and clinician summit. https://core.ac.uk/download/619402116.pdf (accessed on 27th June 2025).

17. Chou, T. F., Edwards, J. E., French, S. W., Gebremariam, T., et al. (2015). Fob1 and Fob2 proteins are virulence determinants of *Rhizopus oryzae* via facilitating iron uptake from ferrioxamine. https://core.ac.uk/download/323079013.pdf (accessed on 27th June 2025).

18. Corzo Leon, D. E., Franco-Cendejas, R., López-Jácome, L. E., Resendiz-Sanchez, F., et al. (2017). Higher *in vitro* proliferation rate of *Rhizopus oryzae* in blood of diabetic individuals in chronic glycemic control compared with non-diabetic individuals. https://core.ac.uk/download/131024048.pdf (accessed on 27th June 2025).

19. El Charkawi, H., & El Sharkawy, O. A. (2022). Management of post COVID-19 mucormycosis with osteomyelitis in the maxilla: New combined consequences of the pandemic (Case report). https://core.ac.uk/download/524992125.pdf (accessed on 27th June 2025).

20. Gopal, M., Parameswaran, S., Pichaivel, M., Samundi, R., et al. (2022). An overview of mucormycosis. https://core.ac.uk/download/542934049.pdf (accessed on 27th June 2025).

21. Hamilos, G., Kontoyiannis, D. P., & Samonis, G. (2012). Recent advances in the use of *Drosophila melanogaster* as a model to study immunopathogenesis of medically important filamentous fungi. https://core.ac.uk/download/pdf/8693944.pdf (accessed on 27th June 2025).

22. Haseli-Mofrad, A., Montazerin, N., Rajavi, Z., Ziaei Ardakani, M., et al. (2023). Ocular manifestations of COVID-19 among patients admitted to the intensive care unit of Khatam-Al-Anbia tertiary center, Tehran, Iran. https://core.ac.uk/download/618356890.pdf (accessed on 27th June 2025).

23. King, J., Lehrnbecher, T., Pana, Z. D., Steinbach, W. J., et al. (2017). Recognition and clinical presentation of invasive fungal disease in neonates and children. https://core.ac.uk/download/131024549.pdf (accessed on 27th June 2025).

24. Kontoyiannis, D. P., Lewis, R. E., Pongas, G. N., Samonis, G., et al. (2009). Voriconazole-associated zygomycotic: A significant consequence of evolving antifungal prophylaxis and immunosuppression practices? https://core.ac.uk/download/pdf/82767841.pdf (accessed on 27th June 2025).

25. Kousser, C. A. (2019). Investigating the impact of polymicrobial interactions on fungal pathogenicity. https://core.ac.uk/download/323305510.pdf (accessed on 27th June 2025).

26. Kumar, B., & Prasad, N. (2022). Mucormycosis of oral cavity: A descriptive case report from a tertiary care hospital. https://core.ac.uk/download/543135934.pdf (accessed on 27th June 2025).

27. Montaño, D. E. (2024). The immune response of human monocytes to *Lichtheimia corymbifera*. https://core.ac.uk/download/642835263.pdf (accessed on 27th June 2025).

28. Nosari, A., Dhouibi, A., Groll, A. H., Pham, A. S., De Pauw, B., Padovani, B., Althoff Souza, C., et al. (2010). Usefulness of molecular biology performed with formaldehyde-fixed paraffin embedded tissue for the diagnosis of combined pulmonary invasive mucormycosis and aspergillosis in an immunocompromised patient. https://core.ac.uk/download/pdf/8379562.pdf (accessed on 27th June 2025).
29. Rauf, A., Chaudhary, A., Conte-Junior, C. A., Lima, C. M. G., Prajapati, P. K., Kumar, P., Sharma, R., et al. (2022). Mucormycosis in the COVID-19 environment: A multifaceted complication. https://core.ac.uk/download/543512942.pdf (accessed on 27th June 2025).
30. Singh, A. P., Singh, A. P., Singh, G., Singh, R., et al. (2021). Mucormycosis (black fungus): A review. https://core.ac.uk/download/482244838.pdf (accessed on 27th June 2025).

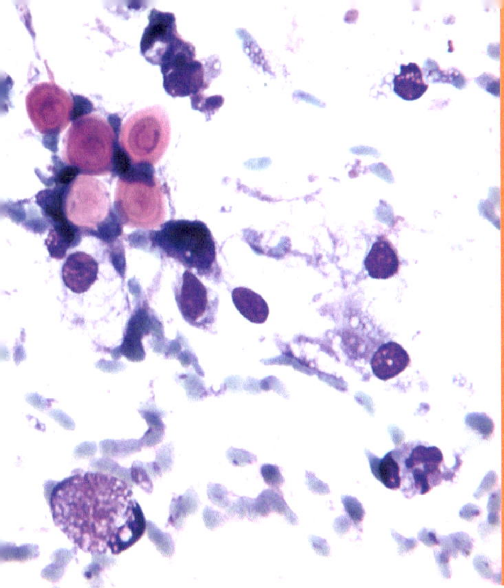

Chapter 11
CRYPTOCOCCOSIS

Contents

Introduction

Cryptococcosis is a serious fungal infection and an important public health issue, most significantly in immunocompromised individuals. The causative organism, *Cryptococcus neoformans*, is an encapsulated yeast that typically acquires entry into the human host by being inhaled in airborne spores. Having once become established within the pulmonary environment, the organism can become disseminated and lead to severe complications such as meningitis. This is especially prevalent with immunocompromised patients, such as those with human immunodeficiency virus (HIV) infection, thereby establishing an even greater need for specifically targeted diagnostic and therapeutic strategies. The interplay between host immunity and fungal virulence determinants elevates the need for greater understanding of cryptococcosis development in various populations and under varied clinical conditions, opening the door to interventions and improved patient outcomes. An understanding of cryptococcosis mechanisms is essential to the formulation of effective treatment protocols. Treatment of the infection includes a complex regimen typically consisting of an induction phase, a consolidation phase, and maintenance therapy. Initial treatment in the majority of instances consists of very powerful fungicidal drugs like amphotericin B combined with flucytosine, both highly effective but in resource-limited settings that often are not available. The shortage increases rates of morbidity and mortality, particularly in highly prevalent HIV areas, in which cryptococcal meningitis is a frequent outcome. Additionally, the systemic infection makes treatment and diagnosis more complicated and necessitates that healthcare systems prioritize preventive as well as curative interventions to combat the escalating burden of cryptococcosis (Parris et al., 2018). It has also identified the phenomenon of cryptococcal immune reconstitution syndrome (IRS) in non-purely immunocompromised hosts. IRS is a condition that manifests when the immune system begins to recover, typically following antiretroviral therapy for HIV-infected patients, triggering inflammation against the established *Cryptococcus* infection. Importantly, novel strategies are being explored to manage IRS, including the use of hydroxychloroquine as an immunomodulatory agent, with favorable outcomes reported in case reports (Banerjee et al., 2011). The approach to the comprehension and treatment of cryptococcosis must therefore shift to optimize for dealing with the sophisticated character of host-fungal interactions, with the aim of total management incorporating both infectious organism and hosts immune response (Figure 11.1).

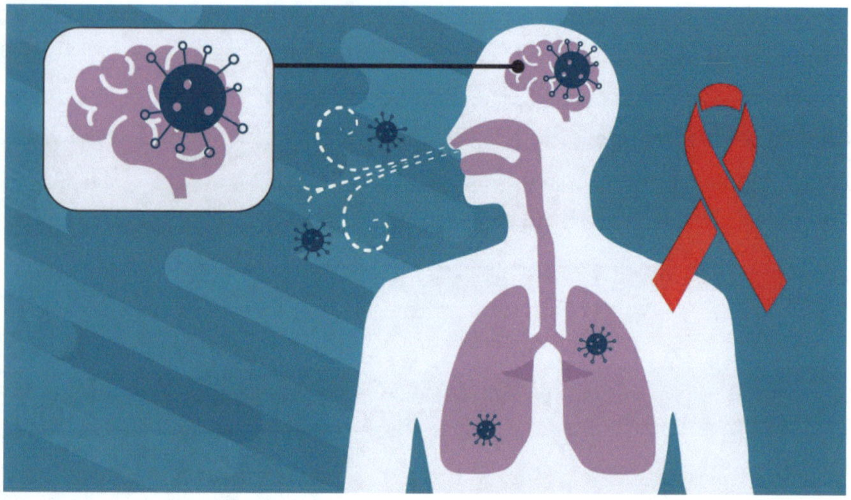

Figure 11.1. Cryptococcosis.

Source: https://www.cdc.gov/cryptococcosis/media/images/2024/05/crypto.jpg.

11.1. Causative Agent

The encapsulated yeast, *Cryptococcus neoformans*, is the principal causative agent of cryptococcosis, a fungus that thrives well in organically rich environments, particularly rotting wood and bird feces. The yeast is very opportunistic and poses high risk to immunocompromised individuals and those with underlying conditions such as human immunodeficiency virus (HIV) infection. Notably, the virulence of *C. neoformans* is aided by its polysaccharide capsule, protective yet deleterious – sheltering it from host immune responses while allowing the development of fulminant disease, such as cryptococcal meningitis in immunocompromised populations. The organism is remarkably adaptable under varied conditions in the environment, solidifying its status as a significant public health concern, notably in tropical and subtropical regions. The pathogenesis of *C. neoformans* is triggered by inhalation of spores in the air, which cause pulmonary infection. The organism, after becoming established in the lungs, has the capacity to counteract host mechanisms of defense and could progress hematogenously to the central nervous system, where fatal and serious complications might follow. The clinical presentation is typically a mix of neurological manifestations like changed mental status, visual disturbances, and confusion, which may initially result in deceptive diagnosis and delayed treatment. For example, in the diagnosis of a man aged 59 years with two weeks' history of headaches, *Cryptococcus* spp. in cerebrospinal fluid was finally found, signifying the challenge to diagnose cryptococcosis early, particularly in non-immunocompromised individuals, as indicated in the report of Faria et al., (2013). Early treatment is critical in cryptococcosis, yet patient prognosis is adversely affected by factors such as late diagnosis and inappropriate initial antifungal therapy. Treatment protocols typically follow standardized procedures involving antifungal medications like amphotericin B and fluconazole, which are effective when administered early. However, host immune response impact factors can affect therapeutic activity and complicate cryptococcosis management strategies in heterogeneous groups of patients. Also, the new studies on new antifungal drugs, such as ravuconazole, show the need for continued study of effective but affordable treatments, particularly in areas with high rates of fungal diseases. Resolving the problems associated with *C. neoformans* as the etiologic agent of cryptococcosis is critical in improving patient outcomes and reducing death caused by this fungus, as it remains a priority concern in international health programs (Ahmed et al., 2014) (Figure 11.2).

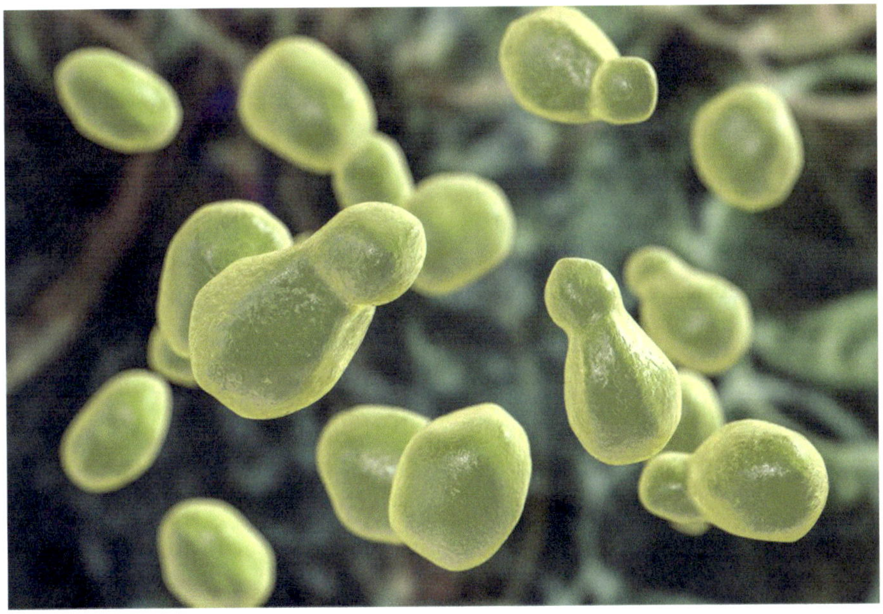

Figure 11.2. The primary causative agent of cryptococcosis is the fungus *Cryptococcus neoformans*, a saprophytic organism that thrives in environments rich in organic matter, particularly within decaying wood and bird droppings.

Source: https://stories.tamu.edu/wp-content/uploads/2024/03/*Cryptococcus*-neoformans-1024x683.jpg.

11.1.1. Description of Cryptococcus neoformans

Understanding the biological and clinical characteristics of *Cryptococcus neoformans* is essential to addressing the growing public health issue of cryptococcosis. *C. neoformans* is a basidiomycetous fungus that is found predominantly in soil and bird feces, and its position at the center of its own epidemiology is key to that. It thrives in fertile organic conditions, and its encapsulated yeast cell is adapted for survival in a broad spectrum of environments, which maximizes its virulence. The most notable feature of *C. neoformans* is the large polysaccharide capsule, which is crucial to the organism's pathogenicity. Not only does this capsule assist in immune evasion, but it is also the hallmark of the organisms' ability to cause local and systemic infections in affected hosts. Greater scrutiny of these features reaffirms the need for aggressive diagnostics and effective treatment regimens for hosts infected with cryptococcosis. *Cryptococcus neoformans* has been serotyped into various different serotypes, with the most prevalent among immunocompromised patients, particularly HIV-infected patients, being serotype A. The variation between the serotypes is significant with regard to virulence, course of disease, and therapeutic response. Serotype A infections, for example, have been described as having more severe outcomes than those caused by serotype D. In a large-scale investigation, it was determined that clinical factors like sex, HIV status, and initial fungal burden were significant determinants of the outcome of cryptococcosis, which is a reflection of the intricate host-pathogen interplay (Amornkul et al., 2007). The virulence of *C. neoformans* to disseminate beyond the lungs into the central nervous system typically indicates severe complications, including cryptococcal meningitis, and this underscores the need for proper early intervention and management protocols. Aside from its biological nature, *Cryptococcus neoformans*' ecological niche is also significant in deliberations on its transmission and impact on animal health. The fungus triggers spontaneous mycosis in various mammals, particularly where grazing animals are exposed in grazing pastures. An illustration of the epidemic prevalence of *C. gattii* in goat flocks in Spain reports the overall ecological factor of cryptococcosis (Alvarado-Ramírez et al., 2018). Such outbreaks demonstrate the species' ability to cause disease not just in human populations but in animals as well, making control an added problem and underscoring the value of public health programs. Public health officials can strategize against risk from this powerful pathogen by identifying the environmental reservoirs of *C. neoformans* and the zoonotic nature of the organism, thereby taking cryptococcosis beyond mere human concerns (Figure 11.3).

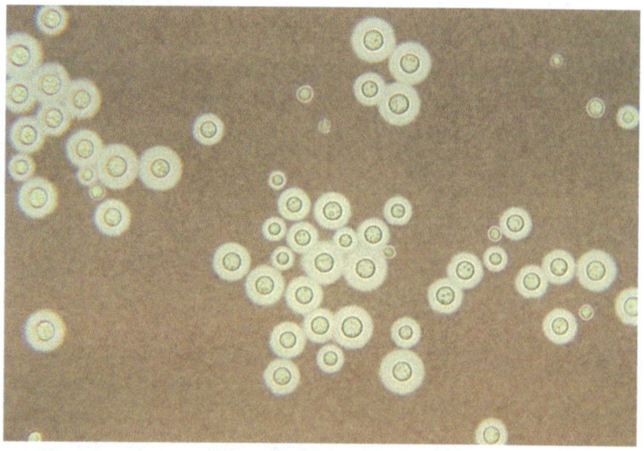

Figure 11.3. *C. neoformans* is a basidiomycetous fungus primarily found in soil and pigeon droppings, which plays a pivotal role in its epidemiology.

Source: https://upload.wikimedia.org/wikipedia/commons/6/6f/*Cryptococcus_*neoformans_using_a_light_India_ink_staining_preparation_PHIL_3771_lores.jpg.

11.1.2. Environmental Sources of the Fungus

Cryptococcus neoformans and *Cryptococcus gattii* environmental reservoirs play significant roles in cryptocoocosis epidemiology. *Cryptococcus neoformans* and *Cryptococcus gattii* are saprophytic fungi yeasts found abundantly in soil, decaying wood, and bird excrement, which they sequester organic matter and nutrients from. Having these organisms present in the environment aids in the examination of transmission dynamics leading to sporadic human infection. Inhalation of dried cells of yeast or particles of spores, typically disrupted by construction or cultivation of soil, subjects the individual to infection. The soil environment facilitates contact with microorganisms, such as amoebae that modulate the survival and virulence of *Cryptococcus* species and allow them to withstand extreme conditions. Such environmental interactions serve not only to highlight the ecological character of such fungi but also to indicate the risk posed by adult populations, particularly immunocompromised individuals and those at risk from opportunistic disease (Aksenov et al., 2017). Additional evidence suggests that the outbreaks of *Cryptococcus gattii* in new environments, particularly temperate climates, pose new public health challenges. Originally recognized as a tropical pathogen, this frequency in the North American Pacific Northwest regions since 1999 is of interest to place in perspective environmental factors involved in its introduction and dispersion. Recent genomic studies indicate that some of the strains among the species complex may have possibly evolved rapidly to fit local ecological niches and possibly benefit from agricultural operations or environmental change brought about by human activity. The aetiology background for the introduction of this pathogen to new environments is biased towards anthropogenic reasons, such as the building of the Panama Canal, which could have aided the facilitation of fungal transmissions from endemic locations (Wanke et al., 2018). The interaction between human activity and reservoir environments provides a two-way scenario that indicates the necessity of monitoring ecosystems in a bid to avoid the spreading of *Cryptococcus*. In addition, information regarding the ecological niches in which *Cryptococcus* species inhabit is not only beneficial to the identification of routes of transmission but also to designing prevention strategies. The role of bird species, including pigeons, in transmitting *C. neoformans* through their excreta is confirmed. The excreta act as a source of nutrient supply for the fungus, hence facilitating its survival and dissemination in urban areas. Residential frequent environmental exposure to these sources highlights public education regarding the dangers of coming in contact with contaminated soil or bird feces. Other climatic variables, for instance, humidity and temperature fluctuations, influence *Cryptococcus* survival of spores in the environment, thus suggesting weather patterns play a key role in its epidemiology. With this information about the environmental reservoirs and their associated risk, public health authorities can make decisions to reduce the occurrence of cryptococcosis among high-risk groups (Aksenov et al., 2017) (Figure 11.4).

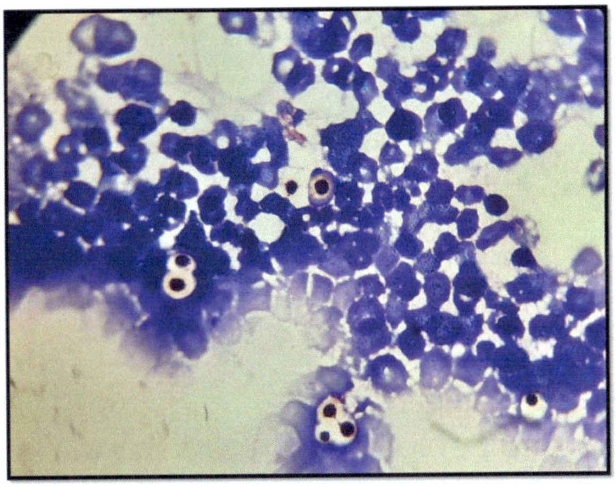

Figure 11.4. The environmental sources of *Cryptococcus*, particularly *Cryptococcus neoformans* and *Cryptococcus gattii*, play a crucial role in understanding cryptocoocosis.

Source: https://www.mdpi.com/biomed/biomed-02-00014/article_deploy/html/images/biomed-02-00014-g001.png.

11.1.3. Pathogenicity and Virulence Factors

The pathogenicity of *Cryptococcus neoformans* is directly related to its environmental adaptability, an ability necessary for the establishment of infection in immunocompromised hosts. The encapsulated organism, best known as a pathogen of cryptococcal meningitis, has evolved various virulence factors to maintain penetration and survival within the host. Of special interest is the polysaccharide capsule, which is not only a physical barrier against phagocytosis but is also essential in regulating the hosts immune response. Additionally, expression of virulence determinants depends on the environmental context of the isolates. Interestingly, clinical strains have greater virulence capacity than environmental strains, suggesting an adaptive process towards immunocompromised status, and this is a proof of the complex nature of its pathogenicity (Buchanan et al., 1998). Hence, the identification of such mechanisms is necessary to designing targeted interventions for cryptococcosis. Ongoing study of virulence factors reveals the multi-pronged strategies employed by *C. neoformans* in order to survive in the host. In addition to the polysaccharide capsule, the fungus also produces melanin, which contributes to the survival of the organism by protecting it against host oxidative stress. Further, the release of specific proteins such as superoxide dismutase and proteases assists in the avoidance of host defense and tissue invasion. Current studies have proven differential gene-expression patterns between clinical and environmental isolates, illustrating an ecological signature in which the virulence of the isolate is determined by its origin (Buchanan et al., 1998). These findings serve to emphasize the relevance of contextual environmental factors in the determination of pathogenic traits of *C. neoformans* and hence reiterating the importance of further studies clarifying such complex interactions.

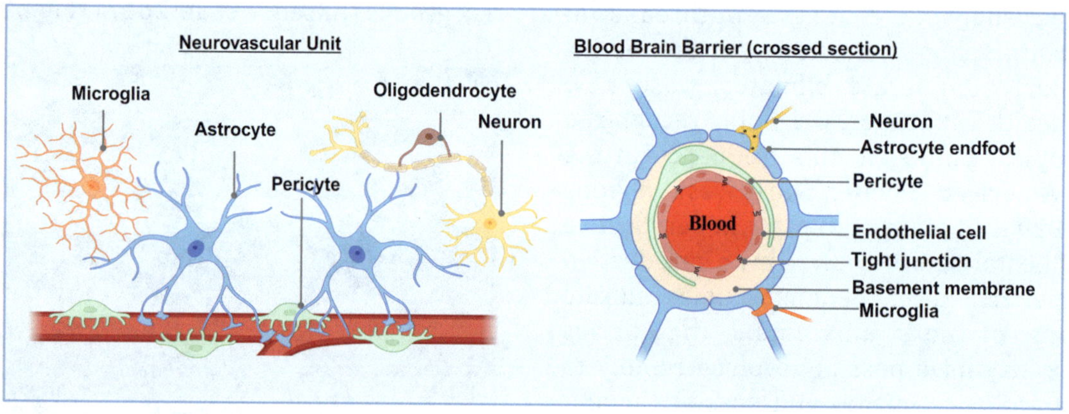

Figure 11.5. The pathogenicity of *Cryptococcus neoformans* is intricately linked to its environmental adaptability, which is crucial for establishing infection in compromised hosts.

Source: https://www.mdpi.com/jof/jof-10-00586/article_deploy/html/images/jof-10-00586-g001.png.

Cryptococcal pathogenicity studies also highlight the role of genetic determinants for virulence. Various transcriptional profiles in various *C. neoformans* lineages have been associated with pathogenicity, adding to the complexity of the organism. Recent evidence suggests that gene ontology categories for cellular biosynthesis and metabolism are overrepresented in clinical isolates, suggesting metabolic adaptation towards host growth conditions. Furthermore, the observation that an overwhelming proportion of the differentially expressed genes in induced environmental isolates are hypothetical proteins presents promise for the identification of novel virulence factors (Phan et al., 2019). Clarifying such genetic determinants not only enhances the knowledge regarding *C. neoformans*' pathogenicity but is most likely to enable the identification of specific therapeutic treatments against cryptococcosis (Figure 11.5).

11.2. Epidemiology

Epidemiology plays a critical role in explaining the distribution and determinants of cryptococcosis, an invasive fungal infection, particularly among at-risk populations. Cryptococcosis is remarkably prevalent in solid organ transplant (SOT) recipients, according to evidence documenting its presence among such individuals. Surveys conducted in a large group of adult recipients of SOT showed cryptococcal infection, although rare, occurred in 0.37% of patients with significant morbidity, including cryptococcal meningitis in 44% of patients. This points towards the necessity of ongoing surveillance and screening practices in transplant recipients to minimize the risks of this infection. Understanding the epidemiology among SOT recipients gives an impetus to interventions that reduce incidence and improve patient outcomes and, in turn, inform clinical practice within transplant medicine (George et al., 2017). The epidemiological environment of cryptococcosis is not only confined among SOT recipients to other groups that are afflicted by immunosuppression, such as those with HIV infection. Geographically, from different regions of the world, including regions like Phnom Penh, Cambodia, the prevalence of cryptococcal infections is largely dependent on the occurrence of HIV/AIDS. Studies assessing the burden of cryptococcosis in these populations define important risk factors, such as profound immunosuppression and low CD4 cell counts, that render the population susceptible to higher rates of infection. Information collected not only inform public health responses in terms of improving HIV care and treatment but are also an integral component of disease control efforts. Such frequent review of epidemiological trends is very important to the delivery of optimal healthcare interventions tailored to the specific conditions of at-risk groups (Amornkul et al., 2010). Temporal factors also influence cryptococcosis epidemiology, particularly concerning the timing after transplantation. Median time to the diagnosis of cryptococcosis varies depending on the category of SOT recipient, reflecting diverse risk profiles. Lung, heart, and liver transplant recipients, for instance, experience an earlier onset of disease, which is quite a difference compared to that of kidney transplant recipients with a median of over 600 days.

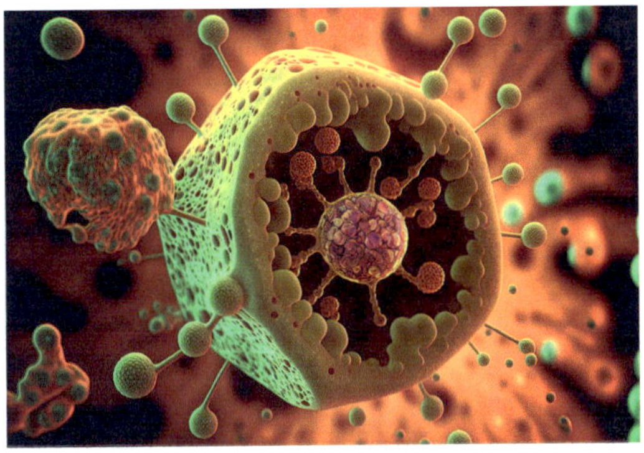

Figure 11.6. Cryptococcosis is notably prevalent among solid organ transplant (SOT) recipients, as indicated by studies highlighting its incidence within this group.

Source: https://s3.amazonaws.com/production.scholastica/article/117277/large/adobestock_580905009.jpeg?1714557349.

That it represents a time-sensitive epidemiological characteristic emphasizes the complexities of predicting and treating cryptococcosis. The lung transplant recipients' high hazard ratios definitively establish the imperative for intense research and effective preventive measures in this population subgroup. By understanding such temporal trends, health practitioners are able to more reliably forecast outbreaks, improve the enhancement of management measures, and ultimately optimize survival rates among patients (George et al., 2017) (Figure 11.6).

11.2.1. Global Distribution of Cryptococcosis

The global spread of cryptococcosis is a manifestation of significant epidemiological patterns influenced by geography, climate, and socio-economic conditions. A high frequency of the fungal infection is largely observed in those regions with high prevalence of the human immunodeficiency virus (HIV). Middle- and low-income countries have particularly predominant levels of cryptococcal meningitis, the most aggressive of the infections, largely due to the limited access to adequate healthcare centers, including antifungal therapy. Under such conditions, individuals with compromised immune systems, particularly those with HIV/AIDS, are disproportionately affected, leading to high rates of morbidity and mortality. As noted, "mortality is unacceptably high," again emphasizing the critical importance of better access to diagnosis and treatment among such at-risk populations (Parris et al., 2018). Accordingly, international health programs should thus emphasize fair resource distribution to be able to control such a public health hazard effectively. Geographic variation in *Cryptococcus neoformans* and *Cryptococcus gattii* species distribution also parallels ecological variation influencing pathogen prevalence. *Cryptococcus neoformans* var. grubii, for instance, is the most prevalent subtype in Singapore, accounting for 95% of disease experienced by HIV patients, who are younger and highly immunocompromised (Barkham et al., 2014). The epidemiological significance of the subtypes is such that the clinical presentation and prognosis of cryptococcosis are quite different. In contrast, *C. gattii* disease, which is less common, manifests in immunocompetent hosts to have a unique clinical picture in the form of pulmonary and neuro involvement. This only demonstrates the necessity for region-based epidemiological surveys to design targeted interventions to alleviate the burden of cryptococcosis in different populations around the world. Recognition of the global spread of cryptococcosis necessitates evaluation of socio-economic conditions that increase health disparities in endemic areas. Access to diagnostics and therapeutic interventions varies starkly, with more affluent countries in most instances being able to provide high-tech care, including antifungal treatment and supportive care, that are too frequently unavailable in resource-limited environments. This discrepancy renders death rates disproportionately elevated in settings of high HIV prevalence since the lack of effective induction therapy exacerbates the effect of the disease.

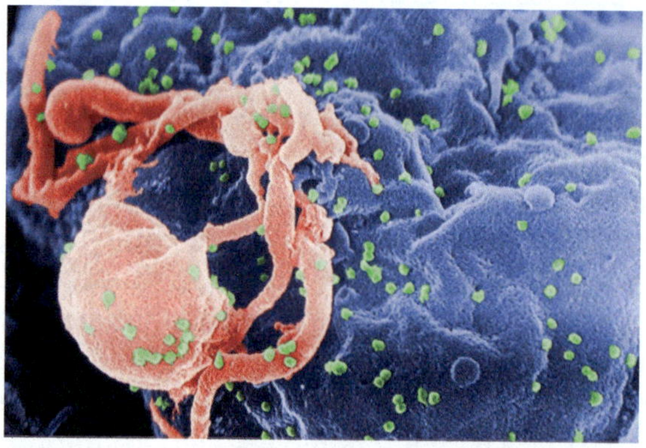

Figure 11.7. High incidences of this fungal disease are primarily observed in regions with a high prevalence of human immunodeficiency virus (HIV).

Source: https://cdn.britannica.com/09/172009-050-312FDA97/Scanning-electron-micrograph-virions-HIV-lymphocyte-bumps.jpg.

Further, early antiretroviral treatment initiation among HIV-infected individuals will significantly reduce cryptococcal disease incidence. Yet, the necessity to develop healthcare infrastructure and programming in a greater form immediately within endemic regions is crucial to counteract the ongoing cryptococcosis threat (Parris et al., 2018). Greater accessibility to the services is not only a health necessity but also an initial step towards achieving global health equity (Figure 11.7).

11.2.2. Populations at Risk

At-risk populations for cryptococcosis are primarily immunocompromised individuals, with HIV/AIDS patients especially vulnerable. Epidemiological data show that patients with very advanced HIV infection are particularly likely to present with cryptococcal meningitis, which is still a leading cause of death in such patients. For instance, there has been evidence of high levels of WHO clinical stage 3 and 4 conditions during early antiretroviral treatment (ART) in settings with limited resources, specifically pointing out the heightened vulnerability to opportunistic infections such as cryptococcosis among the group of individuals (A d'Monforte et al., 2012). Interplay among compromised immune status and environmental contact with *Cryptococcus neoformans* spores enhances the requirement for active screening and management strategies among high-risk populations, especially where HIV infection is endemic. Beyond HIV/AIDS, other groups can be at heightened risk for cryptococcosis. Immunosuppressed individuals, such as patients undergoing chemotherapy, organ transplant recipients, or corticosteroid therapy, are more likely to be infected due to weakened immunity. The risk of cryptococcosis in solid organ transplant recipients additionally warrants regular monitoring because such patients are highly susceptible to opportunistic infection. In addition, emerging guidelines related to HIV testing strategies recognize the importance of increasing prevention, care, and treatment service access among all vulnerable populations. Through identifying risk in individuals at an early stage and encouraging widespread health care access, public health interventions can decrease cryptococcosis burdens and improve outcomes for affected populations. Apart from medially vulnerable populations, certain socioeconomic factors contribute to the risk of cryptococcosis. Individuals residing in poverty environments also face challenges such as inadequate access to health care, insufficient information about preventive interventions, and unsanitary living conditions that provide exposure to *Cryptococcus*. Besides, underprivileged groups, for example, drug injectors, reside under greater health inequalities that make them susceptible to other infections such as cryptococcosis. Therefore, integrating social support systems with medical interventions is necessary in order to address the multisided nature of risk factors among these groups. Through the implementation of community-based health programs, we can foster improved disease prevention and ensure that the individuals at highest risk receive the interventions and information necessary to effectively combat cryptococcosis (Figure 11.8).

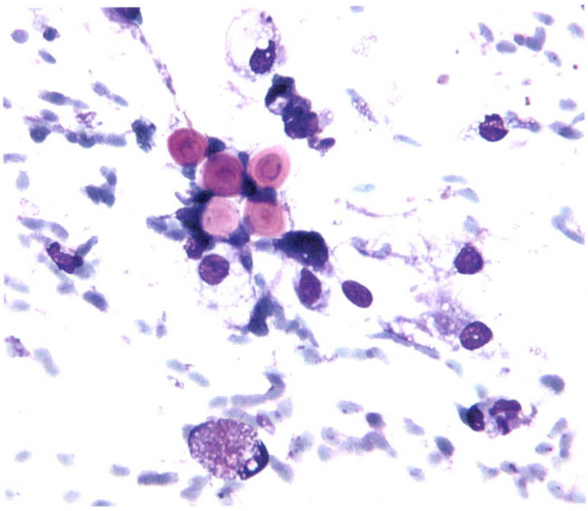

Figure 11.8. Populations at risk for cryptococcosis primarily encompass immunocompromised individuals, with people living with HIV/AIDS being particularly vulnerable.

Source: https://upload.wikimedia.org/wikipedia/commons/thumb/3/36/Cryptococcus.jpg/1200px-Cryptococcus.jpg.

11.2.3. Transmission Routes

Understanding the routes of cryptococcosis transmission is central to comprehending how this fungal infection spreads among human and animal hosts. *Cryptococcus neoformans*, the preponderant causative organism, is a microorganism that is frequently isolated from soil and decaying organic material, particularly where bird droppings are present in large concentrations. Yeast is transmitted via aerosolized particles, and therefore inhalation is the predominant method of transmission among humans. Once inhaled, *Cryptococcus* can evade the hosts immune system, particularly in immunocompromised hosts. This suggests the interplay between host susceptibility and environmental exposure where prior immunodeficiency is likely to exacerbate infection. Research has established that individuals with compromised immunity, such as HIV/AIDS or other immunosuppressive diseases, are at increased risk for developing severe cryptococcosis. In addition, zoonotic transmission from infected animals, especially in veterinary facilities, is an added risk. Companion animals, such as dogs and cats, may also serve as reservoirs for the fungus. In this regard, immunodeficiency among pets, typically due to a range of infectious agents, may also enhance transmission to humans. It has been noted that feline immunodeficiency virus or canine distemper, as examples, may result in immunosuppression, hence the secondary infections such as cryptococcosis. The dynamics of interspecies transmissions of such pathogens expand the range of epidemiological inquiry and highlight the necessity for public health intervention. Recognition of the critical role of animal reservoirs can be applied to inform preventive intervention and clinical management of cryptococcosis in populations. Current advances in the process of reproduction in fungi also apply to transmission and genetic variation within *Cryptococcus* species. Traditionally, fungi, such as *Cryptococcus neoformans*, were considered to be quite asexual. Recent genetic and genomic studies have now recorded sexual reproduction occurring at the population level, influencing transmission patterns. Increased genetic diversity can lead to more virulent strains that may withstand environmental stress or immune response. Moreover, the ability of fungal pathogens to execute outcrossing populations lends a dynamic component to their virulence and evolution. Such observations are reflective of the complexities of transmission routes not merely as a propagation process but as part of an evolutionary process. By integrating data on environmental reservoirs, zoonotic transmission, and fungal reproductive biology, we can design strategic prevention measures against cryptococcosis, especially in immunocompromised patients (Sykes et al., 2010; Carter et al., 2014) (Figure 11.9).

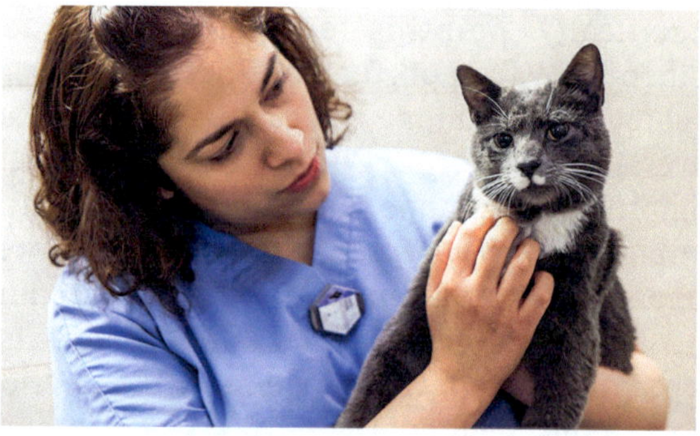

Figure 11.9. Companion animals, such as dogs and cats, may serve as reservoirs for the fungus. In this regard, immunodeficiency in pets, often linked to various infectious agents, may further facilitate transmission to humans.

Source: https://www.aspca.org/sites/default/files/cat-care_cat-diseases_main-image.jpg.

11.3. Clinical Manifestations

The presentation of cryptococcosis is extremely variable depending on the immune status of the hosts and the specific subtype of the pathogen, *Cryptococcus neoformans* or *Cryptococcus gattii*. It must be noted that the majority of cryptococcal infections occur in hosts who are immunocompromised, mainly HIV/AIDS patients. These patients carry the disease most often presented with symptoms like fever, cough, and altered sensorium, thus central nervous system involvement being implicated. It should be noted that *C. neoformans* var. grubii-infected patients have more severe symptoms complicating diagnosis and treatment further. As one of the major subtypes infecting immunocompromised patients, it constitutes a high percentage of cryptococcosis burden globally and is where early diagnosis and treatment are crucial in improving patient outcomes (King et al., 2017). The presentation of patients with cryptococcosis also has peculiar differences based on the subtype. For instance, Singapore statistics show that *C. neoformans* var. grubii infects younger, immunocompromised hosts, particularly individuals with HIV, presenting symptoms that differ from those seen in their immunocompetent counterparts. Specifically, the patients less frequently exhibit altered mental status, which is typically seen in elderly patients, and more frequently show an aggressive disease course with presenting symptoms that require prompt clinical attention. Conversely, *Cryptococcus gattii*, although rare, prefers immunocompetent patients and is associated with pulmonary manifestations that may escalate to disseminated disease (Barkham et al., 2014). Such nuances need to be appreciated by clinicians to personalize their diagnostic and treatment approach accordingly. While neurologic involvement is typical of cryptococcosis, pulmonary manifestations also play a crucial role in the clinical presentation of the disease. In the case of HIV-negative patients, evidence indicates that pulmonary involvement is more common than among HIV-positive subjects. Such differences may affect the timing and mode of diagnosis and initial treatment, resulting in differences in clinical outcomes. Further, use of fluconazole is reportedly far more common in HIV-negative patients, indicating a difference in therapeutic approach based on patient groups and underlying health status. Consequently, effective treatment of cryptococcosis depends on an appreciation of the characteristic clinical manifestation of varying subtypes and host states, underscoring the need for healthcare providers to maintain a high suspicion index among risk populations (Barkham et al., 2014) (Figure 11.10).

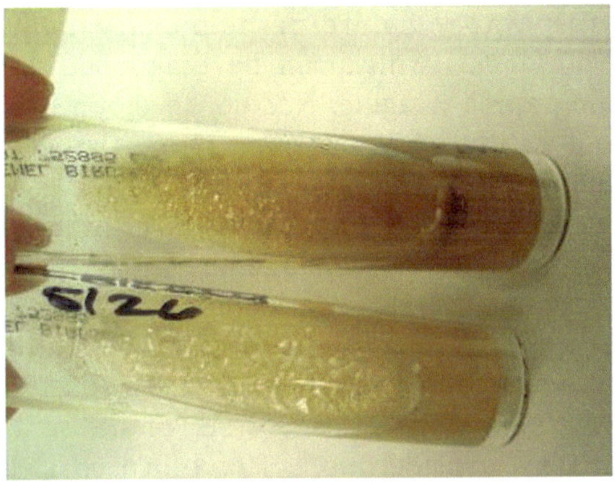

Figure 11.10. *Cryptococcus neoformans* or *Cryptococcus gattii*. It is important to note that the majority of cryptococcal infections occur in immunocompromised individuals, predominantly those with HIV/AIDS.

Source: https://journals.sagepub.com/cms/10.1258/ijsa.2010.010182/asset/ddfee6e9-826b-40e5-b267-07c90e6b9355/assets/images/large/10.1258_ijsa.2010.010182-fig4.jpg.

11.3.1. Symptoms of Pulmonary Cryptococcosis

The clinical presentation of pulmonary cryptococcosis is notoriously protean, a reflection of the disease's complicated pathophysiology. It is not unusual for patients to have an array of respiratory complaints easily confusable with other pulmonary infections. The most common presentations are cough, which can be either dry or productive and is often pleuritic. Dyspnea, shortness of breath, can then follow, particularly in immunocompromised patients. Fever, which is possibly chronic, most often indicates an infectious process underway. The nonspecific nature of such signs may complicate diagnosis, and a high index of suspicion is required, especially in immunocompromised conditions like HIV/AIDS, where opportunistic infections like cryptococcosis are much more likely (King et al., 2017). In more severe cases, pulmonary cryptococcosis can lead to complications of respiratory failure or pulmonary nodule development, which can be diagnosed with radiographic imaging. Nodule development is proof of the bodys attempt at localizing the infection but must be further investigated to rule out malignancies or other infectious etiologies. Curiously, while some patients may be asymptomatic for long periods, those with raised susceptibility may be acute on presentation and need immediate medical attention. This variation highlights the necessity of differential diagnosis consideration of cryptococcosis for pulmonary presentation in high-risk groups, particularly where disease incidence is rising, for instance, owing to higher prevalence of HIV (King et al., 2017).

In addition, the spread of cryptococcal infection at the systemic level aggravates pulmonary symptoms. Constitutional symptoms such as malaise, night sweats, and weight loss can be seen in the patients, suggesting that the infection may have extended into the body beyond the lungs. The correlation between pulmonary and systemic symptoms underscores the necessity of comprehensive clinical evaluations, including serological testing and imaging studies. Diagnosis of pulmonary cryptococcosis is crucial for the use of proper antifungal therapy, which can dramatically alter clinical outcomes. Because cryptococcosis remains a leading cause of death and disability among immunocompromised patients, understanding the complete spectrum of symptoms in the lungs is critical in making early diagnosis and management of this serious infection (Amornkul et al., 2010) (Figure 11.11).

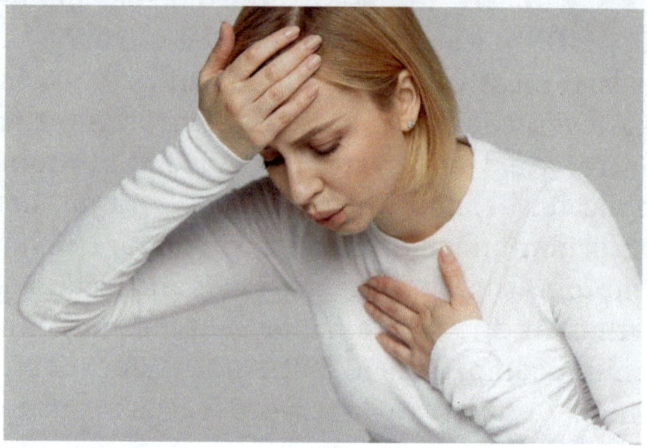

Figure 11.11. Dyspnea.

Source: https://sa1s3optim.patientpop.com/assets/images/provider/photos/2674486.jpg.

11.3.2. Symptoms of Cryptococcal Meningitis

Early symptoms of cryptococcal meningitis may occur subtly and, therefore, early diagnosis is not easily achieved. Symptoms presented by the patients are usually nonspecific and include headaches, fever, and malaise, which can be confused with a usual viral infection. The early presentation is due to an inflammatory response within the central nervous system that is caused by the *Cryptococcus neoformans* yeast. As the infection progresses, the clinical presentation begins to evolve, presenting with additional neurological features such as neck stiffness and photophobia. Interestingly, the symptoms in such cases generally reflect an advanced stage of the disease, pointing towards the urgency of increased awareness among medical personnel, particularly among high-risk individuals, such as those with compromised immune systems, as indicated in studies conducted across various regions, as mentioned in Amornkul et al., (2010). Progressing from initial symptoms, the patient may exhibit profound cognitive alterations and motor dysfunction during the course of cryptococcal meningitis. Mental status changes range from mild confusion to severe disorientation and coma. Furthermore, typical neurological findings such as seizures may be caused by intracranial pressure elevation due to the accumulation of cerebrospinal fluid (CSF). Clinically, the aforementioned signs are proportionate to the bodys physiologic response to the infection, including potential cerebral edema. The importance of accurate diagnosis of this condition is evidenced by cases where patients experienced diagnostic delays due to false-negative outcomes from routine diagnostic testing, pointing to the difficulties in cryptococcal meningitis presentations, as evidenced in the case described in Burnham et al., (2017).

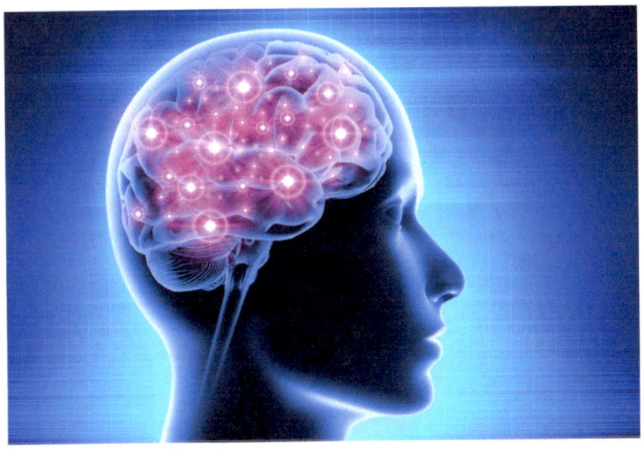

Figure 11.12. Distinctive neurological manifestations such as seizures may arise due to increased intracranial pressure stemming from the accumulation of cerebrospinal fluid (CSF).

Source: https://sensobrain.com/wp-content/uploads/2023/01/featured-image-2.png.

Besides cognitive and physical deterioration, cryptococcal meningitis patients usually complain of persistence symptoms such as nausea and vomiting. These presentations in the gastrointestinal tract can also contribute to the clinical picture, with risk for dehydration and malnutrition. There may also be skin lesions and respiratory manifestations, particularly in the case of advanced disease, as there is a possibility of dissemination of the cryptococcal infection beyond the central nervous system. The clinical profile of cryptococcal meningitis necessitates a holistic approach to management and treatment, emphasizing the necessity of early intervention in the control of acute complications. An awareness of the entire range of symptoms of this disease is important to healthcare workers, especially in view of cryptococcosis burden in the high-risk groups afflicted with co-morbidities, as reiterated in findings of a number of epidemiological research studies, including those in Amornkul et al., (2010) (Figure 11.12).

11.3.3. Other Systemic Manifestations

The systemic presentation of cryptococcosis is outside the central nervous system, indicating the intricacy of the disease. While neurological complications are emphasized, studies have found that cryptococcal infection affects the respiratory, dermatological, and even gastrointestinal systems. For instance, pulmonary cryptococcosis may present as pneumonia, which tends to mimic other common pulmonary infections. Immunocompromised patients, particularly HIV-infected ones, are at higher risk of such a presentation that can complicate diagnosis and treatment. Furthermore, cryptococcosis may also appear with systemic symptoms such as fever, chills, and weight loss, which might be interpreted as other infectious or inflammatory illnesses. Treatment of these manifestations is essential in an effort to create effective management protocols and improve patient outcomes, particularly in highly endemic regions where cryptococcal infection is common (King et al., 2017). The disease can also result in significant dermatological manifestations, again revealing the diseases complex nature. Cutaneous lesions have been experienced in immunocompromised and immunocompetent hosts as papules, nodules, or ulcers. Such lesions can not only be markers of disseminated disease but also themselves be diagnostic pitfalls, easily mistaken for benign entities or other infections. In a retrospective study spanning more than a decade, a significant percentage of patients presented with skin lesions in addition to classical cryptococcosis symptoms, and it follows that dermatologic assessment should be part of the diagnostic workup. Hence, the recognition of the interaction between skin involvement and systemic disease can facilitate earlier detection and successful treatment measures, ultimately reducing morbidity in affected groups. The cryptococcosis process also holds important public health implications, especially among regions with high prevalence rates of attendant risk factors such as HIV infection. The elevated mortality levels for cryptococcal meningitis create a need for more awareness and active screening activities in high-risk groups. In studies examining clinical profiles, evidence reveals an impressive pattern for cryptococcal disease in immunocompromised hosts, with many of the cases occurring in individuals who were previously healthy, disproving the assumption that only severely immunocompromised patients are at risk. This emphasizes the necessity for further study to elucidate the whole spectrum of systemic presentation and to modify public health strategies appropriately. Increased education and monitoring of cryptococcosis can lead to improved clinical outcomes and greater understanding of its epidemiology, particularly in regions with high HIV and other predisposing factors burden (King et al., 2017) (Figure 11.13).

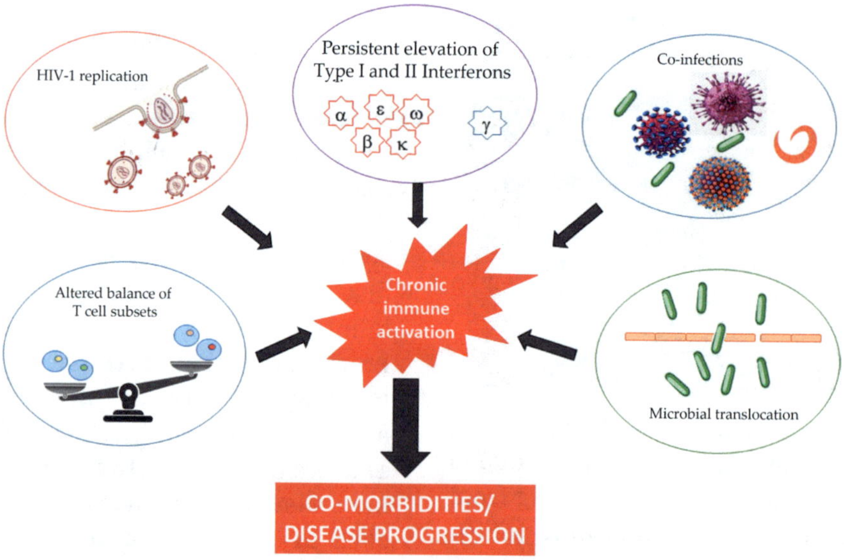

Figure 11.13. Patients with compromised immune systems, particularly those living with HIV, are at greater risk for such presentations, which can complicate diagnosis and treatment.

Source: https://pub.mdpi-res.com/biomedicines/biomedicines-11-00159/article_deploy/html/images/biomedicines-11-00159-g001.png?1673230828.

11.4. Diagnosis

The diagnosis of cryptococcosis presents a great challenge since the disease and its clinical presentation are multifaceted. The key etiologic agent, *Cryptococcus neoformans*, has a tendency to induce opportunistic infections, particularly in immunocompromised individuals such as those with HIV/AIDS. The clinical presentation can range from mild respiratory illness to life-threatening meningoencephalitis, thus complicating its diagnosis. Standard diagnostic procedures, which in most cases are based on culture methods, are tedious and insensitive and hence may delay treatment. In addition, the heterogeneous nature of cryptococcal strains and their possible drug resistance require immediate and precise identification to achieve optimal therapeutic protocols. To cope with these issues, more recent diagnostic tools, such as polymerase chain reaction (PCR) and antigen detection tests, have developed to enhance the efficiency and accuracy of cryptococcal diagnosis with which clinicians are now able to intervene in an appropriate manner. Precise diagnostic methods become even more relevant as the outcome is related to the speed of diagnosis in cryptococcal disease. In low-resource environments, where access to advanced laboratory facilities may be poor, diagnosis in the majority of cases relies on the observation of clinical signs and straightforward laboratory tests. Emerging strategies, involving the integration of next-generation sequencing and proteomics, are set to revolutionize the process of diagnosis. These technologies not only have the potential to increase sensitivity and specificity but also allow for determination of drug resistance profiles, which are critical determinants in the control of treatment regimens of cryptococcal infections. Based on these new approaches, clinicians can address the urgency of cryptococcal disease diagnosis, whereby early treatment intervention can effectively prevent morbidity and mortality of cryptococcosis. (Arastehfar et al., 2019) indicates the necessity for rapid detection and the shortages of current methods, hence the compelling demand for research in this field. Further, the application of routine program data obtained from resource-limited settings has provided insights into cryptococcosis diagnosis as well as its impact on all-cause mortality. The research draws a direct link between early detection and treatment of WHO stage 3 and 4 conditions at diagnosis upon ART start, emphasizing the importance of proper diagnosis on patient outcomes. Healthcare can be improved through systems concentrating on integrating diagnostic data, particularly in high-prevalence settings. For cryptococcosis, their application can facilitate improved monitoring on infection rates and treatment status, ultimately informing better public health programs. From analysis of program data, diagnostic capacity gaps can be revealed, and the necessity for ongoing training and resource investment can be emphasized to enhance healthcare infrastructures. The shared goal is to ensure that diagnostic equipment stays abreast of the epidemiological patterns of diseases in a bid to provide effective care for vulnerable populations. (Athan et al., 2013) emphasizes the importance of accurate and accessible diagnosis in the management of cryptococcosis morbidity in vulnerable patients (Figure 11.14).

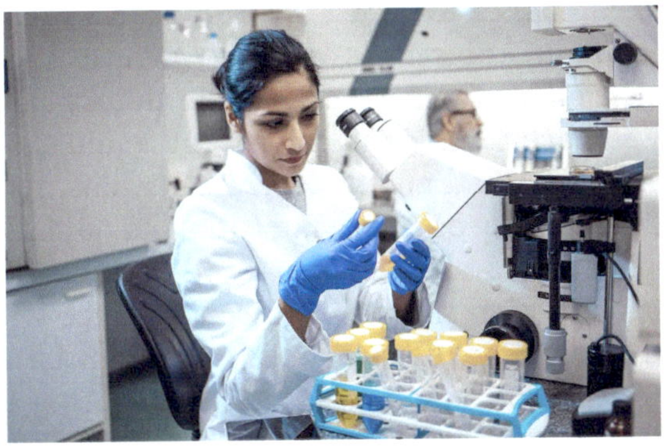

Figure 11.14. In resource-limited settings, where access to advanced laboratory facilities may be restricted, the diagnosis often hinges on reliance on clinical signs and basic laboratory tests.

Source: https://etimg.etb2bimg.com/thumb/msid-108867254,imgsize-61010,width-1200,height=765,overlay-ethealth/diagnostics/the-role-of-regulation-in-strengthening-indias-diagnostic-industry.jpg.

11.4.1. Laboratory Tests for Cryptococcosis

In diagnosing cryptococcosis, there are several laboratory procedures that are essential in confirming the presence of the etiologic agent *Cryptococcus neoformans*. Detection of cryptococcal antigen (CrAg) in serum and cerebrospinal fluid (CSF) is one of the most frequently employed procedures. The procedure employs the specific antibodies that develop against the polysaccharide capsule of *Cryptococcus*. The CrAg test is most useful due to its high sensitivity and specificity, making it useful for screening immunocompromised patients, such as HIV/AIDS. The issue of recent consensus definitions streamlines the categorizations of invasive fungal diseases (IFDs), including cryptococcosis, allowing clinicians to make use of these laboratory tests more accurately and with greater reliability, beyond the constraints faced by patients falling outside the traditionally defined high-risk groups, like the immunocompromised population (Akan et al., 2019). One of the major laboratory developments towards cryptococcosis is the use of the Lateral Flow Assay (CrAg® LFA), which offers rapid results in the detection of cryptococcal antigens. In recent evaluation, CrAg® LFA had an extremely high sensitivity and specificity of 100%, indicating its potential application as a diagnostic agent. Besides that, this assay also showed high concordance with the reference Cryptococcal Antigen Latex Agglutination System (CALAS®), ensuring its reliability in clinic practice. These advances contribute significantly in facilitating early diagnosis and treatment, which ultimately saves cryptococcosis morbidity and mortality, particularly among individuals at high risk. Implementation of these laboratory techniques into everyday practice would significantly enhance the ability of health care providers to treat invasive fungal infections efficiently (Chiller et al., 2017). Cultures and radiological tests, besides antigen detection, augment cryptococcosis laboratory diagnosis. Although culture remains the reference standard for laboratory diagnosis of fungal infections, it is cumbersome and requires specialized laboratory equipment. In addition, imaging studies such as CT and MRI scans are also beneficial in defining potential complications, particularly with CNS involvement. These imaging techniques have the ability to reveal characteristic findings of cryptococcal meningitis, which aid in the decision to treat. The application of an interdisciplinary process that includes antigen testing, culture, and imaging may greatly improve diagnostic accuracy and outcomes among patients. Facilitating early and effective cryptococcosis management involves regular research and development of laboratory diagnostics that not only work, but are available across a range of different healthcare settings (Akan et al., 2019) (Figure 11.15).

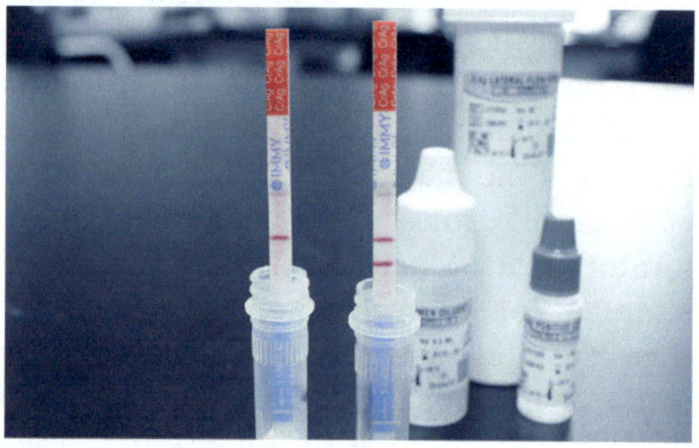

Figure 11.15. One of the most frequently employed methods is the detection of cryptococcal antigen (CrAg) in serum and cerebrospinal fluid (CSF).

Source: https://www.rapidmicrobiology.com/rmbdata/userfiles/suppliers/alpha_laboratories_ltd/2118_Alpha_Cryptococcal_Antigen.jpg.

11.4.2. Imaging Techniques used in Diagnosis

Cryptococcosis is a case of multi-modal diagnosis, with many imaging techniques employed in high percentages to establish spread and nature of the disease. Computed tomography and magnetic resonance imaging are both utilized to ascertain cerebral involvement, particularly when the infection has extended to the central nervous system. CT scans enable the immediate visualization of potential lesions and complications such as cryptococcal meningitis, where meningeal enhancement suggests inflammation or infection. Furthermore, MRIs demonstrate increased detail of the soft tissue structures, significant in making distinctions between cryptococcal lesions and other neurological diseases. Application of these imaging modalities not only helps in definitive diagnosis but also directs treatment and monitoring of therapy in patients, especially immunocompromised individuals with an increased risk for severe disease presentation, as in the case of new classification criteria for invasive fungal diseases (Akan et al., 2019). In pulmonary cryptococcosis, imaging techniques play a valuable role in revealing unique findings that can guide diagnosis. Chest radiography is usually the initial imaging technique that will be applied, to identify pulmonary nodules, consolidation, or cavities typically associated with cryptococcal disease. If the radiographs result in indeterminate results, more advanced imaging techniques like CT scans or even HRCT may define the intricacies of lung involvement. Imaging results can be seen with ground-glass opacities and thickening of interlobular septal septa, which are suggestive of the fungal aetiology of lung lesions. Examination of the same becomes increasingly significant in accordance with the epidemiology of cryptococcosis, particularly where it is seen in immunocompromised patients and differentiating it from malignancy or other infections is essential to treat them adequately (Barkham et al., 2014). Moreover, integration of imaging findings with laboratory diagnosis plays an important role in making a definitive diagnosis of cryptococcosis. Modern imaging techniques could serve as adjuncts to serological tests, such as cryptococcal antigen detection, which detects polysaccharide antigens in serum or cerebrospinal fluid. Interplay between laboratory and imaging results makes it easy for clinicians to classify the disease into probable or proven cases, an inevitable step in the implementation of timely and effective therapy (Akan et al., 2019). Despite altered definitions and strategies, the relevance of imaging has only increased, emphasizing the need for an interdisciplinary treatment of cryptococcosis. Modern practice places a strong premium on early imaging in both the diagnostic and prognostic context, and it draws attention to how these modalities can illuminate the way to better outcome in high-risk patient populations (Barkham et al., 2014) (Figure 11.16).

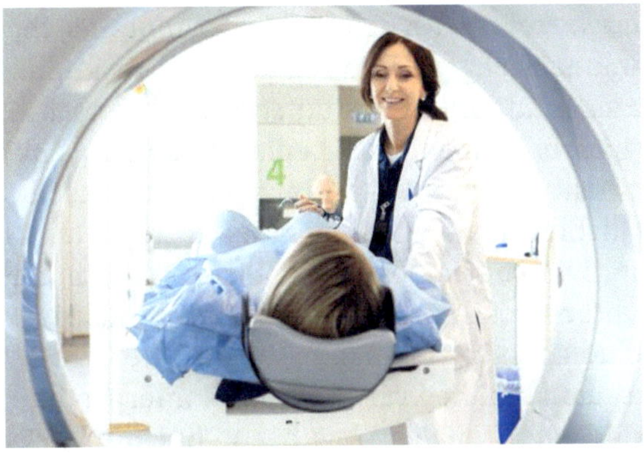

Figure 11.16. Computed tomography (CT) scans and magnetic resonance imaging (MRI) are pivotal in assessing cerebral involvement, particularly in cases where the infection radiates to the central nervous system.

Source: https://tischbraintumorcenter.duke.edu/sites/default/files/styles/3_2_small/public/2023-07/duke_blog_image_july_.jpg?itok=C2eUyJ87.

11.4.3. Differential Diagnosis Considerations

The differential diagnosis of cryptococcosis requires full appreciation of the clinical syndrome associated with the infection, particularly its potential overlap with other conditions. Cryptococcosis is found primarily in immunocompromised patients, particularly those with HIV/AIDS, and signs may be imitated by other central nervous system disorders. Such symptoms as headache, fever, and altered mental status may also be caused by other conditions, so clinicians have to conduct thorough examinations. Imaging studies such as computed tomography (CT) and magnetic resonance imaging (MRI) can facilitate the differentiation from other neurological conditions, thus emphasizing the need for precise diagnostic processes to establish an appropriate treatment regimen. Thus, the coincidence of clinical presentations requires careful attention and use of ancillary diagnostic techniques to minimize misdiagnosis and facilitate effective intervention. In a patient who presents with neurological symptoms, their immune background in relation to their immune status is important in a differential diagnosis. As cryptococcal meningoencephalitis carries a 20% mortality rate in HIV-positive patients, based on available data, early diagnosis is important in improving outcomes. The ability to differentiate cryptococcosis from other causal infectious agents, including bacterial meningitis or other fungi, is based on radiological and clinical interpretation. Radiological imaging has been shown to reveal large lesions associated with cryptococcal meningoencephalitis; thus, clinicians ought to interpret the presence of specific lesions and patterns against disease severity. By obtaining such information, healthcare providers can make an informed choice regarding the patient's underlying illness, which is important towards the ultimate diagnosis and directing proper treatment modalities. Differential diagnosis also encompasses the process of evaluating numerous non-infectious reasons that may present in a similar way as cryptococcosis and therefore complicate the diagnosis. One must include conditions such as tumors, multiple sclerosis, or even new head trauma that can be mimicking classic signs attributed to cryptococcal infections. Additionally, the presence of neurological deficits may require looking for autoimmune disorders or vascular disorders, which underscores the necessity of a widened differential diagnosis to include the entire gamut of potential underlying causes. Having vigil for all these different possibilities ensures treatment not only addresses cryptococcosis specifically but also cures any of the conditions associated with it which contribute to patient morbidity. It is here, as in the ongoing researches on imaging and diagnostic tools, that the convergence of thorough analyses, and the careful observation of the symptoms are essential to the achievement of accurate diagnostic outcomes in cases suspected of cryptococcosis (LeCouteur et al., 1999; Arayawichanont et al., 2008) (Figure 11.17).

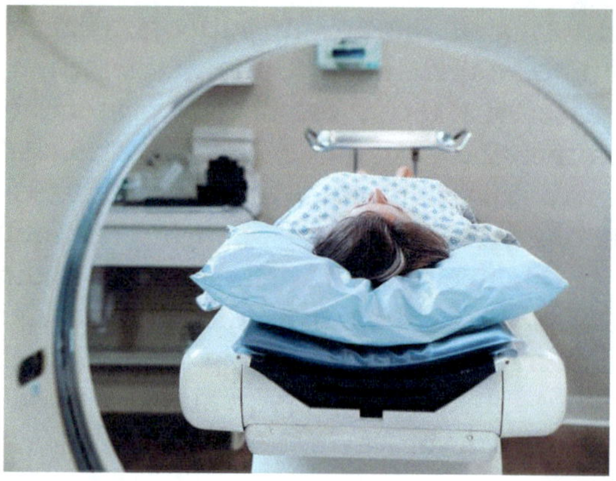

Figure 11.17. Neuroimaging studies, including computed tomography (CT) and magnetic resonance imaging (MRI), can assist in distinguishing cryptococcal infections from other neurological conditions, emphasizing the need for precise diagnostic approaches to develop an effective treatment plan.

Source: https://media.post.rvohealth.io/wp-content/uploads/2020/09/MRI_scan-732x549-thumbnail.jpg.

11.5. Treatment

Effective control of cryptococcosis, and more so cryptococcal meningitis, is critical in reducing morbidity and mortality rates of this lethal fungal infection. The course of treatment is typically split into three distinct phases: induction, consolidation, and maintenance. Induction therapy has predominantly used powerful antifungal agents such as amphotericin B and flucytosine, which are said to significantly reduce the amount of fungus in highly infected individuals. But in those low-resource settings with the greatest burden of disease, access to these essential drugs is typically hindered, resulting in unacceptably high mortality, and thus greater availability and delivery of effective therapy are essential to enhance patient outcomes generally, particularly in areas highly endemic with HIV, since co-infection with immunocompromised infections increases the severity of cryptococcosis (Parris et al., 2018).

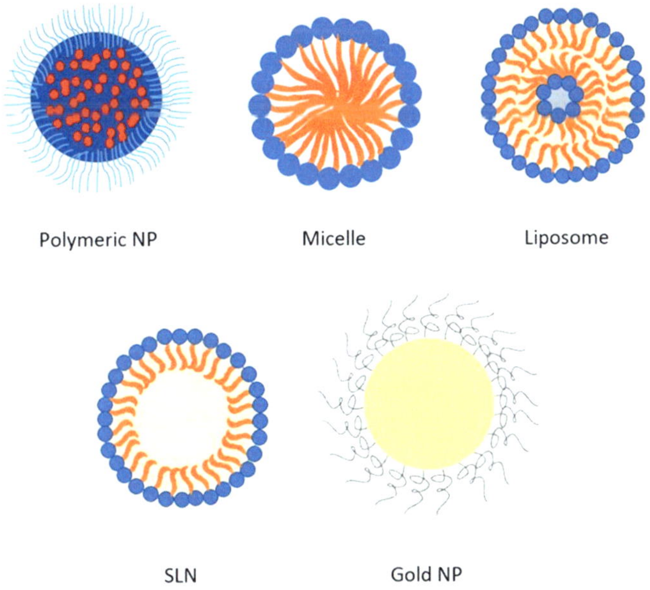

Figure 11.18. First-line therapies typically involve the administration of amphotericin B, a polyene antifungal known for its potent fungicidal properties.

Source: https://pub.mdpi-res.com/pharmaceutics/pharmaceutics-14-01823/article_deploy/html/images/pharmaceutics-14-01823-g001.png?1661850322.

HIV patients are most susceptible to cryptococcosis, particularly in regions such as Sub-Saharan Africa, where the burden of HIV globally is disproportionately concentrated. Under those circumstances, careful control of cryptococcal antigenemia in asymptomatic patients can prevent disease progression while ensuring a timely initiation of antiretroviral therapy. This dual approach not only cures the fungal infection but also boosts the patient's immune against HIV, thereby improving overall health status. The prevalence of the disease necessitates the application of cost-effective and user-friendly diagnostic tools which can be used at the point of care. These technologies are required to counter obstacles posed by the availability of healthcare as well as resource constraints prevalent in most affected locations (Adoga et al., 2014). In conclusion, optimum treatment of cryptococcosis is a multi-pronged approach that entails increased drug access, effective co-morbidity management of the like disease of HIV, and the integration of cutting-edge diagnostic technologies. There is a requirement to mould treatment regimens that not only focus on the immediate eradication of the fungus but also on maintaining patient health with extensive care modalities. While responding to cryptococcosis as an international health community, it is notable to address the associations between drug availability, the socioeconomic determinants of health, and the necessity for strong healthcare systems that can implement relevant interventions. Tackling these issues comprehensively will not only improve patient outcomes at the individual level but also help in serving the greater aim of managing cryptococcosis in high-burden areas (Parris et al., 2018; Adoga et al., 2014) (Figure 11.18).

11.5.1. Antifungal Medications Used

The treatment of cryptococcosis, and particularly cryptococcal meningitis, involves the administration of powerful antifungal medications to combat the opportunistic infection. Initial therapy tends to involve administration of amphotericin B, a polyene antifungal with high fungicidal activity. The medication disrupts the cell membrane integrity of the fungus, thereby killing the cells and consequently reducing the fungal load in patients. In all cases, flucytosine is also given concomitantly with amphotericin B to enhance efficacy during the induction phase. It is a synergistic treatment that is crucial as the combination therapy significantly lessens the mortality rate, especially in immunocompromised patients, including HIV/AIDS patients. However, these drugs' availability varies significantly in poor settings, setting barriers to effective treatment and higher mortality rates in victims of cryptococcosis (Parris et al., 2018). In addition to amphotericin B and flucytosine, consolidation therapy can include azole antifungals such as fluconazole, which is a less toxic, more manageable regimen for extending treatment. This phase is important in preventing relapse after induction therapy. Having effective drug levels in a patient's system, especially in higher-risk groups, means regular monitoring and dosing regimen changes, particularly in patients on antiretroviral drugs for HIV. Such dual management is particularly important in patients that are recovering from COVID-19, who are predisposed to secondary infection like cryptococcosis due to compromised states. The evidence that is arising indicates that patients with a history of previous infection of COVID-19 can develop an increased incidence of cryptococcal infection, and therefore aggressive antifungal prophylaxis and treatment should be implemented with interventions particularly tailored to the risk category of these patients (Agarwal et al., 2021).

Antifungal resistance calls for ongoing research and the formulation of new antifungal agents to broaden the existing treatment range of cryptococcal disease. This is especially so in areas of high endemicity, where the burden of fungal disease, including cryptococcosis, is still high. Inaccessibility to effective antifungal agents, compounded by drug availability and cost factors, contributes to the difficulty in managing cryptococcal infection in the majority of the world. Interventions aimed at improving access to appropriate treatment are essential in an effort to address the high morbidity and mortality rates associated with cryptococcosis, particularly among vulnerable populations. Joint action needs to be witnessed between health professionals and public health authorities in a bid to make sure that patients get appropriate and timely antifungal therapy (Parris et al., 2018).

11.5.2. Treatment Protocols for Different Stages

Management of cryptococcosis involves a multi-modal and stage-specific approach, particularly due to the infection's varied presentations, such as pulmonary and central nervous system. Initial therapy is generally directed towards antifungal treatment, commonly beginning with amphotericin B, which is highly active against *Cryptococcus neoformans*. Subsequent maintenance therapy is often carried out with fluconazole to prevent recurrence. The transition between the phases is significant, as the choice of antifungal treatment is usually both based on the patients clinical condition and the location of the infection. After response to treatment by laboratory observation like cerebrospinal fluid testing or imaging tests enables therapeutic protocol modifications so that patients receive optimal treatment from the treatment regimen (Beretta et al., 2020). As the infection becomes more severe, particularly with central nervous system complications, it is more complicated to treat. In neurological presentation, such as meningitis or cryptococcal granulomas, adjunctive corticosteroid therapy could be used to reduce inflammatory processes as well as mitigate symptoms of pressure effects due to lesions. However, the use of glucocorticoids must be done with care since immunosuppression may lead to unfavorable results under certain circumstances. Moreover, drug resistance is a major concern; therefore, the combination of treatment with flucytosine with triazole antifungals like itraconazole is advisable in advanced disease cases (Sivell et al., 2014). Regular monitoring and clinical assessment permit the timely adjustment of treatment regimens in accordance with clinical outcomes and potential drug interaction. For advanced stages of cryptococcosis, particularly among immunocompromised persons, treatment protocols may need a more aggressive approach.

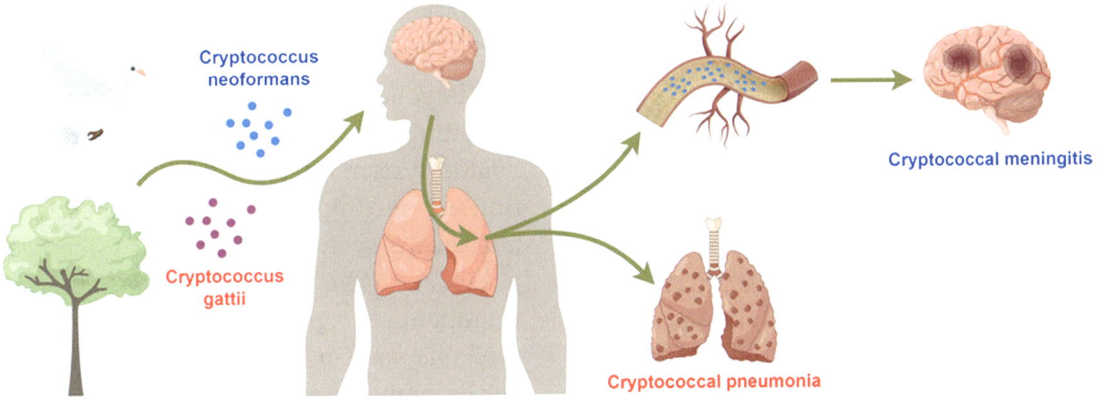

Figure 11.19. For patients presenting with neurological involvement, such as meningitis or cryptococcal granulomas, the adjunctive use of corticosteroids may be considered to help reduce inflammatory responses and alleviate symptoms associated with pressure from lesions.

Source: https://media.springernature.com/lw685/springer-static/image/art%3A10.1007%2Fs00415-024-12193-8/MediaObjects/415_2024_12193_Fig1_HTML.png.

This might include the establishment of combination antifungal therapy and hospitalization to facilitate intensified monitoring and treatment. Parenteral therapy, especially in extremely ill patients with widespread disease, can involve drugs such as voriconazole or micafungin. Maintenance monitoring of host parameters is also necessary; correction of the underlying immunosuppression, for instance, that is seen in HIV/AIDS patients, is crucial for optimal treatment outcome. Multidisciplinary collaboration between clinicians, infectious disease specialists, and microbiologists is required to further streamline these guidelines, underlining the importance of unbroken care pathways to combat the complexity of cryptococcosis (Beretta et al., 2020) (Figure 11.19).

11.5.3. Challenges in Treatment and Drug Resistance

Cryptococcosis is a significant treatment challenge, primarily due to the severity of the illness and the paucity of available therapeutic agents. Treatment with antifungal drugs and amphotericin B and flucytosine is the backbone of therapy for cryptococcal meningitis, although these drugs are not always successful and can cause significant side effects. In addition, use of these agents highlights the imperative problem of drug resistance, especially among patients with weakened immune systems, e.g., HIV-infected individuals. With increased rates of cryptococcal infection in areas with high HIV prevalence, e.g., Sub-Saharan Africa, the imperative need for efficient, affordable drugs is critical. The prevailing healthcare system is prone to running short of the critical medical supplies, and hence, these infections are difficult to manage, leading to higher patient mortality rates. Drug shortages or side effects that lead to breaks in treatment further make cryptococcosis management worse, such that effective care is difficult to obtain. Drug resistance to cryptococcosis itself occurs due to extensive use of the existing antifungal drugs such that, in the long run, the effectiveness of treatment is lost. Resistance mechanisms may include mutations of the fungal pathogen at the genetic level, which can alter its sensitivity to traditional antifungal agents. This is particularly worrisome in HIV/AIDS, as patients are likely to require long-term antifungal therapy due to recurrent infections. The present pharmacological landscape is devoid of new antifungal classes that can overcome resistant forms, and thereby an increasingly greater dependence on existing medications with performance limitations. Furthermore, patient adherence to treatment guidelines is also an issue that aggravates the condition, as inconsistent dosing could cause drug resistance. The dynamic therefore necessitates an interventionist treatment approach that involves not only improved drug formulation but also successful patient education and adherence measures (Adoga et al., 2014).

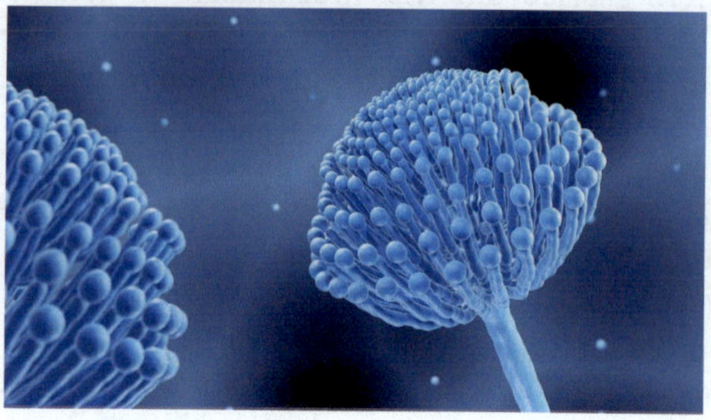

Figure 11.20. Drug resistance in cryptococcosis specifically emerges from the extensive use of available antifungal agents, leading to diminished treatment efficacy over time.

Source: https://asm.org/ASM/media/Article-Images/2022/November/Antifungal-resistance-feature-879x492.jpg?ext=.jpg.

Beyond this, countering the issue of drug resistance in cryptococcosis entails broader health system issues, specifically in resource-limited settings. In most of these regions, healthcare systems are placed under extreme pressures that hinder timely detection and treatment of cryptococcal infections. Insufficient available point-of-care diagnostics, as uncovered by the requirement for streamlined monitoring and testing, may weaken interventions, and the infection tends to develop and become resistant. In addition, the lack of trained healthcare personnel also tends to complicate control over cryptococcosis, with fewer opportunities for early detection and appropriate adjustment of treatment. This is particularly poignant in Sub-Saharan Africa, where well-equipped treatment centers are woefully underdeveloped (Adoga et al., 2014). It will take coordinated effort on the part of health systems to ensure that patients see integrative, timely, and effective treatment of cryptococcosis, not just the treatment itself but resolving the system issues themselves (Adoga et al., 2014) (Figure 11.20).

SUMMARY

Cryptococcosis is predominantly caused by the yeast *Cryptococcus neoformans*, its var. grubii being the most frequent etiologic agent of cryptococcal meningitis globally. The disease occurs most frequently in individuals with profoundly compromised immune systems, such as HIV/AIDS patients. Recent studies, however, have shown an increase in the detection of *C. neoformans* var. grubii infections in even immunocompetent individuals, for example, in Vietnam and China. This shift necessitates a greater understanding of the pathogenic potential of specific strains, such as the MLST ST5 lineage, that have been observed to exhibit more phenotypic heterogeneity and immune response tolerance in certain contexts. It is significant to examine the reason why such variation would expose otherwise healthy persons to CNS infections caused by cryptococcosis, a topic still under active research in mycology and infectious disease research (Lam et al., 2018). It is worth exploring the role of the immune system in cryptococcosis to comprehend its clinical relevance. The interleukin-12 (IL-12) cytokine family plays a fundamental role in mediating intracellular pathogen immunity with cellular immunity, such as the *Cryptococcus* genus. Of particular importance is IL-23, which has come to be regarded as an or cheating cytokine to orchestrate protective immunity to fungal infection with a chronic character. Studies describe the role of endogenous and exogenous IL-23 in survival rates and outcomes of infection in murine models. For instance, IL-23-deficient mice had reduced survival and impaired immune response when compared to their treated counterparts with recombinant IL-23. This indicated a subtle role for IL-23 in modulation of immunity in cryptococcosis, which had implications for therapeutic exploitation and vaccine therapy (Kleinschek et al., 2006). Lastly, strain pathogenicity as well as host immune response are key factors to take note of in cryptococcosis epidemiology and treatment. The unique genetic makeup of some *C. neoformans* isolates, such as ST5, might account for the inconsistent outcomes among infected patients and highlight the need for personalized therapeutic strategies. Meanwhile, the cytokine dynamics, particularly with regards to IL-12 and IL-23, illustrate the complexity of the immune process and suggest that therapeutic interventions augmenting these mechanisms might improve the outcome in the patients. With ongoing discoveries of the interaction between these factors, accrued knowledge will play a critical role in the development of more effective diagnostic, prevention, and treatment strategies against cryptococcosis. The shifting epidemiology of the disease necessitates ongoing vigilance and innovative efforts to counter the emerging and evolving threat (Lam et al., 2018; Kleinschek et al., 2006).

A CLOSER LOOK

CELLULAR IMMUNITY

Cellular immunity, or cell-mediated immunity, is a branch of the immune response that involves T cells in defending the body against intracellular pathogens like viruses, some bacteria, and cancer cells. Unlike humoral immunity based on antibodies, cellular immunity acts directly against infected or abnormal cells. Key players are cytotoxic T cells, which destroy infected cells, and helper T cells, which activate other immune cells. This immune response is important for killing pathogens that live within cells, where they are inaccessible to antibodies.

REFERENCES

1. Adoga, M. P., Agwale, S. M., & Aleku, G. A. (2014). HIV point of care diagnostics: Meeting the special needs of Sub-Saharan Africa. https://core.ac.uk/download/74132837.pdf (accessed on 27th June 2025).
2. Agarwal, R., Asija, R., Sharma, A., Tanwar, S., et al. (2021). Fungal infections associated with COVID-19. https://core.ac.uk/download/482241778.pdf (accessed on 27th June 2025).
3. Ahmed, S. A., Duncanson, F., Fahal, A. H., Hoog, G. S. de, et al. (2014). *Madurella mycetomatis* is highly susceptible to ravuconazole. https://core.ac.uk/download/43291204.pdf (accessed on 27th June 2025).
4. Akan, H., Alexander, B. D., Andes, D., Azoulay, E., et al. (2019). Revision and update of the consensus definitions of invasive fungal disease from the European Organization for Research and Treatment of Cancer and the Mycoses Study Group Education and Research Consortium. https://core.ac.uk/download/287649722.pdf (accessed on 27th June 2025).
5. Aksenov, S., Cherniak, R., Dykstra, C., Ellis, D., et al. (2017). Nutritional requirements and their importance for virulence of pathogenic *Cryptococcus* species. https://core.ac.uk/download/96767909.pdf (accessed on 27th June 2025).
6. Alanio, A., Alffenaar, J. W., Ayanlowo, O. O., Beardsley, J., et al. (2024). Global guideline for the diagnosis and management of cryptococcosis: An initiative of the ECMM and ISHAM in cooperation with the ASM. https://core.ac.uk/download/619688613.pdf (accessed on 27th June 2025).
7. Ali, N., Gilbert, R., & Pervaiz, M. (2018). The prevalence and under-reporting of needle-stick injuries among dental healthcare workers in Pakistan: A systematic review. https://core.ac.uk/download/159074647.pdf (accessed on 27th June 2025).
8. Alvarado-Ramírez, E., Mendoza, M. H. de, Segura-Roca, G., Torres-Rodríguez, J. M., et al. (2018). Cryptococcosis by *Cryptococcus gattii* in immunocompetent goats in Spain and review of the literature. https://core.ac.uk/download/303976616.pdf (accessed on 27th June 2025).
9. Amornkul, P. N., Antinori, A., Bennett, J. E., Bland, S., Bottone, E., Brouwer, A., et al. (2007). Determinants of disease presentation and outcome during cryptococcosis: The Crypto A/D study. https://core.ac.uk/download/pdf/7550813.pdf (accessed on 27th June 2025).
10. Amornkul, P. N., Antinori, A., Chariyalertsak, S., Chhin, S., Darras-Joly, C., Dromer, F., French, N., et al. (2010). Cryptococcal meningitis in HIV-infected patients: A longitudinal study in Cambodia. https://core.ac.uk/download/pdf/9417833.pdf (accessed on 27th June 2025).
11. Arastehfar, A., Boekhout, T., Buda De Cesare, G., Butler, G., et al. (2019). Recent trends in molecular diagnostics of yeast infections: From PCR to NGS. https://core.ac.uk/download/286086540.pdf (accessed on 27th June 2025).
12. Arayawichanont, A., Ruiz, A., Troncoso, A., Venkataramana, A., Zuger, A., Fontanet, A., Charlier, C., et al. (2008). Cryptococcal neuroradiological lesions correlate with severity during cryptococcal meningoencephalitis in HIV-positive patients in the HAART era. https://core.ac.uk/download/pdf/7973497.pdf (accessed on 27th June 2025).
13. Athan, E., Casas, E. C., Curtis, A. J., da Fonseca, M. S., et al. (2013). Impact of HIV-associated conditions on mortality in people commencing anti-retroviral therapy in resource-limited settings. https://core.ac.uk/download/pdf/18409718.pdf (accessed on 27th June 2025).

14. Bakker-Woudenberg, I. A. J. M., Bergers, E., van Etten, E. W. M., Hagen, F., et al. (1995). Liposomes as delivery systems in the prevention and treatment of infectious diseases. https://core.ac.uk/download/43317636.pdf (accessed on 27th June 2025).

15. Banerjee, C., Holt, P. A., & Narayanan, S. (2011). Cryptococcal immune reconstitution syndrome during steroid withdrawal treated with hydroxychloroquine. https://core.ac.uk/download/pdf/82157465.pdf (accessed on 27th June 2025).

16. Barkham, T., Chan, M., Chow, A., Lye, D., et al. (2014). Clinical and microbiological characteristics of cryptococcosis in Singapore: Predominance of *Cryptococcus neoformans* compared with *Cryptococcus gattii*. https://core.ac.uk/download/pdf/81965217.pdf (accessed on 27th June 2025).

17. Beretta, J. S., Ehlers, L. P., Rodrigues, R., Slaviero, R., et al. (2020). Cats with central nervous system cryptococcosis. https://core.ac.uk/download/388592681.pdf (accessed on 27th June 2025).

18. Bigna, J. J., Cohen, J. F., Dromer, F., Harrison, T. S., et al. (2018). Impact of routine cryptococcal antigen screening and targeted pre-emptive fluconazole therapy in antiretroviral-naive HIV-infected adults with less than 100 CD4 cells/μL: A systematic review and meta-analysis. https://core.ac.uk/download/161257182.pdf (accessed on 27th June 2025).

19. Bonifaz, A., Bruder-Nascimento, A., Lindenberg, A., Silva-Hernández, A. G., Tichellio, A. G., Roe, C. C., Hepp, C. M., Engelthaler, D. M., Overy, D. P., DeBess, E., et al. (2018). Dating the *Cryptococcus gattii* dispersal to the North American Pacific Northwest. https://core.ac.uk/download/323069956.pdf (accessed on 27th June 2025).

20. Buchanan, K. L., & Murphy, J. W. (1998). What makes *Cryptococcus neoformans* a pathogen? https://core.ac.uk/download/pdf/8248837.pdf (accessed on 27th June 2025).

21. Burnham, C. A., Dubberke, E., Franklin, A., Lainhart, W., et al. (2017). Pitfalls associated with the use of molecular diagnostic panels in the diagnosis of cryptococcal meningitis. https://core.ac.uk/download/212862559.pdf (accessed on 27th June 2025).

22. Carter, D. A., Dyer, P. S., Heitman, J., Soll, D. R., et al. (2014). Sexual reproduction of human fungal pathogens. https://core.ac.uk/download/42494447.pdf (accessed on 27th June 2025).

23. Casadevall, A. (1996). Antibody-based therapies for emerging infectious diseases. https://core.ac.uk/download/pdf/8248041.pdf (accessed on 27th June 2025).

24. Chiller, T., Cáceres, D. H., González, Á., Gómez, B. L., et al. (2017). Evaluation of a cryptococcal antigen lateral flow assay in serum and cerebrospinal fluid for rapid diagnosis of cryptococcosis in Colombia. https://core.ac.uk/download/268294974.pdf (accessed on 27th June 2025).

25. d'Arminio Monforte, A., Miranda, A., Curtis, A. J., Walker, A. S., Castelnuovo, B., Ledergerber, B., Marshall, C. S., et al. (2012). Incidence of WHO stage 3 and 4 conditions following initiation of anti-retroviral therapy in resource-limited settings. https://core.ac.uk/download/pdf/10674401.pdf (accessed on 27th June 2025).

26. De Beaudrap, P., Harrison, T. S., Kunda, J., Lortholary, O., et al. (2017). Long-term mortality and disability in cryptococcal meningitis: A systematic literature review. https://core.ac.uk/download/131246049.pdf (accessed on 27th June 2025).

27. Faria, D., Ferreira, R., Louro, R., Monteiro, M., et al. (2013). Fungal meningitis in an immunocompetent patient. https://core.ac.uk/download/70639903.pdf (accessed on 27th June 2025).

28. George, I. A., Olsen, M. A., Powderly, W. G., Santos, C. A. Q., et al. (2017). Epidemiology of cryptococcosis and cryptococcal meningitis in a large retrospective cohort of patients after solid organ transplantation. https://core.ac.uk/download/83101140.pdf (accessed on 27th June 2025).

29. King, J., Lehrnbecher, T., Pana, Z. D., Steinbach, W. J., et al. (2017). Recognition and clinical presentation of invasive fungal disease in neonates and children. https://core.ac.uk/download/131024549.pdf (accessed on 27th June 2025).

30. Kleinschek, M. (2006). Beyond Th1 and Th2: A non-classical immune pathway induced by interleukin (IL)-23 complements IL-12 in immunity to *Cryptococcus neoformans* infection. https://core.ac.uk/download/226096402.pdf (accessed on 27th June 2025).

31. Lam, T. T. (2018). Characterization of the virulence and determinants of virulence of *Cryptococcus neoformans* var. *grubii* genotypes from HIV infected and uninfected patients in Vietnam. https://core.ac.uk/download/159107971.pdf (accessed on 27th June 2025).

32. LeCouteur, R. A., & Vernau, K. M. (1999). Feline vestibular disorders. Part II: Diagnostic approach and differential diagnosis. https://core.ac.uk/download/323068734.pdf (accessed on 27th June 2025).

33. Levinsky, N. G., University Hospital, Evans Memorial Department of Clinical Research and Preventive Medicine. (1989). *Evans medicine*. https://core.ac.uk/download/142079169.pdf (accessed on 27th June 2025).

34. Mesa-Arango, A. C., Fusco-Almeida, A. M., de Oliveira, H. C., Werther, K., Scorzoni, L., Mendes-Giannini, M. J. S., Trevijano-Contador, N., et al. (2016). Impact of resistance to fluconazole on virulence and morphological aspects of *Cryptococcus neoformans* and *Cryptococcus gattii* isolates. https://core.ac.uk/download/pdf/82870130.pdf (accessed on 27th June 2025).

35. Parris, V., & Sloan, D. J. (2018). Cryptococcal meningitis: Epidemiology and therapeutic options. https://core.ac.uk/download/153533112.pdf (accessed on 27th June 2025).

36. Phan, H. T. (2019). Ecology of *Cryptococcus neoformans* in Vietnam. https://core.ac.uk/download/224959271.pdf (accessed on 27th June 2025).

37. Sivell, M. (2014). Cryptococcosis: A proteomic investigation of an emerging fungal disease. https://core.ac.uk/download/41237841.pdf (accessed on 27th June 2025).

38. Sykes, J. (2010). Immunodeficiencies caused by infectious diseases. https://core.ac.uk/download/323070119.pdf (accessed on 27th June 2025).

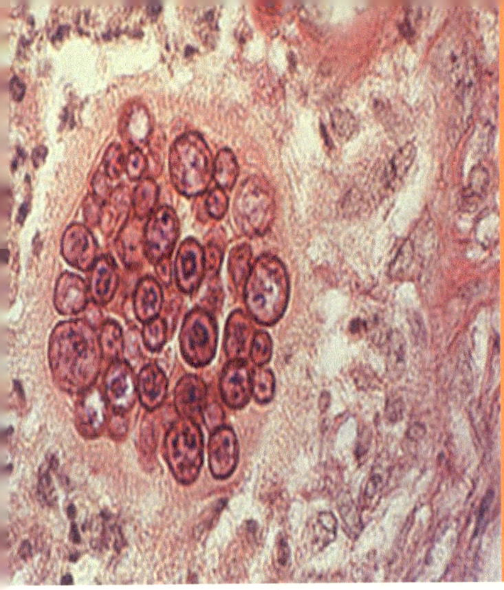

Chapter 12
COCCIDIOIDOMYCOSIS

Contents

Introduction

Coccidioidomycosis, or Valley fever, is a fungal infection caused by inhalation of spores of the fungi *Coccidioides immitis* and *Coccidioides posadasii*, among others in this group. The disease is specifically endemic to the United States Southwest, Mexico, and parts of Central and South America. The clinical significance of coccidioidomycosis is both in its ability to cause severe respiratory disease and in its broader public health impact. While more movement of populations has been taking place as a result of globalization, the epidemiological pattern of fungal infections like coccidioidomycosis is also evolving. The evolution highlights the importance of enhanced awareness and understanding among physicians, particularly in regions where such infections are gaining prevalence, and highlights the necessity for ongoing research in their pathogenesis and management (Ampel et al., 2012). A proper understanding of coccidioidomycosis entails a study of its historical and geographical context. The advent of modern times and associated movements toward urbanization and population migration have further spread the endemic disease. While people move into previously unexposed areas, they are often immunologically naive and thus extremely vulnerable to the pathogen. In addition, socioeconomic factors like agricultural activities and environmental changes are facilitators of *Coccidioides* spore spread. These dynamic relationships underscore the importance of epidemiological studies that assess the impact of changing environmental parameters and human behavior on infection transmission and incidence, including coccidioidomycosis (Homei et al., 2020). As the medical community wrestles with controlling the menace of coccidioidomycosis, research into diagnostic and therapeutic management becomes essential. There is new technology, such as the design of systems that identify antigens and better antifungal medications, enhancing clinical outcomes in fungal pneumonias. All this is a consequence of increased knowledge regarding the genomics and cellular morphology of fungi, facilitating easy and correct diagnosis. Accordingly, medical practitioners are able to employ timely intervention, lowering morbidity and mortality from coccidioidomycosis. Additionally, an awareness of the development of antibiotic resistance and its impact on treatment effectiveness is imperative in the fight against fungal infections. Thus, an integrated approach involving research, clinical practice, and public health interventions continues to be vital to control and prevent the effects of coccidioidomycosis effectively (Ampel et al., 2012) (Figure 12.1).

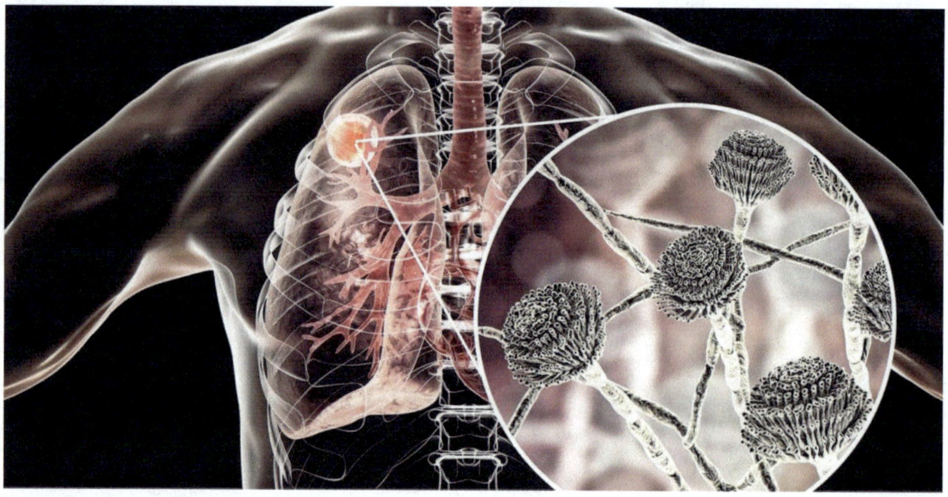

Figure 12.1. Coccidioidomycosis.

Source: https://respiratory-therapy.com/wp-content/uploads/2020/01/3d-lung-fungal-infection-2k-1280x640.jpg.

12.1. Causative Agent

The causative organism of coccidioidomycosis is a soil-inhabiting fungus known as *Coccidioides* species, primarily composed of *Coccidioides immitis* and *Coccidioides posadasii*. These fungi are present in arid environments prevalent in the northwestern region of the Southwestern United States, Mexico, and certain areas of Central and South America. *Coccidioides*' life cycle involves developing arthroconidia, which are infective spores released by the mycelium when the soil is disturbed. On inhalation, such spores can germinate in the respiratory tract and cause pulmonary infection. As spores disseminate within the earth, they present a vital site of overlap among environmental parameters and public health, placing special emphasis on sustained research in soil microbiomes and their implications for human susceptibility to disease, particularly with regards to at-risk populations that might be exposed to aerosolized pathogens emanating from dust storms or worksites (Lee et al., 2011). The role of *Coccidioides* spp. extends beyond mere infection; it is a serious threat to health, particularly in immunocompromised patients. *Coccidioides* is an opportunistic pathogen, and it may exploit abnormalities in defense mechanisms of the host to produce disseminated infection. Certain characteristics of *Coccidioides*, such as its capacity to modulate the immune response and to become accustomed to the host environment, are accountable for the virulence of coccidioidomycosis. Of particular concern is that the clinical presentation of infection will imitate other respiratory diseases, posing difficulties in making a timely diagnosis and treatment. Furthermore, as seen in veterinary research, for example, in research on feline populations within endemic areas, the infection is not solely human-specific, and this speaks to its ubiquitous nature, prompting further investigation into the ecological and epidemiological patterns of *Coccidioides* (Arbona et al., 2020).

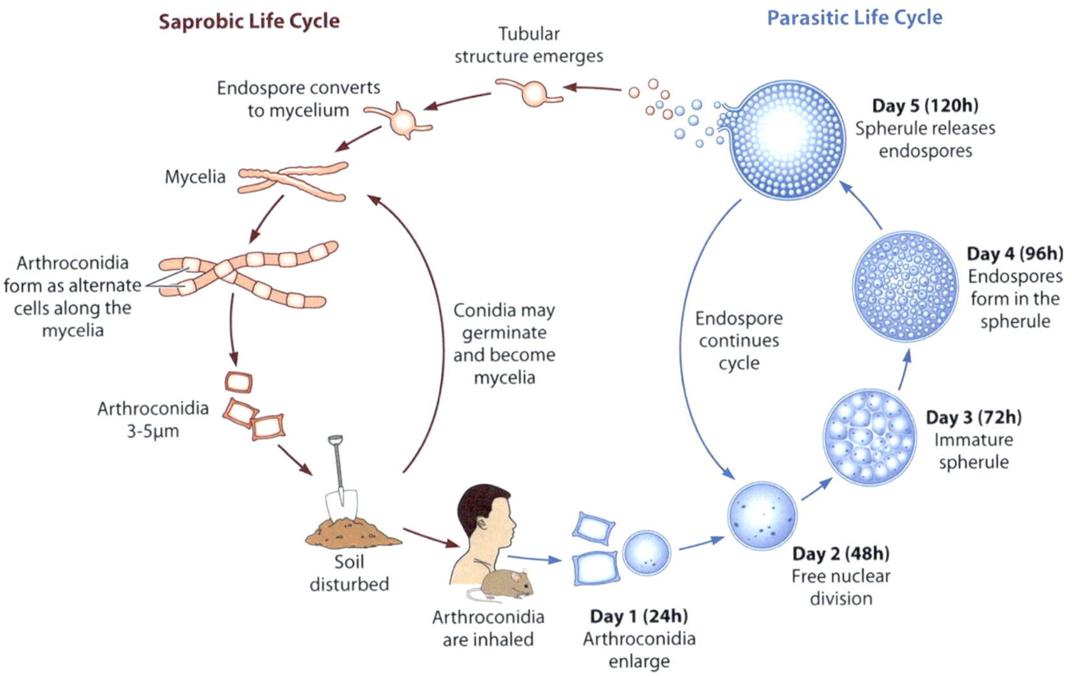

Figure 12.2. The life cycle of *Coccidioides* involves the production of airborne arthroconidia, which are infectious spores released from the mycelium following disturbance of the soil.

Source: https://journals.asm.org/cms/10.1128/cmr.00112-19/asset/fc73603b-0016-4b6c-9359-a670a7ae3aad/assets/graphic/cmr.00112-19-f0001.jpeg.

The ecologic occurrence of *Coccidioides* species is also responsible for raising pertinent issues regarding land use and environmental interactions that influence disease patterns. For instance, soil disruption through agricultural activities or urban expansion might increase the likelihood of spore aerosolization. Therefore, it is crucial to understand the ecologic factors favoring transmission of this fungal pathogen to implement effective public health interventions. With additional evidence of increasing cases of coccidioidomycosis, particularly in areas where climate change impacts are being experienced, public health authorities must develop a strong surveillance system. Such systems must encompass the animal and human domain by monitoring the environment's prevalence of *Coccidioides* spp. in order to provide proactive intervention to reduce exposure risk and improve health outcomes (Lee et al., 2011) (Figure 12.2).

12.1.1. Description of Coccidioides Fungi

The genus *Coccidioides* comprises two principal species, *C. immitis* and *C. posadasii*, both of which produce coccidioidomycosis, also known as valley fever. The fungi have become proficient in inhabiting dry and semi-dry regions, and even more so in the southwestern United States, i.e., California and Arizona, and extend their habitat into Central and South American regions. *Coccidioides* fungi differ from other fungi in that they may be saprophytes in the ground, which form airborne arthroconidia, the infective form which may become aerosolized and inhaled by animal and human hosts. This ecological niche in arid habitats provides the foundation for their virulence, as environmental factors like temperature and humidity play vital roles in fungal growth and sporulation. Understanding ecological resistances and life cycles of *Coccidioides* fungi is essential in assessing the public health relevance of coccidioidomycosis, especially with respect to climatic modification that affects their spread in non-endemic areas (Arathoon et al., 2016). Molecular biology has also revealed the evolutionary history and population structure of *Coccidioides* species and how the two exhibit comprehensive genetic divergence from one another. Phylogenetic studies reveal that *C. posadasii* is the older species, which has a speculated origin in the southern Arizona-northern Mexico area. Genetic diversity within *C. posadasii* indicates strong mechanisms of adaptation, allowing the species to inhabit varied ecological niches outside its classical ranges. Notably, new evidence suggests that the geographic distribution of coccidioidomycosis is not fixed; it has extended to non-endemic regions, which is a matter of concern in terms of the likelihood of increased infection incidence. The existence of distinct geographic clades in *C. posadasii* also indicates the complex interplay between environmental forces and evolutionary processes of these fungi, and further research should be done to comprehend their population dynamics and processes of dispersal (Arathoon et al., 2016).

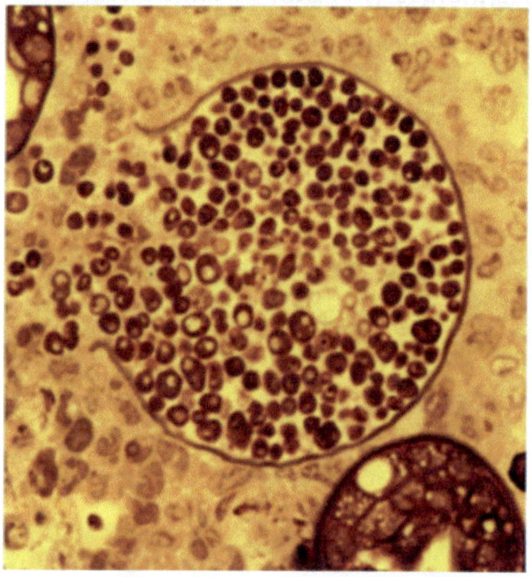

Figure 12.3. The genus *Coccidioides* comprises two primary species, *C. immitis* and *C. posadasii,* both of which are responsible for coccidioidomycosis, commonly known as valley fever.

Source: https://ars.els-cdn.com/content/image/3-s2.0-B9780128012383023990-f02399-03-9780128117361.jpg.

Beyond their ecological and epidemiological significance, *Coccidioides* fungi have been found to infect a variety of mammals, reptiles, and birds and, by this inference, have suggested a broader ecological complex involved in their life cycle. Existing literature indicates that the fungus possesses reservoir animals of various species, which facilitate its transmission and which further highlight the significance of learning about its habitat and ecology as a whole. The taxonomy of *Coccidioides* spp. since halotolerant organisms signifies their adaptability in various saline environments; however, their dependency on animal reservoirs underlines a critical aspect of their life cycle. The association also highlights wildlife's interdependence with environmental conditions and human health in coccidioidomycosis. As this disease continues to manifest and expand geographically, there is a need to dismantle the complexities of these hosts' involvement in promoting the survival and spread of *Coccidioides* fungi (Figure 12.3).

12.1.2. Life Cycle and Environmental Conditions

The causative fungi of Coccidioidomycosis, *Coccidioides* species, possess a life cycle directly associated with specific environmental conditions that are favorable for their growth and replication. The fungi thrive and develop in semi-arid and dry locations, such as the Southwestern United States, where they largely reside in the soil. Under favorable environmental conditions—i.e., hot and dry climates—*Coccidioides* exhibits a life cycle of asexual reproduction, producing arthroconidia, which are hardened and resistant to poor environmental conditions in the ground. Upon disturbance, the spores release into the environment and can be inhaled by man where there is high dust exposure, hence environmental factors are of essential concern in public health for Coccidioidomycosis.

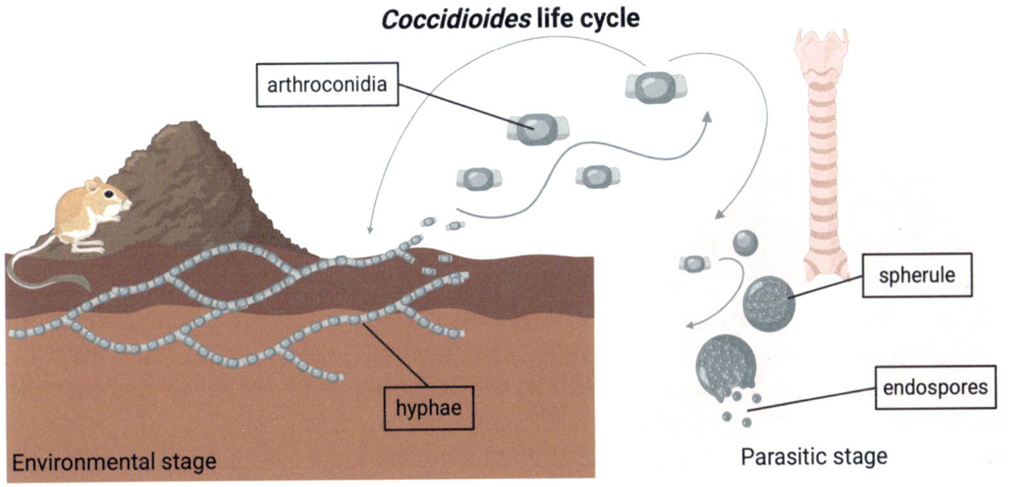

Figure 12.4. The ambient environmental conditions greatly influence the viability and distribution of *Coccidioides*, as these fungi are particularly affected by soil composition, humidity, and seasonal weather patterns.

Source: https://www.mdpi.com/jof/jof-11-00309/article_deploy/html/images/jof-11-00309-g001.png.

The environmental conditions in the surrounding area play a huge role in the habitat and viability of *Coccidioides* because these fungi are sensitive to soil chemistry, water content, and the time of the year. Soil health, including its microbial diversity and organic matter, also plays a role in the life cycle of the fungi, which can be explained in the context of soil biodiversity. In this case, the soils are not just homes for *Coccidioides* but also reservoirs of pathogenic and non-pathogenic microorganisms. Despite the fact that most soil-borne microbes are innocuous and contribute to ecosystem services, the presence of *Coccidioides* adds a pathogenic spin, illustrating the dynamic interrelationship between environmental factors and public health problems associated with soil-borne disease (Lee et al., 2011). Besides that, the significance of dust in the air in the spread of *Coccidioides* cannot be overstated. Particles of soil can float for miles on dust storms, enhancing the risk of exposure to human beings by such spores of disease. The connection between dust and lung health is significant in that breathing dusty air will enhance the number of incidences of Coccidioidomycosis, particularly in vulnerable people. Coordinated regional efforts in monitoring and regulating dust exposure will be necessary to limit the spread of this fungal disease. In addition, applying soil conservation and land management practices that minimize dust generation will be necessary in keeping cases of the disease low and protecting public health security, demonstrating how environmental stewardship directly translates to mitigating the risk of Coccidioidomycosis (Baklanov et al., 2021) (Figure 12.4).

12.1.3. Geographic Distribution of the Fungi

The geographic distribution of the fungi *Coccidioides immitis* and *C. posadasii*, causative agents of coccidioidomycosis, is an expression of the evolutionary adaptation and ecological plasticity of these etiologic agents. Endemic predominantly to dry regions of the Southwestern United States, namely Arizona and California, these fungi have adapted to the dry, sandy soils of these regions. The spores are aerosolizable and therefore a public health concern in areas of endemic involvement. Recent epidemiologic studies have illuminated the alarming trend of expanding geographic range. New groups of coccidioidomycosis have been reported beyond traditional boundaries, including within Washington state, raising questions about environmental processes and human activity potentially driving this dissemination. This shifting distribution needs to be understood to plan public health and effective response strategies, as the incidence of this fungal infection plays an effective role in influencing local communities (Arathoon et al., 2016). Population genetic work has been instrumental in defining the geographic extent of *Coccidioides* species. Genome analysis-based research indicates strong population structure in *C. posadasii*, with distinct geographic clades focused primarily in central and southern Arizona, and Texas, Mexico, and Central and South American populations. Such findings accentuate the complexity of fungal dissemination patterns and suggest an ancestral origin in southern Arizona and northern Mexico. The heterogeneity of climate conditions and soil quality between these locations might be accountable for the diverse ecological niches occupied by these fungi. This not only influences local epidemiology but, due to this geographic heterogeneity, transmission of disease and pathogenesis in human populations exposed to such a fungus becomes even more challenging (Arathoon et al., 2016). Furthermore, the clinical significance of the geographic distribution of the *Coccidioides* species extends into clinical practice, particularly among high-risk populations such as recipients of solid organ and hematopoietic cell transplants. According to findings of a multicenter surveillance study, coccidioidomycosis infections among these groups, while uncommon, are dire in outcome, including death. The study quoted a cumulative incidence of coccidioidomycosis of 12 months in transplant recipients, validating the use of geographic epidemiology in pre-transplant evaluation and post-operative care protocols. With endemically occurring mycoses like coccidioidomycosis continuing to emerge and spread, practitioners should be aware of the nuanced geographic determinants influencing availability and access to prevention and treatment. Appreciation thereof may go to serve to significantly improve clinical outcomes in at-risk populations (Figure 12.5).

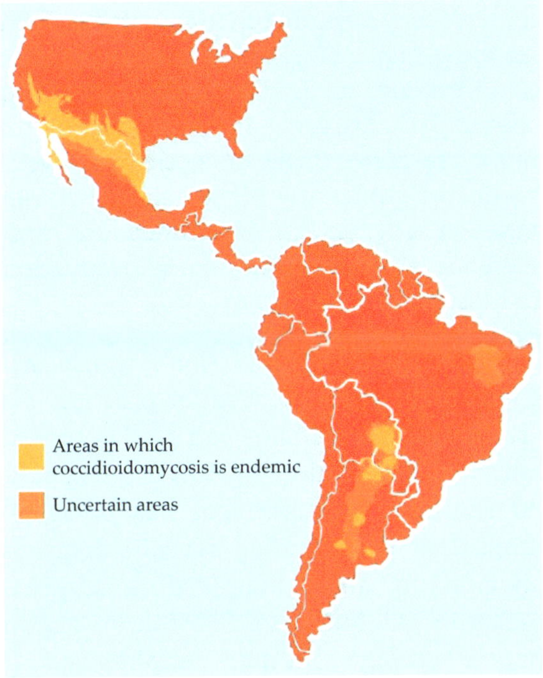

Figure 12.5. Primarily endemic to arid regions of the Southwestern United States, particularly Arizona and California, these fungi thrive in dry, sandy soils.

Source: https://www.researchgate.net/publication/8036876/figure/fig1/AS:281212523434005@1444057698422/Geographic-Distribution-of-Coccidioidomycosis.png.

12.2. Transmission and Infection

The dissemination of coccidioidomycosis, which is due to the presence of fungi *Coccidioides immitis* and *C. posadasii*, is primarily through the inhalation of arthroconidia, environmental infectious spores. The spores are commonly present in the soil within the arid and semi-arid regions of North America where the fungi are present. These spores, when disrupted from the soil, such as by construction, farming, or natural occurrences such as windstorms, release them into the air and make them breathable for humans and animals. Once inhaled, the spores can change to spherules in the body of the host, resulting in infection. The reliance of such fungi on environmental conditions emphasizes the way in which human activities will unwittingly increase the risk for transmission, particularly in endemic areas (Mehrkens et al., 2016). In addition to human infection, coccidioidomycosis is also a risk for other mammals and animals, including pets in domestic settings. Research indicates that dogs can develop serious health complications due to this fungal disease, including protein-losing nephropathy with immune complex glomerulonephritis (ICGN). In infected dog studies, high rates possessed renal histopathological changes, demonstrating that *Coccidioides* spp. are capable of having significant impacts not only on one's respiratory tract but also their kidneys (Mehrkens et al., 2016). This cross-species transmission teaches us something regarding the ecological subtlety of coccidioidomycosis that provokes questions regarding the role of various animals in adding to the life cycle of the fungus and if they are reservoirs or disseminators in their respective environments (Mart et al., 2016). Understanding the transmission dynamics of coccidioidomycosis is both essential in public health as well as veterinary medicine. The etiology of this disease has been linked to changed environmental settings, which allows an increased occurrence of infection in humans and animals. Secondly, understanding the natural reservoirs and potential disseminators of *Coccidioides* spp. is increasingly important in disease control interventions. Additional research is required to explore the environmental interfaces that facilitate the spread of these fungi, particularly as a result of climate change and loss of habitat potentially changing the range of infected animal populations (Mehrkens et al., 2016; Mart et al., 2016). Combined, these points emphasize the complex interrelationship between environment, reservoir animals, and human health in the case of coccidioidomycosis and demand a multidisciplinary approach to mitigation and management (Figure 12.6).

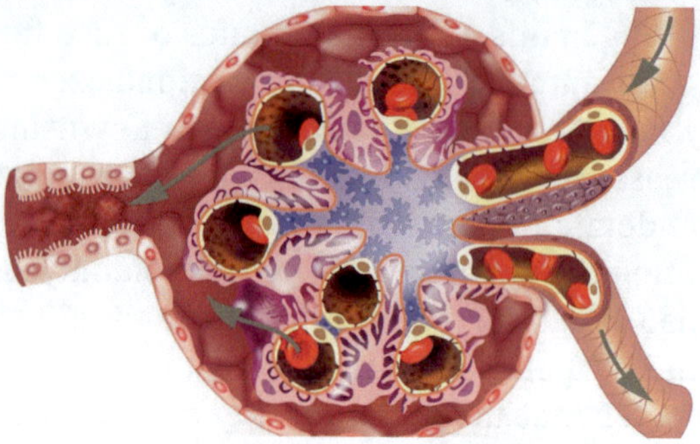

Figure 12.6. Immune complex glomerulonephritis (ICGN).

Source: https://cdn.royalcanin-weshare-online.io/ZufminYBaPOZra8qy5zA/v1/vf-feline-renal-proteinuria-430-800.

12.2.1. Modes of Transmission to Humans

Understanding the modes of transmission of coccidioidomycosis is essential to both public health action and individual attitude. Valley fever or coccidioidomycosis is most frequently caused by the inhalation of spores of the fungus *Coccidioides* in the air, which, in turn, occurs in arid and semi-arid zones, most prominently in the southwestern United States and some parts of Central and South America. The spores may be suspended in the air through dust storms or soil disturbances, where the fungus naturally occurs. Upon inhalation, spores can lead to respiratory infections, demonstrating how environmental factors have a determining influence on the transmission patterns of this fungal infection. This aerial transmission highlights the importance of learning not only about the pathogen itself but also about the environmental and meteorological conditions facilitating its spread because they directly influence the risk of infection in susceptible populations. Occupational exposure is a central factor in the transmission of coccidioidomycosis, particularly for workers in agriculture, building, or other occupational activities outdoors away from the ground. Workers in such occupations are more likely to inhale the disease-causing spores, especially during dry weather when dust is more prevalent. Cases of coccidioidomycosis have been significantly higher among workers engaged in activities that have contributed to soil disturbances, thus making some occupational activities major risk factors.

This occupational dimension of transmission suggests that targeted prevention practices, such as respiratory protection and risk occupation public health education, can lower the infection risk. Therefore, occupational risk prevention is important to stemming coccidioidomycosis transmission and safeguarding high-risk population public health. The role of regional climatic change further emphasizes the evolving patterns of coccidioidomycosis transmission to humans. With climate change modifying precipitation regimes and elevating temperatures, the spatial range of *Coccidioides* spores could extend, thus exposing additional populations to infection. Such dynamic change necessitates elaborate surveillance systems to track environmental factors favorable to spore dispersal. Researchers have established prioritization strategies that assess many factors, including environmental ones, to identify most vulnerable pathogens due to climate change, coccidioidomycosis being a notable example (Cox et al., 2013). Such observations highlight the importance of incorporating climatic information in public health strategies to mitigate the effects of coccidioidomycosis. As the climate shifts, adaptive measures must be planned to counteract this change, thus marking the connectivity of infection prevention and environmental health (Figure 12.7).

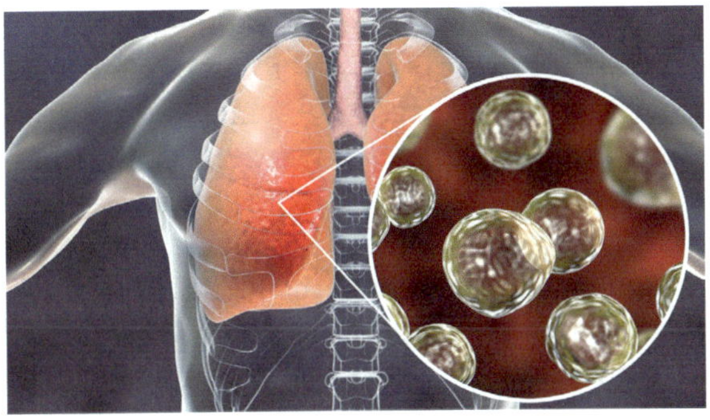

Figure 12.7. Occupational exposure contributes significantly to the transmission of coccidioidomycosis, particularly among individuals working in agriculture, construction, or other outdoor jobs that disturb the soil.

Source: https://i0.wp.com/www.sciencenews.org/wp-content/uploads/2023/01/010923_TI_fungal_QA_feat.jpg.

12.2.2. Risk Factors for Infection

Coccidioidomycosis, or Valley fever, is a type of fungus infection by the *Coccidioides* fungi that occur in some geographic locations, primarily the southwestern part of the United States. Understanding the risk factors for infection is necessary for prevention and treatment. Individuals living or working in endemic areas, particularly those with outdoor jobs like construction, farming, and landscaping, are at greater risk of exposure to the fungal spores. Environmental situations, including dust storms and drought, add to the risk of exposure to the spores. Historical and geographic information of *Coccidioides* ecology, therefore, is not just informative for public health policy but also dictates individual protective measures among workers in high-risk occupations (Dzialowski et al., 2021). Demographics also appear as a key factor in susceptibility to coccidioidomycosis. Evidence indicates that certain populations, particularly those with compromised immune systems, such as HIV/AIDS patients, diabetics, or undergoing immunosuppressive therapy, are at a greater risk of developing severe forms of the disease. Hispanics, African Americans, or Filipinos also seem to have higher dissemination rates of coccidioidomycosis, which can lead to lethal outcomes (Bays et al., 2018). This increased risk underscores the necessity of heightened caution and close surveillance in these specific groups to allow earlier diagnosis and treatment, potentially averting adverse outcomes. Socioeconomic determinants could also affect infection rates and access to medical care among those with coccidioidomycosis. Groups with limited healthcare resources may face challenges in accessing adequate diagnostics and treatment, which can perpetuate increased disease burden among such groups. Moreover, socioeconomic status can be lower as a correlate with increased endemic area exposure and limited access to preventive interventions, such as adequate respiratory protection in work-related activities. Consequently, public health programs must mitigate these inequalities so that risk factor education and available health resources are extended to these vulnerable populations (Dzialowski et al., 2021). Focusing interventions on the right targets will result in decreased incidence and severity of coccidioidomycosis, ultimately enhancing health results in infected populations (Figure 12.8).

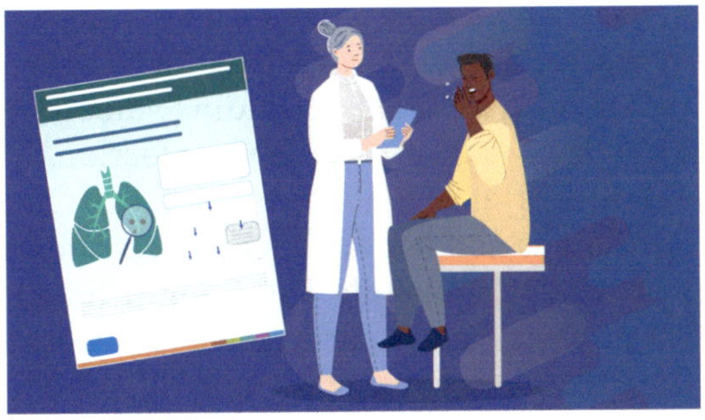

Figure 12.8. Socioeconomic factors can further influence infection rates and access to medical care for individuals affected by coccidioidomycosis.

Source: https://www.cdc.gov/valley-fever/media/images/2025/04/24_350798-A_Lutfy_Fungal_Disease_Awareness_Week_2024_notext_16x9_Fungal_Pneumonias_GP.png.

12.2.3. Incubation Period and Initial Symptoms

Incubation period of coccidioidomycosis, or the disease that is brought about by the pathogen *Coccidioides immitis*, is a critical time that impacts diagnosis and treatment. This is generally one to three weeks after exposure to the spores but can be prolonged in some. The diversity makes it challenging for physicians as signs and symptoms are non-specific and can be similar to other more common respiratory conditions. Consequently, diagnosis of coccidioidomycosis early is often complicated and can lead to misdiagnosis. Moreover, there are subclinical infections, and the patient remains asymptomatic, which emphasizes the need for greater awareness in areas where the disease is endemic and the likelihood of exposure is higher, most prominently for patients who work in outdoor or construction-related occupations. The early presentation of coccidioidomycosis may be a carbon copy of a typical viral respiratory infection, and therefore it is extremely important to remember the specific context of potential exposure. Patients may present with fever, cough, and fatigue, and headache and myalgia, all of which together may lead to uncertainty of the etiology. In other cases, patients may have more severe respiratory symptoms, including chest pain and dyspnea, with progressing infection. The presence of erythema nodosum, which is tender erythematous nodules on the lower extremities, can be a distinguishing symptom, though it is not present in all patients. It is necessary for healthcare providers to understand these heterogeneous presenting symptoms since early intervention and diagnosis are crucial factors in how patient outcomes and complications can be reduced. Also, symptom development during the incubation period can assist clinicians in assessing severity of coccidioidomycosis. Studies indicate that serologic responses assist clinicians in understanding the course of infection because titers may mirror the bodys response to defense. For example, maximum complement fixation titers are seen at 31 days following onset of initial serologic reactivity, which is a critical time for intervention. The patient classes have had varying median maximum titers, and those that have established pulmonary and disseminated infection patterns have had more severe serologic responses. The data indicates the significance of observing patients closely in the early stages with signs pointing toward coccidioidomycosis, given timely diagnosis is an important factor in assisting in the prevention of any complications associated with the disease (Belay et al., 2018; Lamerato et al., 2018) (Figure 12.9).

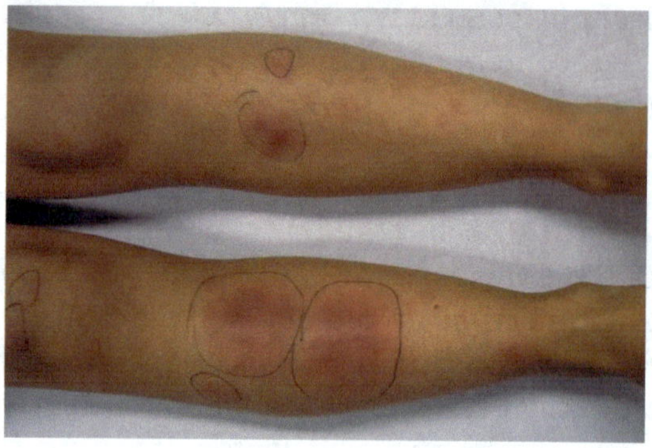

Figure 12.9. The presence of erythema nodosum, characterized by painful red nodules on the lower extremities, can serve as a distinguishing symptom, though it is not experienced by all patients.

Source: https://img.lb.wbmdstatic.com/vim/live/webmd/consumer_assets/site_images/article_thumbnails/BigBead/erythema_nodosum_bigbead/1800x1200_erythema_nodosum_bigbead.jpg?resize=750px:*&output-quality=75.

12.3. Clinical Manifestations

The clinical manifestations of coccidioidomycosis are highly diverse, and they form a spectrum of illness from asymptomatic infection to severe, disseminated disease. Patients typically acquire flu-like illness, which is manifested as cough, fever, malaise, and chest pain, that may mimic other respiratory infections. Notably, about 60% of patients with coccidioidomycosis acquire self-limited pulmonary disease, or pulmonary uncomplicated coccidioidomycosis (PUC). Despite the benign symptomatology, serologic typing of patients with these symptoms indicates disparate immune responses, with maximum titers of complement fixation differing considerably across disease groups, defining the place of clinical evaluation in defining therapy (Bays et al., 2018). Interestingly, almost 25.4% of PUC patients may have undetectable titers, hence making it harder in terms of diagnosis, with close monitoring of serologic markers on the course of the disease (Bays et al., 2018). Also, chronic pulmonary manifestations can be seen in about 10% of the infected, which is defined as pulmonary chronic coccidioidomycosis (PCC). The chronic manifestation typically presents with long-standing conditions such as persistent cough, weight loss, and hemoptysis, so it is likely to be confused with other pulmonary conditions. Clinical studies indicate that PCC patients typically have elevated fixed complement titers (1:24) of uncomplicated disease, reflecting increased systemic action of the disease. In addition, the serological recovery is delayed in such patients because median titers are rising at a rate of 112 days per dilution. Such prolonged durations of symptoms necessitate individualized therapeutic interventions and underscore the need for ongoing clinical monitoring and titration of antifungal therapy to maximize outcomes in the infected (Bays et al., 2018). Acute presentations of coccidioidomycosis result from the spread of infection by the lung system into other organs such as bones, skin, and less commonly, the central nervous system, resulting in coccidioidal meningitis (CM). Such individuals typically present with a more complex clinical picture with neurological symptoms, cutaneous lesions, and musculoskeletal complaints. The diagnostic challenges of disseminated coccidioidomycosis (DC) are rooted in the variety of presentations and the significant fluctuation of serologic titers, which have a median peak of 1:128 for DC cases. Moreover, serologic recurrences in this group are exceedingly high with about 50% of patients experiencing fluctuation in their complement fixation titers after initial treatment. This is complicated by a multi-dimensional diagnosis and management assessment, for example, the application of serologic testing to quantify disease severity and predict complications (Figure 12.10).

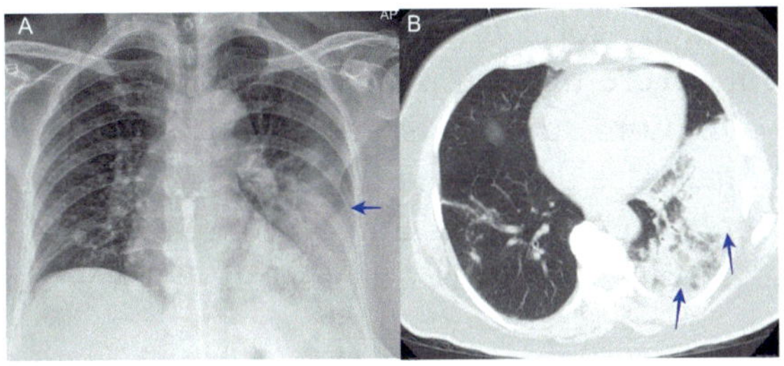

Figure 12.10. Pulmonary uncomplicated coccidioidomycosis (PUC).

Source: https://www.mdpi.com/jof/jof-10-00724/article_deploy/html/images/jof-10-00724-g005.png.

12.3.1. Common Symptoms of Coccidioidomycosis

Coccidioidomycosis or valley fever is primarily characterized by an array of respiratory presentations that are similar to those found in other respiratory infections. Acute presentation is usually characterized by cough, fever, chest pain, and weakness, simulating a flu-like illness. There may be asymptomatic or mild clinical findings in most cases, but some patients present with severe manifestations as the disease progresses. The heterogeneity of the symptom severity is extreme; therefore, patients with compromised immune systems or patients residing in endemic zones can have heightened responses, and complications such as pneumonia can ensue. This is the case because it brings out the aesthetics of the diseases, where the geographic location and immune state could affect the presentation of the symptoms and overall health effects, with a focus on keen vigilance to potential infection by those infected (Calvert et al., 2014). In certain instances, coccidioidomycosis has extrapulmonary manifestations, where the infection spreads beyond the lungs to other body systems. Its manifestations may be characterized by joint pain, particularly of the knees, rashes, and systemic complaints that resemble other illnesses. The acute onset of such symptoms is likely to lead to misdiagnosis, as seen in two case presentations involving patients with isolated knee pain, originally diagnosed as potential neoplastic processes. Surgical biopsies were revealed with large spherules compatible with coccidioidal infection, showing the importance of greater awareness of atypical presentation of symptoms among doctors. For disseminated disease, the clinical presentation is more complex and may frequently necessitate serologic diagnosis and better patient evaluation (Calvert et al., 2014). Serological testing is also crucial in defining the severity of coccidioidomycosis and guiding treatment decisions. Serological categories recognize differential symptom profiles associated with various levels of severity of infection. For instance, uncomplicated pulmonary coccidioidomycosis patients usually have smaller complement fixation titers than patients with severe disseminated versions of the disease. Such a relationship indicates that quantitation of symptom severity is possible by serological tests, which further helps in clinical management. Clinical care during the treatment of coccidioidomycosis is highly facilitated by awareness of such symptom correlations along with serological dynamics and thus yields improved health outcomes, particularly for high-risk patients (Figure 12.11).

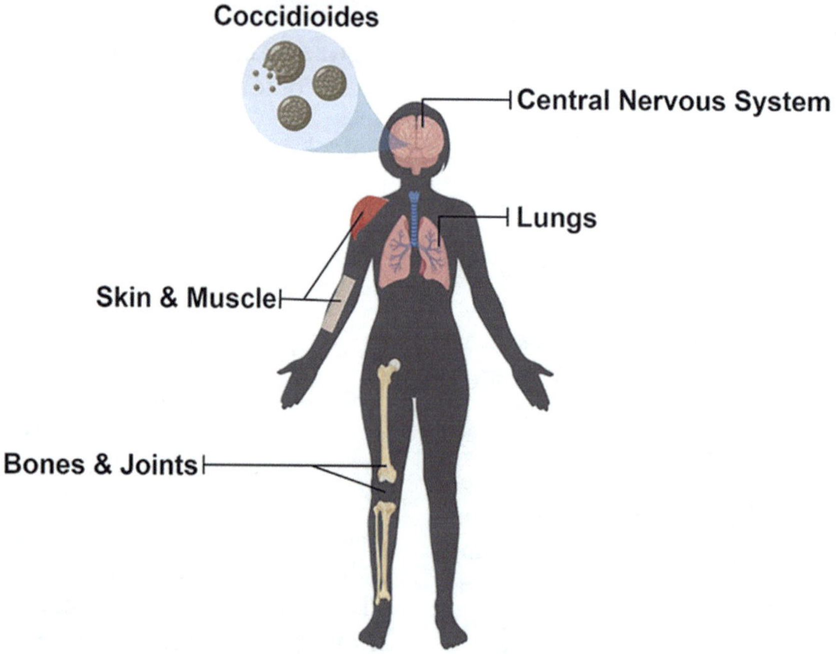

Figure 12.11. In certain cases, coccidioidomycosis can lead to extrapulmonary manifestations, where the infection spreads beyond the lungs, affecting other body systems.

Source: https://www.frontiersin.org/files/Articles/484838/fimmu-10-02188-HTML/image_m/fimmu-10-02188-g001.jpg.

12.3.2. Severe Cases and Complications

The implications of severe coccidioidomycosis extend beyond primary infection and produce severe health problems for the patient. While the majority of infections present with mild symptoms or are asymptomatic, approximately 3 to 5% of infections develop into chronic pulmonary disease or disseminate to extrapulmonary organs. These severe forms complicate the clinical presentation because chronic pulmonary coccidioidomycosis can present similarly to tuberculosis or lung cancer and therefore complicates diagnosis and treatment. Additionally, in endemic areas, the prevalence of primary pulmonary coccidioidomycosis has not only increased but also constitutes almost 29% of cases of community-acquired pneumonia. As more patients with these conditions appear before healthcare providers, knowing the range of the disease is crucial in enhancing patient outcomes and implementing effective treatment patterns (Thompson et al., 2015). Perhaps most importantly, morbidity and mortality due to coccidioidomycosis mostly arise in patients who have severe presentation. Extrapulmonary complications, including meningitis, osteomyelitis, and cutaneous coccidioidomycosis, reflect the systemic nature of the condition. Recent research has shown that patients presenting with disseminated disease are at increased risk for serious health outcomes, necessitating prolonged hospitalization and intensive care. These individuals might need to be managed with multidimensional therapy beyond antifungal therapy, including immunosuppressive agents and close monitoring. The challenge is not only in the management of these severe manifestations but also long-term follow-up to attempt to treat sequelae that can worsen quality of life (Thompson et al., 2015). Beyond the direct medical effects of severe coccidioidomycosis, the disease complications burden healthcare resources significantly. Involved patients typically need multidisciplinary treatment from different specialists since the disease has a very broad range of manifestations, ranging from infectious disease experts to pulmonologists. It needs a general management strategy including both medical management of the illness and supportive therapy in involved complications. Surveillance and intensity of care in the patients with disseminated disease remain critical for those waging the fight against the chronic effects of infection, eventually dictating clinical outcomes and healthcare costs. As scientists strive towards advancement in treatment protocols, the complexity of coccidioidomycosis and its complications justify the instant use of healthcare interventions in severe cases (Figure 12.12).

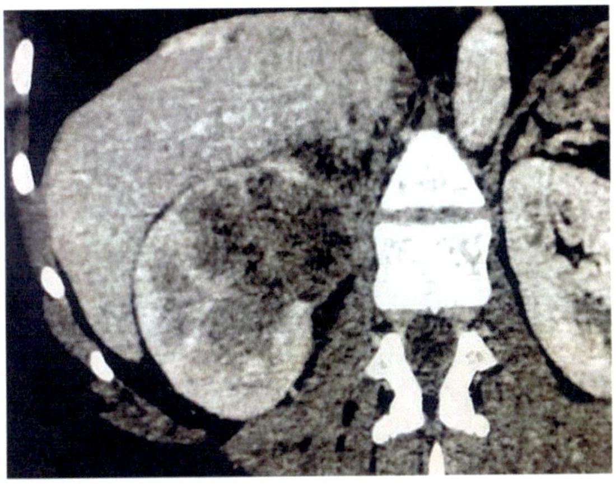

Figure 12.12. Tuberculosis mimicking.

Source: https://media.springernature.com/lw685/springer-static/image/art%3A10.1186%2Fs13256-019-2073-0/MediaObjects/13256_2019_2073_Fig1_HTML.png.

12.3.3. Differences in Symptoms Among Populations

Coccidioidomycosis, or valley fever, exhibits a wide range of symptoms, whose severity and intensity differ among groups. Severity and expression of these symptoms are influenced by numerous factors such as geographic location, socioeconomic status, and underlying health status. In immunocompromised patients, the illness progresses to disseminated coccidioidomycosis and may manifest with severe manifestations affecting more than one organ. Healthy persons have milder respiratory symptoms that can resemble influenza, including cough, fever, and fatigue. This distinction suggests that immune response is a key determinant of symptom severity.

It would be necessary to explore more in terms of how demographic and biological determinants can contribute to disease outcomes. Studies show that some groups, such as those residing in endemic areas or with underlying health conditions, present specific symptom patterns for coccidioidomycosis. For example, African or Filipino patients are said to have increased rates of severe cases among ethnic groups. Such differences could result from genetic susceptibility or differences in healthcare access and education about the disease. Further, the lack of testing leads to underdiagnosis and underestimation of disease incidence, as pointed out by Bartlett et al., (2008). This gap in diagnosis impacts the treatment and control of the disease, hence the need for specific public health interventions among high-risk groups to mitigate the burden of coccidioidomycosis. Socio-economic factors further play a critical role in determining health outcomes for coccidioidomycosis. Poor socioeconomic groups may have limited access to healthcare units and information about the disease, which may worsen their symptoms and progress of the disease. These individuals are less likely to report for early infection in a timely manner, thus more likely to be complicated. Poor living conditions also tend to expose patients to native fungal spores to their environment, thereby increasing their risk. The relationship between these socio-economic forces highlights the necessity to eradicate health disparities to minimize the difference in symptoms and outcomes across groups. Greater sensitivity and resource allocation directed towards high-risk groups are essential as a lack of testing can lead to underdiagnosis and underestimation of disease, as per (Douglas et al., 1996) (Figure 12.13).

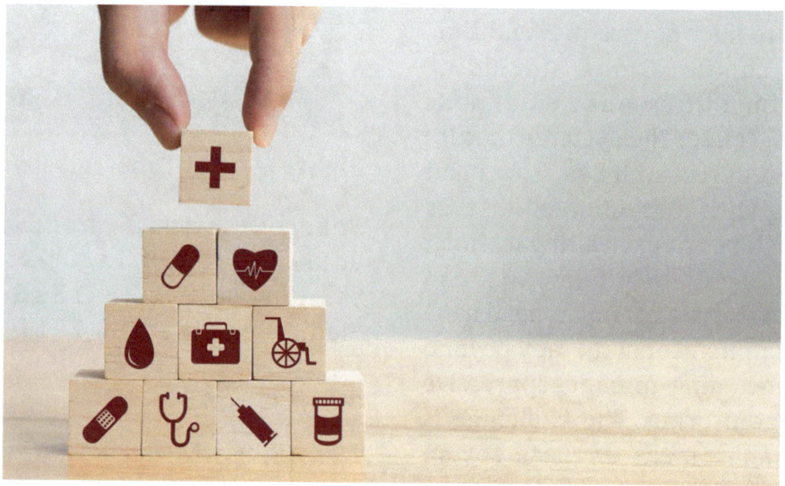

Figure 12.13. Populations in low-income areas may have limited access to healthcare resources and education about the disease, which can exacerbate the progression and severity of symptoms.

Source: https://nationalhealthcouncil.org/wp-content/uploads/2022/05/shutterstock_1021932094-scaled.jpg.

12.4. Diagnosis

The coccidioidomycosis diagnosis, or Valley fever as it is better known, requires a multidisciplinary strategy because of the varied clinical presentation of the disease. The diagnosis initially depends on the patients clinical presentation, especially the geographic exposure of the patient to endemic areas of *Coccidioides* fungi. In those with symptoms, like pulmonary infection, the laboratory plays an important role. Serological testing, specifically complement fixation (CF) titer measurement, has been the gold standard for diagnosis. Elevated levels of CF titers may indicate the severity of infection; for instance, in cases of disseminated coccidioidomycosis (DC), the median highest CF titer is considerably greater than in patients with pulmonary uncomplicated coccidioidomycosis (PUC) or pulmonary chronic coccidioidomycosis (PCC) (Mehrkens et al., 2016). Thus, prompt serological assessment is paramount to successful clinical management and treatment decision-making. Besides serology, histopathological results can further enhance the diagnostic yield in coccidioidomycosis, especially in atypical cases. For instance, a study among dogs with coccidioidomycosis presented evidence of immune complex glomerulonephritis (ICGN) with the disease, indicating a potential renal expression of the disease. 54% of the canines, in this retrospective case series, showed renal histopathologic lesions, thereby stressing the necessity of adding coccidioidomycosis to the differential diagnosis of renal disease (Mehrkens et al., 2016). It is stressing the necessity for clinicians to utilize an array of diagnostic tools, including urine analysis and tissue histopathology, combined with serological tests, especially in presentation with organ-specific complications or atypical symptoms. The ephemeral nature of serological reactions in coccidioidomycosis complicates the interpretation of diagnostic tests. Studies have disclosed variability in antibody production, particularly in patients with different severities of disease. For example, while 25.4% of patients with PUC did not develop measurable titers, the rates dropped in patients with more severe disease such as coccidioidal meningitis (CM) (Bays et al., 2018). This difference calls for an understanding that a negative serologic test does not exclude diagnosis, particularly in moderate to severe illness. Therefore, clinicians must adopt a rigorous diagnostic process that integrates clinical evaluation, serologic testing, and histopathological examinations. This tactic is crucial in order to prevent mistaken diagnosis and inappropriate therapy of coccidioidomycosis, particularly as the presentation of the disease in patients may be different (Figure 12.14).

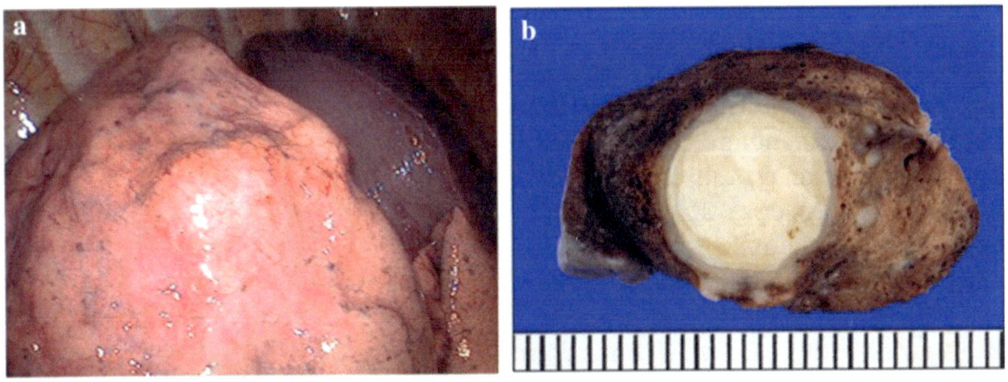

Figure 12.14. Pulmonary chronic coccidioidomycosis (PCC).

Source: https://media.springernature.com/lw685/springer-static/image/art%3A10.1007%2Fs00595-023-02736-3/MediaObjects/595_2023_2736_Fig2_HTML.jpg.

12.4.1. Clinical Evaluation and Patient History

The clinical evaluation of coccidioidomycosis calls for complete knowledge of patient history, as it is of vital significance to diagnosis as well as treatment plan. Providers in areas of endemicity should maintain a high level of suspicion for the disease, particularly in patients who have respiratory disease or recent exposure to dust in regions where *Coccidioides* species are endemic. Detailed patient histories must cover symptoms such as cough, fever, and chest pain, as well as prior travel or residence in endemic regions. By meticulous recording of patient history, health care providers can detect coccidioidomycosis cases at an earlier point so that timely intervention and improved patient outcomes can be achieved. Serologic examinations are of key importance in the clinical diagnosis of coccidioidomycosis, and complement fixation (CF) titers are the most significant diagnostic tool. The CF titers are typically expressed according to the patients clinical classification: pulmonary uncomplicated, pulmonary chronic, disseminated, or coccidioidal meningitis. There is an interesting point that certain titers are linked with varying severities of the disease, as illustrated in a study where the patients were classified depending on their CF levels. These dynamics not only allow clinicians to diagnose coccidioidomycosis but also determine disease progression and response to therapy. The use of serological results as part of clinical assessment highlights the importance of continued patient assessment and close follow-up, which are critical to manage this complicated infection successfully (Bays et al., 2018). Beyond standard evaluation procedures, patient history might identify unique cases that highlight the importance of early diagnosis and treatment. A particularly noteworthy case was that of a pregnant woman who came in with massive hemoptysis and grave pulmonary complications related to coccidioidomycosis. This case highlights the necessity to acknowledge the rapid deterioration potential of coccidioidomycosis, especially with the additional vascular concerns of pregnancy. In this case, close observation and the reengineering of clinical management methods became mandatory in order to treat both the acute infection as well as the patient's pregnancy adequately. These examples are used to highlight that a detailed recording of clinical history is not an ivory-tower activity; it has concrete treatment pathway and patient safety implications, illustrating the intricate interplay between patient history and clinical practice in coccidioidomycosis (Burns et al., 2016) (Figure 12.15).

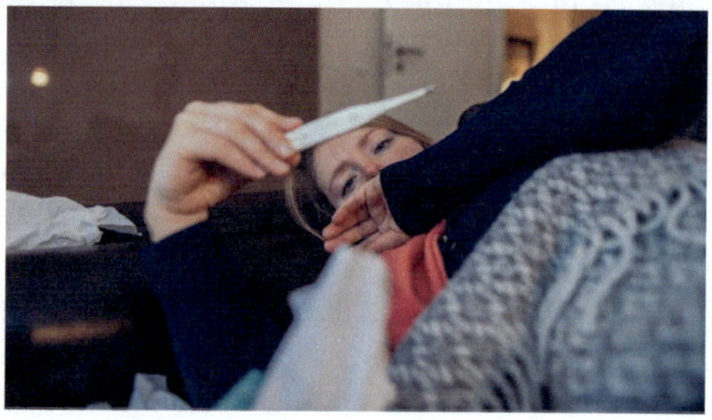

Figure 12.15. Detailed patient histories should encompass symptoms such as cough, fever, and chest pain, as well as any prior travel or residence in endemic zones.

Source: https://i0.wp.com/post.healthline.com/wp-content/uploads/2020/06/cough-sick-fever-1296x728-header.jpg?w=1155&h=1528.

12.4.2. Laboratory Tests and Imaging Techniques

In diagnosis of coccidioidomycosis, laboratory and imaging investigations are crucial in helping differentiate this infection from other potential diseases. Serological investigations to establish the presence of anti-*Coccidioides immitis* antibodies are widely employed, with a relatively speedy identification process. While enzyme immunoassays of IgM and IgG antibodies yield results informing clinical decisions, their interpretation must be provided in keeping with patients clinical presentation as well as epidemiologic context. Radiology is also used in diagnosis, particularly when the disease presents pulmonary symptoms. X-rays of the chest are able to detect infiltrates, and CT scans are able to reveal more accurate images of pulmonary lesions so that extrapulmonary manifestations, which are capable of mimicking other diseases and making diagnosis complicated (Calvert et al., 2014), are observable. Imaging modalities not only prove useful in the diagnosis of coccidioidomycosis but are also helpful in follow up of disease course or response to treatment. In the situation of suspected extrapulmonary disease, particularly in such presentations with solitary lesions, more advanced imaging modalities such as MRI are of immense value. For instance, bone lesions can be confused with neoplasm, as demonstrated in clinical experience where solitary lytic lesions were actually diagnosed to be extrapulmonary coccidioidomycosis by histopathological examination (Calvert et al., 2014). The diagnostic uncertainty highlights the importance of an integrative approach in which imaging features are combined with laboratory findings in order to make an accurate diagnosis. Continued advances in imaging technology could further enhance the likelihood of identification of such rare presentations of coccidioidomycosis, with effective and timely management. Improved diagnostic process for fungal infections, including coccidioidomycosis, has been facilitated by advances in new laboratory techniques. Molecular epidemiological techniques have gained importance, allowing rapid and precise identification of the fungal genome, which enhances diagnosis in comparison to the traditional culture technique. The development of new antigen detection systems has proven useful in the diagnosis of pulmonary fungal infections, with the potential of solutions allowing tests to be completed easily from serum or bronchoalveolar lavage fluid. These developments speak to the necessity for the introduction of new laboratory techniques alongside standard imaging and serological testing to support enhanced patient outcomes. With ongoing advances in science, the convergence of these divergent diagnostic modalities will likely provide an even more advanced and beneficial paradigm for the management of coccidioidomycosis and its varied complications (Figure 12.16).

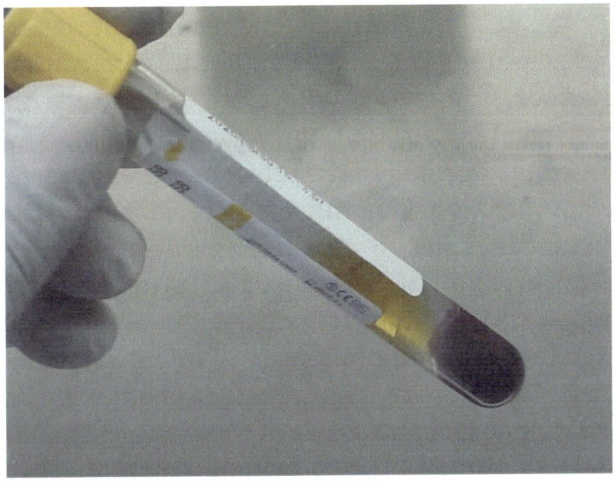

Figure 12.16. Serological tests that detect antibodies against *Coccidioides immitis* are widely utilized, offering a relatively quick means of identification.

Source: https://medicallabnotes.com/wp-content/uploads/2025/03/*Coccidioides*-Antibody-Testing-Introduction-Clinical-Significance-Test-methods-Result-Interpretation-and-Additional-Information.jpg.

12.4.3. Differential Diagnosis with Other Diseases

Upon diagnosing coccidioidomycosis, clinicians need to keep a wide differential diagnosis list in mind due to the non-specific presentation of the disease. The patients classically present with pneumonia-like or upper respiratory tract infection-like respiratory symptoms. Additionally, extrapulmonary disease will create further confusion since manifestations may be mimicked by a number of malignancies or granulomatous diseases. This overlap demands careful scrutiny of the patient's clinical background, including potential exposure to endemic regions, when evaluating imaging examinations that could initially indicate more sinister diagnoses. Ultimately, distinguishing coccidioidomycosis from these diagnoses is critical in order to administer appropriate treatment and management, lest failure to do so results in misdiagnosis and delay in treatment for the patient. Radiographic manifestations in coccidioidomycosis also complicate differential diagnosis. Imaging will often present with nonspecific lung or bone lesions, which may be inappropriately attributed to neoplasms or other infection. Illustratively, in certain reported instances, solitary patellar lytic lesions have been inaccurately diagnosed as primary bony neoplasms, leading to referral for orthopedic oncologic consultation prior to being correctly diagnosed. Particularly in regions of endemicity, the radiologic appearance of such lesions should raise the differential to include fungal disease like coccidioidomycosis. Orthopedic surgeons and radiologists should be vigilant for such imaging findings, including awareness, which can facilitate early diagnosis of such infections and thus improve patient outcomes, forming the basis of a successful clinical practice in regions where the etiologic pathogen is endemic. The importance of accurate patient assessment cannot be overlooked in making an accurate diagnosis for coccidioidomycosis. Particularly, inclusion of travel history and risk evaluation of exposure is helpful. A case was reported where a patient presented to the UK with nonspecific respiratory symptoms but was subsequently diagnosed with coccidioidomycosis, illustrating the risk of misdiagnosis outside of an endemic region. These lectures emphasize the importance of an end-to-end strategy of clinical assessment, appropriate imaging, and lab workup to confirm the diagnosis. Additionally, a growing awareness of how coccidioidomycosis manifests as a component of other disease syndromes can allow clinicians to make educated decisions that minimize the likelihood of misdiagnosis and provide optimal care and management for patients (Figure 12.17).

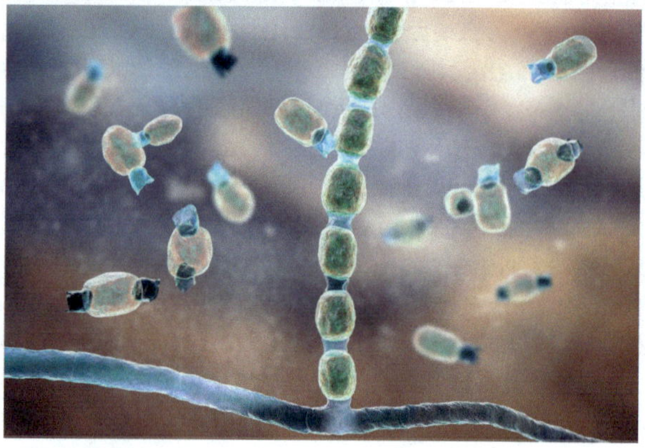

Figure 12.17. The importance of thorough patient evaluation cannot be overstated when it comes to establishing a correct diagnosis for coccidioidomycosis.

Source: https://www.rollingstone.com/wp-content/uploads/2023/02/valley-fever-*Coccidioides*.jpg?w=1581&h=1054&crop=1.

SUMMARY

Coccidioidomycosis, or Valley Fever, is an infection caused by inhaling the spores of *Coccidioides*, most commonly in dry regions of the south-west United States. Illness appears in a variety of forms, ranging from benign respiratory illness to severe pulmonary disease or disseminated disease. Diagnosis is most commonly accomplished through serologic testing, which quantitates the immune response to the fungus. Studies have shown that serologic screening is particularly necessary in the immunocompromised group as they are likely to have a decreased response, making the infection difficult to detect. Testing has been more effective and precise with the use of multiple diagnostic tools among such risk groups, thus validating the rationale for targeted intervention in clinical practice (Ana et al., 2006). Climatic factors play a significant part in coccidioidomycosis epidemiology, impacting the cases' distribution and seasonality of epidemics. Climate, soil, and dispersal of *Coccidioides* spores have been demonstrated to be implicated in a complex interaction as a determinant for disease patterns. Bimodal seasonality in coccidioidomycosis was not reported in the literature until now, based on analyses. Of specific interest, desiccating fore summer rainfall, even several years prior to an outbreak, was found to be a significant predictor of infection rates (Andrew et al., 2005). This illustrates the significance of environmental drivers in ascertaining the risk of coccidioidomycosis for individuals residing in high-risk areas. Lastly, the inclusion of climatic data into predictive models provides useful insight into trends in coccidioidomycosis and supports public health intervention. Both antecedent and concurrent climatic influences must be taken into account for accurate forecasting, as evidenced by models explaining up to 80% of disease incidence variance. Such predictive ability allows the implementation of targeted surveillance and prevention efforts, particularly during recognized high-risk periods. Furthermore, the integration of ecologic study with clinical knowledge of serologic responses enables presenting coccidioidomycosis holistically in the end, resulting in better patient outcomes and efficient resource usage within healthcare facilities.

A CLOSER LOOK

COCCIDIOIDES POSADASII

Coccidioides posadasii is a species of fungus that belongs to the genus Coccidioides and is responsible for causing coccidioidomycosis, commonly known as Valley Fever. This pathogenic fungus is primarily found in arid and semi-arid regions of the southwestern United States, parts of Mexico, and Central and South America. The fungus thrives in the soil, particularly in areas with warm temperatures and low rainfall. In its environmental state, C. posadasii exists as a mold that produces microscopic spores called arthroconidia. These spores become airborne when disturbed, and when inhaled by humans or animals, they can infect the lungs, leading to respiratory symptoms such as coughing, chest pain, and fever.

Infection with C. posadasii may result in asymptomatic disease, but it can also progress to severe forms, such as pulmonary coccidioidomycosis or disseminated coccidioidomycosis, where the fungus spreads beyond the lungs to other organs. Risk factors for severe disease include weakened immune systems, such as in individuals with HIV/AIDS or those undergoing immunosuppressive treatments. Diagnosis typically involves serological tests, culture, or molecular methods to detect the presence of the fungus. Treatment usually involves antifungal medications, such as fluconazole or itraconazole, depending on the severity of the infection.

REFERENCES

1. Abu-Elmagd, K., Demetris, A., Fung, J. J., Furukawa, H., et al. (1994). Three years clinical experience with intestinal transplantation. https://core.ac.uk/download/12205033.pdf (accessed on 27th June 2025).
2. Adenis, A., Arathoon, E., Araujo, P., Flores, B., et al. (2022). Current situation of endemic mycosis in the Americas and the Caribbean: Proceedings of the first international meeting on endemic mycoses of the Americas (IMEMA). https://core.ac.uk/download/572931512.pdf (accessed on 27th June 2025).
3. Alexander, B. D., Anaissie, E. J., Andes, D. R., Baddley, J., et al. (2014). Endemic fungal infections in solid organ and hematopoietic cell transplant recipients enrolled in the Transplant-Associated Infection Surveillance Network (TRANSNET). https://deepblue.lib.umich.edu/bitstream/2027.42/106980/1/tid12186.pdf (accessed on 27th June 2025).
4. Al-Obaidi, M. M., Nix, D. E., & Ostrosky-Zeichner, L. (2023). Trends of azole antifungal prescription in the United States: Medicare Part D provider utilization and payment data analysis. https://core.ac.uk/download/604669181.pdf (accessed on 27th June 2025).
5. AMCLI Mycology Committee, Angheben, A., Conte, M., D'Aleo, F., et al. (2023). Endemic systemic mycoses in Italy: A systematic review of literature and a practical update. https://core.ac.uk/download/614217516.pdf (accessed on 27th June 2025).
6. Ampel, N. M., Anstead, G. M., Babady, N. E., Baddley, J. W., Bariola, J. R., Ben-Ami, R., Bialek, R., et al. (2012). Pulmonary fungal infections. http://deepblue.lib.umich.edu/bitstream/2027.42/92435/1/j.1440-1843.2012.02150.x.pdf (accessed on 27th June 2025).
7. Arathoon, E., Barker, B., Chiller, T., Driebe, E., et al. (2016). Local population structure and patterns of Western Hemisphere dispersal for *Coccidioides* spp., the fungal cause of Valley Fever. https://core.ac.uk/download/323069894.pdf (accessed on 27th June 2025).
8. Arbona, N., Butkiewicz, C., Keyes, M., Shubitz, L., et al. (2020). Clinical features of cats diagnosed with coccidioidomycosis in Arizona, 2004–2018. https://core.ac.uk/download/288175168.pdf (accessed on 27th June 2025).
9. Baaj, A. A., Galgiani, J. N., Martirosyan, N. L., Skoch, J. M., Zaninovich, O., & Zoccali, C. (2015). A paradigm for the evaluation and management of spinal coccidioidomycosis. https://core.ac.uk/download/577169683.pdf (accessed on 27th June 2025).
10. Baklanov, A., Barker, B. M., Castillo, J., Gassó, S., et al. (2021). Health and safety effects of airborne soil dust in the Americas and beyond. https://core.ac.uk/download/539648047.pdf (accessed on 27th June 2025).
11. Bandeira, S. P., Camargo, Z. P., Rocha, F. A., Castelo-Branco, C. M., et al. (2012). Biochemical characterization of an in-house *Coccidioides* antigen: Perspectives for the immunodiagnostic of coccidioidomycosis. https://core.ac.uk/download/37738337.pdf (accessed on 27th June 2025).
12. Bartlett, B. J., Park, B. J., Chiller, T. M., Engelthaler, D. M., Dodge, D. C., Chang, D. C., Galgiani, J. N., et al. (2008). Testing for coccidioidomycosis among patients with community-acquired pneumonia. https://core.ac.uk/download/pdf/8227271.pdf (accessed on 27th June 2025).
13. Bays, D., Dinh, B. T. N., McHardy, I. H., Pappagianis, D., et al. (2018). Coccidioidomycosis complement fixation titer trends in the age of antifungals. https://core.ac.uk/download/323071342.pdf (accessed on 27th June 2025).

14. Bergen, M. E. (2020). *Valley Fever: Education for Primary Care Providers and Allied Health Care Professionals*. https://core.ac.uk/download/368317161.pdf (accessed on 27th June 2025).
15. Bille, J., Devriese, L., Dominguez, J., Greub, G., et al. (2018). *Enterococcus cecorum* septicemia in a malnourished adult patient. https://core.ac.uk/download/159151706.pdf (accessed on 27th June 2025).
16. Burns, C., Carrillo, M., Flores-Guardado, J., Hampton, B., et al. (2016). Coccidioidomycosis in pregnancy: Case report and literature review of associated placental lesions. https://core.ac.uk/download/pdf/82774540.pdf (accessed on 27th June 2025).
17. Calvert, G., Hanrahan, C. J., Jones, K. B., Li, X., et al. (2014). Coccidioidomycosis infection of the patella mimicking a neoplasm: Two case reports. https://core.ac.uk/download/323070868.pdf (accessed on 27th June 2025).
18. Chang, D. C., Anderson, S., Wannemuehler, K., Engelthaler, D. M., Erhart, L., Sunenshine, R. H., Burwell, L. A., et al. (1996). Testing for coccidioidomycosis among patients with community-acquired pneumonia. https://core.ac.uk/download/pdf/8227271.pdf (accessed on 27th June 2025).
19. Comrie, A. C., CDC, Kerrick, S. S., Kolivras, K. N., Komatsu, K., & Maddy, K. (2005). Climate factors influencing coccidioidomycosis seasonality and outbreaks. https://core.ac.uk/download/pdf/3779261.pdf (accessed on 27th June 2025).
20. Cox, R., Revie, C. W., & Sanchez, J. (2013). Multi-criteria decision analysis tools for prioritizing emerging or re-emerging infectious diseases associated with climate change in Canada. https://core.ac.uk/download/158370208.pdf (accessed on 27th June 2025).
21. Cunliffe, L. J., & Renwick, I. (2017). Valley fever in the UK? –The importance of a travel history. https://core.ac.uk/download/74225319.pdf (accessed on 27th June 2025).
22. Dzialowski, K. (2021). *Coccidioidomycosis (Valley Fever) awareness*. https://core.ac.uk/download/482122685.pdf (accessed on 27th June 2025).
23. Healy, J. R., Kraft, W. K., & Moore, J. N. (2015). Pharmacologic and clinical evaluation of posaconazole. https://core.ac.uk/download/46974003.pdf (accessed on 27th June 2025).
24. Homei, A., & Worboys, M. (2020). Chapter 4 Endemic mycoses and allergies. https://core.ac.uk/download/478142798.pdf (accessed on 27th June 2025).
25. Homei, A., & Worboys, M. (2020). Chapter bibliography. https://core.ac.uk/download/478137736.pdf (accessed on 27th June 2025).
26. Iqbal, H., Jones, K., Mehmood, B. F., Roytman, D., et al. (2024). Fungal infections in liver cirrhosis. https://core.ac.uk/download/617036237.pdf (accessed on 27th June 2025).
27. Kafatos, M., Laniado-Laborin, R., & Sarafoglou, N. (2019). Coccidioidomycosis: Medical and spatio-temporal perspectives. https://core.ac.uk/download/324197992.pdf (accessed on 27th June 2025).
28. Kafatos, M., Laniado-Laborin, R., Sarafoglou, N., Sprigg, W. A., et al. (2020). Interdisciplinary science to confront coccidioidomycosis. https://core.ac.uk/download/324197920.pdf (accessed on 27th June 2025).
29. Kauffman, C. A., & Terpenning, M. S. (1988). Deep fungal infections in the elderly. https://deepblue.lib.umich.edu/bitstream/2027.42/111183/1/j.1532-5415.1988.tb04028.x.pdf (accessed on 27th June 2025).

30. Lee, J. S., & van der Putten, W. (2011). *Soil Borne Human Diseases*. https://core.ac.uk/download/38621779.pdf (accessed on 27th June 2025).

31. Martínez-Herrera, E., Duarte-Escalante, E., Ocaña-Monroy, J. L., Pérez-Huitrón, M. A., Reyes-Montes, M. del R., Frías-De-León, M. G., & Arenas, R. (2016). The habitat of *Coccidioides* spp. and the role of animals as reservoirs and disseminators in nature. https://core.ac.uk/download/pdf/81918935.pdf (accessed on 27th June 2025).

32. Mehrkens, L. R., Mohr, F. C., & Sykes, J. E. (2016). Clinicopathologic and histopathologic renal abnormalities in dogs with coccidioidomycosis. https://core.ac.uk/download/323070128.pdf (accessed on 27th June 2025).

33. Panackal, A. A., Breternitz, J., Cairns, M., Centers for Disease Control and Prevention, Barton, C., Dennis, D. T., Warnock, D. W., et al. (2004). Coccidioidomycosis among workers at an archeological site, Northeastern Utah. https://core.ac.uk/download/pdf/8708429.pdf (accessed on 27th June 2025).

34. Santelli, A. C., Coakley, B., Smith, C. E., Pappagianis, D., Palmer, D. F., et al. (2006). Serologic testing for symptomatic coccidioidomycosis in immunocompetent and immunosuppressed hosts. https://core.ac.uk/download/pdf/8351188.pdf (accessed on 27th June 2025).

35. Sher, A., & Kumar, R. (2014). Epidemiology of coccidioidomycosis in Missouri. https://core.ac.uk/download/77954647.pdf (accessed on 27th June 2025).

36. Thompson, G., & Twarog, M. (2015). Coccidioidomycosis: Recent updates. https://core.ac.uk/download/pdf/144850390.pdf (accessed on 27th June 2025).

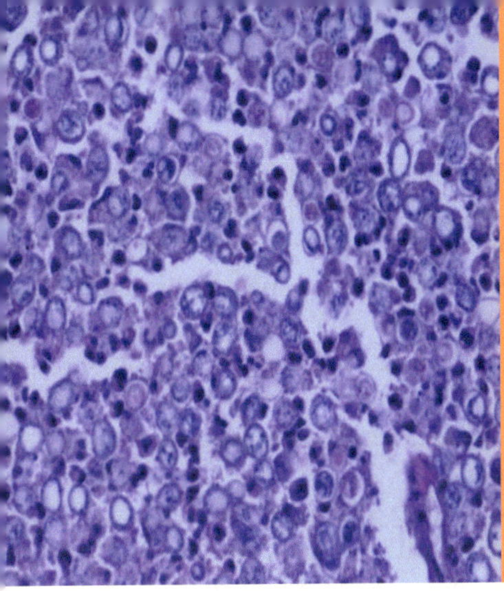

Chapter 13

BLASTOMYCOSIS

Contents

Introduction

Blastomycosis is a systemic mycosis resulting from the dimorphic fungus *Blastomyces dermatitidis* and is most frequently found in certain geographic regions, specifically regions surrounding the Great Lakes, the Ohio River Valley, and portions of Canada. The organism exists in mold and yeast forms, with the mold form being aerial, rendering the spores respirable by host susceptible individuals. Infection is usually seen after exposure to contaminated soil or rotting organic matter. Blastomycosis clinical presentation can be highly variable, including asymptomatic infections to severe respiratory disease, thus making it challenging to diagnose. This variability in nature highlights the value of epidemiological awareness and clinical suspicion, especially in endemic areas, where early detection and treatment are essential for patient outcome optimization (Mohammad et al., 2025). Symptomatic patients might present with pneumonia that has cough, chest pain, and fever, which is indistinguishable from other respiratory illnesses and therefore causes misdiagnoses. The incubation period between exposure and development of symptoms might also be highly variable, and it is challenging to establish a clear temporal relationship between environment and disease. Moreover, the disease course of blastomycosis can result in disseminated infection in multiple organ systems, like the skin and bones, in immunocompromised individuals. The diagnostic challenges of blastomycosis underscore the significance of heightened awareness by clinicians, especially in cases of having nonspecific respiratory symptoms combined with exposure history to endemic areas (Larsson et al., 2024). Recent developments in diagnostic techniques, such as molecular technology and antigen testing, have increased our ability to diagnose a case of blastomycosis and separate it from other fungi. While with this development, treatment is primarily antifungal therapy, with the medications itraconazole and amphotericin B being the main treatment. Treatment would depend on the severity of infection and patient's overall health status. A good understanding of the epidemiology, clinical manifestation, and diagnostic strategy of blastomycosis is essential when dealing with this disease, which remains a key public health concern in certain regions. Therefore, ongoing studies are important to maximize therapeutic regimens as well as increase diagnostic capacity, hence maximizing the management of the disease in affected patients (Figure 13.1).

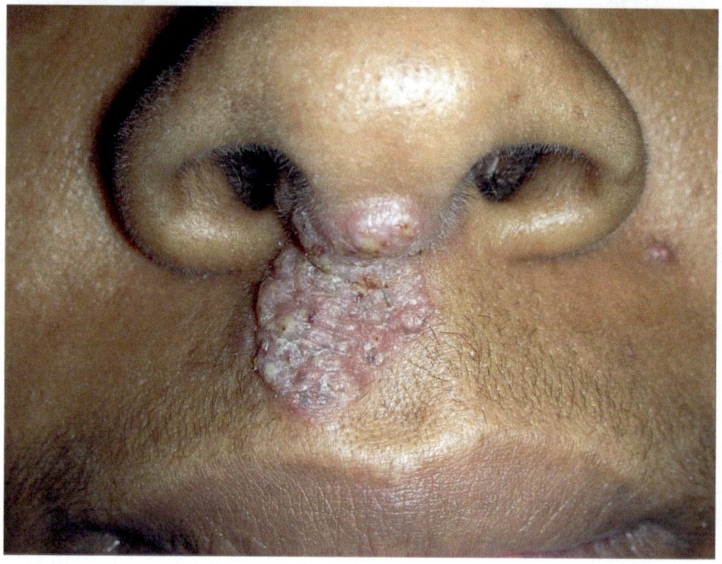

Figure 13.1. Blastomycosis.

Source: https://www.dermatologyadvisor.com/wp-content/uploads/sites/20/2019/03/ch784.fig1_.jpg.

13.1. Causative Agent

The causative agent of blastomycosis is the dimorphic fungus *Blastomyces dermatitidis*, which occurs most frequently in moist, organic soils, particularly in areas near water sources. This pathogen exhibits temperature-dependent morphologic variation; it exists as a mold in nature and converts to a yeast form at body temperature. The habitat of *Blastomyces dermatitidis* usually exists in close relation with decaying materials, such as wood and leaves that have fallen, and therefore sites with abundant vegetation become suitable for its growth. The interaction of external conditions with the biological properties of the fungus greatly influences its infectability. Studies highlight that while many microorganisms present in soils play significant ecological roles, others like *Blastomyces dermatitidis* can cause serious diseases, particularly among individuals with weakened lung functions or the immunocompromised individuals, thereby illustrating the two-edged sword character of soil diversity (Lee et al., 2011). Blastoymycosis is spread by primary inhalation of spores of *Blastomyces dermatitidis*, which will lead to pulmonary infection. Inhalation of polluted dust most often happens through extrinsic activities such as mining, trekking, or even domestic renovation in the endemic area. Upon inhalation, the spores could transform into yeast form that could disseminate throughout the body, causing an array of symptoms ranging from minor respiratory compromise to severe pneumonia. Early detection of early signs of this infection is crucial since delayed diagnosis could complicate the treatment outcome. Advances in diagnostic technology, such as antigen detection systems, have facilitated the detection of blastomycosis in medical practice. This has made it possible to obtain faster and more accurate diagnostic functions, which can significantly increase the morbidity levels of the disease, reflecting a required advancement in our management and understanding of mycotic infections (Ampel et al., 2012). Understanding the ecological niche and pathogenicity of *Blastomyces dermatitidis* is not only critical to the control of blastomycosis but sheds light on the broader importance of fungal infection in relation to environmental determinants. When habitat modification via human activity such as land use and tillage is on the rise, so potentially is exposure to this pathogen. Soil-districting land management practices such as construction or deforestation can potentially drive spore dispersal into the air. Concurrently, the emergence of drug resistance among certain fungal pathogens underlines the necessity for ongoing monitoring and investigation into blastomycosis and other fungal infections. Change detection in incidence rates or blastomycosis patterns using improved epidemiological methods is vital for public health intervention and successful prevention among high-risk groups, finally resolving the complexities of fungal disease in human populations (Lee et al., 2011) (Figure 13.2).

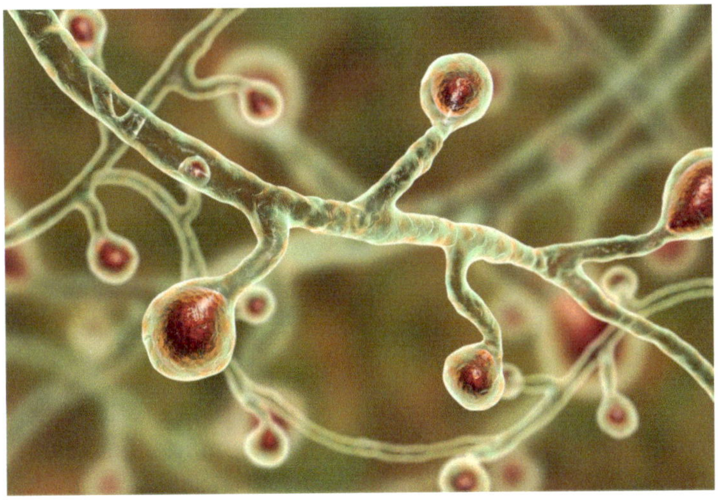

Figure 13.2. The causative agent of blastomycosis is the dimorphic fungus *Blastomyces dermatitidis*, which predominantly resides in moist, organic-rich soils, particularly in areas near water bodies.

Source: https://www.news-medical.net/images/Article_Images/ImageForArticle_22022_16430214615164084.jpg.

13.1.1. Description of Blastomyces dermatitidis

Blastomyces dermatitidis fungus is responsible for causing blastomycosis, which is a significant systemic mycosis endemic primarily in North America. It exhibits yeast morphology in tissues and mold form in the environment and also possesses a unique ability to adapt to diverse conditions. *B. dermatitidis*, inhaled from infested soil or organic matter, transform to yeasts once inside the warm, humid environment of the lung. This is necessary to its pathogenicity because the yeast form is more adapted for survival and dissemination in the host. Its distinctive morphology, where the thick-walled yeast cells are typically in a "broad-based bud," makes it easier to identify the organism in clinical specimens and histopathological preparations, ultimately leading to identifying blastomycosis effectively. Geographically, *Blastomyces dermatitidis* distribution is primarily concentrated in specific areas in the United States, around the Mississippi and Ohio River basins. Current epidemiological studies have documented the frequency of blastomycosis and hospitalization rates, with some states, of which Wisconsin is a notable example, having the highest age-adjusted hospitalization incidence of the disease (Amy et al., 2014). It has a disproportionate impact on men with a median age of 53 years among hospitalized cases, which indicates the most affected groups. The variation in incidence rates across states indicates ecological causes affecting the prevalence of this pathogen and, therefore, the need for targeted public health measures in such areas. Understanding regional characteristics of *B. dermatitidis* will contribute significantly to awareness and readiness against this potentially virulent fungal infection.

Biochemical properties of *Blastomyces dermatitidis* also contribute significantly to the identification and confirmation of the pathogenicity of this fungus. Experiments have determined that polysaccharides obtained from the organism have certain antigenic properties, capable of inducing some immune responses in hosts (Knight et al., 2007). The polysaccharides, especially those produced in greater amounts in the culture broth than in yeast-phase cells, are of utmost significance in developing skin test antigens that could aid in diagnosing blastomycosis. Certain antigenic activity of *B. dermatitidis* and that it cross-reacts with *Histoplasma capsulatum* indicate the complexity of diagnosing fungal infections. Further, research on the antigenic nature of *B. dermatitidis* is enlightening towards the future prospects of vaccine development as well as immunological interventions that can limit the transmission and efficacy of the disease in endemic regions (Figure 13.3).

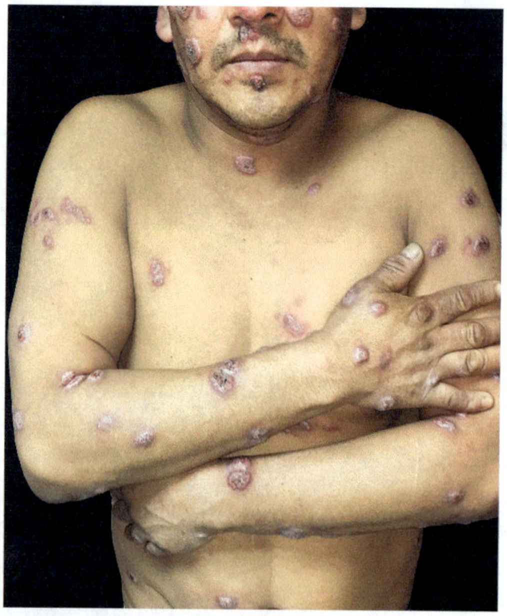

Figure 13.3. The conidia of *B. dermatitidis*, which are inhaled from contaminated soil or organic matter, transform into yeasts upon entering the warm, humid environment of the lungs.

Source: https://www.nejm.org/cms/10.1056/NEJMicm1706238/asset/8117b9ad-b7ba-4909-8152-f9860ecdd58e/assets/images/large/nejmicm1706238_f1.jpg.

13.1.2. Life Cycle and Environmental Conditions

The life cycle of *Blastomyces dermatitidis*, the causative agent of blastomycosis, is deeply intertwined with its environmental environment. The fungus likes to exist most frequently in moist soil and decaying organic debris, particularly where vegetation is dense, such as in forests and swamps. Under such conditions, *B. dermatitidis* exists as a mycelial organism, a filamentous form that can withstand environmental stresses. When soil conditions are suitable, that is, moisture and temperature for growth, mycelium develops to its pathogenic form, yeast. This dimorphism is part of the organism, infecting hosts, humans in this instance, incidentally by laboring in the fungus-infested soil, tending to the garden, or digging in infected soil, emphasizing environmental factors in controlling its life cycle. Environmental factors not only influence the life cycle of *B. dermatitidis* but also its spread and outbreak patterns. Climate change has been found to modify the occurrence and geographic distribution of many fungal pathogens, including *B. dermatitidis*. Global warming and precipitation change are likely to augment the proliferation of the fungus in certain regions, thus enhancing exposure among humans.

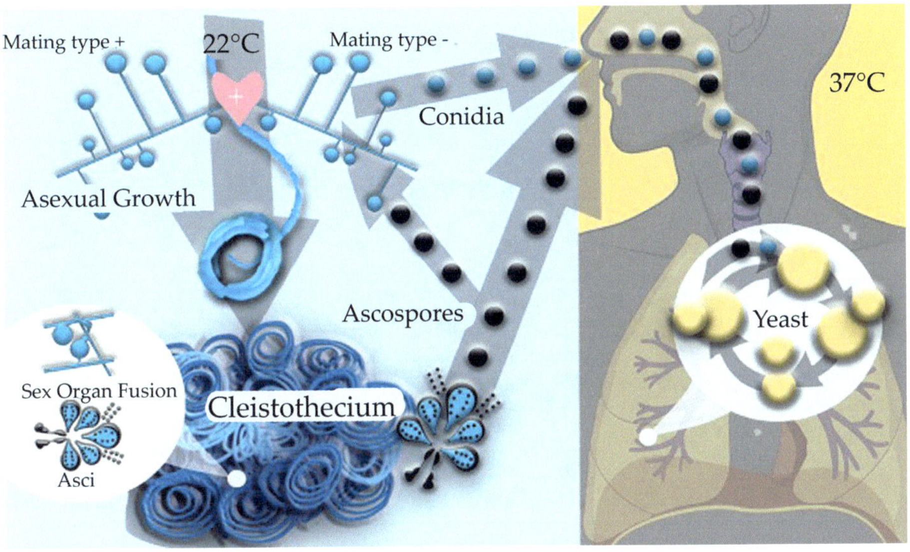

Figure 13.4. The life cycle of *Blastomyces dermatitidis*, the etiological agent of blastomycosis, is intricately linked to its environmental conditions.

Source: https://ars.els-cdn.com/content/image/1-s2.0-S1087184523000282-gr3.jpg.

Consequently, it is necessary to understand the relationship between climatic variables and fungal processes to forecast the probability of outbreaks of blastomycosis. Public health interventions may need to modify when these environmental components vary, underlining the interconnectedness of animal illness, health in the ecosystem, and human illness, a dynamic reinforced by One Health theory, which recognizes the interconnected nature of human, animal, and environmental health (Andrade et al., 2023). Furthermore, the soil microbiome assists with the life cycle of blastomycosis by acting as a reservoir for the pathogen and altering its pathogenicity. Highly organic matter soils, which support high microbial diversity, are able to support opportunistic pathogens like *B. dermatitidis* in addition to those with ecological functions. While most of the microorganisms in soil function beneficially in the workings of the ecosystem, there are others that are virulent to immunocompromised hosts, hence the implication of richness of soil health. Soil health and interactions of fungal pathogens are the most critical component of an ecosystem, as there are certain soil management techniques that can either reduce or enhance this threat. Improved understanding of these interactions, along with empirical evidence of soil-borne disease, is crucial in developing strategies for the prevention of infection, reducing risks of infection with *B. dermatitidis*, and improving public health outcomes (Lee et al., 2011) (Figure 13.4).

13.1.3. Geographic Distribution of the Fungus

The geographical location of *Blastomyces dermatitidis*, the causative agent of blastomycosis, is highly correlated with some ecological conditions conducive to its survival and reproduction. Research has indicated that the fungus is most commonly found in areas with high moisture levels, particularly near streams and regions with well-suited soil composition. In Wisconsin, where blastomycosis is more prevalent, maximum entropy modeling showed that most cases had their origin in northern counties and the western lake shore of Lake Michigan.

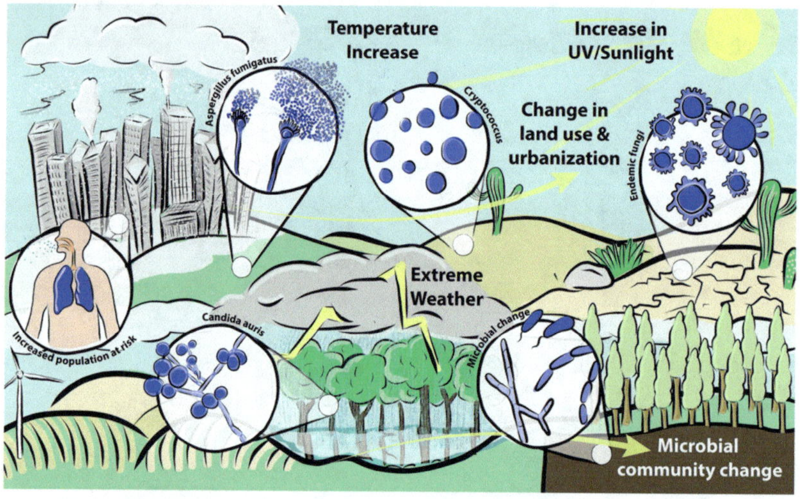

Figure 13.5. The geographic distribution of *Blastomyces dermatitidis*, the causative agent of blastomycosis, is notably linked to specific ecological conditions conducive to its survival and proliferation.

Source: https://pub.mdpi-res.com/jof/jof-07-00367/article_deploy/html/images/jof-07-00367-g001.png?1620478548.

These regions have climate and environmental conditions that are favorable for the survival of *B. dermatitidis* in the environment, highlighting the importance of taking regional geographical features into account when assessing risk for exposure to the pathogen (Bakerspigel et al., 2008). On this basis, these results inform evidence-based targeted public health strategies aimed at decreasing infection rates within vulnerable populations. Ecologically favorable conditions exist for *B. dermatitidis* are not restricted to rural or undeveloped regions alone; urban regions too possess characteristics that can potentially allow the growth of the fungus. Such habitat flexibility suggests that the geographical spread of blastomycosis may be broader than is generally thought to exist, and a larger surveillance system would be required. As seen, urban regions with adequate drainage systems, parks, and surrounding bodies of water can also help in the occurrence of outbreaks, thereby complicating diagnosis and treatment. Moreover, misdiagnosis risks of blastomycosis, as well as other endemic mycoses such as coccidioidomycosis and histoplasmosis, even more emphasize the necessity of enhanced awareness among health professionals regarding the epidemiology of these conditions. Therefore, the detection and monitoring of habitat variability are also relevant for developing effective diagnostic protocols and public health campaigns. Geographic distribution awareness of *B. dermatitidis* directly affects public health responses as well as educational initiatives in relation to blastomycosis. Surveillance of the fungus's endemic regions can be applied in order to discover populations at risk, particularly in regions where exposure is more likely. Greater public awareness can lead to early medical intervention that can increase recovery among infected patients with the fungus. Targeting resources where environmental conditions conducive to the development of blastomycosis are seen helps health authorities target screening and educational campaigns more strategically against populations at increased risk. Additionally, ongoing research must be aimed at clarifying our knowledge of the environmental determinants affecting the stability and transmission of *B. dermatitidis*, thus enabling preventive action to minimize the impact of this potentially debilitating disease on public health (Bakerspigel et al., 2008) (Figure 13.5).

13.2. Transmission and Infection

Understanding of the transmission and infectious mechanism is crucial in knowing blastomycosis, an infection caused by *Blastomyces dermatitidis*, a fungus. The parasite lives primarily in moist soil and decaying organic matter, so locations with abundant these are potential reservoirs for infection. Primarily through inhalation of aerosolized spores, infection through pulmonary entry to the human respiratory system may occur. Geographical area, climate, and soil contribute significantly to the environmental presence of *Blastomyces dermatitidis*. Therefore, individuals with outdoor activity exposure in endemic regions have a higher risk, emphasizing the importance of environmental surveillance in infection avoidance. The interplay of numerous variables within the environment and host susceptibility are significant factors in the incidence of blastomycosis. Certain groups, such as men aged 30-50 and individuals with compromised immune function, present with enhanced susceptibility to this infection. Additionally, the prevalence of blastomycosis typically is related to soil heterogeneity and the conditions that allow survival for the causative fungus. According to recent research, soil ecosystems contain various microbes that are both potential pathogens as well as useful organisms in the maintenance of ecological balance (Lee et al., 2011). Such dual role necessitates public health strategies for conservation as well as exposure risks so that blastomycosis transmission can be managed effectively. Along with this, spatial analysis can also be used to further enhance our understanding of the epidemic outbreaks of blastomycosis and geographical extent. Systematic review of outbreak investigations revealed a fairly low application of spatial methods in infectious disease analysis, with only about 0.4% of published cases applying these techniques (Bull et al., 2015). Spatial tools such as geographic information systems can provide useful information on the environmental drivers of outbreaks and map at-risk areas. By correlating transmission data with spatial analysis, researchers are able to make better predictions and deal with oncoming cases of blastomycosis, thus enabling focused interventions based on the particular ecological characteristics of the affected population (Figure 13.6).

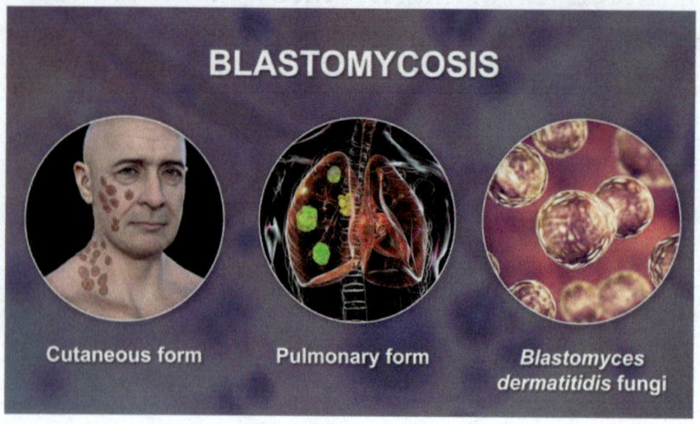

Figure 13.6. Transmission occurs primarily through inhalation of aerosolized spores, which can lead to pulmonary infection upon entering the human respiratory system.

Source: https://www.leading-medicine-guide.com/cms/image/u6454/AdobeStock_703242217.jpg.

13.2.1. Modes of Transmission to Humans

The infection spreads in man primarily because of spore inhalation in an aerosolized form, produced by the fungus *Blastomyces dermatitidis* that grows in specific environmental settings. The spores are found in damp, forested areas, particularly where the ground has been disturbed, such as in the construction of buildings or agricultural activities. Those who go out of doors for sports like hiking, gardening, or camping in regions where the disease is endemic are at greater risk of exposure. Inhalation is an important mode of entry since, after the spores have been inhaled into the lungs, they can convert to a yeast that is more virulent and lead to the development of pulmonary blastomycosis. Understanding these modes of transmission is relevant to public health personnel in order to create awareness and elicit preventive actions among high-risk individuals. Transmission is not limited to respiratory exposure alone; environmental factors play a considerable role in the life cycle of *Blastomyces dermatitidis*. The organism prefers to be solitary within decomposing organic matter, such as leaves and wood, that are rich in humid environments to grow. Disturbances in these ecosystems due to human activity can amplify spore dissemination. Certain occupations such as forestry, construction, and farming can result in wholesale soil disturbance and thereby threaten airborne infectious spores. Temporal and climatic fluctuations also contribute to the distribution of Blastomyces in that more infections occur during warm weather when outdoor activity is greatest.

Public health intervention would then be directed towards educating workers in high-risk occupations about the potential for exposure risk in these environments and promoting preventive practice such as suitable respiratory protection. Individuals who are infected can transmit the fungus through a number of mechanisms, though transmission from person-to-person has not been a proven route. While Blastomycosis attacks the lungs, it also has a tendency to spread to other organs, like the skin and bones, and form disseminated disease. There must be ongoing public health surveillance in order to observe outbreak trends and intervene, particularly where there are large environmental risk factors. In addition, recognizing the relationship between free-roaming domestic cats and zoonotic diseases is significant because cat systems can overlap with disease-endemic ecosystems where Blastomyces is known to be present and can transmit disease among human communities. The social structure of unowned cat populations reflects an expanded public health concern that needs holistic initiatives to prevent not only Blastomycosis but other vector-borne diseases too, as recent research indicates (Halls et al., 2022) (Figure 13.7).

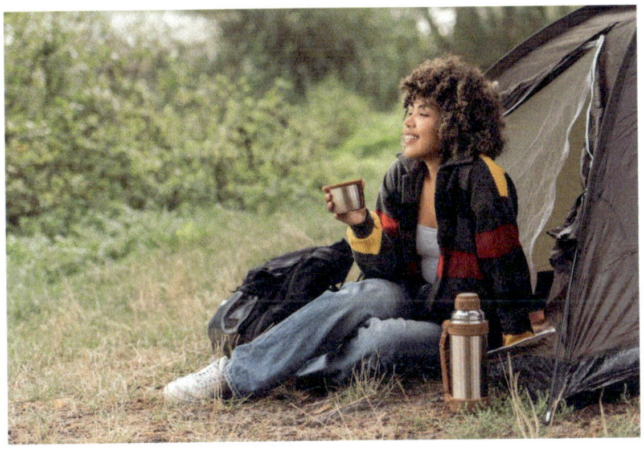

Figure 13.7. Individuals who engage in outdoor activities like hiking, gardening, or camping in endemic areas are at increased risk of exposure.

Source: https://campinggears.ph/wp-content/uploads/2024/08/freepik-export-20240802035956mRWu-scaled.jpeg.

13.2.2. Risk Factors for Infection

Knowledge of the risk factors for infection is important in managing the occurrence of blastomycosis, a fungal illness brought on by *Blastomyces dermatitidis*. Where one resides is important, as the organism is found in areas like the Midwestern and Southeastern United States and Canada. People who reside or spend time in such places, especially near forests, riverbanks, and ground, are more likely to be exposed. Besides, occupational exposure is also a critical issue; workers engaged in activities like forestry, agriculture, or construction, where soil is being upturned, are more likely to inhale the spores. Identification of such geographical and occupational risk factors facilitates planning specific prevention measures among such exposed communities and workplaces and thus decreases cases of this otherwise serious infection. Demographics, more so immune status and age, contribute significantly to the susceptibility of an individual toward blastomycosis. The greatest risk lies with individuals aged 30 to 60 years, most probably due to greater exposure outdoors compared to other decades. Of greatest importance, however, are immunocompromised patients, such as HIV/AIDS victims, cancer victims, or those receiving immunosuppressive therapy, which show higher susceptibility as their body's infection-fighting ability is significantly diminished. The significance of these factors indicates the necessity of enhanced awareness and vigilance among high-risk populations. Education of this group through public health initiatives on symptoms and preventive measures should be the top priority to facilitate early diagnosis and treatment of the disease. Enhanced awareness and prompt intervention can substantially reduce morbidity and mortality from blastomycosis in high-risk groups. Environmental factors also have a pivotal role to play in the enhancement of the risk of blastomycosis infection, and hence a complete knowledge of such parameters is necessary for control.

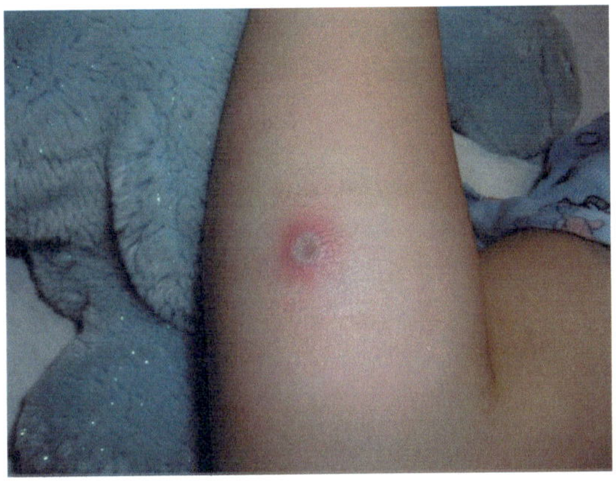

Figure 13.8. Enhanced awareness and prompt intervention can significantly reduce morbidity and mortality associated with blastomycosis in at-risk populations.

Source: https://www.jaad.org/cms/10.1016/j.jaad.2018.04.059/asset/a521168c-be4c-4885-8353-7c78ac716114/main.assets/gr2_lrg.jpg.

The site must be damp and wooded with rich organic debris, which provides a congenial setting for *Blastomyces dermatitidis* to grow. Soil-perturbing or aerosol-generating operations such as construction or agriculture also lead to increased exposure. Therefore, being up to date with local outbreaks becomes necessary; clinicians in Ontario, for example, would have to understand symptoms and areas endemic (Armstrong et al., 2006). This encourages a demand for consistent monitoring of environmental trends and public health alerts, prompting preventive action as well as education among populations affected. By recognizing and acting on these environmental risk factors, we are able to limit the burden of blastomycosis and maximize health outcomes for individuals at risk of infection (Figure 13.8).

13.2.3. Pathogenesis of Blastomycosis

Understanding the pathogenesis of blastomycosis necessitates an exploration of its etiologic agent, *Blastomyces dermatitidis*. The naturally occurring dimorphic fungus typically exists in the form of a mold, particularly in moist, organic debris-rich soil and decaying wood. It grows into yeast upon the introduction of its inhalational conidia into the host organism's body temperature environment. This morphological change is necessary for infection since the yeast phase is more effective at evading the host immune system, thereby worsening the diseases condition.

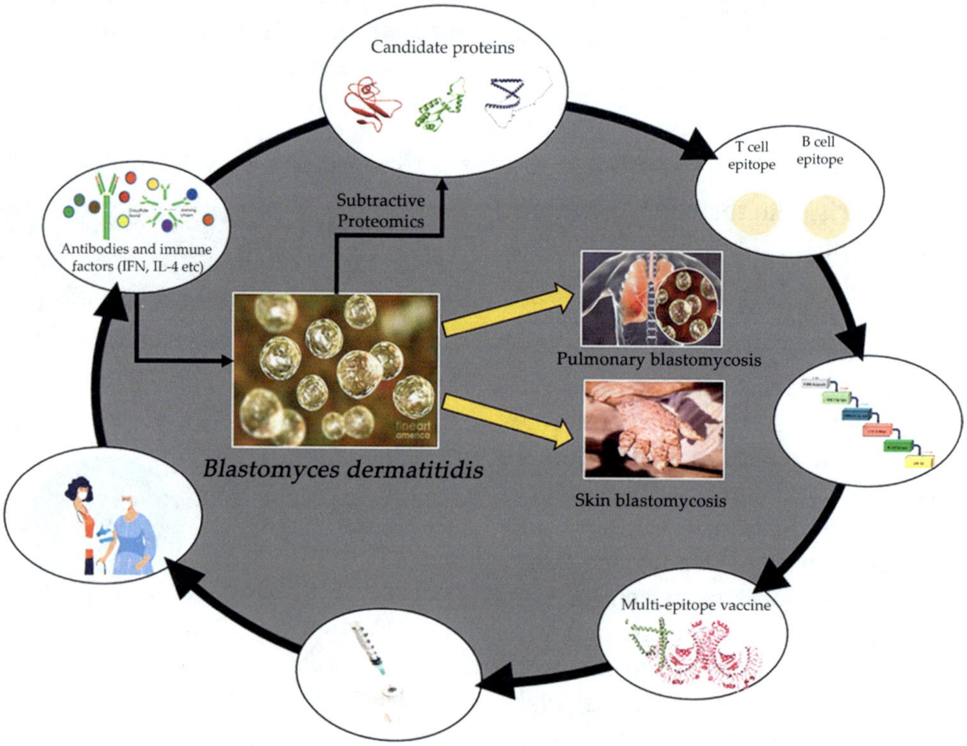

Figure 13.9. Pathogenesis of blastomycosis.

Source: https://www.cell.com/cms/10.1016/j.heliyon.2024.e36153/asset/8f71f0bc-c930-4b2a-8b3a-02aab7e206fa/main.assets/ga1_lrg.jpg.

The immune status of the host is one factor among others that causes successful infection, with immunocompromised hosts being more susceptible. The interplay of these factors is the secret to the ecological niches that are conducive to the organisms life cycle and also its pathogenicity, which makes a complete understanding of the fungus vital in the bid to control the disease (Kauffman et al., 1988).

Subsequent to the initial inhalation of conidia, the involved immunological response plays a pivotal role in understanding the pathogenesis of blastomycosis. Its neutrophils and alveolar macrophages play a role in initial protection against the inhalation of the fungus. *Blastomyces dermatitidis* can, however, escape such immune cells through mechanisms like phenotypic switch and the production of virulence factors like glycoproteins that suppress phagocytosis. The inflammatory response that follows may lead to pulmonary lesions and spread to other organs. Chronic infection patients often present granulomatous inflammation, reflecting the immune response's attempt to encapsulate the infection. The very complex interrelationship between the pathogen and host defense mechanisms emphasizes the importance of further research in identifying specific pathways in which the fungus establishes infection and evades immune responses. Clinical presentation of blastomycosis is also directly correlated with its pathogenesis. The disease spectrum is from asymptomatic pulmonary infections to severe disseminated infections involving the skin, bones, and central nervous system. The symptoms usually appear weeks to months after exposure and may initially be indistinguishable from other pulmonary infections, making diagnosis difficult. Notably, dissemination is not only a function of the virulence of *Blastomyces dermatitidis* but also of the immune competence of the host. Chronic pulmonary blastomycosis becomes highly risky in case of lack of timely treatment and emphasizes the necessity for timely treatment and awareness about the disease process. Investigation into pathogenesis gives valuable hints to the potential therapeutic measures, including antifungal treatment and immunomodulation, which may have been beneficial to the victims (Kauffman et al., 1988) (Figure 13.9).

13.3. Symptoms and Clinical Manifestations

The clinical presentation of blastomycosis is typically insidious and can present a dilemma in diagnosis. The presentation would typically be that of flu or another infection of the respiratory system, hence risking misdiagnosis. Cough, fever, night sweats, and lethargy are symptoms most frequently reported. Weight loss and chest pain on breathing have been observed in some patients. This nonspecific presentation is also aggravated by the absence of certain and prompt diagnostic techniques for acute cases, which requires a high index of suspicion from health workers, particularly for those who reside in or are travelers to endemic areas. The slow development of these symptoms can cloud the underlying fungal disease, thus predisposing to delay in optimal treatment and worsening of clinical outcomes, highlighting the importance of suspicion of potential cases of blastomycosis among high-risk groups (Kauffman et al., 1988). As the disease evolves, more severe signs can manifest, especially if the infection is neglected or improperly treated. Pulmonary blastomycosis can cause severe complications including necrotizing bronchopneumonia, mediastinal lymphadenitis, and chronic lung disease presented as tree-in-bud reticulonodularity on imaging. A unique case is reported in recent literature to demonstrate this sequence in an otherwise healthy young adult who, after initial presentation with flu-like illness, progressed to severe lung disease and was treated with antifungals for cure (Britto et al., 2018). Development of pleural effusion in such circumstances suggests the potential for serious complications in the event that early detection and appropriate antifungal treatment are not implemented. These presentations underscore the importance of early diagnosis and management in achieving effective control of blastomycosis. Diagnosis of blastomycosis is based on a synergy of clinical evaluation, imaging studies, and laboratory diagnosis, which in concert determine the nature of the infection. Where the patient is not responding to conventional antibiotic therapy, further investigation is warranted. For instance, transbronchial needle aspiration cytology and bronchoalveolar lavage are helpful in demonstrating the presence of *Blastomyces dermatitidis*. The problem, however, lies in that without heightened sensitivity to the disease's characteristics and presentation, doctors may belittle the fatal fungal infection and command delayed diagnosis and worse outcome. This underscores the value of education and training beyond residency in the recognition of the diverse clinical presentation of blastomycosis, particularly where the fungus has a focal area of endemicity and among groups at higher risk for serious disease (Kauffman et al., 1988) (Figure 13.10).

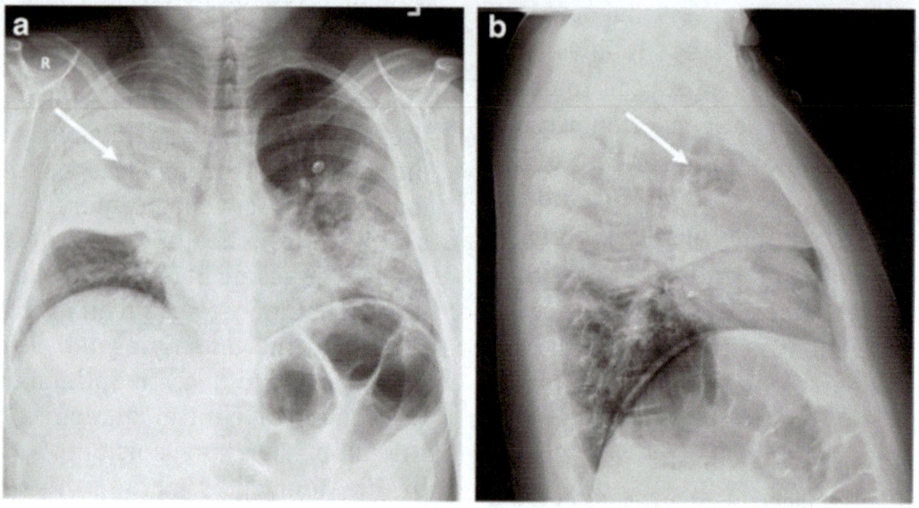

Figure 13.10. Pulmonary blastomycosis can lead to significant complications, including necrotizing bronchopneumonia, mediastinal lymphadenopathy, and chronic lung disease characterized by tree-in-bud reticulonodularity on radiographic imaging.

Source: https://media.springernature.com/lw685/springer-static/image/art%3A10.1007%2Fs00247-022-05402-x/MediaObjects/247_2022_5402_Fig3_HTML.png.

13.3.1. Common Symptoms of Acute Blastomycosis

In describing the general presentation of acute Blastomycosis, its broad clinical spectrum must be recognized because it has a tendency to imitate other respiratory diseases. Most patients enter with flu-like illness, or fever, chills, and malaise, obscuring the chronic nature of the disease. Where individuals have travelled to endemic areas or are themselves from such areas, the common symptomatology with influenza can lead to misdiagnosis and unnecessary delay in treatment. The onset of respiratory distress, cough, and chest pain assumes a greater role, since these symptoms not only enhance the initial clinical presentation but become crucial for differential diagnosis absolutely. Therefore, heightened alertness for common and unusual manifestations is essential on the part of health care providers to enable timely intervention. With the progression of the illness, pulmonary presentation may become worse, resulting in more severe respiratory impairment. In a case study in depth, a patient with acute pulmonary blastomycosis presented with an association of consolidation of the left lung and mediastinal lymphadenopathy. This deterioration was associated with development towards necrotizing bronchopneumonia and pleural effusion, emphasizing the point that symptoms can dramatically deteriorate in the absence of treatment. On radiological images, tree-in-bud reticulonodularity is a feature of late lung involvement. These findings underscore the importance of clinicians developing a high degree of suspicion in the presence of refractory cases that do not respond to standard antibiotic therapy because failure to achieve an early diagnosis will predispose to increased severe clinical sequelae, as attested by the above case study (Britto et al., 2018). Those patients with acute Blastomycosis also have systemic manifestations in the form of night sweats, weight loss, and cutaneous lesions, as these are less common in the initial phases. Cutaneous manifestations in the form of papules or ulcers occur as the disease progresses from the lungs to other tissues, evidence of the multifaceted nature of this fungal disease.

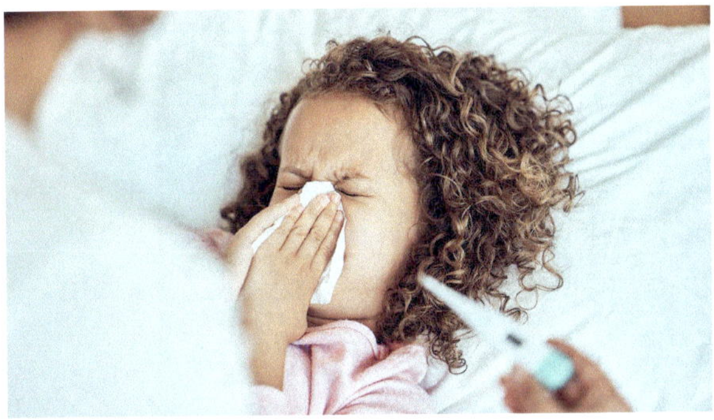

Figure 13.11. Patients typically present with flu-like symptoms, including fever, chills, and fatigue, which may obscure the chronic nature of the disease.

Source: https://www.childrenscolorado.org/globalassets/parenting-advice/articles/cold-vs-flu-article-image_1280x720.jpeg?v=4a556a.

This level of involvement is indicative of the transition from localized respiratory findings to a state where it has generalized, which must alert clinicians of the possibility of blastomycosis in patients with unusual skin findings along with respiratory findings. Early clinical diagnosis and antifungal treatment are necessary to avoid clinical morbidity, as seen in cases where early intervention led to significant recovery and healing of lung lesions (Kauffman et al., 1988). As such, the identification of the variety of acute blastomycosis manifestations is central to maximizing patient outcomes (Figure 13.11).

13.3.2. Chronic Forms and Complications

Chronic blastomycosis often goes along with serious respiratory sequelae, heavily affecting quality of life. Patients may present with a chronic cough, chest pain, and progressive dyspnea, showing the subclinical characteristics of the infections. The pulmonary blastomycosis presentation can be mimicked by other chronic lung infections, such as tuberculosis and lung cancer, and hence may prove to be challenging to diagnose. In cases where the infection is chronic, there is broncholithiasis and diffuse fibrosis. These chronic presentations have the fungus evading the host's immune system, resulting in a long-lasting infection that can result in irreparable lung damage. The chronic pulmonary impairment requires long-term management therapy, typically consisting of antifungal therapy and close monitoring for decompensation. The possibility of fatal complications underscores the importance of early detection of chronic blastomycosis and implementation of optimal treatment regimens in accordance with the patient's clinical status. In addition to respiratory infections, chronic blastomycosis can lead to other complications, including disseminated illness that involves multiple organ systems. Central nervous system, bone, and skin involvement symptoms can be encountered by the patients since the fungus is able to hematogenously disseminate. Of particular mention in this case are the skin, where chronic forms of blastomycosis most often present, as chronic ulcers or chronic lesions, potentially mistaken for other dermatologic conditions. The possibility of chronic cutaneous complications, including those resembling necrobiosis or granulomatous disease, demonstrates the diversified clinical presentation of this mycosis. Systemic infection is feasible and can progress unchecked with existing therapy, resulting in significant morbidity. The multifactorial character of the complications of chronic blastomycosis necessitates an integrative treatment approach, consisting of both antifungal therapy and potential supportive treatment. Understanding of these complications is a requirement for patient outcome enhancement and future research interest guidance. The chronic nature of blastomycosis also presents significant issues with long-term treatment and management efficacy. New evidence indicates that antifungal treatment alone may not be fully effective at managing the diverse range of complications associated with ongoing infection. The application of biologic agents, like those used in the treatment of conditions such as acrodermatitis continua of Hallopeau, can offer new methods for managing chronic cases and preventing irreversible injury such as osteitis or onychodystrophy, as seen in some chronic skin conditions. While there is a standard method for treatment, studies must be conducted to determine better management protocols for chronic blastomycosis. With the potential for severe, long-term sequelae from the disease, encouraging a multidisciplinary approach with both infectious diseases specialists and dermatologists can maximize outcomes. Subsequent studies will need to attempt to define the subtleties of chronic blastomycosis and offer evidence-based treatment recommendations, again supporting the importance of individualized therapeutic care in diverse patient populations (Network, 1957; Beck et al., 2019) (Figure 13.12).

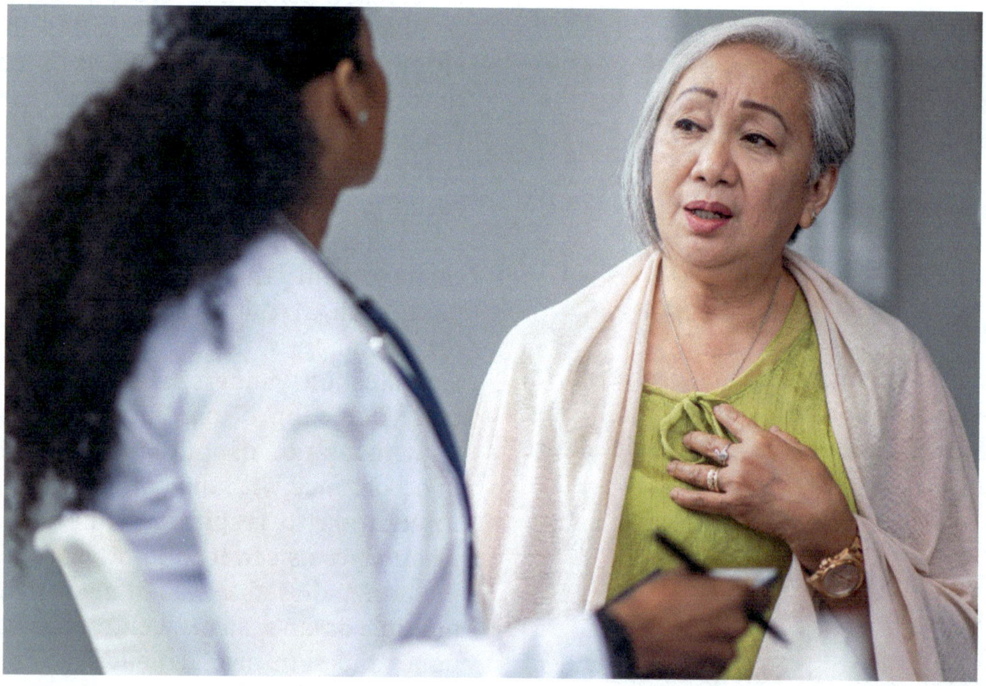

Figure 13.12. Patients may present with a long-standing cough, chest pain, and progressive dyspnea, reflecting the infections insidious nature.

Source: https://images.ctfassets.net/222znibi5gto/RoxvYP9Y7Dr8qtE0Nq3DQ/9c337b7d08128ca5191232ba078e880b/senior-patient-complaining-of-chest-pain-GettyImages-1348111919-3000x2000.jpg.

13.3.3. Differences in Symptoms Based on Demographics

The clinical manifestation of blastomycosis can vary significantly based on demographic factors such as age, gender, and underlying health status. Research indicates that certain populations, particularly those that are immunocompromised, have increased susceptibility to severe manifestations of the disease. For instance, individuals with autoimmune disease or those undergoing immunosuppressive therapy exhibit heightened susceptibility to blastomycosis. These patients may have atypical presentations, including disseminated disease with involvement not only of the lungs but also of extrapulmonary sites like skin and bones, highlighting demographic factors in the manifestation of this fungal infection. Such information is thus a key clinician's tool in diagnosis and in planning therapy. Age groups particularly influence the symptomology of blastomycosis, with older individuals experiencing more severe symptoms than younger individuals.

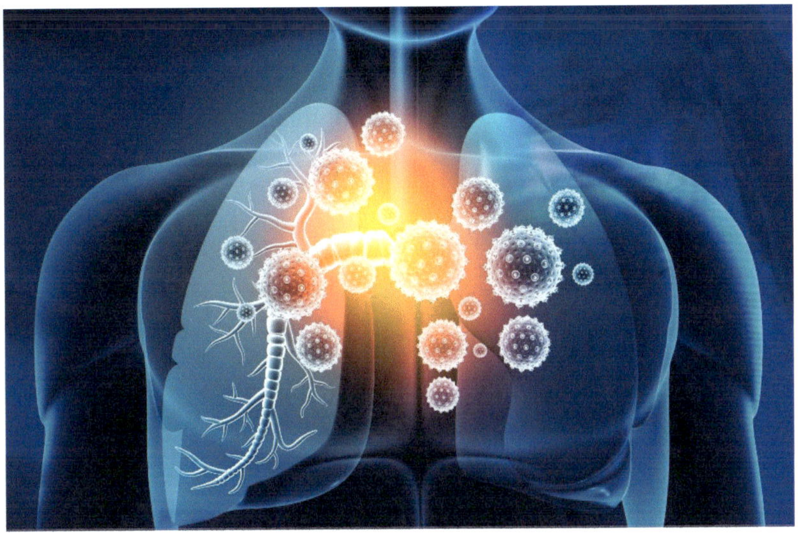

Figure 13.13. Individuals with autoimmune disorders or those undergoing immunosuppressive therapies exhibit heightened vulnerability to blastomycosis.

Source: https://www.news-medical.net/images/news/ImageForNews_734648_16723203205328165.jpg.

Weakened immune status that accompanies advancing age likely raises the risk of complication of blastomycosis. Clinical experience shows that the elderly typically develop acute respiratory distress and disseminated infection more frequently than do younger individuals, which would be consistent with a possibly lower tolerance for the disease. Furthermore, the nature of exposure to the endemic environment, as may be characteristic of outdoor activities in older adults, enhances their risk and, along with variations in symptom severity based on prior health status or concurrent disease states such as diabetes mellitus or chronic lung disease, is responsible for variation in expression (Bariola et al., 2022). These all serve to underscore the interaction between age and the clinical presentation of blastomycosis. Gender differences also emerge through the examination of the symptoms of blastomycosis, with studies revealing that men are more often diagnosed compared to women. This may be attributed to lifestyle, as men are likely to engage in more high-risk outdoor activities that expose them to the fungi that are responsible for the disease. In addition, demographic studies have concluded that men infected with blastomycosis are likely to have more severe pulmonary symptoms than women due to differences in respiratory status and immunity. Aside from this, the presence of comorbidities like smoking or occupational exposure may further complicate the clinical presentation among men, which emphasizes the need for personalized prevention and treatment approaches based on demographics (Bariola et al., 2022). In doing so, understanding such gender differences can assist healthcare providers in treating blastomycosis better (Figure 13.13).

13.4. Diagnosis

Diagnosis of blastomycosis is a sophisticated process, given that its clinical presentation can most often mimic other diseases and lead to the risk of misdiagnosis. The key diagnostic modalities include radiographic imaging, serologic tests, and histopathological examination. Detailed history and physical examination are necessary, particularly regarding potential exposure to environments in which *Blastomyces dermatitidis*, the etiologic agent, is more prevalent. Serological assays can test for the presence of particular antibodies, while cultures of respiratory secretions or tissue biopsies remain the gold standard for certain diagnosis. Interestingly, the tests may be sensitive depending on the stage of disease, and so early testing is important in suspected cases (Hauk et al., 2019). The nuances of diagnosis require an interdisciplinary cooperation of medical practitioners to afford appropriate identification and urgent treatment. Blastomycosis diagnosis is critically dependent on radiological imaging due to its ability to present characteristic pulmonary and extrapulmonary lesions. Whole-body positron emission with fluorine-18-fluorodeoxyglucose has been found highly useful in the identification of fungal lesions. This method is particularly beneficial as the vigorous uptake of FDG by Blastomyces-associated lesions can mimic malignancy, thus making diagnosis difficult (Matwichuk et al., 2001). The challenge is that differentiation between fungal infection and malignancy may be difficult, and hence careful consideration of the severity and pattern of uptake on imaging studies is essential. Such discrimination is not only necessary for diagnosis but also plays a significant role in the subsequent management and therapeutic strategies utilized by the patient. In addition, histopathological examination of biopsy specimens provides direct identification of *Blastomyces dermatitidis*, enabling accurate diagnosis.

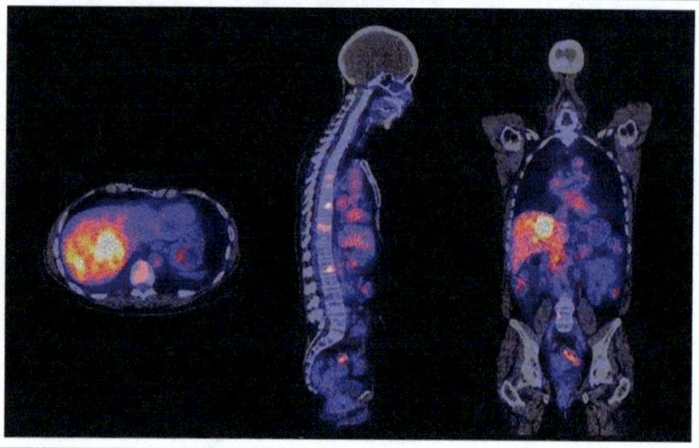

Figure 13.14. Whole-body positron emission tomography (PET) utilizing fluorine-18-fluorodeoxyglucose (FDG) has demonstrated significant utility in detecting fungal lesions.

Source: https://ascopubs.org/cms/10.1200/JCO.2014.57.8278/asset/8be2715b-e515-4007-a23e-4b5826625c4d/assets/graphic/zlj9991051100002.jpeg.

Detection of typical forms of yeast forms within tissue, as displayed by special stain techniques, aids pathologists in demonstrating blastomycosis. In some instances, polymerase chain reaction (PCR) assay is also able to yield rapid and sensitive detection of fungal DNA from clinical specimens. Such molecular tests, though promising, however, are not readily practiced and can require special laboratory facilities (Hauk et al., 2019). Thus, a combination of multiple diagnostic modalities—radiological, serological, and histopathological—is required for a comprehensive assessment of blastomycosis. Early diagnosis and correct diagnosis are important not only in control of the acute infection but also to minimize complications from advanced or misdiagnosed cases of this illness (Figure 13.14).

13.4.1. Clinical Evaluation and Patient History

Understand the clinical evaluation and history of the patient in blastomycosis is critical to make accurate diagnosis and management. The patients come up with a range of complains, including chronic cough, fever, and weight loss, which are similar to any other pulmonary infections, thereby highlighting the challenge of distinguishing blastomycosis from pneumonia. Serious patient history that includes documented exposure to endemic areas, particularly those areas around water bodies where *Blastomyces dermatitidis* is endemic, must be employed in clinical decision-making. Serious interview questioning of work and leisure activities, particularly in northern Wisconsin and adjacent areas bordering Lake Michigan, can enlighten regarding potential risk exposure, as these geographic locations have been found to have high disease rates. This context allows clinicians to design appropriate diagnostic approaches and treatment plans tailor-made to the individual patient's context. The incorporation of advanced diagnostic techniques enhances clinical evaluation of suspected blastomycosis cases. Whole-body positron emission tomography (PET) is a valuable tool that can differentiate between Blastomyces granulomas and neoplastic disease based on its ability to detect high levels of fluorodeoxyglucose (FDG) uptake in Blastomyces infection. Research indicates that FDG uptake by blastomycosis lesions is comparable to that of malignant tumors, thereby illustrating the necessity to cautiously interpret these imaging results to avoid misdiagnosis (Matwichuk et al., 2001). Therefore, when evaluating patients, clinicians must be mindful of imaging and symptom findings indicating blastomycosis, and PET scanning can be a helpful adjunct that helps identify disease distribution and progression, which can dictate treatments that can range from antifungal therapy to surgical intervention. Patient history is also essential to long-term management of blastomycosis. Understanding the patients' basic state of health and immunocompromised status may exclude them from responding to treatment as well as test for complications.

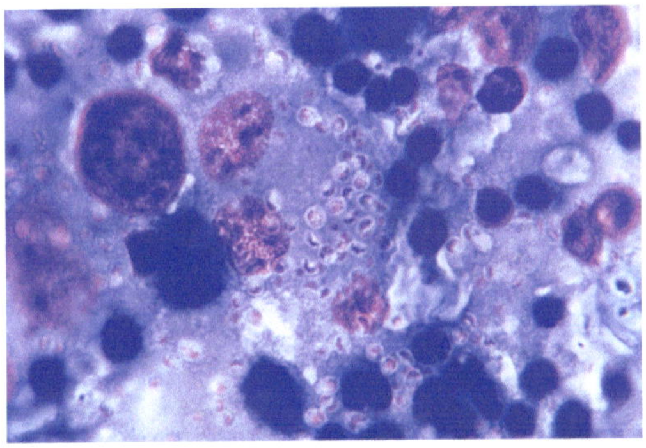

Figure 13.15. The ecology of *Blastomyces dermatitidis* suggests a complex relationship between the pathogen and environmental factors; thus, patient histories that reflect geographical and environmental exposure can enrich clinical insights and inform ongoing public health initiatives.

Source: https://ecuadoctors.com/wp-content/uploads/h5p/content/6/images/file-5aa0926e801fe.jpg.

The ecology of *Blastomyces dermatitidis* suggests a complex interaction between environmental component and pathogen; therefore, patient histories that take into account geographical and environmental exposure can add clinical understanding and inform current public health policy (Bakerspigel et al., 2008). For instance, data demonstrating common environmental settings in which the fungus's survival is probable can guide public health messages and encourage prevention where it has been shown to occur. An integrated patient history and clinical evaluation therefore not only aid in expedient diagnosis and treatment but advance the overall effort toward determining and eliminating the risk factors of blastomycosis (Figure 13.15).

13.4.2. Laboratory Tests and Imaging Techniques

Accurate diagnosis of blastomycosis, a fungal infection caused by *Blastomyces dermatitidis*, relies heavily on the integration of laboratory diagnostic tests with imaging to assess for the disease and degree of infection. Initial diagnosis is occasionally followed by serologic studies to detect antibodies to Blastomyces. Such tests are inconsistent and may necessitate confirmatory lab tests. Direct visualization of the organism by culture from tissue biopsies and body fluids remains the gold standard for definitive diagnosis. In a case of suspected pulmonary involvement, imaging procedures like chest X-ray or CT scan are valuable to identify abnormal pulmonary patterns, such as nodules or infiltrative lesions that may present masquerading other lung pathology. All these imaging and laboratory modalities are indispensable to the attainment of an early diagnosis and then proper therapy in patients, particularly in the endemic environment. In a remarkable case report, a previously healthy adult presented with flu-like symptoms that were not responsive to standard antibiotic therapy, ending in a diagnosis of progressive acute pulmonary blastomycosis. Radiologic findings, as part of transbronchial needle aspiration cytology and bronchoalveolar lavage cultures, were instrumental in diagnosing the infection. Radiologic imaging techniques showed diffuse pulmonary alterations of tree-in-bud reticulonodularity and mediastinal lymphadenopathy that served to differentiate blastomycosis from other infections. The ability of imaging studies to follow disease progression is noteworthy in that mediastinal lymphadenopathy and pleural effusions may signify infection dissemination. Thus, frequent radiographic follow-up, along with laboratory examination, is crucial to optimize patient care and prevent treatment complications. Newer imaging modalities such as Gallium-67 scans have also demonstrated promise in the work-up of blastomycosis. While these nuclear medicine techniques were traditionally utilized in the diagnosis of other fungal infections, they have been found helpful in assessing the extent of pulmonary impairment in patients with blastomycosis. Gallium-67 scanning can be used in correlation with the disease course and mark those sites of active infection, thereby assisting in better prognosis of the patient. This synergy between noninvasive imaging and laboratory tests underscores the value of a multidisciplinary approach to managing blastomycosis. The application of these integrative technologies introduces early diagnosis as well as directs treatment and ultimately results in good clinical outcomes. With advances in laboratory procedures and imaging modalities, clinicians can currently detect and manage this potentially lethal fungal infection better (Figure 13.16).

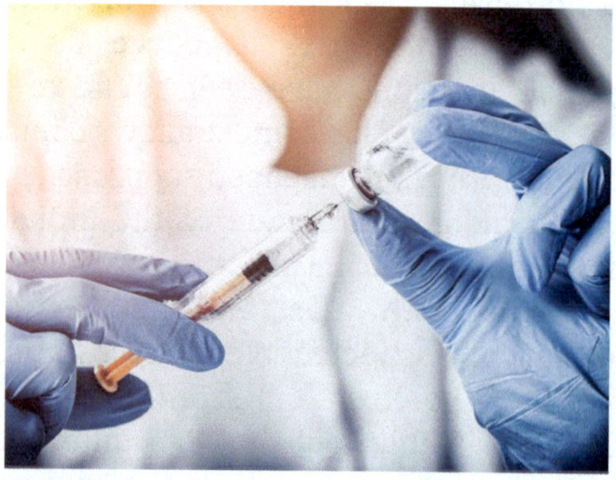

Figure 13.16. Gallium-67 scans.

Source: https://media.post.rvohealth.io/wp-content/uploads/2020/08/gallium-scan_thumb-1-732x549.jpg.

13.4.3. Differential Diagnosis with Other Diseases

With reference to blastomycosis diagnosis, a differential diagnosis incorporating several infectious as well as non-infectious diseases needs to be kept in mind. Conditions such as histoplasmosis, coccidioidomycosis, and other systemic mycoses bear close resemblance to blastomycosis due to overlapping clinical presentation in the form of respiratory and systemic disease. These conditions present with fever, malaise, and chest pain, further complicating the diagnosis. The mere existence of specific geographic exposures and immunocompromised status can serve to limit the differential. A prime example is the shared endemic occurrence of blastomycosis and histoplasmosis in the Midwest, requiring fine-sliced consideration of patient history and lab findings to distinguish between these well-established mycoses. Discrimination against bacterial infections such as pneumonia must also be made because of the difference in treatment approaches required by these conditions. While pneumonia can also present with respiratory findings, diagnostic radiography and microbiological tests including sputum culture and blood cultures help clinicians distinguish these entities better. In blastomycosis, radiographic findings can similarly detect a characteristic imaging pattern of pulmonary nodules and cavitation, emphasizing the need for a diligent diagnostic workup. Clinical setting and response to initial therapies can similarly be the hallmark features in distinguishing blastomycosis from other respiratory illnesses, especially in patients with atypical presentation which may mimic more common diseases. Finally, non-infectious disease such as sarcoidosis and granulomatosis with polyangiitis must also be considered in the differential diagnosis of blastomycosis. Both illnesses can yield granulomatous inflammation, thereby causing pulmonary disease and extrapulmonary manifestations that are the same as those of blastomycosis. For example, patients with sarcoidosis will have pulmonary nodules, adenopathy, and constitutional symptoms, as this underscores the importance of histological documentation to make a proper diagnosis. Diagnostic imaging and tissue biopsies are essential parts of this process wherein histopathological study has the potential to show unequivocal patterns characteristic of blastomycosis and thereby differentiate it from other granulomatous disorders such as those in patients with certain malignancies or systemic disorders such as that documented in Buikstra et al. (1978) and Anwer et al. (2018) (Figure 13.17).

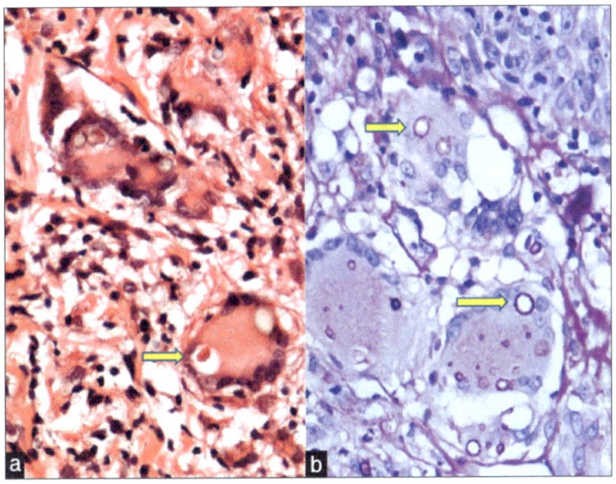

Figure 13.17. Diagnostic imaging alongside tissue biopsies plays an integral role in this process, as histopathological examination can reveal distinct patterns characteristic of blastomycosis.

Source: https://ijdvl.com/content/126/2013/79/1/Images/ijdvl_2013_79_1_92_104676_f4.jpg.

13.5. Treatment Options

The treatment modes for blastomycosis are typically dependent on the severity of the infection and the patient's health status. In plain cases, especially asymptomatic or mild cases, mere observation would suffice. But moderate to severe cases oftentimes require antifungal therapy. The most common mode of treatment is most frequently itraconazole, which has been found effective against the fungal pathogen *Blastomyces dermatitidis*. In severely ill or immunocompromised individuals, intravenous amphotericin B would be the treatment of choice due to its more thorough antifungal action and rapid onset. The treatment thus hinges on a wise assessment of presentation and patient-related factors, indicating the necessity for individualized treatment protocols in the management of this disseminated fungal infection. Improved treatment regimens in development are promising for patients with treatment-resistant blastomycosis. These particularly include those that do not respond to standard antifungal treatment. Recent evidence suggests these could be helped by the use of adjunct therapies in the form of immunomodulatory agents, with the effectiveness of treatment increased. Examples include cases of blastomycosis-like pyoderma that have had satisfactory outcomes with treatment modalities such as acitretin, especially where patients present with co-morbidities such as diabetes or immunosuppression making it complicated to utilize the standard treatment modality. Literature confirms that despite the shortcomings of conventional treatments, the addition of new modalities of treatment can bring dramatic improvement, but guidelines need to be developed based on further research on these difficult cases (Adişen et al., 2011).

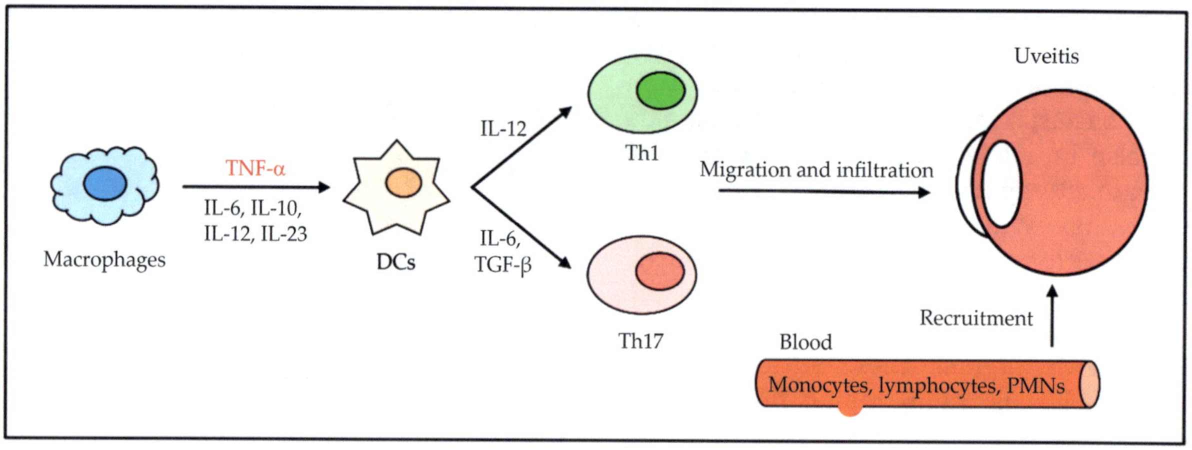

Figure 13.18. Agents such as anti-tumor necrosis factor candidates have been employed in similar inflammatory skin conditions, leading to promising outcomes.

Source: https://www.mdpi.com/ijms/ijms-22-02719/article_deploy/html/images/ijms-22-02719-g005.png.

Also, biologic agents are being more and more considered for the treatment of complicated fungal infections, though specifics concerning blastomycosis are scarce. The effectiveness of some biologics in the management of conditions like acrodermatitis continua of Hallopeau indicates the promise for long-term application in fungal infections. Medications such as anti-tumor necrosis factor agents have found application in similar inflammatory cutaneous disorders with acceptable outcomes. The application of biologics to treat blastomycosis, however, needs to be researched thoroughly with the use of large clinical trials to confirm their safety and effectiveness. The field is changing, and the integration of infectious disease specialists and dermatologists has the potential to pave the way for new treatment protocols, ultimately improving patient outcomes (Beck et al., 2019) (Figure 13.18).

13.5.1. Antifungal Medications and Their Effectiveness

Treatment of blastomycosis, the systemic fungal disease that is caused predominantly by the organism *Blastomyces dermatitidis*, relies almost entirely on antifungal medications, which are the cornerstone of treatment of the disease. The key pharmacologic agents available for treatment are itraconazole and amphotericin B, with drug choice depending on the severity of the disease. Itraconazole is most commonly employed for its oral form to permit outpatient treatment for mild to moderate disease. Conversely, amphotericin B is mostly reserved for severe infections due to its very potent activity, yet it produces a higher rate of adverse reactions. The drugs' pharmacodynamics reveal their modes of action, i.e., disruption of fungal cell membranes or inhibition of essential biosynthetic processes. Such an individualized method of antifungal therapy emphasizes the importance of expedient clinical intervention as untreated blastomycosis is highly morbific. In addition to conventional antifungal therapy, recent advances in topical antifungal preparations have broadened therapy for cutaneous blastomycosis and related infections.

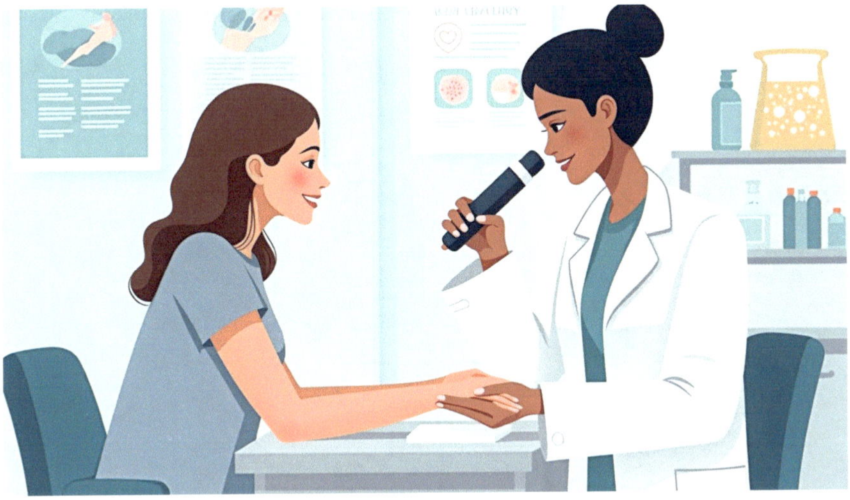

Figure 13.19. Impaired immune function in these patients necessitates a meticulous approach to antifungal therapy, often requiring careful monitoring and adjustment of treatment regimens.

Source: https://www.kaya.in/media/mageplaza/blog/post/b/e/betamethasone-uses-benefits-side-effects-guide.jpg.

New studies have explored new cream vehicles that contain more than one antifungal ingredient, such as garlic oil and clove oil, which have synergistic activity. Topical therapy has been effective, particularly in the treatment of localized disease with fewer side effects at the systemic level associated with oral or intravenous drugs. The process of development relies on modifying the creams physicochemical characteristics to achieve the best drug delivery and efficacy. (Rana et al., 2022) illustrates this through a detailed analysis of a cream containing active pharmaceutical ingredients combined with emulsifiers and additives aimed at promoting skin health, which would prove to be more beneficial for patients with dermatological conditions caused by blastomycosis.

Also, the effectiveness of antifungal medications may be checked among specific patient groups, i.e., lung transplant recipients, who are highly susceptible to fungal infections such as those caused by *Blastomyces dermatitidis.* (Escamilla et al., 2023) also highlights the significance of early diagnosis and treatment because these types of fungal infections in the mentioned population can have catastrophic results ranging from damage to allograft. Impaired immune function in these patients necessitates a judicious antifungal treatment strategy, which, in most cases, requires close monitoring and titration of therapeutic regimens. This focused therapy not only works against the immediate danger presented by fungal infection but also helps to prevent the long-term complications of chronic lung allograft dysfunction, further defining the indispensable role that effective antifungal regimens play in high-risk populations suffering from blastomycosis and other invasive fungal diseases (Figure 13.19).

13.5.2. Duration and Management of Treatment

Therapy of blastomycosis involves a structured process that is complemented with appropriate diagnosis and early treatment. The course of therapy commonly adopted for uncomplicated pulmonary blastomycosis typically starts with the administration of antifungal drugs in the form of itraconazole, which is typically prolonged to six to twelve months.

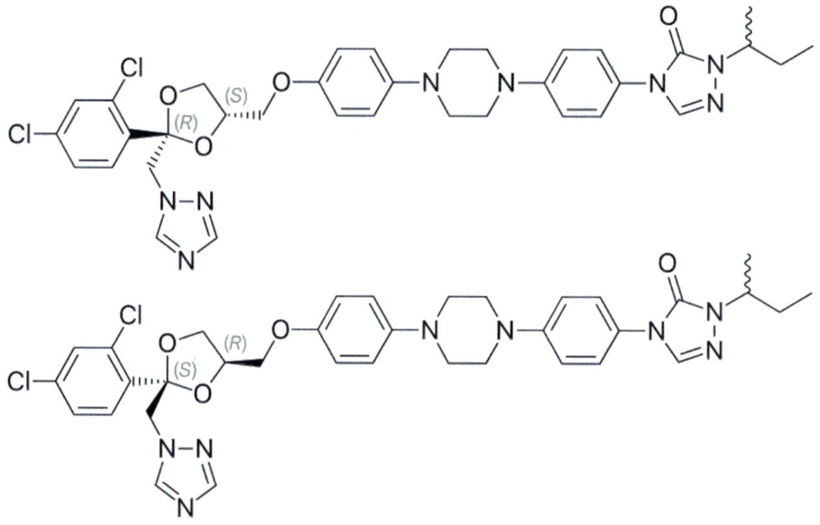

Figure 13.20. Itraconazole.

Source: https://upload.wikimedia.org/wikipedia/commons/thumb/0/0d/Itraconazole.svg/1920px-Itraconazole.svg.png.

Besides being essential for the remission of symptoms, this duration is also important for mycological eradication. But when the infection is more extensive or disseminated, treatment may progress to the administration of amphotericin B as the initial treatment, and then the extended duration on itraconazole. Most apparent in this case is the observer variation of treatment duration due to patients' immune responses and the patients' own health status, to point towards optimizing the duration based on clinical improvement to enhance outcomes by individualizing the treatment courses. The management of blastomycosis extends beyond mere pharmacological control; it requires strict monitoring across the treatment phase to evaluate effectiveness and tolerance. Duration of treatment is a relevant factor because the longer the duration of treatment, the more favorable the patient outcomes, particularly in immunocompromised patients who are at risk of developing complications. Follow-up evaluation comes into play in determining whether to extend the course of treatment since the majority of the patients may still have residual signs or laboratory findings of infection despite initial treatment. This adaptive approach is concordant with guidelines for invasive fungal infection management, which emphasize not only the completion of regular treatment protocols but also the adaptable plan based on particular patient factors like underlying illness and fungal load severity (Escamilla et al., 2023).

The complexity of blastomycosis treatment dictates the convergence of highly educated practice protocols tending towards empiric antifungal therapy while mandating individual risk determinations. Existing reviews have underlined the gaps in standardization particularly regarding empirical antifungal therapy for mold disease and other blastomycosis (Cockle et al., 2016). One of the primary concerns is in determining when to discontinue empirical and institute targeted therapy based on test findings and response to treatment. Recommendations from existing clinical practice guidelines indicate heterogeneity in the quality of process and specificity regarding termination of antifungal treatment. These differences represent an acute requirement for additional research to enhance management strategies and maximize the efficacy of treatment regimens, thus ensuring both guideline adherence and optimal patient outcomes in the management of blastomycosis (Figure 13.20).

13.5.3. Role of Supportive Care in Recovery

Supportive care plays a significant role in the management of patients diagnosed with blastomycosis, given the multidimensional nature of the fungal infection. Blastomycosis may present as diverse symptoms, including respiratory insufficiency and systemic illness, which necessitate extensive management strategies. Supportive care constitutes a variety of interventions, ranging from oxygen therapy, fluid hydration, to enteral nutrition, all aimed at enhancing the patient's general resilience while undergoing treatment. These supportive measures not only help in the management of the symptoms but also facilitate the body to react best to antifungal therapy, maximizing the success of recovery. The inclusion of support care in clinical pathways legitimates the importance of a whole-person treatment approach and the realization that vanquishing the infection itself is inadequate without allowance for the surrounding needs of the patient's health and wellness. Immunocompromised individuals with blastomycosis require tailored supportive therapy measures that not only target the infection but also treat predisposing conditions for adverse outcomes. Double-directional focus is crucial because secondary infection or complications can occur when the immune system is weakened. For instance, in pediatrics where invasive fungal infection is presented, prescriptions are made for some antifungal treatments accompanied by support such as vitamins and anti-inflammatory drugs to boost immune function (Cockle et al., 2016). Similarly, use of prophylactic measures among immunocompromised individuals is crucial because maximal health is able to lower secondary infection risk by a great extent as well as facilitate overall recovery from blastomycosis. Therefore, doctors must adopt an integrated strategy in a manner that secondary prophylactic procedures are aptly integrated with the treatment regime of the patient to ease the recovery process. Aside from drug treatments, emotional care and counseling for the patient are also of great significance. Patients recovered from blastomycosis generally undergo great psychological stress, which can jeopardize their physical recovery. There must be incorporation of psychosocial support systems like counseling and education about the disease, treatment expectations, and self-care mechanisms in creating an environment that is healing and supportive. For example, as was demonstrated in cases of deep pyoderma where supportive therapy, such as vitamins, was continued to facilitate recovery, the same integrative approaches may be applied to blastomycosis (Damhuri et al., 2024). By focusing on both the emotional and medical aspects of patients, supportive care ultimately enhances treatment compliance and overall outcomes, placing its importance prominently in the total care model of this complex infection (Figure 13.21).

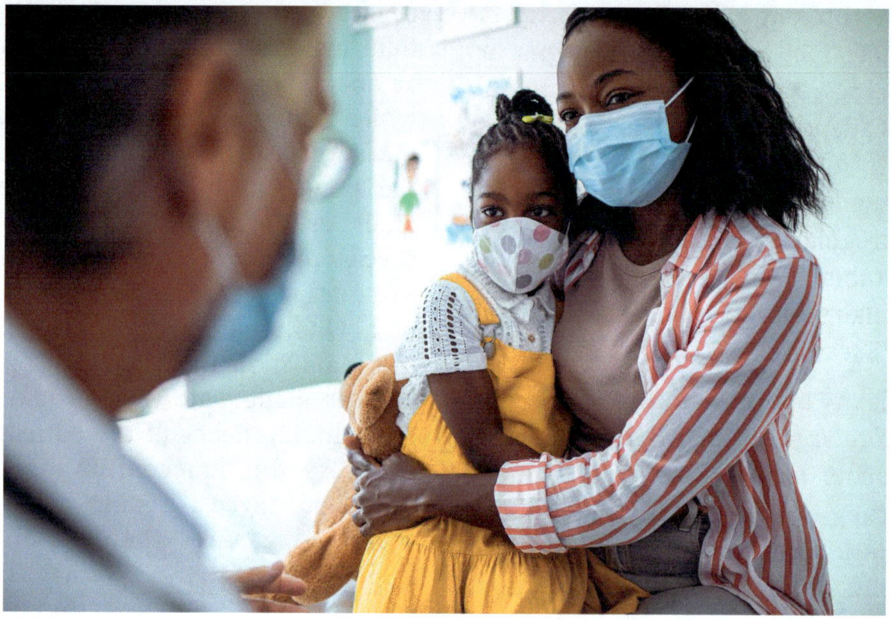

Figure 13.21. Supportive care plays a crucial role in the recovery of patients diagnosed with blastomycosis, particularly due to the multifaceted nature of this fungal infection.

Source: https://www.verywellhealth.com/thmb/N4dHE7I-GahTeskCR75Pyhg69-A=/1500x0/filters:no_upscale():max_bytes(150000):strip_icc()/GettyImages-1266645987-794e994a28604f73ae14d3d256d2d521.jpg.

SUMMARY

The clinical presentation of blastomycosis, an infection of *Blastomyces dermatitidis*, highlights the key problems in treating it. Areas of controversy in recent years have revolved around identifying new antifungal drugs that have novel mechanisms of action. Such therapy is currently thwarted by issues regarding toxicity, potential drug interactions, and the emergence of resistance. New antifungal drug developments, including glucan synthesis inhibitors ibrexafungerp and rezafungin, are potential alternatives to traditional therapy. New formulations and treatments also aim to improve safety profiles with decreased interaction, thereby achieving more efficient treatment of infections like blastomycosis. Research into such treatment developments is important as they provide an insight into overcoming the hurdles posed by existing treatment regimens, and thus promising hope for patients stricken by this debilitating fungal infection (Coler-Reilly et al., 2020). Another important area of discourse in the field of blastomycosis is the nature of accurate diagnosis, which forms the cornerstone of effective treatment outcomes. Because the diseases present differently, it is particularly challenging to differentiate blastomycosis from other respiratory infections. The prognosis of the patient largely relies on early detection, and as such, more sophisticated methods of diagnosis are required. Current molecular methods, such as polymerase chain reaction (PCR) testing, can possibly accelerate detection of *Blastomyces dermatitidis* in samples, thereby enabling early treatment. Moreover, information regarding the epidemiologic trends of blastomycosis can inform public health policy and promote the awareness of healthcare practitioners. These measures must be taken in endemic areas so that there is early diagnosis and treatment of infection, which is crucial to prevent morbidity and mortality from the disease (Hanson et al., 2000). The ongoing evolution in diagnosis and treatment of blastomycosis contains a bigger story regarding the co-evolution between humans and pathogens. While scientists venture into the complexities of fungal infections, it is obvious that the understanding of the past of such diseases enriches today's practice of medicine. Through the analysis of the skeletons of historical populations, paleopathologists have illustrated the ways in which human beings have even in the past lived in co-existence with different pathogens. This understanding reveals how contemporary populations could respond to infections like blastomycosis. Hence, the integration of conclusions obtained from contemporary medicine and paleopathology can lead to a revolutionized strategy in the management of fungal infections. Through the understanding of how the infections were widespread among ancient populations, researchers can make comparisons that can inform future epidemiological studies and treatment plans, for the sake of the overall management of blastomycosis (Coler-Reilly et al., 2020).

A CLOSER LOOK

GALLIUM-67 SCANS

Gallium-67 scans are another type of nuclear medicine imaging used to detect inflammation, infection, and certain tumors. Gallium-67 is a radiopharmaceutical that complexes with transferrin and localizes in areas of ongoing inflammation or actively growing tumors. The patient is imaged with a gamma camera several hours to days following intravenous injection, depending on the rationale for the study. These scans work particularly well in disease diagnosis like lymphoma, osteomyelitis, and sarcoidosis. However, more advanced imaging modalities like PET scans are coming into popularity quickly due to higher resolution and specificity.

REFERENCES

1. Adişen, A., Bianchi, B., Brinkmeier, C., Choi, D., Dutta, H., Harish, H., Hegarty, A., et al. (2011). Blastomycosis-like pyoderma with good response to acitretin. https://core.ac.uk/download/pdf/8610222.pdf (accessed on 27th June 2025).
2. Agrawal, V., Brinda, B. J., & Farag, S. S. (2020). *Histoplasma capsulatum* infection in an allogeneic hematopoietic stem cell transplant patient receiving voriconazole prophylaxis. https://core.ac.uk/download/299809034.pdf (accessed on 27th June 2025).
3. Ali, N., Gilbert, R., & Pervaiz, M. (2018). The prevalence and under-reporting of needle-stick injuries among dental healthcare workers in Pakistan: A systematic review. https://core.ac.uk/download/159074647.pdf (accessed on 27th June 2025).
4. Ampel, A., Anstead, G., Babady, N., Baddley, J., Bariola, J., Ben-Ami, R., Bialek, R., et al. (2012). Pulmonary fungal infections. http://deepblue.lib.umich.edu/bitstream/2027.42/92435/1/j.1440-1843.2012.02150.x.pdf (accessed on 27th June 2025).
5. Andrade, E. de, Sabino, R., & Simões, D. (2023). Fungi in a one health perspective. https://core.ac.uk/download/599463930.pdf (accessed on 27th June 2025).
6. Anwer, A., Armao, D., Atlas, S., Beck, J., Bourekas, E., Canal, C., Celli, R., et al. (2018). Imaging diagnosis: Magnetic resonance imaging of diffuse leptomeningeal oligodendrogliomatosis in a dog with "dural tail sign." https://core.ac.uk/download/77600867.pdf (accessed on 27th June 2025).
7. Armstrong, C., Bakerspigel, A., Baumgardner, D., Bernstein, H., Bialek, R., Limerick, B., Bradsher, R., et al. (2006). Blastomycosis in Ontario, 1994–2003. https://core.ac.uk/download/pdf/8738882.pdf (accessed on 27th June 2025).
8. Bakerspigel, A., Peterson, A. T., DiSalvo, A. F., Hirzel, A. H., MacEachren, A. M., Peterson, A. T., Peterson, A. T., et al. (2008). Ecologic niche modeling of *Blastomyces dermatitidis* in Wisconsin. https://core.ac.uk/download/pdf/8001225.pdf (accessed on 27th June 2025).
9. Bariola, J. R., Dare, R., Krishnan, G., Power, J., et al. (2022). Comparison of indirect fungal diagnostic tests in patients with proven histoplasmosis. https://core.ac.uk/download/551626375.pdf (accessed on 27th June 2025).
10. Beck, K. M., Bhutani, T., Liao, W., Ly, K., et al. (2019). Acrodermatitis continua of Hallopeau: Clinical perspectives. https://core.ac.uk/download/323063230.pdf (accessed on 27th June 2025).
11. Britto, J. (2018). Non-resolving community acquired pneumonia (CAP) due to *Blastomyces dermatitidis* (pulmonary blastomycosis): Case report and review of literature. https://core.ac.uk/download/217211048.pdf (accessed on 27th June 2025).
12. Buikstra, J. E., & Cook, D. C. (1978). Pre-Columbian tuberculosis: An epidemiological approach. https://core.ac.uk/download/51294881.pdf (accessed on 27th June 2025).
13. Bull, M., Fry, H., Hayward, A. C., & Le Comber, S. C. (2015). Spatial methods for infectious disease outbreak investigations: Systematic literature review. https://core.ac.uk/download/77039456.pdf (accessed on 27th June 2025).
14. Camargo, E. E., De Lima, M. C. L., Etchebehere, E. C. S. D. C., Pires, B. C., Ramos, C. D., Santos, A. D. O., Teixeira, A. B. M. D. J., et al. (2015). Gallium-67 imaging in a patient with Para

coccidioidomycosis: A case report. https://core.ac.uk/download/296634560.pdf (accessed on 27th June 2025).

15. Cheang, M., Choptiany, M., Embil, J. M., Hammond, G., et al. (2016). Risk factors for acquisition of endemic blastomycosis. https://core.ac.uk/download/644030943.pdf (accessed on 27th June 2025).
16. Chen, L., Li, M., Roberts, C. A., Zhao, H., et al. (2019). A male adult skeleton from the Han Dynasty in Shaanxi, China (202 BC–220 AD) with bone changes that possibly represent spinal tuberculosis. https://core.ac.uk/download/578096638.pdf (accessed on 27th June 2025).
17. Cockle, J. V., Hassan, H., James, B., Lethaby, L., et al. (2016). Critical review of current clinical practice guidelines for antifungal therapy in pediatric hematology and oncology. https://core.ac.uk/download/74235423.pdf (accessed on 27th June 2025).
18. Coler-Reilly, A., Larson, L., Rauseo, A. M., Spec, A., et al. (2020). Hope on the horizon: Novel fungal treatments in development. https://core.ac.uk/download/287888129.pdf (accessed on 27th June 2025).
19. Damhuri, D., Insulistyowati, A., Ningsih, A. T., Safitri, R., et al. (2024). Diagnosis and treatment of deep pyoderma in a Maine Coon cat. https://core.ac.uk/download/641649909.pdf (accessed on 27th June 2025).
20. Escamilla, J. E., January, S. E., & Vazquez Guillamet, R. (2023). Diagnosis and treatment of fungal infections in lung transplant recipients. https://core.ac.uk/download/572691204.pdf (accessed on 27th June 2025).
21. Halls, V., Kohn, B., Krämer, F., Lappin, M., et al. (2022). Vector-borne and other pathogens of potential relevance disseminated by relocated cats. https://core.ac.uk/download/553570211.pdf (accessed on 27th June 2025).
22. Hanson, A. J. (2000). Skeletal evidence of tuberculosis and treponematosis in a prehistoric population from west-central Illinois. https://core.ac.uk/download/212829224.pdf (accessed on 27th June 2025).
23. Hauk, E. (2019). Evaluation of an outpatient parenteral antimicrobial therapy program in a specialty clinic setting. https://core.ac.uk/download/228020196.pdf (accessed on 27th June 2025).
24. Kauffman, C. A., & Terpenning, M. S. (1988). Deep fungal infections in the elderly. https://deepblue.lib.umich.edu/bitstream/2027.42/111183/1/j.1532-5415.1988.tb04028.x.pdf (accessed on 27th June 2025).
25. Khrais, M. Z., Smith, J., Gandhi, T., Arif, S., & Rico, J. C. (2025). A cautionary tale of false-positive histoplasma urine antigen in an HIV patient: A case report. *Access Microbiology, 7*. https://www.semanticscholar.org/paper/989313cda5a174bed58c86d22cb2d8befd0ca134 (accessed on 27th June 2025).
26. Knight, R. A. (2007). *PhD* [Doctoral dissertation]. https://core.ac.uk/download/276268298.pdf (accessed on 27th June 2025).
27. Larsson, A. E., Renlund, H., Andréasson, B., Holmberg, H., Liljeholm, M., & Själander, A. (2024). Myelofibrosis therapies and risk of major bleeding, thrombotic events and mortality, a matched nationwide population-based study. *Blood*. https://www.semanticscholar.org/paper/5eb7384321e58638e03db0c98bc0ae8d5713713c (accessed on 27th June 2025).

28. Lee, J. S., & Van Der Putten, W. (2011). *Soil Borne Human Diseases*. https://core.ac.uk/download/38621779.pdf (accessed on 27th June 2025).

29. Lehigh Valley Health Network. (1957). *Journal of the Allentown Hospital*. https://core.ac.uk/download/267859779.pdf (accessed on 27th June 2025).

30. Matwichuk, C. L. (2001). Characterization of fluorine-18-fluorodeoxyglucose accumulation in *Blastomyces dermatitidis*-associated inflammation. https://core.ac.uk/download/588288269.pdf (accessed on 27th June 2025).

31. Rana, A., Saxena, C., Singh, D., Paul, P., Kumar, P., & Pandey, R. K. (2022). The role of herbal drugs for the management of fungal skin diseases: A review. https://core.ac.uk/download/603898073.pdf (accessed on 27th June 2025).

32. Seitz, A. E., Watts, B., Klein, B. S., Klein, B. S., Hage, C. A., Steiner, C. A., Baumgardner, D., et al. (2014). Incidence and trends of blastomycosis-associated hospitalizations in the United States. https://core.ac.uk/download/230775531.pdf (accessed on 27th June 2025).

33. Sims, E. (2021). Important canine zoonoses from a public health perspective and the introduction of companion animal surveillance in the Prairie Provinces of Canada. https://core.ac.uk/download/482717861.pdf (accessed on 27th June 2025).

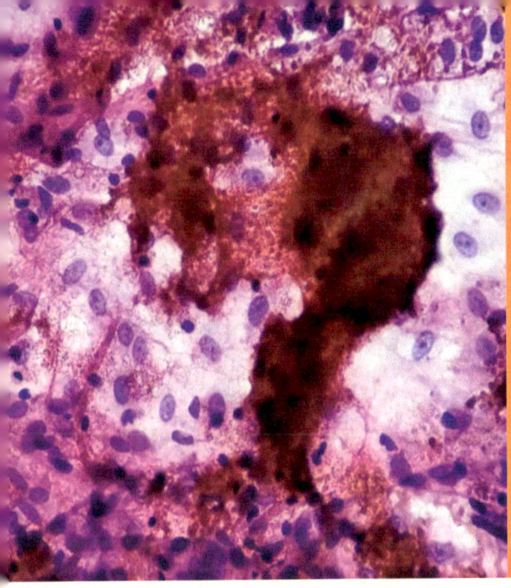

Chapter 14
HISTOPLASMOSIS

Contents

Introduction

Histoplasmosis, due to the fungus *Histoplasma capsulatum*, is a significant public health issue in most regions of the world, particularly in the Americas. The organism inhabits environments rich in bird and bat droppings, typically in soil under old buildings and caves. Pulmonary infection is the most frequent presentation, and most are asymptomatic or have minimal symptoms. In immunocompromised individuals, infection can be serious and lead to disseminated disease and respiratory impairment. Understanding epidemiology of histoplasmosis is critical to effective prevention and control. Because of its multisystem presentation and capacity to exert extreme effects on health, healthcare providers must remain vigilant to diagnose and treat the fungal infection. Histoplasmosis is diagnosed but complicated by having multiple presentations. Histoplasmosis can have presentations that are similar to those of other pulmonary conditions, and this can render it misdiagnosed by clinicians who lack knowledge of its presentation. This necessitates a clear understanding of its pathophysiology, e.g., immune responses evoked during infection. In cases of chronic lung diseases or conditions requiring prolonged antibacterial treatment, histoplasmosis may be a causative factor of respiratory distress. Chronic low-grade inflammation has been said to play a central role in the pathogenesis of the disease, and thus additional research into the immunological determinants is needed to determine effective treatments (Hügle et al., 2011). Last but not least, the global ramifications of histoplasmosis attest to the necessity of increased awareness on the part of medical providers, particularly in the endemic regions. As more worldwide travel and migration occur, a greater threat of histoplasmosis exists beyond its traditional geographical areas. According to literature that reports travel medicine, physicians can make an effort to identify infectious and environmental threats of travel in the form of disease such as fungal disease in the form of histoplasmosis. As the disease knowledge evolves, further research and education are necessary in reducing its impact on public health. By encouraging awareness and improving diagnostic protocols, the end result is yet to encourage improved patient outcomes and prevent the severe consequences associated with histoplasmosis (Figure 14.1).

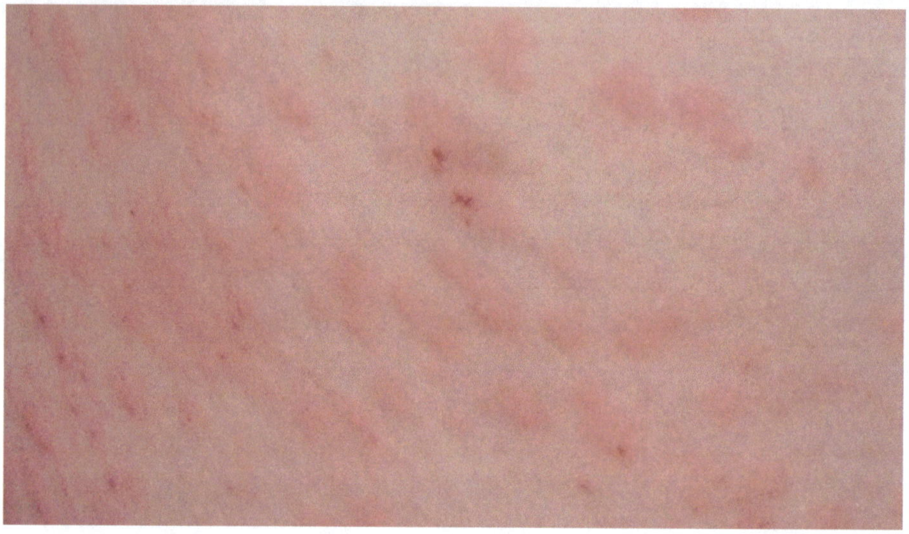

Figure 14.1. Histoplasmosis.

Source: https://i0.wp.com/images-prod.healthline.com/hlcmsresource/images/Clinical-Large-Images/648x364_Histoplasmosis.jpg?w=1155&h=764.

14.1. Causative Agent

The etiologic agent of histoplasmosis is the *Histoplasma capsulatum* fungus that develops in various soil environments, particularly in nitrogen-rich ones such as those with bird and bat fecal material. This opportunistic pathogen exists in two forms: a mycelium form in soil and a yeast form in the body of the host. The environmental conditions favorable to the growth of *H. capsulatum* make certain geographic areas particularly susceptible to histoplasmosis epidemics. Certain studies suggest that this organism can survive for extended periods in soil, awaiting contact with hosts that disturb its habitat, including human beings involved in construction or ecological rehabilitation processes. The life cycle of the pathogen emphasizes the complex interaction between human behavior and environmental stimuli that can lead to disease outbreaks, illustrating the imperative necessity of vigilance and prevention among high-risk groups (Lee et al., 2011). Pathologically, being a pathogen, *H. capsulatum* is one of serious threat, particularly to immunocompromised patients. Once inhaled, the spores turn into yeasts and can evade the host immune system by replicating within macrophages. This characteristic allows the disease pathogen not only to survive but also to travel throughout the body, even producing life-threatening forms of the disease, such as disseminated histoplasmosis. For residents in endemic areas, the environmental reservoirs of *H. capsulatum* constitute an ever-present danger. Understand and awareness of the mechanisms have the potential to be the basis for public health strategies for reducing exposure in at-risk populations. Understanding the causative agent justifies itself beyond the individual infections, with significant implications for broader epidemiologic investigation and intervention (Aklilu et al., 2016). Investigations of *H. capsulatum* have revealed intricate interactions between ecology in the environment and human disease. Soil ecosystems, which are highly diverse, contain multiple microorganisms that interact with *H. capsulatum* and impact its pathogenicity. Most notably, although most soil organisms benefit ecosystem processes, opportunistic pathogens such as *H. capsulatum* take advantage of compromised host immunity, making it even more challenging to deal with soil-borne disease dynamics. It therefore becomes a necessity to perform interdisciplinary research focusing on land management activities and their effects on histoplasmosis outbreaks. These are agricultural management, urbanization, and land cover changes, which can affect the prevalence rate of *H. capsulatum* in soil, later justifying further studies to avoid threats. This focus on the etiologic agent not only supports public health readiness but also sustainable environmental resource management to prevent soil-transmitted diseases emergence (Lee et al., 2011) (Figure 14.2).

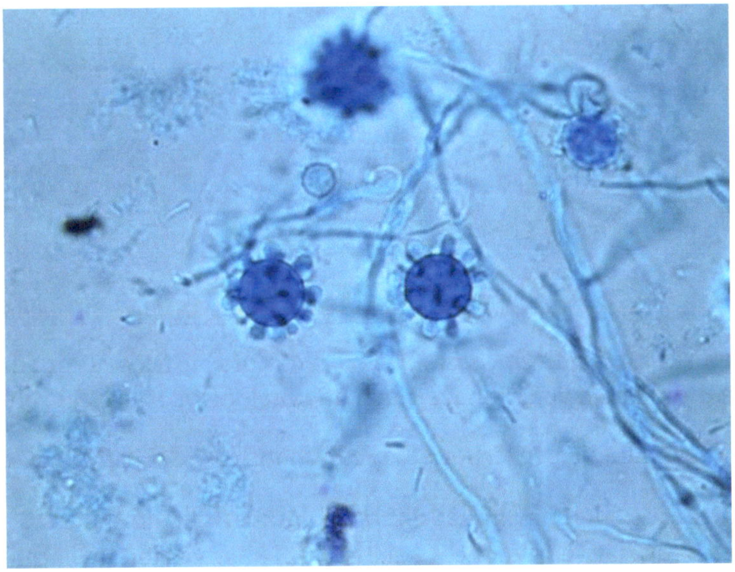

Figure 14.2. The causative agent of histoplasmosis is the fungus *Histoplasma capsulatum*, which thrives in various soil environments, particularly in nitrogen-rich ecosystems such as those enriched by bird and bat droppings.

Source: https://media.npr.org/assets/img/2013/10/24/histo-43340f08510fdb9d11a0a1e9e4c260541a35ad06.jpg?s=1100&c=50&f=jpeg.

14.1.1. Description of Histoplasma capsulatum

The disease-causing agent *Histoplasma capsulatum* is a dimorphic fungus that has a complex life cycle with a mold and a yeast phase, both which are part of its virulence. It is present as a mold in the environment, in soil that is high in organic matter found in bat and bird droppings. The morphology of the mold, when it forms conidia, is aerosolizable and inhalable and represents the primary route of infection to humans. The conidia, upon invading the host, are converted into a yeast phase, which possesses the ability to be resistant to the immune system. This form-switching ability is essential to survival within tissue within hosts, most notably under conditions of immunocompromise, where fulfilment of critical pulmonary infections can occur. These characteristics highlight the virulence and adaptability of *H. capsulatum* and make it a significant public health concern in endemic regions (Mohammed et al., 2024). Ongoing research on *Histoplasma capsulatum* discovers notable heterogeneity among strains, which has implications for both virulence and the immunogenic response of the host.

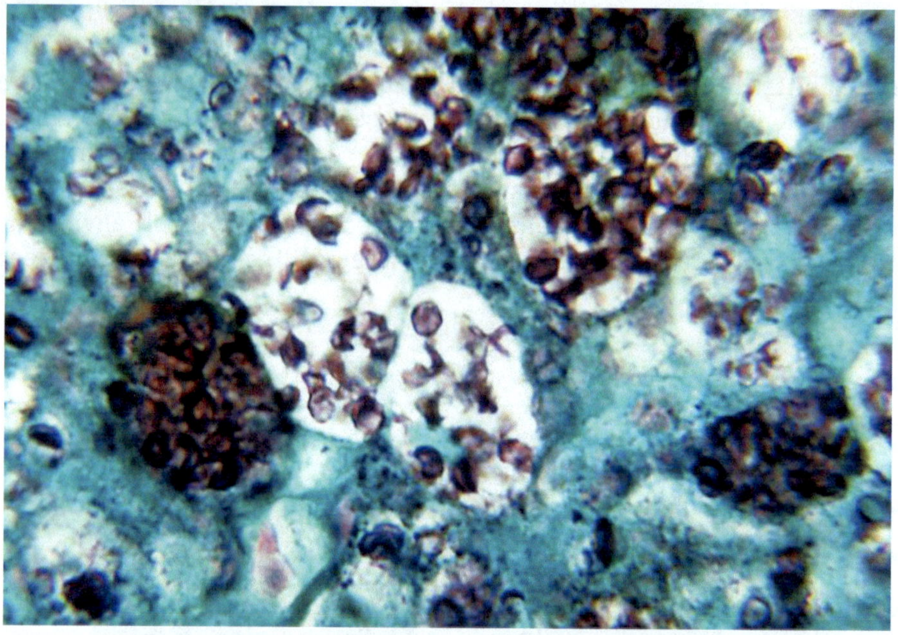

Figure 14.3. The organism *Histoplasma capsulatum* is a dimorphic fungus that displays a complex life cycle involving both a mold and a yeast phase, each of which plays a critical role in its pathogenicity.

Source: https://upload.wikimedia.org/wikipedia/commons/4/42/Histoplasmosis_capsulatum.jpg.

There have been works depicting similar characteristics among different strains in macroscopic appearance, spore size, and relative virulence as measurable parameters by lethal dose through model organisms. For instance, certain strains like G10 and G17M have demonstrated equal immunogenic potential when compared for protection efficacy in immunized subjects, while strains like 3154 are highly virulent (Anderson et al., 2007). Such diversity is not only important to achieve the ecological niche of *H. capsulatum* but also to design targeted vaccines and therapeutic strategies. The public health significance of strain characteristics encompasses continued monitoring of environmental populations of *H. capsulatum* for forecasting imminent outbreaks. The virulence mechanisms of

Histoplasma capsulatum are a complex balance between the fungus and the immune response of the host. Upon inhalation, the organism encounters alveolar macrophages, wherein it employs host cellular machinery for supporting its internalization and replication. The ability of *H. capsulatum* to die and multiply within macrophages is an inherent component of its virulence. The disease can manipulate immune reactions and escape being destroyed by the ability to regulate host cell responses. This can be very unsettling in immunocompromised patients, who are found to be highly susceptible to disseminated histoplasmosis, contributing to a risk factor in poor outcomes from the disease. Identification of these interactions is important for the development of effective treatment protocols and prophylactic intervention, especially in high-risk groups where the disease burden is disproportionately high (Mohammed et al., 2024) (Figure 14.3).

14.1.2. Life Cycle and Reproduction of the Fungus

The life cycle of fungi, particularly those species responsible for histoplasmosis, suggests the complex interrelationship in their ecosystems. *Histoplasma capsulatum* has a unique dimorphic life cycle since it develops as mold and yeast, depending on the environment. The fungus develops in mycelium form in soil, particularly the rich organic soil like that of bird or bat guano, develops asexually by the development of conidia. These spores are expelled into the air, which they become inhaled by their prospective hosts.

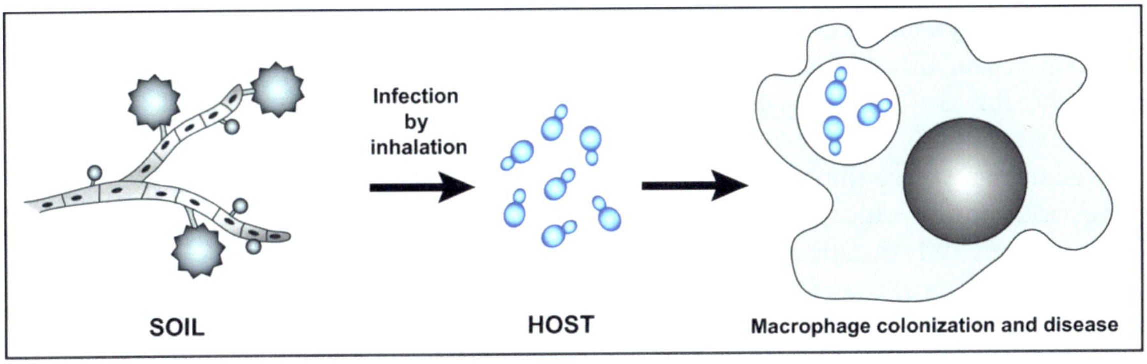

Figure 14.4. *Histoplasma capsulatum* demonstrates a unique dimorphic life cycle, existing as both a mold and yeast, depending on environmental conditions.

Source: https://media.springernature.com/lw1200/springer-static/image/art%3A10.1186%2F1471-2180-11-216/MediaObjects/12866_2011_Article_1517_Fig1_HTML.jpg.

The transformation from the mold to yeast phase typically occurs on inhalation, where the spores are inhaled and then germinate within the warm, nutrient-rich environment of the lungs. Understanding this life cycle is critical, as it demonstrates how the environmental aspects lead to the pathogenicity of the fungus and how it infects, particularly immunocompromised, hosts. *H. capsulatum* has a primarily asexual reproduction, a significant determinant of its epidemiology. Reproduction in the soil environment results in spores via a process of conidiation, in which the fungus forms conidia, or asexual spores. This mode of reproduction allows the organism to develop extremely fast under good conditions, namely where organic matter is plentiful. Furthermore, the capability of the organism to develop within harsh environments allows it to live within soil, thus presenting prolonged exposure threats to humans. This resistance underscores the fungus's opportunistic infection potential because infected individuals can inadvertently breathe in the spores when engaging in routine activities, such as gardening or spelunking where bats reside. Thus, an understanding of its reproductive process is paramount to public health education and prevention in endemic areas. Overall, *H. capsulatum*'s intricate life cycle and reproductive processes are all why histoplasmosis is known. The ability of the fungus to alternate between yeast and mold forms under different conditions plays a significant role in its pathogenicity and infectivity. Notably, the ecological niche established by nutrient soils assures the organisms survival and reproduction fitness, enabling it to establish itself in differing geographic ranges. Additionally, understanding these life cycle dynamics makes preventive interventions against histoplasmosis possible, particularly for susceptible populations. Endemic residents are advised to avoid high-risk environments where the spores are most likely to occur, in line with the importance of raising awareness and education in minimizing the impact of this fungal disease on health (Lee et al., 2011; Cernat et al., 2023) (Figure 14.4).

14.1.3. Environmental Conditions Favoring Growth

The environmental conditions favoring *Histoplasma capsulatum* growth, the causative fungus of histoplasmosis, are strongly linked with specific ecological niches. *Histoplasma capsulatum* is a heat-loving, moist-preferring fungus and accordingly is normally found in environments where organic matter, mostly feces of birds or bats, accumulate. Fungal development in such substrate is optimum since the decaying organic material provides it with essential nutrients. Urban areas, where the habitats are fragmented, are likely to host the bird populations that adapt to the new environment and thus are at risk of coming into contact with spores released into the environment. Environmental fragmentation, besides encouraging growth in avian species, encourages the spreading of the fungus, which increases the risk of histoplasmosis among adjacent human populations (Armstrong et al., 2016). Thus, understanding these ecological interdependencies is of paramount importance in the design of effective public health interventions. Apart from substrate availability, humidity and temperature are just as critical in the life cycle of *Histoplasma capsulatum*. The fungus most favors climates with high temperature and humidity, where spore germination and growth take place. It has been noted that regions with mild winters and warm seasons are particularly suitable for the pathogen's spread. The interaction of animal populations with their environment impacts these environmental factors very strongly. For instance, the presence of specific bird populations, such as pigeons and sparrows, has been linked to an increase in fungal spore density in urban areas, thus impacting wildlife and human health ultimately (Ronanki, 2024). These findings highlight that environmental factors need to be tracked to predict outbreaks as well as effectively control public health. Besides, recognition of the changes in the environment and the evolution of histoplasmosis highlights the necessity for the conservation of the environment. Through human activity as a cause of habitat modification and landscape disruption, the dynamics of environmental health, wildlife behavior, and fungal growth become more complicated. Conservation activities aimed at maintaining natural habitats can deter the agents that favor Histoplasma growth by limiting exposure to birds' and their habitats' disturbance. This policy not only assists in the prevention of histoplasmosis epidemics but also preserves biodiversity since it ensures that the ecosystem remains stable. Additionally, the combination of public health practices and environmental protection can help us learn more about how ecosystems function and how they impact human health (Armstrong et al., 2016). Through this, encouraging an interdisciplinary nexus that combines ecology, public health, and conservation has the potential to enhance our ability to tackle the challenge of histoplasmosis more efficiently (Figure 14.5).

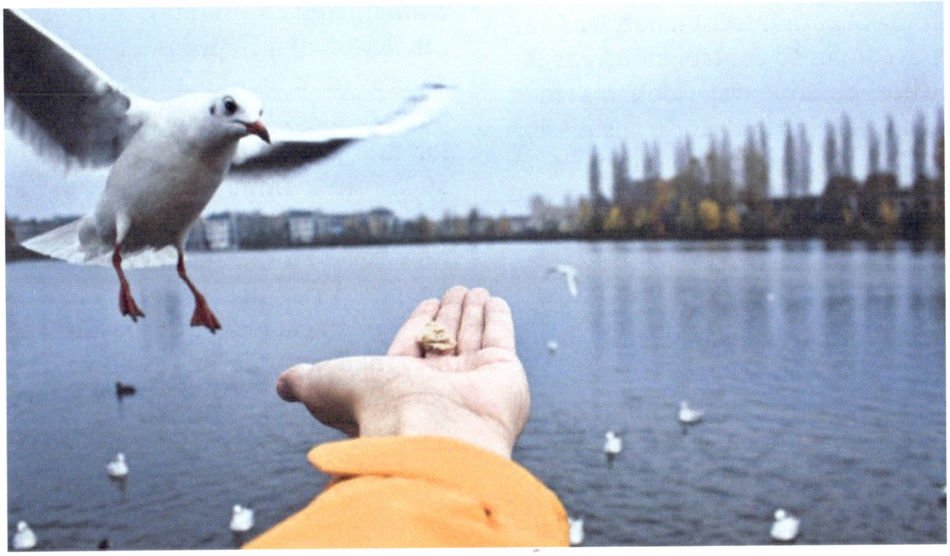

Figure 14.5. Urban areas, where habitats are fragmented, often concentrate bird populations that adapt to their new surroundings, thereby increasing the likelihood of exposure to the spores released into the environment.

Source: https://media.springernature.com/lw685/springer-static/image/chp%3A10.1007%2F978-3-319-91689-7_13/MediaObjects/440107_1_En_13_Fig4_HTML.jpg.

14.2. Transmission and Infection

Transmission of Histoplasmosis, caused primarily by the dimorphic fungus *Histoplasma capsulatum*, results from inhalation of spores that are airborne. It is endemic in various locations, particularly where the soil is contaminated with bats' and birds' fecal pellets, which are its natural reservoirs. On inhalation, the spores can transform from the mold stage to a yeast stage in the host's body, where they are able to grow and cause infection. Clinical presentation of primary pulmonary histoplasmosis is occasionally nonspecific; the patient typically develops fever, chills, malaise, and cough. The severity of infection is dependent chiefly on the number of spores inhaled and the patient's immune status. For instance, immunocompromised patients are at a risk of more extensive disease progression, whose clear exposure risk comprehension and transmission process is critical (Mohammed et al., 2024). Immunocompetent patients tend to present with asymptomatic infection, and acute pulmonary histoplasmosis also leads primarily as a result of extreme exposure to spores. Interestingly, the majority of the cases resolve on their own or with extremely minimal antifungal treatment. Yet, in the immunocompromised, the infection tends to progress rapidly and develop into disseminated histoplasmosis with a high fatality rate unless treated. Diagnosis usually involves combining clinical presentation with laboratory findings that can detect the presence of *H.*

capsulatum. The difficulties of timely and correct diagnosis highlight the need for geographical areas of proven endemism of the fungus and patient history of suspected exposure to be taken into consideration. Hence, there should be an understanding of both infection patterns and transmission dynamics to control and treat the disease in the best possible way (Mohammed et al., 2024). The relationship between transmission rates and infection rates highlights the need for strict public health measures and individual vigilance, particularly in endemic areas. Risk training on exposure to bat or bird droppings can play a pivotal role in disease prevention. With additional information available regarding the pathogenesis and immune response elicited by *H. capsulatum*, treatment regimens are being developed to better control histoplasmosis. This is particularly relevant in light of how immunocompromised patients respond differently than their immunocompetent counterparts. Continuous funding and research efforts, such as those offered by the MRC Centre for Medical Mycology, are imperative to influence our understanding of histoplasmosis transmission and infection control procedures towards improved patient care (Figure 14.6).

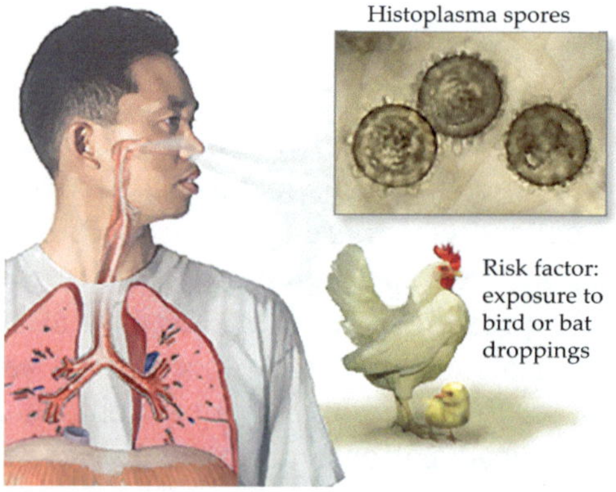

Figure 14.6. The severity of the infection largely depends on the quantity of spores inhaled and the immune status of the individual.

Source: https://ssl.adam.com/graphics/images/en/17222.jpg.

14.2.1. Modes of Transmission to Humans

Histoplasmosis, brought about by fungus *Histoplasma capsulatum*, is predominantly transmitted to human beings through the inhalation of air-spores. The spores often occur where there is a high concentration of bird or bat excrement, which are good environments for the growth of fungi. Activities that disrupt such environments, such as construction activities, farming, or caving, have the tendency to aerosolize the spores and consequently put people at risk of inhalation. When inhaled, the spores can get lodged in the lungs and transform into their yeast form, leading to infection in the end. In regions where Histoplasma is endemic, such as the Ohio and Mississippi River basins, individuals who engage in activities that expose them to these habitats are most susceptible to the disease, and thus the importance of being well-informed about the modes of transmission to better prevent and control it. Cutaneously, Histoplasma infects humans by direct contact with infected material, but much less so than with inhalation. For instance, occupational contact in persons working with soil or in bat colonies can accidentally give rise to skin infection. These infections occur in cutaneous histoplasmosis as localized lesions that appear where the inoculation was made. The partial study has provided evidence in different animal populations, such as horses, of Histoplasma DNA presence in blood and pus samples, which indicates potential transmission routes through contact with animals. The veterinary implications here can inform human exposure and illustrate the interconnectedness of environmental health and zoonotic diseases and more affirm the dynamics of complexity in transmission (Aklilu et al., 2016). Beyond cutaneous and respiratory dissemination, symptomatic presentations of histoplasmosis occasionally follow ingestion of contaminated food or water, but this is less well explained. Clinical presentations range from mild flu-like illness to fulfilment acute respiratory failure in case reports of patients with acute histoplasmosis presenting with nausea, vomiting, and gastrointestinal symptoms alongside classic pulmonary findings (Cole et al., 2014). This range of routes of transmission highlights public awareness and understanding of histoplasmosis, particularly in endemic regions, where common activities that disturb possible sources of contamination are prevalent. Therefore, follow-up education on prevention strategies is essential in order to minimize the risk of transmission, illustrating the role of community health programs in the battle against this fungal infection (Figure 14.7).

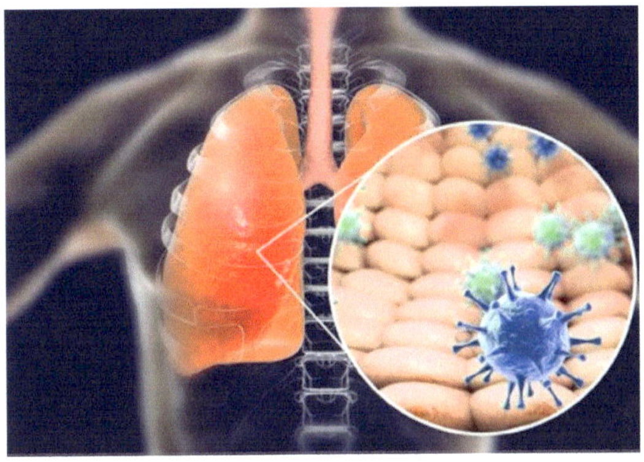

Figure 14.7. Clinical presentations range from mild flu-like symptoms to severe respiratory distress, as indicated in case reports of individuals with acute histoplasmosis who presented with nausea, vomiting, and gastrointestinal symptoms alongside typical pulmonary signs.

Source: https://images.medicinenet.com/images/article/main_image/wuhan-coronavirus.jpg.

14.2.2. Risk Factors for Infection

It is important to know the risk factors of the infection in treating histoplasmosis, a fungal infection resulting from the inhalation of spores of *Histoplasma capsulatum*. There are populations in which individuals who are immunocompromised are at an exceptionally high risk of developing severe complications from this infection. Interestingly, those who are infected with HIV are more likely to develop more severe opportunistic infections, with histoplasmosis being no exception. A Guatemalan study identified that of the HIV-positive patients evaluated, a significant 25.3% had an AIDS-defining illness (ADI) at presentation, and histoplasmosis was the fourth most common ADI in 11.4% of patients. This connection underscores the necessity of surveillance for histoplasmosis among HIV patients, especially given that most of them are marked by increased morbidity because of increased opportunistic infections, which can complicate their clinical presentation and outcome (Cordon et al., 2017). Geographic distribution is also crucial in maintaining the risk of histoplasmosis infection. Environmental factors such as soil composition, weather, and bird or bat droppings all contribute significantly to spore viability and human exposure. Individuals living in rural areas are more susceptible as evidenced through findings of the Guatemalan cohort study which indicated that histoplasmosis was more frequently diagnosed among patients living in rural areas. These settings are likely to establish conditions favorable to the growth of histoplasmosis spores, particularly in regions where agriculture activity breaks up the ground and increases human contact with contaminated settings. This fact indicates the need for targeted public health interventions in areas notorious for causing histoplasmosis infections, with an aim to sensitizing vulnerable populations on the risk posed by particular settings (Cordon et al., 2017). Furthermore, occupational exposure is a primary risk factor for histoplasmosis infection, particularly for individuals conducting work that stirs up large quantities of soil or organic matter. Construction work, agricultural work, and landscaping work all naturally increase the risk of contracting infectious spores. Medical evidence suggests healthcare workers also carry greater risk when caring for patients with severe immunocompromisation or outbreak situations. Secondly, the retrospective cohort study identifies the significance of understanding occupational exposure since some occupational activities carry higher risk for heightened histoplasmosis incidences. This understanding is important to the formulation of preventive interventions considering environmental and occupational risk factors among high-risk groups, hence boosting effective public health interventions and education programs aimed at suppressing histoplasmosis infection (Figure 14.8).

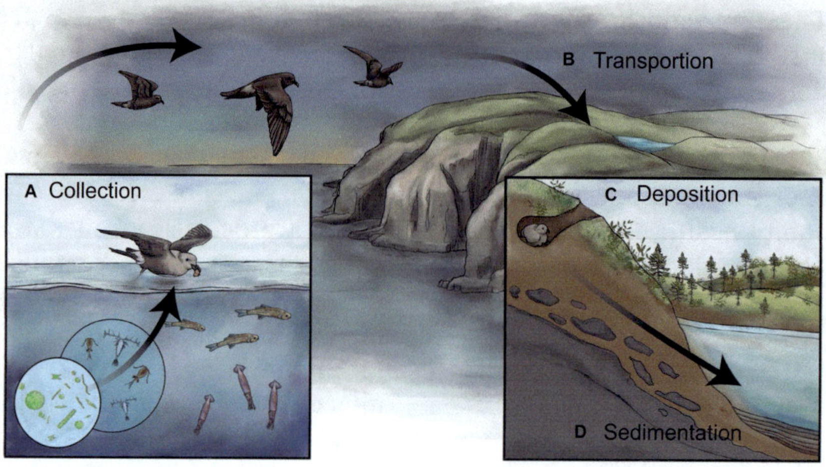

Figure 14.8. Environmental factors such as soil composition, climate, and the presence of bird or bat droppings contribute significantly to spore viability and human exposure.

Source: https://www.frontiersin.org/files/Articles/698175/fevo-09-698175-HTML/image_m/fevo-09-698175-g001.jpg.

14.2.3. Populations at Higher Risk

Having knowledge of the populations with higher risk of acquiring histoplasmosis will be beneficial for effective public health intervention and planning. People with compromised immune status, for instance, individuals with HIV/AIDS, are significantly at risk of contracting severe histoplasmosis. This is because they have an immunosuppressive status that hinders them from combating fungal infection, hence leaving them susceptible. In various studies, the authors have observed that prevalence of histoplasmosis in HIV-infected patients is relative to their health status and nutritional levels, showing a serious correlation between the systemic diseases and opportunistic fungal infections. There are other susceptibilities that are triggered by populations with social stigmatization of their ailments, resulting in a decrease in their intent for preventive and curative care interventions. Also, a few socio-economic and demographic factors increase susceptibility to histoplasmosis in specific populations. For instance, Hispanic populations are highly impacted, particularly where traditional cultures have very high levels of contact with environments with high levels of histoplasma fungi, such as bird or bat guano-infested regions. Research has established that obesity and diabetes are rampant in these communities, even further complicating conditions since those with the conditions have already been placed at higher risk due to many diseases, including histoplasmosis. The cultural beliefs of the body image and health in these communities tend to make them reluctant to alter lifestyle habits because most individuals equate weight loss with disease rather than with health gain, thereby dominating critical health education that assists in reducing the prevalence of histoplasmosis and other infections among vulnerable populations (Abel et al., 2019). Lastly, the lack of proper monitoring in regions with high burdens of fungal infections is a significant barrier to understanding and control of risks associated with histoplasmosis. In Central and South America, where the epidemiology of histoplasmosis in combination with other serious fungal infections is not well investigated, at-risk groups are largely unsupervised. This gap in data collection limits public health measures and incapacitates the development of productive interventions to meet the requirements of these populations. Lacking mandatory reporting and national surveillance of fungal diseases, health systems could not effectively allocate resources or raise awareness on preventive measures necessary for high-risk populations, including those with compromised immunity or who reside in endemic regions (Chaudhuri et al., 2022). Urging an organized attack on these gaps in surveillance and intervention is key to reducing morbidity from histoplasmosis in high-risk populations (Figure 14.9).

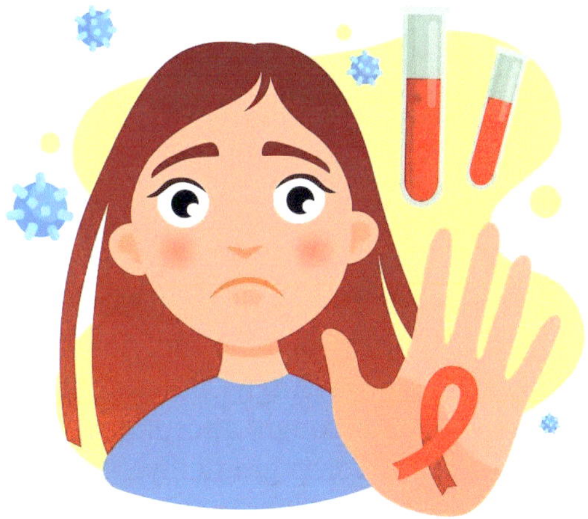

Figure 14.9. Individuals with compromised immune systems, such as those living with HIV/AIDS, face a significantly elevated risk of contracting severe histoplasmosis.

Source: https://www.mylabbox.com/wp-content/uploads/2017/03/picture-hiv-aids-young-woman-with-hiv-ribbon.webp.

14.3. Symptoms and Clinical Manifestations

Histoplasmosis, caused predominantly by the fungus *Histoplasma capsulatum*, has a spectrum of presentations ranging from asymptomatic respiratory infection to fulminant systemic disease. The presenting illness usually includes fever, chills, cough, and weakness, which may easily mimic other diseases of the respiratory tract. The nonspecific symptoms may be responsible for delaying diagnosis, particularly in immunocompetent individuals who may recover spontaneously without any intervention. There should be a high suspicion by the healthcare provider in regions of endemicity, especially in a patient with chronic respiratory complaints not responsive to standard therapy. As the disease worsens, complications can be severe and consist of chest pain, hemoptysis, and respiratory failure, particularly in patients with pre-existing lung disease or immunocompromised status. The extremely immunocompromised, such as recipients of allogeneic stem cell transplant, are at high risk of developing severe histoplasmosis. In the immunocompromised patient, the illness can be more severe and have a shorter onset, including fever, night sweats, and weight loss, and can represent a disseminated infection. Counterintuitively, even in the setting of antifungal prophylaxis, e.g., voriconazole, there can be substantial infection. A reported case showed that a patient developed Histoplasma pneumonia despite therapeutic antifungal levels, with proof of the challenges in treating histoplasmosis among immunocompromised individuals. Early diagnosis and early treatment with appropriate antifungals, e.g., itraconazole, may lead to great clinical improvement, with high alertness being highlighted in these high-risk patients (Agrawal et al., 2020). Besides respiratory manifestations, systemic disease may be seen with advanced histoplasmosis, such as organ disease and granulomatous inflammation. Lymphadenopathy, hepatosplenomegaly, and skin rash may appear, reflecting the diseases potential for dissemination from the lungs. Such nonspecific systemic symptoms must be closely clinically evaluated, particularly in endemic individuals or those with relevant risk factors. The diagnostic challenges arise not only due to the similar symptoms with other infections but also due to the heterogeneity in the clinical presentations. It is thus important for clinicians to employ the appropriate diagnostic tests, such as fungal cultures or antigen detection, in order to diagnose histoplasmosis in order to implement appropriate and timely treatment (Kauffman et al., 1988) (Figure 14.10).

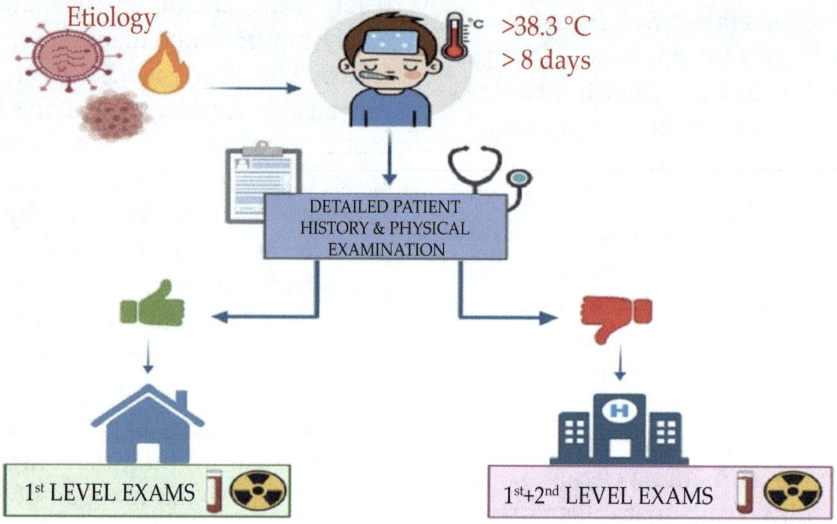

Figure 14.10. In endemic areas, healthcare providers must maintain a high index of suspicion, especially in patients presenting with persistent respiratory symptoms that do not resolve with standard therapy.

Source: https://pub.mdpi-res.com/children/children-11-00020/article_deploy/html/images/children-11-00020-ag.png?1703641638.

14.3.1. Acute Histoplasmosis Symptoms

Acute histoplasmosis is an acute infectious illness due to exposure to the fungus *Histoplasma capsulatum*, typically found in soil with a high content of bird or bat droppings. Individuals who are acutely infected may have a range of symptoms, which may be surprisingly indistinguishable from other respiratory illnesses. They may typically present with fever, cough, and pleuritic pain, as well as fatigue, myalgia, and arthralgia. Typically, symptoms may develop gradually over weeks after exposure, thereby the delay in diagnosis. Acute histoplasmosis is, in its severe form, capable of triggering acute respiratory distress syndrome, complicating the clinical presentation on misdiagnosis as pneumonia or other respiratory infections. Typical of acute histoplasmosis is also the fact that it is capable of mimicking other diseases, making diagnosis and treatment difficult. For instance, studies highlight that patients may have an overlapping of a large number of symptoms, e.g., community-acquired pneumonia or even rheumatological manifestations, particularly in the presence of systemic presentations such as weight loss and malaise. A patient, in one such case report, came with dry cough, chest tightness, and exertional dyspnea, which initially misguided the diagnosis until histoplasmosis was diagnosed by radiologic and cytologic examination. It draws attention to the importance of including histoplasmosis in differential diagnoses among patients with respiratory symptoms, especially within endemic regions where natives are most likely to be exposed (Britto et al., 2018). The implications of accurate diagnosis of acute histoplasmosis are severe since early antifungal medication treatment will yield significant clinical improvement. For example, failure of patients to respond to broad-spectrum antibiotics should prompt clinicians to have a high index of suspicion for histoplasmosis, particularly in endemic areas. The case reports show that the patients typically improve remarkably once they receive appropriate antifungal therapy, emphasizing the importance of the clinician to be aware of the early manifestations and perform appropriate diagnostic workups. Further, methods such as endobronchial ultrasound-guided bronchoscopy can also aid in confirmation of diagnosis in the case of high clinical suspicion, allowing for an effective treatment approach that can significantly enhance patient outcomes (Agrawal et al., 2020) (Figure 14.11).

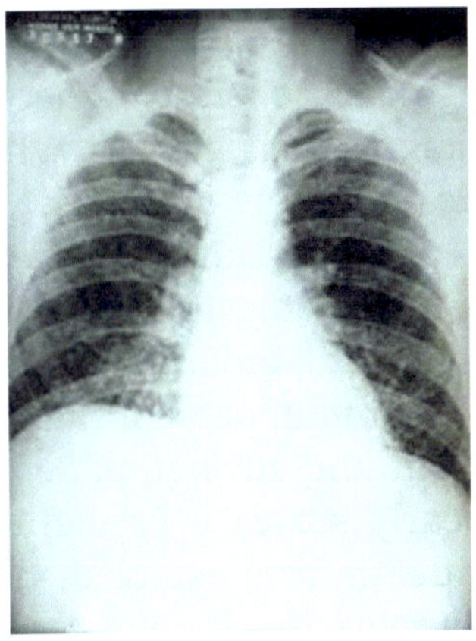

Figure 14.11. Acute histoplasmosis is an infectious disease resulting from exposure to the fungus *Histoplasma capsulatum*, often found in soil enriched with bird or bat droppings.

Source: https://encrypted-tbn0.gstatic.com/images?q=tbn:ANd9GcTmtUiT1yCalkeTXqEdk28YOsTPxEKlmo7KTYftQlO3E6Q1OfmmxPXbVof8geRyiVBvZX4&usqp=CAU.

14.3.2. Chronic Histoplasmosis Symptoms

Chronic histoplasmosis is associated with a broad range of symptoms that can severely impact individuals, particularly those with compromised immune systems. Unlike other forms of the disease, chronic histoplasmosis can develop gradually, leading to chronic respiratory symptoms like tuberculosis or another lung infection. Symptoms can range from chronic cough, weakness, fever, and loss of weight that may be mistaken for other chronic respiratory conditions. The insidious nature of these symptoms can hinder diagnosis and treatment, which causes further complications. During the development of the disease, patients can also acquire the production of sputum that may be bloody, which shows the gravity of the condition and how important proper diagnosis is when it happens in endemic areas. Other than pulmonary complications, chronic histoplasmosis can affect other extrapulmonary tissues, forming extrapulmonary symptoms that show its severity. The patients may develop lymphadenopathy, hepatosplenomegaly, and dermatosis as infection progresses more in immunocompromised patients, for instance, those on allogeneic stem cell transplantation. Clinical presentation of chronic histoplasmosis is thus multifaceted, often requiring complete evaluation to differentiate from other infectious and inflammatory diseases. For instance, among antifungal prophylaxis patients, such as those taking voriconazole, development of histoplasmosis becomes a possibility even at therapeutic levels, pointing to the importance of caution and case-specific assessment strategies, especially in regions where the causative agent is endemic (Agrawal et al., 2020). The challenge in diagnosis of chronic histoplasmosis lies in the fact that its symptoms closely mimic those of other respiratory conditions. Physicians often are forced to base a diagnosis on a combination of clinical evaluation, chest radiographs, and serologic testing. In some cases, lung biopsies may be necessary to identify the *Histoplasma capsulatum* organism itself. The most common treatment is prolonged antifungal therapy, and itraconazole is often used as initial therapy. However, effectiveness of treatments may vary, especially in immunocompromised patients. Therefore, it is important that ongoing research on best management practices be pursued. As has been observed, such patients with chronic symptoms but who are given appropriate and timely therapy can be indeed greatly improved clinically, and awareness and active management strategies development in risk populations is increasingly supported (Kauffman et al., 1988) (Figure 14.12).

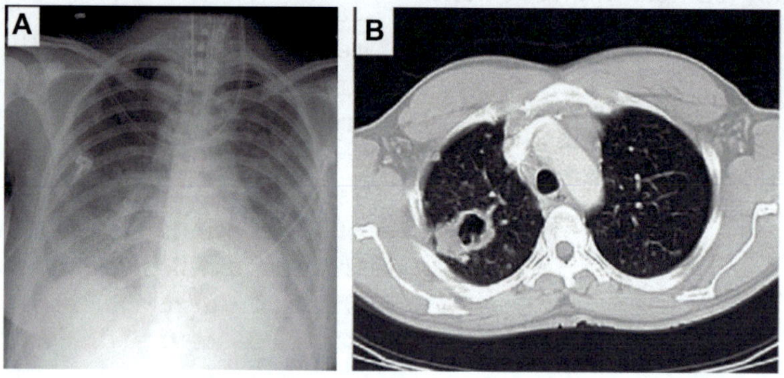

Figure 14.12. In addition to pulmonary issues, chronic histoplasmosis can affect various extrapulmonary sites, leading to systemic symptoms that reflect its severity.

Source: https://www.id.theclinics.com/cms/10.1016/j.idc.2021.03.011/asset/2833a6d2-85e6-45fe-aa69-f09e1f789e95/main.assets/gr2_lrg.jpg.

14.3.3. Disseminated Histoplasmosis Symptoms

Disseminated histoplasmosis is an severe form of histoplasmosis, typically encountered in immunocompromised patients or inhabitants of endemic regions. It can present with systemic findings and be very protean and hence diagnostic. The classical findings are fever, weight loss, fatigue, and nocturnal sweats, which, though nonspecific, imply a disseminated infection. Patients may also have respiratory manifestations of cough and dyspnea since the fungus may spread to other organs from the lung and create complications in the form of pneumonia. The clinical scenario may also be complicated by opportunistic infection, especially in immunocompromised patients, that is responsible for unnecessary delay in appropriate treatment and adverse patient outcomes (Agrawal et al., 2020). Recognition of these symptoms in the early stages is crucial in the early management of disseminated histoplasmosis, thereby reducing death from established disease. In addition to symptoms in the respiratory tract, gastrointestinal symptoms are also observed in patients presenting with disseminated histoplasmosis, including abdominal pain, diarrhea, and dysphagia. These represent manifestations of the effect of the histoplasma organism in the gastrointestinal tract, which typically results in ulcerative lesions and malabsorption. Cutaneous manifestations can include rashes or ulcerations, most often in chronic cases when the immune system is compromised. Neurologic presentation can arise, particularly if histoplasmosis reaches the central nervous system and presents with headache, seizures, or altered mental status. As mentioned, central nervous system (CNS) histoplasmosis diagnosis can be highly difficult. While cerebrospinal fluid (CSF) (1,3)-β-d-glucan (BDG) tests may aid in diagnosis, they are not very sensitive, and multifactorial analysis is needed for proper assessment (Albers et al., 2018). Disseminated histoplasmosis clinical course can lead to life-threatening complications if not well managed. More severe cases may develop multi-organ failure of the liver and spleen, which may lead to extensive morbidity and mortality. Risk of severe presentation is particularly prevalent in immunocompromised patients, such as those undergoing allogeneic stem cell transplantation. In these patients, a lower threshold for evaluation is recommended, regardless of antifungal prophylaxis, since the usual treatment may not be sufficient for those residing in endemic areas (Agrawal et al., 2020). Consequently, health care providers must have an increased index of suspicion for disseminated histoplasmosis manifestations and pursue vigorous diagnostic workup to enable swift and appropriate treatment, which is of critical value in maintaining patient prognosis and quality of life (Figure 14.13).

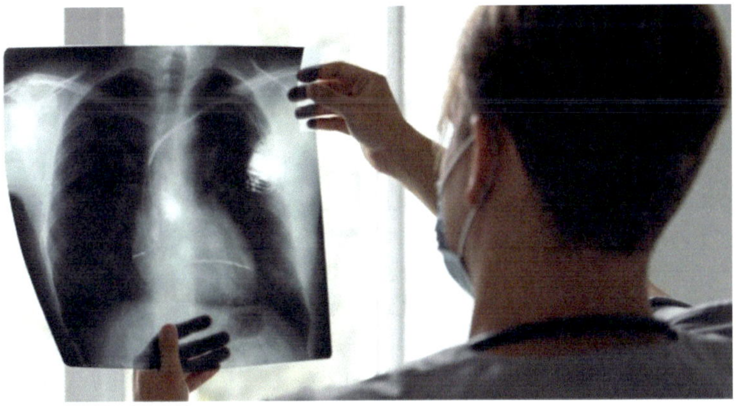

Figure 14.13. Patients may also present with respiratory symptoms, such as cough and shortness of breath, as the fungus can spread from the lungs to other organs, leading to complications like pneumonia.

Source: https://max-website20-images.s3.ap-south-1.amazonaws.com/Pneumonia_d7585eafca.jpg.

14.4. Diagnosis

The diagnosis of histoplasmosis is replete with unique challenges, primarily due to the non-specificity of its clinical presentation. The manifestations are typically indistinguishable from those of other respiratory illnesses, which creates the likelihood for misdiagnosis and deferment of treatment. The clinicians have to resort to a combination of clinical evaluation and laboratory testing for a diagnosis of histoplasmosis. Among the diagnostic methods, serologic testing to detect antibodies against the *Histoplasma capsulatum* organism are common, though their sensitivity is extremely heterogeneous. In the endemic area, a high index of suspicion is to be maintained and, specifically in immunocompromised patients, an early diagnosis must be achieved to prevent disastrous outcomes. Through increased attention to the epidemiologic context and the patient's presentation, clinicians can more successfully traverse the nuances of diagnosing this fungal infection. A novel method for the diagnosis of histoplasmosis has come from the use of cerebrospinal fluid (CSF) markers, namely (1,3)-β-d-glucan (BDG). While this biological marker has been useful in the identification of fungal infections within the central nervous system (CNS), its usefulness as a diagnostic tool in histoplasmosis is still under research. Evidence indicates that CNS histoplasmosis patients have elevated levels of CSF BDG, whose median concentration is notably greater than in controls with other fungal infections. One study had 53.2% detection for BDG, which, as informative as it is, underscores the need for adjunct diagnostic methods due to its lack of specificity. In histoplasmosis, application of CSF BDG in a multi-fold diagnostic strategy can enhance total accuracy and assist with timely intervention (Albers et al., 2018). With all the advances that have been made in diagnosis, challenges remain, the primary one being the discrimination between histoplasmosis and other diseases characterized by similar symptomatology. For example, the overlapping clinical presentations with other fungal infections complicate diagnosis. Application of a combination of imaging, serology, and molecular tests may increase rates of diagnosis. Further research into CSF BDG's diagnostic potential may eventually result in improved guidelines on its use. Current programs to fund research, such as the MRC Centre for Medical Mycology's provision, aim to continue to elucidate these diagnostic concerns and facilitate the establishment of standard criteria for the diagnosis of histoplasmosis. With ongoing research continuing to define the utility and limitations of existing tests, doctors will be better placed to meet the challenges of histoplasmosis diagnosis in the field (MacInnes et al., 2021) (Figure 14.14).

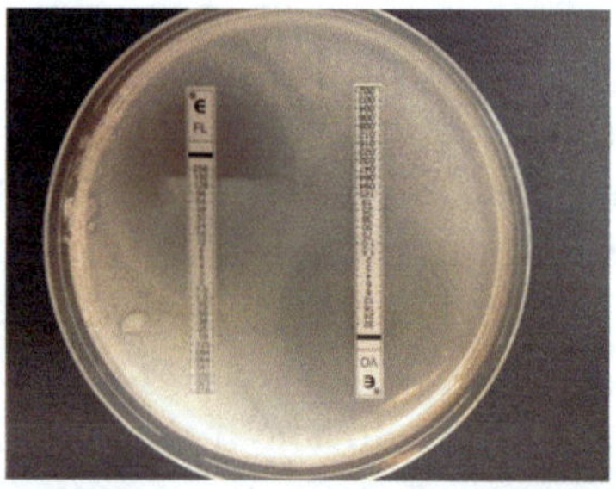

Figure 14.14. An innovative approach to diagnosing histoplasmosis has emerged through the utilization of cerebrospinal fluid (CSF) markers, specifically (1,3)-β-d-glucan (BDG).

Source: https://i0.wp.com/thoracickey.com/wp-content/uploads/2016/09/A64602_2_En_13_Fig9_HTML.gif?fit=326%2C245&ssl=1.

14.4.1. Clinical Evaluation and Patient History

The clinical evaluation of patients who present with symptoms resembling histoplasmosis needs a rigorous approach, particularly in the knowledge of their patient profile. The doctors need to ask them extensively regarding potential exposure to endemic areas that have *Histoplasma capsulatum* as the causative agent. Symptoms such as cough, chest discomfort, and fever can be mimicry of numerous respiratory ailments, and hence diagnosis is difficult. A complete history of the patient should cover not just recent residence or travel, but also leisure and work activities that may increase exposure, such as gardening, building activity, or visits to bird roosts. Since symptoms are frequently non-specific, recording a timeline of onset and duration can go a long way in helping the clinicians in pursuing appropriate diagnostic measures. Thus, effective patient history-taking is a basic element in arriving at clinical suspicion for histoplasmosis. Aside from localization of exposure, other clinical signs are also significant when evaluating a suspected case of histoplasmosis. Awareness of the patients overall condition of health, including immunocompromised conditions or underlying respiratory illnesses, can also inform the diagnostic process. For example, a patient who presents with polyarthralgia, myalgia, and a chronic cough, as in the case of a patient from a Kentucky case report, can initially be diagnosed with overlapping symptoms of other diseases like community-acquired pneumonia or autoimmune disease. It is an indication of the importance of high suspicion on the part of healthcare providers, more so in areas of endemism, where there is greater chance of histoplasmosis. Furthermore, the nature of histoplasmosis diagnosis calls for pertinent differential diagnosis consideration, necessitating comprehensive laboratory workup, imaging, and, in certain instances, invasive diagnostic interventions with the purpose of determining the presence of the disease and its impact on pulmonary function (Britto et al., 2018). Following a comprehensive clinical evaluation, effective diagnosis of histoplasmosis can improve clinical outcomes through timely treatment. When the patient does not respond to the initial antibiotic treatment, i.e., in the present case, precise radiological and histological findings become vital in diagnosis. Cytological diagnosis of necrotizing granulomas can be positive for histoplasmosis diagnosis and can steer the correct antifungal therapy. Precise clinical assessment along with a detailed patient history is thus not only helpful in diagnosis but also in the planning of treatment. Early treatment and diagnosis of histoplasmosis can enable good prognosis, thus strict analysis in clinical practice becomes relevant. Clinicians should, therefore, be extremely cautious with both the history and clinical presentation of their patients to guide them in the right direction to good diagnosis and cure (Ramesh et al.). (Figure 14.15).

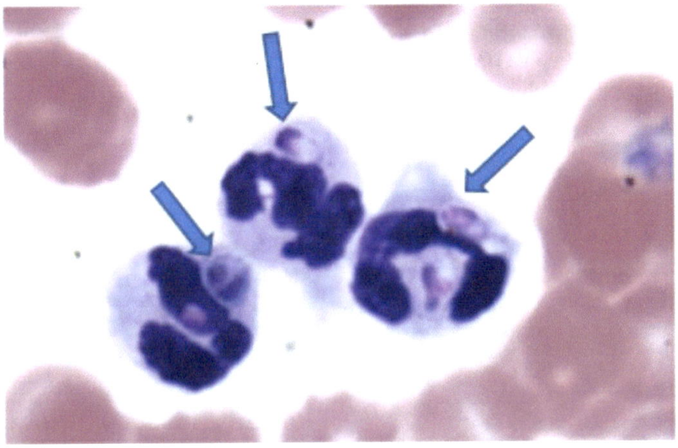

Figure 14.15. Physicians must delve into a detailed inquiry regarding potential exposure to endemic areas known for *Histoplasma capsulatum*, the organism that causes the infection.

Source: https://vhc.missouri.edu/wp-content/uploads/2017/08/diagnose2.jpg.

14.4.2. Laboratory Tests and Imaging Techniques

Effective diagnosis of histoplasmosis is largely based on laboratory studies and imaging methods combined, which enable the identification of the etiologic agent, *Histoplasma capsulatum*. Among the most frequent laboratory tests is the cultivation of body fluids or tissues, which is time-consuming but capable of absolute results. Other useful testing is via histopathological examination identifying the characteristic yeast form of the fungus in tissue biopsies. In addition, serological assays such as immunodiffusion and enzyme-linked immunosorbent assays are used to detect antibodies that are elicited after the infection. These methods can also offer faster results and therefore be of greater assistance towards early diagnosis of histoplasmosis, especially in subjects with past history of exposure to regions where the disease is prevalent. The combination of these laboratory tests is critical in arriving at the correct diagnosis, particularly when the clinical presentation is nonspecific. Imaging techniques are also crucial in the diagnostic process of histoplasmosis, particularly in distinguishing pulmonary manifestations from other respiratory infections such as lung cancer. Radiological studies, including chest X-rays and computed tomography (CT) scans, are typically characterized by pulmonary nodules or infiltrates that can mimic neoplastic disorders.

A retrospective review confirmed that many histoplasmosis patients were found to have lesions very closely resembling metastases, necessitating interpreting imaging findings with caution (Bello et al., 2013). The imaging modalities not only enable the differentiation of histoplasmosis and malignancy but also aid in identifying the degree of advancement of disease and involvement of other organ systems. Imaging is therefore a part of a multiglobal approach to accurately diagnose histoplasmosis and guide its subsequent management. Coupled with clinical evaluations, laboratory diagnostic testing and imaging modality provide a systematized approach in which to interpret the course of histoplasmosis.

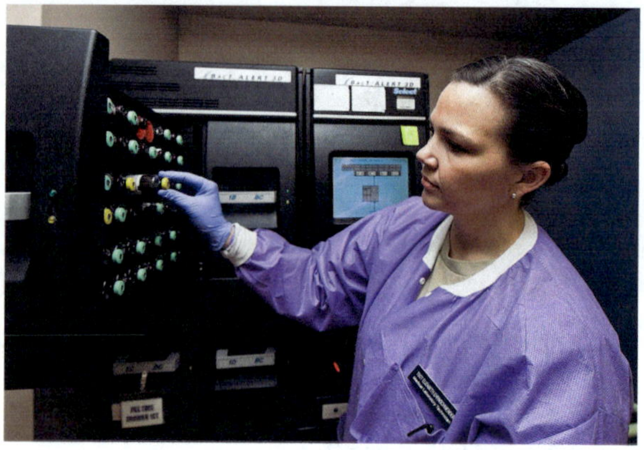

Figure 14.16. Among the most widely used laboratory procedures is the culture of body fluids or tissues, which, although time-consuming, can provide definitive results.

Source: https://upload.wikimedia.org/wikipedia/commons/thumb/f/ff/National_Lab_Week_130410-F-TT327-090.jpg/1200px-National_Lab_Week_130410-F-TT327-090.jpg.

Interpenetration of serologic tests, culture results, and imaging data provides differential diagnosis between histoplasmosis and other mimicking diseases. For instance, the atypical radiologic features observed in immunocompromised hosts can only be managed with an robust diagnostic arsenal to diagnose correctly underlying infections (Mohammed et al., 2024). Further, knowledge of the geographic distribution of *H. capsulatum* and certain clinical syndromes enhances diagnostic specificity such that clinicians can include histoplasmosis in a differential diagnosis in appropriate populations. Ultimately, the integration of laboratory and imaging techniques enhances diagnostic performance and, by extension, benefits patients through timely and cost-effective therapeutic interventions (Figure 14.16).

14.4.3. Differential Diagnosis

It is crucial to medical providers to understand the differential diagnosis of histoplasmosis, particularly since it is misdiagnosed for other serious diseases. It is not easy to identify histoplasmosis since it presents with a broad spectrum of nonspecific clinical features. To illustrate, fever, weight loss, and anorexia are all characteristic of both histoplasmosis and certain malignancies, and thus granulomatous infection must be included along with neoplastic disease. The presentation of disseminated histoplasmosis can be indistinguishable from septic shock in individuals with advanced HIV disease and will lead to multiorgan failure without inducing respiratory failure. Clinicians must therefore maintain a high degree of suspicion for histoplasmosis in individuals with these clinical features, especially in endemic areas, emphasizing the necessity of early and accurate diagnosis for proper treatment (Correia et al., 2023). Apart from infectious diseases like histoplasmosis, the clinical presentation of other conditions can be comparable and thus needs differentiating based on patient history and clinical presentation. For example, histoplasmosis patients may present with lesions that also resemble malignancies, thus also making diagnosis more difficult. An article highlights that certain patients have radiographic findings that seem to be lung cancer but are instead diagnosed with histoplasmosis. The differentiating criteria consist of thorough imaging tests and, if necessary, tissue biopsy. One recent paper reminded us of the case of misdiagnosed cancer-induced histoplasmosis with lesions, reminding us again that granulomatous infections are part of the differential diagnosis of lung nodules or masses. Such information is crucial in order to avoid misdiagnosis and appropriate therapeutic maneuvers are implemented (Bello et al., 2013). To enhance alertness regarding histoplasmosis, there is a need to educate medical professionals on its potential presentations and mimicking symptoms.

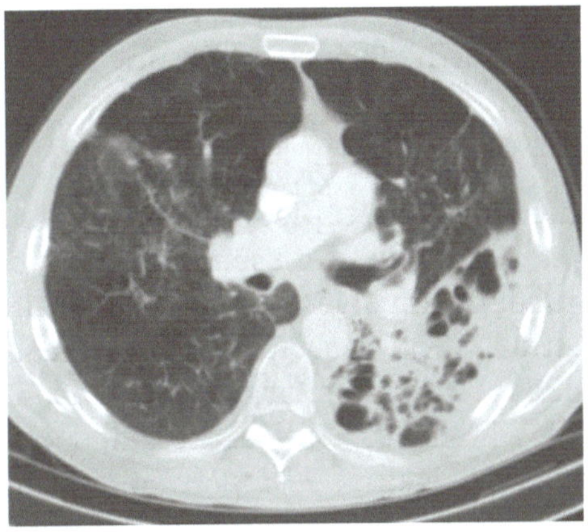

Figure 14.17. Histoplasmosis can present with a variety of nonspecific symptoms, complicating its identification.

Source: https://www.mdpi.com/jof/jof-09-00236/article_deploy/html/images/jof-09-00236-g006-550.jpg.

Geographical exposure, immunocompromised state, and radiological presentation should be considered in differential diagnosis. Clinicians need to be sensitive to consider patients who have long-standing pulmonary symptoms, especially those with established history of exposure to bird or bat dropping-rich environments. In addition, as certain patients might arrive with acute severe illness, such as septic shock, early identification of histoplasmosis can have a major impact on outcomes and lower mortality rates. Hence, having a complete understanding of differential diagnosis pathways not only helps to detect histoplasmosis at the correct time but also enhances overall patient care and management (Correia et al., 2023; Bello et al., 2013) (Figure 14.17).

14.5. Treatment Options

Treatment of histoplasmosis is markedly variable based on infection severity and immune status of the patient. No therapy is needed in most immunocompetent individuals who have mild to moderate pulmonary histoplasmosis as the infection tends to self-resolve. Antifungal medication is, however, necessary in those with persistent symptoms or in those who are at risk of developing complications, such as those with chronic pulmonary illnesses. The primary management of acute or chronic pulmonary histoplasmosis is the administration of itraconazole, which is a triazole antifungal medication that effectively reduces fungal burden and symptoms. For patients with disseminated histoplasmosis, particularly in immunocompromised patients, more aggressive treatment with amphotericin B is provided initially before being switched to itraconazole for long-term suppression of the fungus (Mohammed et al., 2024). This therapeutic strategy stresses individualized treatment according to clinical presentation and patient factors. Apart from antifungal medication, management of underlying disease is crucial to improve the course of patients with histoplasmosis, particularly those with immunodeficiency. In HIV-infected patients, disseminated histoplasmosis is a significant contributor to morbidity and mortality and is normally linked with insidious courses that mimic other infectious diseases like tuberculosis (Garner et al., 2020). The therapeutic approach is complicated by the common clinical overlap, and accurate diagnosis should be obtained by extensive diagnostic workup to differentiate between the conditions effectively. Following the first therapy, it is important to subject patients to close observation for relapse, particularly in immunocompromised individuals who may need prolonged antifungal therapy to prevent recurrences. This precautionary approach highlights the importance of both therapeutic management and ongoing monitoring to ensure the best outcome for patients with histoplasmosis.

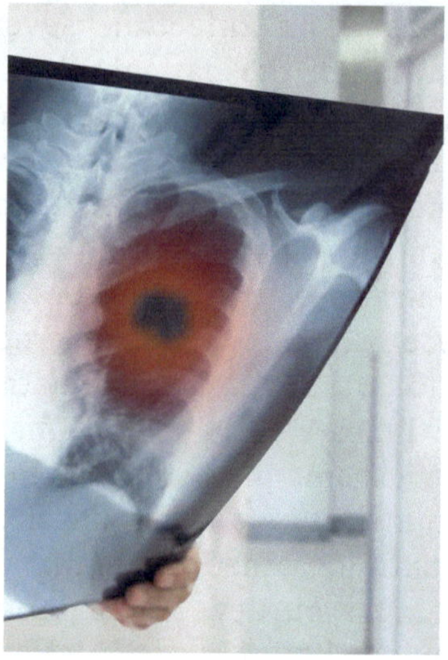

Figure 14.18. The primary treatment for severe or chronic pulmonary histoplasmosis involves the use of itraconazole, a triazole antifungal that effectively reduces fungal burden and alleviates symptoms.

Source: https://cdnintech.com/books/9487/1713443628-1958903706/cover.jpg.

New understanding of histoplasmosis pathogenesis and immune evasion strategies of *Histoplasma capsulatum* has opened new avenues for drug development. Clinical research into immune-modulating treatment, including the use of checkpoint inhibitors, is underway and may provide new promise for those experiencing treatment failure with conventional antifungal therapy. Lastly, greater education and awareness on the part of healthcare providers about the heterogeneous presentation and management strategy of histoplasmosis are crucial. As outlined in clinical practice guidelines, the implementation of evidence-based recommendations into practice can lead to improved control of this fungal infection in various populations, particularly where it is endemic (Garner et al., 2020). This will eventually lead to enhanced clinical outcomes and reduction in histoplasmosis-associated morbidity and mortality, highlighting the need for an integrated approach to managing this critical public health issue (Figure 14.18).

14.5.1. Antifungal Medications

Treatment of histoplasmosis, particularly when it occurs in a disseminated or severe form, usually involves the use of antifungal medications. The most commonly prescribed medicines are amphotericin B and itraconazole, both of which are well established in their effectiveness against *Histoplasma capsulatum*, the causative agent. Amphotericin B is frequently applied in acute infections due to its broad-spectrum antifungal activity, which renders it suitable for life-threatening diseases. Once a patient is stabilized, the treatment may be converted to itraconazole, which is preferably utilized for both severe and moderate forms and long-term maintenance therapy. The shift from amphotericin B to itraconazole is particularly found to reduce the incidence of side effects associated with the long-term use of the latter. It is crucial to know the pharmacological profiles of the drugs for the optimization of patient benefits and customization of therapeutic interventions in histoplasmosis therapy. Duration of antifungal drug therapy in histoplasmosis varies with clinical presentation and severity. Acute pulmonary histoplasmosis is treated for a duration of three to six months of antifungal therapy based on the patient's immunocompetence and clinical response. But patients with disseminated disease can be treated for a more extended period of time, sometimes longer than one year in order to prevent relapse. The need for long-term antifungal treatment draws substantial attention to the need for routine assessment of potential toxicities such as nephrotoxicity from amphotericin B and hepatotoxicity from itraconazole. Drug interactions are also to be considered, especially in immunocompromised patients receiving multiple drugs. Thus, proper care during antifungal therapy is essential to prevent complications while allowing therapeutic efficacy. Mounting evidence of trends in antifungal resistance is alerting to a growing threat to the therapy of fungal infection, including histoplasmosis. Indications are that there may be a reduced susceptibility of *Histoplasma capsulatum* strains to systemic antifungals due to improper use or over-reliance on certain agents. This emerging fact necessitates further research to enhance treatment algorithms and define new antifungal agents with enhanced effectiveness against resistant pathogens. According to epidemiological evidence, serious fungal infections, including histoplasmosis, disproportionately affect vulnerable groups, and this makes it necessary to have appropriate national surveillance (Chaudhuri et al., 2022). It is not only crucial for prevalence estimation but also determining the efficacy of treatment strategies and in formulating public health policies. Hence, further research and monitoring are imperative in order to tackle the challenge of antifungal resistance to combat fungal infections (Figure 14.19).

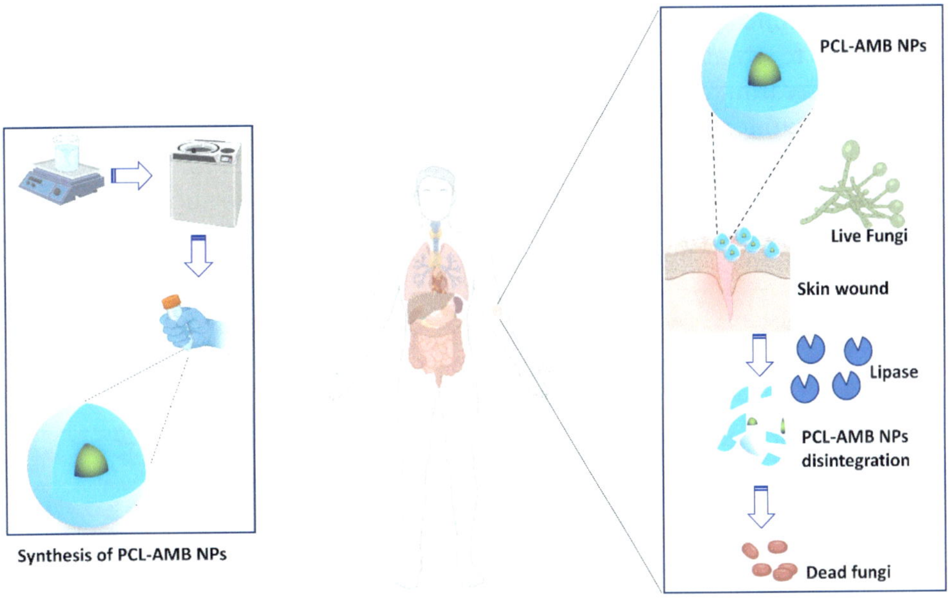

Figure 14.19. Amphotericin B is often utilized in acute situations due to its broad-spectrum antifungal activity, making it suitable for life-threatening infections.

Source: https://pub.mdpi-res.com/nanomaterials/nanomaterials-13-00155/article_deploy/html/images/nanomaterials-13-00155-ag.png?1672393155.

14.5.2. Supportive Care and Management

Supplementary treatment and management form part of the general treatment of histoplasmosis, particularly in severe cases or immune-compromised subjects. Proper management is important because the disease presents in varying clinical manifestations, including acute pulmonary, chronic pulmonary, and disseminated histoplasmosis. Each of these presentations may have different clinical demands. For instance, while antifungal therapy remains the cornerstone of therapy, with agents such as itraconazole, supportive interventions such as oxygenation, hydration, and nutrition are important in patients with respiratory compromise or systemic disease. Early recognition and management of complications are also essential, especially in immunocompromised individuals, such as those undergoing hematopoietic stem cell transplants, where risk of histoplasmosis is elevated within endemic areas (Agrawal et al., 2020). Secondly, enhancing the quality of life for histoplasmosis patients is also a priority. This not only involves treating physiological issues in the short run but also emotional and psychological needs. The chronicity of the disease has the ability to lead to anxiety and depression, particularly in those who have long-standing health problems. Multidisciplinary approaches that include counseling, disease education, and support group attendance are therefore crucial in this setting. Implementation of such psychosocial support systems may play an important role in patient adherence to treatment regimens and quality of life. With the continuous need for holistic management, supportive care also emphasizes the need to address the patient holistically rather than dealing with the infection alone. In special populations, such as those with co-infections such as HIV or receiving treatment for other infectious diseases, personalized supportive care matters. For individuals on antiretroviral therapy, histoplasmosis treatment is more complicated with increased danger for immunocompromised patients and unpredictable results to standard treatments. Continuous education of medical professionals about the nuances of treating concurrent infections in the context of histoplasmosis is necessary in order to address treatment challenges. As the literature has identified, management of both the physical and psychological aspects of care can enhance outcomes for the patient and enhance the effectiveness of management (Ramesh et al.). Ultimately, effective supportive care will require an interdisciplinary approach to deliver overall treatment personally tailored to address specific patient needs (Figure 14.20).

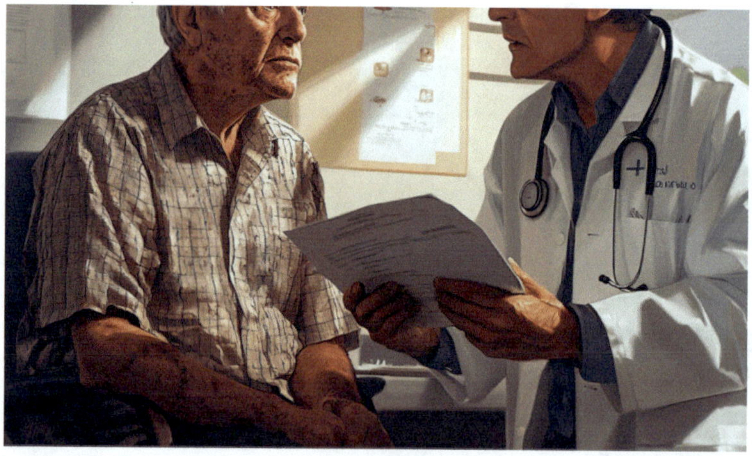

Figure 14.20. Supportive care and management play a crucial role in the comprehensive treatment of histoplasmosis, particularly in patients with severe cases or those with immune compromise.

Source: https://cdn-ilcfhpf.nitrocdn.com/MpIMYOcylyDEZXHWnnskFLOpgiNlSrBN/assets/images/optimized/rev-f673c3a/mdsearchlight.com/wp-content/uploads/2024/11/28906-1731467784582-728x420.png.

14.5.3. Treatment for Severe Cases

In the management of severe histoplasmosis, treatment is typically followed on a course where giving antifungal medications is given priority, particularly in cases of disseminated forms of the disease. Liposomal amphotericin B has become a first-line therapy, especially in severe cases, where prompt treatment is necessary. This form of drug delivery allows for higher drug levels to be delivered to the fungal infection and restricts renal toxicity, which is a restrictive factor for conventional amphotericin preparation. Current clinical trials have demonstrated that the administration of a single initial dose of liposomal amphotericin B can significantly enhance patient outcomes, paving the way for the subsequent treatment with itraconazole as consolidation therapy. Such strategies point towards the necessity for new treatment patterns to provide better and lower toxicity options for patients presenting with life-threatening infections (Bahr et al., 2023). The rationale behind this approach shows a growing recognition of the importance of early and aggressive treatment in severe forms of histoplasmosis. Severe forms of histoplasmosis usually occur in immunocompromised patients, particularly in patients with HIV/AIDS. Clinical presentation in these patients is generally very subtle as the presentation could closely mimic the presentation of other infections, e.g., disseminated tuberculosis (Garner et al., 2020).

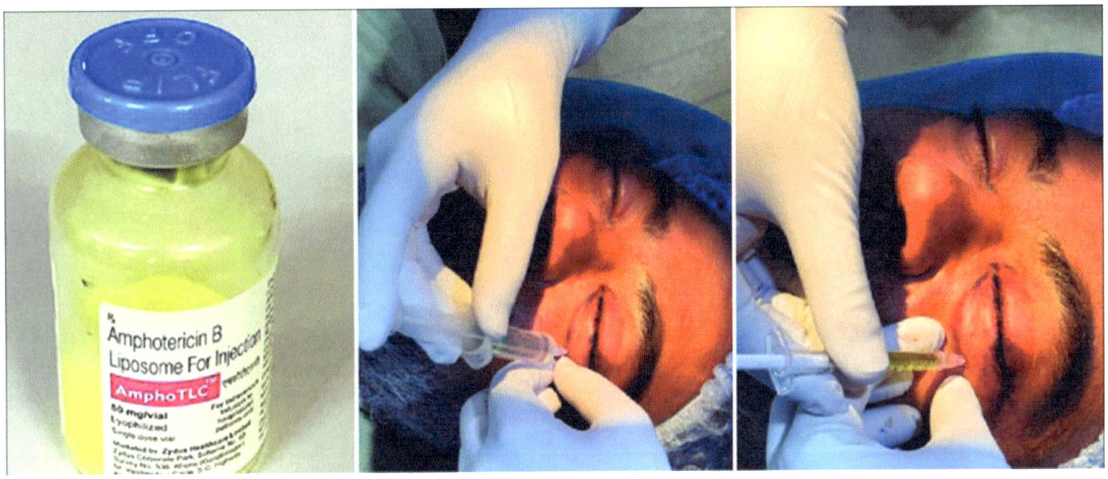

Figure 14.21. Liposomal amphotericin B has emerged as a frontline therapy, especially in severe cases, where immediate intervention is crucial.

Source: https://www.researchgate.net/publication/381861010/figure/fig1/AS:11431281257618419@1719844846316/a-Liposomal-amphotericin-B-50-mg-ml-which-was-used-for-preparing-TRAMB-injection-b.png.

Hence, precise diagnostic tests and timely initiation of treatment are crucial in an attempt to maximize survival. In such patients, the administration of a combination therapy of amphotericin B and subsequent itraconazole treatment has been encouraging to prevent disease advancement and reduce mortality. The agents' application is justified based on their proven efficacy against *Histoplasma capsulatum*, the causative organism of opportunistic infections in vulnerable patients. Therefore, it is the job of clinicians to know the symptoms of acute histoplasmosis and act quickly to administer effective treatment to enhance patient outcomes and prevent the disease complications. Besides the first therapeutic regimens, ongoing research continues to alter treatment regimens and discover new antifungal drugs that can offer enhanced efficacy with negligible side effects. Those newly explored options, such as isavuconazole, present inherent advantages to patient care, but further enhance the arsenal aimed at histoplasmosis and other endemics. With rising incidence, particularly in previously considered low-risk regions, healthcare systems become obligated to revise and redesign treatment regimens. Continued studies on drug efficacy and safety profiles are crucial, especially in high-risk populations like immunocompromised hosts (Bahr et al., 2023). Enhanced treatment effectiveness can be realized through the evolution of antifungal therapy, ultimately resulting in enhanced clinical outcomes and mitigation of the case fatality rate of critical histoplasmosis in different populations (Figure 14.21).

SUMMARY

Histoplasmosis is a systemic infection produced most often by the fungus *Histoplasma capsulatum*, a saprotrophic organism that thrives in environments rich in organic matter, particularly where large quantities of bird or bat droppings are present. The disease is typically limited to the lung after inhalation of spores and leads to a spectrum of clinical syndromes that range from being clinically benign to severe respiratory illness. Weakened immune systems of high-risk populations are most susceptible to disseminated histoplasmosis, which underscores the importance of early diagnosis and treatment. Both geographical instances and ecological environments where the fungus occurs affect disease presence significantly, with certain areas of the United States experiencing higher incidence rates due to favorable microecologies for fungus development. Understanding the pathophysiology of histoplasmosis is important for effective management and treatment. The innate immunity of the body is important in keeping the infection at bay, with macrophages attempting to engulf and kill the fungal spores. However, Histoplasma has devised mechanisms to ensure its survival through evading death, allowing it to survive and multiply within host cells. The interaction can lead to chronic pulmonary disease or systemic infection if not effectively controlled. As with current research, new treatment options are in the pipeline with antifungal agents and immunomodulators to enhance patient outcomes. Coming together of results from various studies brings a better understanding of histoplasmosis, resulting in the development of interventions tailored to certain groups of patients and their respective health conditions. Finally, prevention measures are extremely crucial through public health for histoplasmosis, particularly in areas where this fungus is endemic. Training on the risk of exposure to contaminated environments is important, especially for workers who participate in activities like demolition, construction, or cleanup of bird and bat roosting colonies. Regular monitoring and surveillance could identify high-risk sites and populations and guide preventive practices like personal protective equipment use and strategic vaccination when it is available. Ultimately, collaborative efforts among healthcare professionals, researchers, and environmental agencies will be more comprehensive in bringing about a control and containment of the incidence of histoplasmosis, with significant benefits to public health (Camacho et al., 2011; Brown et al., 2015).

A CLOSER LOOK

IMMUNOMODULATORS

Immunomodulators are medications that alter the immune system's activity, either suppressing or enhancing it, to manage many conditions. They can either be natural or man-made and used in instances where the immune response needs leveling, for example, in autoimmune diseases, infections, or cancer. Examples include corticosteroids (suppressive of immune activity), biologics like TNF inhibitors (used in rheumatoid arthritis), and drugs like interferons (used in multiple sclerosis). Immunomodulators are mostly concerned with restoring immune balance and improving patient outcomes in immune-related disorders.

REFERENCES

1. Abel, J. W., Allen, O., Bullock, D., Finley, et al. (2019). "I don't want to look sick skinny": Perceptions of body image and weight loss in Hispanics living with HIV in South Texas. https://digitalscholarship.unlv.edu/cgi/viewcontent.cgi?article=1875&context=jhdrp (accessed on 27th June 2025).
2. Agrawal, V., Brinda, B. J., & Farag, S. S. (2020). *Histoplasma capsulatum* infection in an allogeneic hematopoietic stem cell transplant patient receiving voriconazole prophylaxis. https://core.ac.uk/download/299809034.pdf (accessed on 27th June 2025).
3. Aklilu, N., Ashine, T., Christley, R., et al. (2016). Development and evaluation of a molecular diagnostic method to rapidly detect *Histoplasma capsulatum* var. *farciminosum*, the causative agent of epizootic lymphangitis, in equine clinical samples. https://core.ac.uk/download/80778446.pdf (accessed on 27th June 2025).
4. Albers, A., Bloch, K. C., Chow, F. C., et al. (2018). Detection of (1,3)-β-d-glucan in cerebrospinal fluid in histoplasma meningitis. https://core.ac.uk/download/227054295.pdf (accessed on 27th June 2025).
5. Anderson, K. L. (2007). Immunity to histoplasmosis induced in mice by components of *Histoplasma capsulatum*. https://core.ac.uk/download/276269419.pdf (accessed on 27th June 2025).
6. Armstrong, B., Burchett, M., Irga, P. J., et al. (2016). Correspondence between urban bird roosts and the presence of aerosolized fungal pathogens. https://opus.lib.uts.edu.au/bitstream/10453/44033/1/Irga%20et%20al%20Mycopathologia%202016.pdf (accessed on 27th June 2025).
7. Bahr, N., & Thompson, G. (2023). Endemic mycoses–are we making progress in management? https://core.ac.uk/download/631293001.pdf (accessed on 27th June 2025).
8. Baker, S., Denning, D. W., Mutapi, F., et al. (2021). Determining the burden of fungal infections in Zimbabwe. https://core.ac.uk/download/478175636.pdf (accessed on 27th June 2025).
9. Bhat, R., Maheshwari, S. K., & Saha, S. (2025). Treating HIV/AIDS patients in India with antiretroviral therapy: A management challenge. https://core.ac.uk/download/pdf/6443480.pdf (accessed on 27th June 2025).
10. Bonnet, Buxton, Centers for Disease Control and Prevention, Dennison, D., et al. (2003). Severe histoplasmosis in travelers to Nicaragua. https://core.ac.uk/download/pdf/8522669.pdf (accessed on 27th June 2025).
11. Britto, J. (2018). Pulmonary histoplasmosis in a patient with cough, dyspnea, pulmonary nodule and rheumatologic manifestations: Case report and review. https://core.ac.uk/download/217211020.pdf (accessed on 27th June 2025).
12. Brown, G. D., Chen, W. Y., Chu, C. L., et al. (2015). CR3 and Dectin-1 collaborate in macrophage cytokine response through association on lipid rafts and activation of Syk-JNK-AP-1 pathway. https://core.ac.uk/download/30435723.pdf (accessed on 27th June 2025).
13. Camacho, D., Cebrián Ramos, M., Granados Fontecha, A., et al. (2011). Reducing the loss of information through annealing text distortion. https://repositorio.uam.es/bitstream/10486/663413/3/reducing_granados_ITNDE_2011_ps.pdf (accessed on 27th June 2025).

14. Cernat, R. C., Dumea, E., & Efrim, N. D. (2023). Epidemiology of histoplasmosis. https://core.ac.uk/download/568374135.pdf (accessed on 27th June 2025).

15. Chaudhuri, U. (2022). Fungal burden of disease in Central and South America. https://core.ac.uk/download/621349787.pdf (accessed on 27th June 2025).

16. Cole, E., & Katta, N. (2014). A 41-year-old man with gastrointestinal symptoms and an unusual exposure history. https://core.ac.uk/download/159354435.pdf (accessed on 27th June 2025).

17. Cordon, A. A., Melendez, J., Powderly, W. G., et al. (2017). AIDS-defining illnesses at initial diagnosis of HIV in a large Guatemalan cohort. https://core.ac.uk/download/212862036.pdf (accessed on 27th June 2025).

18. Correia, A. S., Ernande, B. C. S., Fernandes, C. L. L., et al. (2023). Septic shock, hyperferritinemic syndrome, and multiple organ dysfunction without respiratory failure in a patient with disseminated histoplasmosis and advanced HIV disease. https://core.ac.uk/download/568067009.pdf (accessed on 27th June 2025).

19. Deppen, S. A., Dittus, R. S., Grogan, E. L., et al. (2011). Thoracic operations for pulmonary nodules are frequently not futile in patients with benign disease. https://core.ac.uk/download/pdf/82089076.pdf (accessed on 27th June 2025).

20. Eddy, T. A. (1995). A strategy for integrating principles and concepts of wildlife damage control into the school curriculum. https://core.ac.uk/download/17229383.pdf (accessed on 27th June 2025).

21. Fatima, A., Fatima, A., Hussain, S. A., S., et al. (2025). Conventional cervical smears disclose histoplasmosis: A case report. https://core.ac.uk/download/655504339.pdf (accessed on 27th June 2025).

22. Fernandes, T. A., Gerhard, E. S., Leitão, T. do M. J. S., et al. (2010). Clinical and evolutionary characteristics of 134 patients with disseminated histoplasmosis associated with AIDS in the State of Ceará. https://core.ac.uk/download/37708961.pdf (accessed on 27th June 2025).

23. Garner, P., Global HIV, Hepatitis and Sexually Transmitted Infections Programmers, Hine, P., Murray, et al. (2020). Guidelines for diagnosing and managing disseminated histoplasmosis among people living with HIV. https://core.ac.uk/download/326707128.pdf (accessed on 27th June 2025).

24. Homei, A., & Worboys, M. (2020). Chapter introduction. https://core.ac.uk/download/478128193.pdf (accessed on 27th June 2025).

25. Hügle, T. (2011). Immunology of fibrotic lung disease: Managing infections whilst preventing autoimmunity? https://core.ac.uk/download/pdf/8645097.pdf (accessed on 27th June 2025).

26. Kauffman, C. A., & Terpenning, M. S. (1988). Deep fungal infections in the elderly. https://deepblue.lib.umich.edu/bitstream/2027.42/111183/1/j.1532-5415.1988.tb04028.x.pdf (accessed on 27th June 2025).

27. Lee, J. S., & Van Der Putten, W. (2011). Soil borne human diseases. https://core.ac.uk/download/38621779.pdf (accessed on 27th June 2025).

28. MacInnes, R., & Warris, A. (2021). Pediatric histoplasmosis 2000–2019: A review of 83 cases. https://core.ac.uk/download/443939576.pdf (accessed on 27th June 2025).

29. Mohammed, N. A. (2024). A review of *Histoplasma capsulatum* associated with pulmonary histoplasmosis. https://core.ac.uk/download/620857201.pdf (accessed on 27th June 2025).

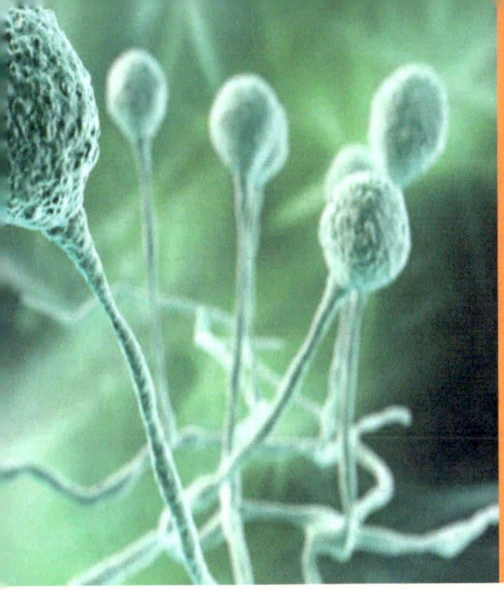

Chapter 15
PARACOCCIDIOIDOMYCOSIS

Contents

Introduction

The pathogenesis of Paracoccidioidomycosis (PCM) calls for the in-depth understanding of its etiology, epidemiology, and clinical presentation. Etiologically caused by the dimorphic fungus *Paracoccidioides brasiliensis*, PCM is primarily endemic to South America, particularly Brazil, and has its main effect on rural communities. A public health concern, the systemic fungal infection has its prevalence linked to various socio-economic determinants and environmental conditions. They start asymptomatically and eventually lead to granulomatous disease affecting greater than one organ system. Dental professionals, and especially dental workers, have a vital role in early identification through the diagnosis of oral lesions that can be observed prior to other systemic signs and symptoms. This introduction will traverse these aspects, having a glimpse into the need to grasp PCM as a severe health concern in the involved locations, hence pointing towards an increased awareness and efficient public health strategies (Almeida et al., 2023). It is important to understand the epidemiological trends of PCM so as to design tailored public health interventions. Middle-aged men are the main victims of the disease, particularly those in agricultural occupations, and this aids in the association between occupational exposure and risk of infection. Rural communities are more vulnerable since environmental exposure to the etiological fungus is greater, with soil tillage and forest clearance further boosting the risk of transmission. As an endemic disease, PCM is likely to have a widespread impact on the quality of life among patients, leading to long-term health complications and chronic management. In coming up with these epidemiological patterns, the integration of qualitative and quantitative research is important and can then inform healthcare providers about populations at risk. This awareness will ultimately facilitate the implementation of targeted awareness programs and prevention strategies for reducing the PCM burden (Camargo et al., 2018). The clinical manifestations of PCM are widespread and reinforce the importance of multidisciplinary collaboration in healthcare settings. Oral lesions are frequently the first indication of the disease, and the contribution of dental professionals cannot, therefore, be overstated in the diagnosis. They can have extensive mucosal involvement and are crucial in proper identification of the disease and treatment planning. They can also be confused with other granulomatous conditions that may mimic PCM, posing a diagnostic challenge to clinicians during clinical assessments. It is therefore imperative that physicians learn about the different manifestations of PCM and in what situations they may occur. In this regard, timely and proper interventions can be administered, thereby ensuring better outcomes for the patients and averting the wider public health implications attributed to this systemic fungal disease (Almeida et al., 2023; Camargo et al., 2018) (Figure 15.1).

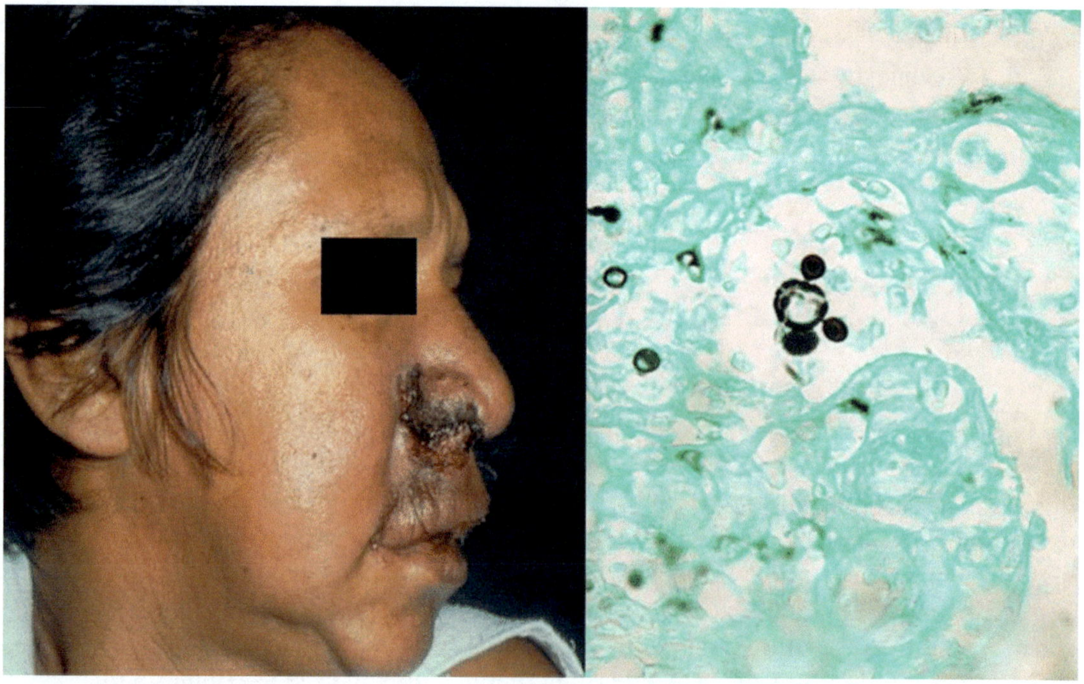

Figure 15.1. Paracoccidioidomycosis.

Source: https://www.researchgate.net/publication/309724565/figure/fig2/AS:434445699293185@1480591334727/Paracoccidioidomycosis-Multiple-budding-of-*Paracoccidioides*-brasiliensis-cells-in-biopsy.png.

15.1. Etiology

Understanding the etiology of paracoccidioidomycosis is essential in order to create effective prevention and treatment measures. The most significant etiologic agent of this mycosis is the dimorphic fungus *Paracoccidioides brasiliensis*, which is predominantly found in Latin America, and more precisely in Brazil, Argentina, and Colombia. The pathogenicity of the disease is determined when spores are inhaled, which leads to pulmonary infection, which can progress to extrapulmonary presentations. The environmental factors favoring the growth of this fungus are warm and humid climates, prevalent in agricultural fields. The climate is not only favorable for the survival of *P. brasiliensis* but also raises occupational exposure among individuals who are working in agriculture. Thus, awareness regarding these environmental and occupational risk factors is essential while tackling the epidemiology of diseases and carrying out focused public health interventions. The role of zoonotic transmission in the etiology of paracoccidioidomycosis cannot be undervalued. Cryptic mycoses have been brought into focus in regions where human and animal habitats are contiguous, with the resultant risk of zoonotic transmission. Although *P. brasiliensis* is fundamentally a human pathogen, domestic mammals may play a role in its ecology and transmission patterns. Existing works reveal that the public health implications of zoonotic fungal infections in poor countries remain uninvestigated and consequently intensive investigations in affected regions are warranted. Nigerian accounts underscore the significance of zoonotic fungi to cause morbidity and mortality among animals and humans as well and thereby indicating the complexity of fungal etiology and transmission dynamics in different ecological environments (Adebiyi et al., 2019).

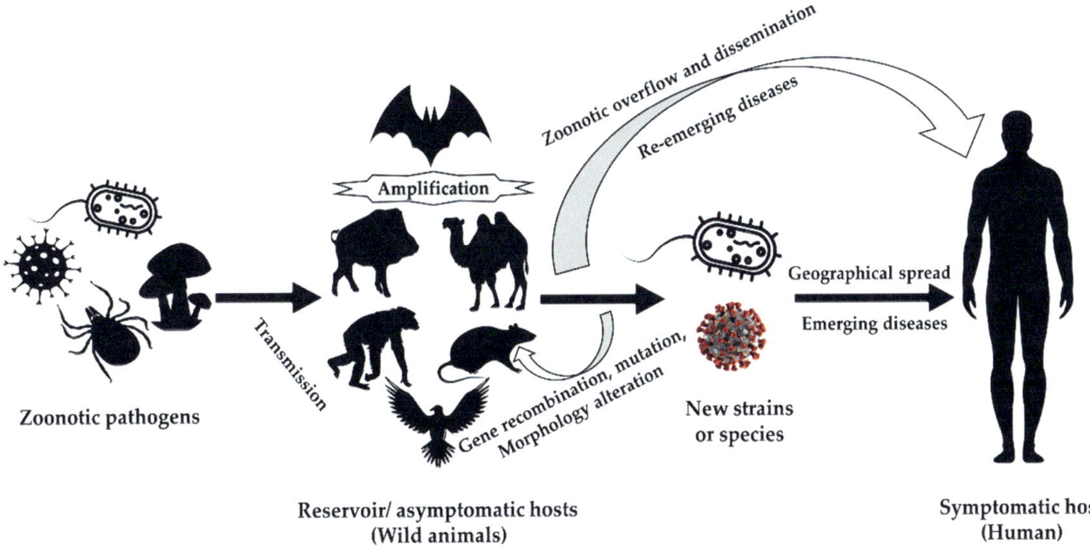

Figure 15.2. The role of zoonotic transmission in the etiology of paracoccidioidomycosis cannot be overlooked.

Source: https://www.mdpi.com/microorganisms/microorganisms-08-01405/article_deploy/html/images/microorganisms-08-01405-g001.png.

While researchers continue to establish a stronger etiologic basis for paracoccidioidomycosis, advances in molecular techniques and diagnostics are required. More advanced diagnostic equipment, such as serologic assays and molecular techniques, are capable of early detection of the disease and treatment, particularly in endemic nations. Lacking are adequate epidemiologic data, which are a significant barrier to healthcare practitioners in endemic nations, denying the introduction of effective intervention strategies. BY prioritizing research to establish the incidence and prevalence of paracoccidioidomycosis, researchers are able to more clearly outline the environmental reservoirs and transmission modes of *P. brasiliensis*. Such a focus on overall research is warranted, as it aligns with international health programs aimed to reduce the burden of the neglected tropical diseases by outlining their fundamental etiologies and improving health outcomes (Fahal et al., 2014) (Figure 15.2).

15.1.1. Causative Agent: Paracoccidioides brasiliensis

Paracoccidioides brasiliensis, the etiologic agent of paracoccidioidomycosis, is a dimorphic fungus inhabitant basically in endemic zones of South and Central America. In the environment, it exists in filamentous form, but becomes yeast-like morphology upon entering the human host, which is critical for pathogenicity. This shape-shifting capability enables the organism to thrive under host conditions of varied nature, posing challenging problems towards treatment and identification. One new way of identifying strains of this fungus is through the use of matrix-assisted laser desorption ionization-time of flight mass spectrometry (MALDI-TOF MS). This approach has proved to be useful in the differentiation of all species in the *Paracoccidioides* genus, facilitating enhanced epidemiological studies and understanding the diversity of the fungi and its application towards paracoccidioidomycosis (Almeida et al., 2015).

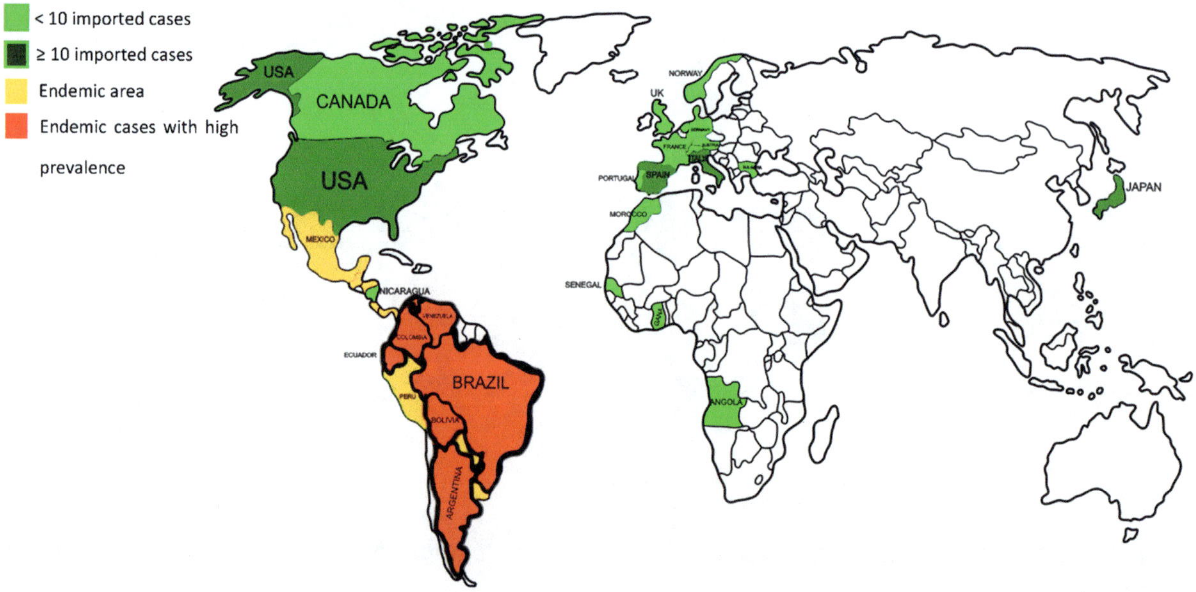

Figure 15.3. The causative agent of paracoccidioidomycosis, *Paracoccidioides brasiliensis*, is a dimorphic fungus primarily found in endemic regions of South and Central America.

Source: https://pub.mdpi-res.com/jof/jof-08-01098/article_deploy/html/images/jof-08-01098-g001.png?1666084058.

Immunological response elicited by *Paracoccidioides brasiliensis* is another subject of study in the ongoing research on paracoccidioidomycosis. Studies that examine the anti-*P. brasiliensis* immunoglobulin isotypes demonstrated variable antibody reactivity in patients with acute and chronic forms of the disease. Notably, immunoglobulin levels responded more intensely towards complete antigens compared to chemically modified antigens, offering critical information about the immune system's recognition and adaptation mechanisms. For instance, the acute form of the disease exhibits a higher IgG and IgM response, yet chronic forms present higher IgA levels, suggesting various immunological conditions. These findings pave the way for improved diagnostic approaches, since the understanding of these immune responses can allow the creation of new therapies. To conceive effective public health interventions in endemic regions, understanding the biology and pathogenicity of *Paracoccidioides brasiliensis* is essential. The environmental reservoirs of *P. brasiliensis* indicate that raising awareness regarding its transmission and conditions conducive to infection is of significant value. In addition, more sophisticated molecular identification techniques like MALDI-TOF MS can inform epidemiological data and lead to expedient public health interventions. Similarly, increased understanding of the immune response can assist in the development of vaccines and immunotherapies. Thus, ongoing research into the causative agent of paracoccidioidomycosis not only aids in the treatment of patients but also makes significant contributions to broader public health schemes aimed at preventing the impact of this debilitating fungal disease among infected people (Figure 15.3).

15.1.2. Environmental Factors Contributing to Infection

The interface between the environmental factors and infectious disease is most evocative in the tropics and subtropics, where conditions are optimal for the development of pathogens. In Paracoccidioidomycosis, the convergence of climate, land use, and biodiversity contributes to the infection prevalence most significantly. For instance, deforestation in the Amazon basin not only eliminates the ecological balance but also alters the habitat of various species that may act as reservoirs or vectors of infectious agents. Destruction of the habitat, leading to loss of biodiversity, has been linked to disease outbreaks because damaged ecosystems are likely to lack the capacity to harbor the natural enemies of pathogens, hence spreading them with ease. This has significant implications for public health, especially in areas where environmental degradation is extensive, and thus it is significant to be aware of these interactions while trying to combat Paracoccidioidomycosis and other infectious diseases (Almeida et al., 2020). Also, some environmental conditions, such as humidity and temperature, play a crucial role in the lifecycle of the fungus *Paracoccidioides brasiliensis* responsible for Paracoccidioidomycosis. The fungus thrives in hot and humid environments, which are typically found where agricultural activities like animal husbandry and agriculture are prevalent. Agricultural activities may contribute to creating an environment that is conducive to infection, given that soil disturbance has the tendency to enhance fungal spore dispersal and human exposure. The intricate interdependence of land use changes and the spread of *Paracoccidioides brasiliensis* is an evident proof of the need for an integrated One Health approach considering environmental, animal, and human health interactions. Emphasis on such environmental factors is key to carrying out effective disease-control strategies and minimizing its impacts on infected populations (Fortes et al., 2009). In addition, socio-economic factors can aggravate the environmental situation that favors Paracoccidioidomycosis infection. Certain groups of people in impoverished places do not receive medical treatment and adequate education on how to avoid infection, and as a result, morbidity can be on the rise. Environmental degradation usually exacerbates these issues since groups that rely on agriculture are more vulnerable to climate change and ecological instability. Furthermore, the interlinked relationship between ecosystem health and human wellbeing emphasizes the need for joined-up policies that address environmental sustainability as much as they address health promotion. By increasing community awareness and developing infrastructures for health, it is possible to develop resilience to environmental stressors as well as to infectious disease, hence reducing the burden of Paracoccidioidomycosis and enhancing public health outcomes in vulnerable populations (Almeida et al., 2020; Fortes et al., 2009) (Figure 15.4).

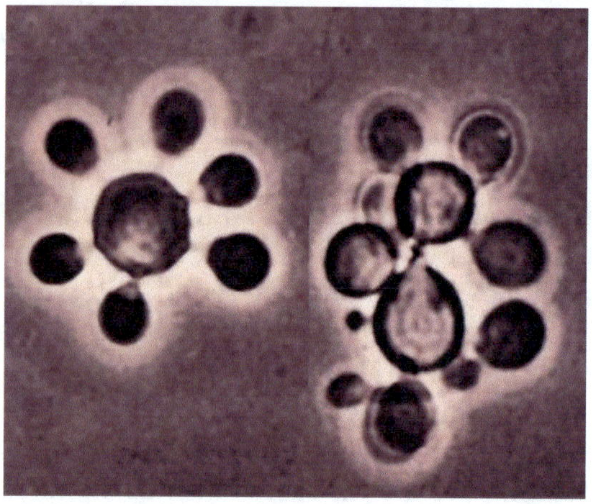

Figure 15.4. *Paracoccidioides brasiliensis.*

Source: https://botit.botany.wisc.edu/toms_fungi/images/paraco1.jpg.

15.1.3. Geographic Distribution of the Fungus

The geographical distribution of *Paracoccidioides brasiliensis*, the etiological fungus of paracoccidioidomycosis, is highly biased towards Latin America, particularly Brazil, where the disease takes on great public health significance. Paracoccidioidomycosis is relatively high in rural settings, suggesting a strong correlation between environmental factors and disease prevalence. These rural settings generally offer the most favorable habitat for fungus growth, particularly in subtropical and tropical areas. This fact needs to be considered while making arrangements for prevention and control measures. In Brazil, epidemiological data indicate that certain areas, such as the South and Southeast, have consistently had a greater mortality rate for this disease, with evidence of localized endemicity. This distributional trend underscores the importance of determining the ecological and environmental dynamics underlying the dissemination of the fungus in these regions and thus of creating adequate public health policies. A mortality study of paracoccidioidomycosis in Brazil from 1980 to 1995 is a reflection of the enormous morbidity of the disease, emphasizing the geographical distribution. The research concluded that paracoccidioidomycosis was the eighth leading infectious disease cause of death with 1.45 deaths per million inhabitants and a clearly unbalanced spatial pattern across the country. The Southern region recorded the highest death rates, the second being the Central West region, hence making it essential regions to be watched. As indicated by the data, approximately 22.71% of the municipalities in Brazil recorded deaths due to this disease. These findings point toward specific public health interventions in endemic regions, and the utility of epidemiological surveillance in explaining patterns of geographic spread as a strategy to contain the impact of such a fungal infection. Wildlife study is also another option compared to knowledge of the ecological distribution of *P. brasiliensis*, pointing toward varying reservoirs of animals that can facilitate transmission of the fungus in various areas. A recent study showed that wildlife killed on the roads were effective in the detection of the presence of some fungal pathogens such as *P. brasiliensis* using PCR methods. Such research highlights the future ecological relationships and the potential roles various animal species can play as reservoirs or vectors of the fungus, especially as researchers learn how these interactions affect the paracoccidioidomycosis epidemiology. By understanding the geographic distribution of fungi in the environment, public health workers can more effectively forecast future outbreaks and develop plans for disease monitoring and control among human and animal populations, hence enhancing health outcomes within affected areas (Bagagli et al., 2010) (Figure 15.5).

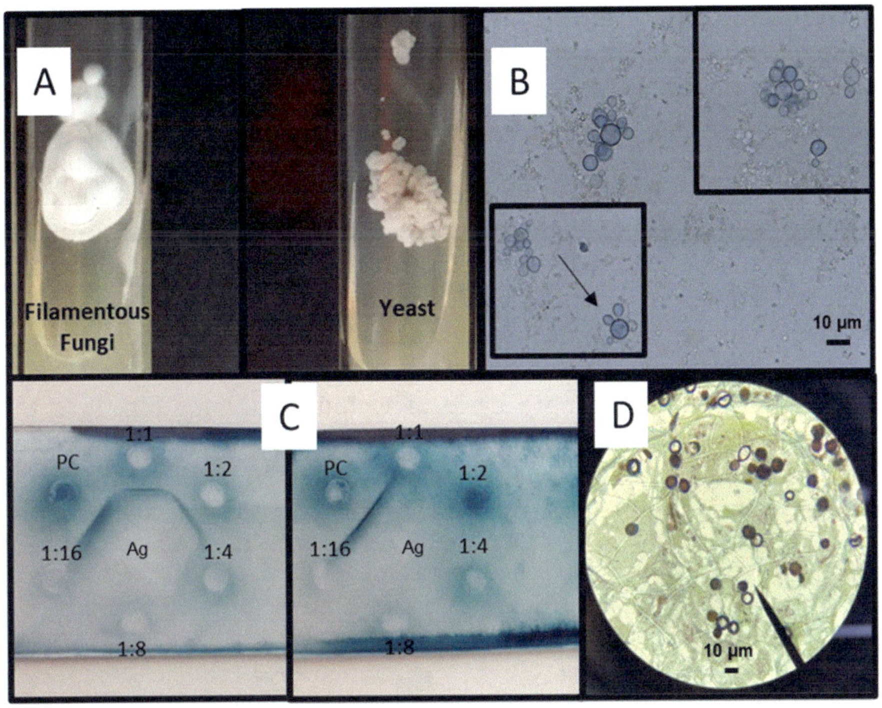

Figure 15.5. The incidence of paracoccidioidomycosis is notably high in rural areas, suggesting a strong correlation between environmental factors and disease prevalence.

Source: https://pub.mdpi-res.com/jof/jof-08-01098/article_deploy/html/images/jof-08-01098-g003.png?1666084053.

15.2. Pathophysiology

The pathophysiology of paracoccidioidomycosis (PCM), the endemic mycosis caused by the dimorphic fungus *Paracoccidioides brasiliensis*, is a highly complex interaction between the immune system of the host and the pathogen. Following inhalation of the fungus spores, the pathogen transforms into the yeast form with a tendency to colonize the lung tissue. The initial immune response is characterized by the activation of alveolar macrophages and the release of pro-inflammatory cytokines. It should be noted that the production of cytokines IL-6 and TNF-α is accountable for the recruitment of immune cells to the infectious site, making possible an efficient local inflammatory reaction. Such immune response dysregulation could lead to a chronic disease when the host is unable to present an efficient immune response, resulting in progressive pulmonary and systemic PCM manifestations. The balance between the virulence factors of the fungi and the host defense mechanisms plays an important role in determining the clinical course of the infected patient. The immune response in PCM patients is also delicate and typically manifested as a predominance of CD8+ T lymphocytes in BALF. The presence of the T cells shows that there is an adaptive immune response specially tailored to combat the infection due to the fungus. It is proven by evidence that pro-inflammatory mediators such as MIP-1α, released by activated alveolar macrophages, play a key role in recruitment of CD8+ T cells to the lungs (Ledeboer et al., 2013). The recruitment plays a crucial role in the elimination of the causative fungus but leads to tissue injury and the pathogenesis of the diseases through excessive or chronic immune response. Moreover, certain host genetic determinants in the immune system could have the potential to influence susceptibility to PCM, highlighting the importance of an understanding of host-pathogen interactions in the pathophysiological paradigm. The understanding of the pathophysiological mechanisms of PCM demands not only the study of immunity but also the involvement of signaling pathways in chronic inflammatory diseases. For instance, studies have found that Toll-like receptor (TLR) signaling pathways are involved in mediating neuropathic pain responses, potentially reflecting the inflammatory pain syndromes experienced by PCM patients (Ledeboer et al., 2013). TLR signaling findings on PCM pathology are of special interest since they might modulate the intensity of the immune response and subsequent disease progression. Elevated levels of inflammatory cytokines lead to increased tissue injury, creating a cycle of vicious inflammation. It is thus essential to understand the intricate mechanisms in order to develop specific therapeutic interventions that can modulate the inflammatory load and also facilitate effective antifungal immunity in patients with paracoccidioidomycosis (Figure 15.6).

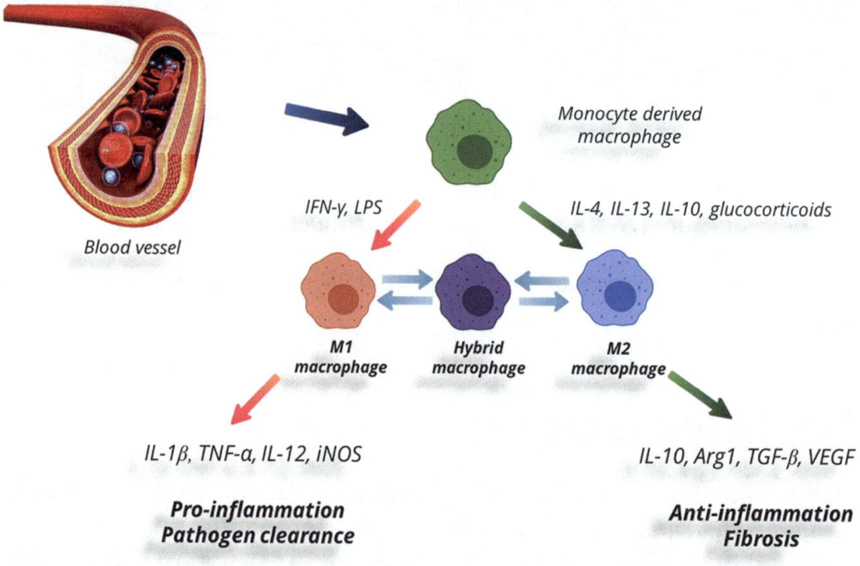

Figure 15.6. The initial immune response is characterized by the activation of alveolar macrophages and the release of pro-inflammatory cytokines.

Source: https://images-provider.frontiersin.org/api/ipx/w=1200&f=png/https://www.frontiersin.org/files/Articles/682871/fimmu-12-682871-HTML/image_m/fimmu-12-682871-g001.jpg.

15.2.1. Mechanism of Infection and Immune Response

The infection process due to *Paracoccidioides brasiliensis*, the causative agent of paracoccidioidomycosis (PCM), is triggered by spore inhalation with subsequent morphological transition into pathogenic yeast forms in the lung of the host. Once established in the pulmonary compartment, the organism exploits its property of immune evasion, primarily through the generation of immunomodulatory compounds. These include the 43 kDa glycoprotein antigen, among others, which play a crucial role in dictating the immune status of the infected host. Particularly, the P10 peptide is a T-cell epitope that evokes a protective immune response, as opposed to the P4 and P23 peptides, which suppress macrophage function and modulate inflammation, ensuring the organisms survival. The ability of such peptides to modulate immune cell activity points towards the pathogenic mechanism employed by *P. brasiliensis* to survive under an apparently destructive immune environment (Feitosa et al., 2012).

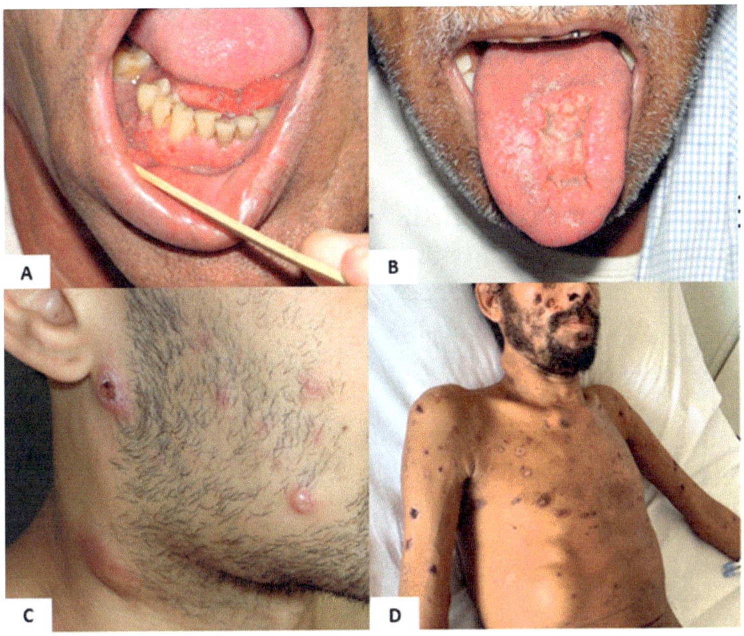

Figure 15.7. The initiation of infection by *Paracoccidioides brasiliensis*, the fungal agent of paracoccidioidomycosis (PCM), begins through the inhalation of spores, which subsequently undergoes morphological transformation into pathogenic yeast forms within the hosts lungs.

Source: https://www.mdpi.com/jof/jof-08-01098/article_deploy/html/images/jof-08-01098-g002.png.

The resultant immune response against *P. brasiliensis* is multicomponent and tends to be characterized by a granulomatous response through Th1 responses. However, in the infection, there is a shift away from a Th2-mediated response, triggered by cytokines such as IL-4, which has the capacity to prevent disease progress. Pre-exposure to cell-free antigens (CFA) prior to infection has, in recent studies, been reported to induce disorganized granuloma formation and increased fungal replication within the host organs. The subsequent rise in IL-4 is linked with enhanced vulnerability to the fungal infection. In models that are deficient in IL-4, the typical pathogenesis of PCM, including fungal colonization and granuloma size, is dramatically impaired. This finding suggests that immunoregulation by IL-4 following CFA exposure is crucial to the extent of PCM and demonstrates the dynamic interplay between immune modulation and fungal virulence (Pina et al., 2011). Interplay between innate and adaptive immunity also explains host responses to the *P. brasiliensis* mechanisms more effectively. Notably, concentration and timing of specific peptides have been shown to skew immune responses towards pro-inflammatory or anti-inflammatory states. In model systems, P4 and P23 peptide administration resulted in significant reductions of inflammatory cytokine production, such as TNF-alpha and IL-6, and elevated IL-10 levels associated with immunosuppression. These mechanisms promote a state conducive to fungal growth and tissue invasion. Lastly, understanding how *P. brasiliensis* modulates the immune response is central to understanding PCM pathogenesis and, by extension, therapeutic intervention into re-establishing the balance of immune activation and tolerance and reinforcing the hosts immunity against this chronic infection (Feitosa et al., 2012) (Figure 15.7).

15.2.2. Clinical Manifestations of the Disease

The clinical presentation of paracoccidioidomycosis (PCM) is mainly an expression of the systemic character of the disease, which results from infection with the dimorphic fungus *Paracoccidioides brasiliensis*. The illness is remarkably endemic in South America, most prominently in Brazil, and predominantly involves middle-aged male individuals residing in rural settlements. Among the earliest symptoms of PCM, mucosal lesions of the oral cavity stand out particularly because they may represent the earliest detectable signs of infection, which, in turn, may appear before pulmonary symptoms. The lesions not only serve to facilitate earliest diagnosis but also pinpoint the role of dentists in the identification and management of such a disorder. The clinical presentation of such lesions can also vary from one single abnormal lesion to many ulcers, depending on the severity and progression of the disease in challenging the immune system of the host (Almeida et al., 2023). In viewing the clinical presentation of PCM, it is essential to take into account the different symptoms observed in different geographical regions. Although predominantly endemic in Brazil, cases of the disease occurring outside endemic areas have been detected, which underlines the requirement for clinical vigilance. In such regions, such as the Northeast of Brazil, patients typically present with distinctive oral lesions, such as multiple ulcers or solitary lesions on the hard palate and buccal mucosa. A study conducted between 2000 and 2017 remarked that all cases reported involved male patients with a mean age of 53.8 years, showing the trends in the population of PCM. The trend verifies the necessity of increased awareness of PCM, particularly for differential diagnoses of chronic oral conditions, which typically would involve squamous cell carcinoma as one of the possibilities (Bonan et al., 2019). Histopathological features of PCM are all that help to explain its clinical manifestation. The patients present with hyperplastic epithelium and intraepithelial microabscesses along with a granulomatous chronic inflammation reaction in the connective tissue. It is essential to recognize the pathogen, as yeasts are visible intra- and extracellularly, often in multinucleated giant cells. Such intricate implication not only shows the systemic progression of the disease but also points to the bodys resistance to infection. All these histological alterations allow us to make essential conclusions regarding the progression of disease and aid in differentiating PCM from other oral conditions. The more skilled clinicians are in recognizing the clinical and histological appearance of these features, the earlier diagnosis and effective therapy become feasible, and ultimately patient outcomes improve (Almeida et al., 2023) (Figure 15.8).

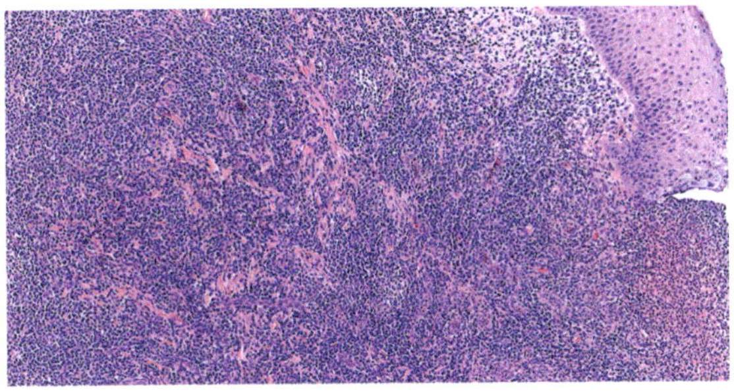

Figure 15.8. The histopathological features of PCM are integral to understanding its clinical manifestations. Patients commonly display hyperplastic epithelium and intraepithelial microabscesses, alongside a granulomatous chronic inflammatory response within the connective tissue.

Source: https://www.researchgate.net/publication/364093119/figure/fig2/AS:1143128110304305 3@1669588318508/Histopathological-features-of-PCM-a-H-E-stain-revealed-the-presence-of-a-subepithelial.jpg.

15.2.3. Complications Associated with Paracoccidioidomycosis

Complications associated with Paracoccidioidomycosis (PCM) are widespread and have the ability to significantly impact patients quality of life. Most prevalent among complications is the development of oral lesions, and these are often the first and most noticeable signs of disease. These lesions most commonly appear on the oral mucosa and are very painful, leading to difficulty eating and speaking. Further, if left untreated, such lesions may progress to more severe forms with potential secondary infection and systemic dissemination of the fungal agent. Dentists and oral health professionals play central roles in diagnosing such presentations early enough to facilitate early intervention that can buffer subsequent complications and guarantee better health outcomes (Almeida et al., 2023). Besides oral manifestations, PCM may also lead to severe pulmonary complications. The respiratory system is usually affected, and the fungus causes chronic granulomatous infections that are imitable for tuberculosis. It presents with chronic cough, hemoptysis, and dyspnea, which can evolve to respiratory failure if the infection is not properly controlled. Chronic pulmonary complications can result in long-term loss of lung function, which can severely impact the patients respiratory status and quality of life. Furthermore, secondary bacterial infection risk in patients with compromised pulmonary function increases, and it needs vigilant monitoring and management (Almeida et al., 2023). Other than oral and respiratory symptoms, PCM can be linked with extra-pulmonary involvement, which affects various organs such as lymph nodes, skin, and even the central nervous system.

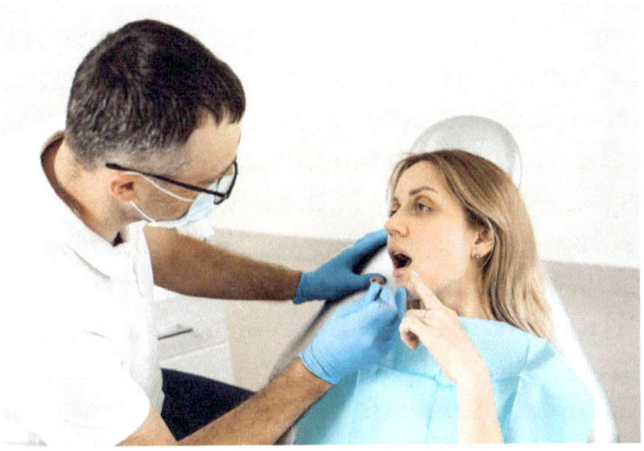

Figure 15.9. Dentists and oral health professionals play a critical role in diagnosing these manifestations early, allowing for timely intervention that can mitigate further complications and promote better health outcomes.

Source: https://cdn.prod.website-files.com/66a29d804d1aff27a2f2ead2/67c86f43f489dfc5f665e105_6759cfa829d93ebdc6d0c7b4_dentistis-and-oral-cancer-prevention.png.

The symptoms can lead to serious systemic complications, including lymphadenopathy, skin lesions, and neurological damage. Of these, neurological involvement is particularly injurious, as it may result in cognitive impairments and neurological disease. Systemic nature of PCM makes the aforementioned complications complicate not only treatment approaches but also endemic areas' public health measures. Awareness of PCMs varied complications is important for healthcare personnel since early diagnosis and treatment can significantly improve patient prognosis (Figure 15.9).

15.3. Diagnosis

Diagnosis of paracoccidioidomycosis (PCM) is beset by numerous challenges due to the overlap of signs and symptoms with other lung diseases. Presentation of the disease can readily mimic such more common conditions as tuberculosis or pneumonia, which necessitates precise identification in order to receive appropriate and timely treatment. In endemic regions, particularly in Latin America where PCM is endemic, clinicians must have a high degree of suspicion, especially in those with occupational history of exposure to *Paracoccidioides brasiliensis* fungus. With the vast agricultural activity present in these countries, a complete patient history and clinical assessment are crucial in shortlisting differential diagnosis,. The use of clinical specimens obtained from other locations, including the oral cavity and lungs, is a required step in establishing the disease and differentiating it from respiratory illnesses, aided by the high rate of samples derived from such areas (Biolowons et al., 2021). Laboratory detection of PCM involves a multifaceted process involving mycologic and serologic tests. Culture methods have long been the gold standard of diagnosis but are frequently time-consuming and in some cases provide false-negative reports. An attempt to overcome these limitations has arrived in the form of the use of antibody detection along with antigen assays, which has significantly enhanced diagnostic sensitivity. The more recent tests, including the gp43 and gp70 antigen detection tests, provide greater reproducibility and sensitivity for PCM identification even in complicated central nervous system and pulmonary cases (Camargo et al., 2008). Health care providers and laboratory professionals need to know the advantages and limitations of these diagnostic tests to maximize patient outcomes, particularly in the event of possible disease progression in undiagnosed infections. Lastly, a successful paracoccidioidomycosis diagnosis relies on a partnership between clinical know-how and advanced laboratory equipment. Research continues to emphasize the importance of an integrated diagnostic strategy that mixes standard histopathology with modern serological methods.

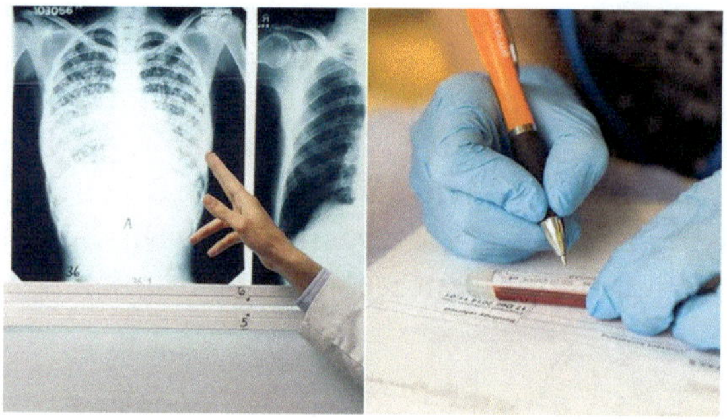

Figure 15.10. The clinical presentation can often mimic more common conditions such as tuberculosis or pneumonia, making accurate identification crucial to ensure timely and effective treatment.

Source: https://images.everydayhealth.com/images/lung-respiratory/tuberculosis/tuberculosis-diagnostic-tests-rm-722x406.jpg?sfvrsn=fe764e81_1.

For instance, the use of antigen detection in body fluids, such as cerebrospinal fluid and bronchoalveolar lavage fluid, can greatly improve diagnostic sensitivity to allow for earlier treatment initiation. Such a multi-faceted approach is particularly crucial in endemic regions, where misdiagnosis can lead to excessive morbidity and mortality. Through rationalization of diagnostic tests and increased awareness of PCMs diverse clinical presentations, clinicians can optimize both diagnostic yield and treatment efficacy regimens (Camargo et al., 2008) (Figure 15.10).

15.3.1. Clinical Assessment and Symptom Evaluation

Clinical examination and symptom assessment are critical components in the diagnosis and treatment of paracoccidioidomycosis (PCM), a fungal infection endemic to certain regions of Latin America. Effective clinical assessment begins with an adequate patient history that targets work exposure and geographical risk factors that could potentially predispose an individual to the infection. Symptoms typically develop variably, with pulmonary disease as the most common presenting symptom, e.g., cough, sputum, and dyspnea. Moreover, the occurrence of oral signs—e.g., mulberry-shaped ulcerations—is an alerting signal for clinicians to seek out potential PCM cases. Because of the multidimensional involvement of the immunological components, especially in immunocompromised patients, meticulous clinical assessment is most critical in order to eliminate other infectious diseases and to institute prompt intervention, which has an ultimate impact on patient outcomes. The significance of a thorough physical examination cannot be overemphasized. Clinicians ought to examine the aforementioned sites most frequently affected by PCM, including the oral cavity and lungs, to find characteristic lesions. Findings reveal that out of individuals diagnosed with oral PCM, the gingiva and alveolar ridge are the locations most often affected, which constitute a prime target for clinicians during examinations. Boolean search techniques in most databases have clarified the clinicopathological features and epidemiological features of PCM, indicating the male predominance and age groups predominantly affected. This cyclical process of clinical examination is helpful in stabilizing a differential diagnosis, particularly since PCM has features overlapping with other neoplastic and infectious conditions. Determination of these facts during primary evaluations can thus revolutionally alter the course of diagnosis and treatment. In addition, symptom assessment of PCM is important in guiding therapeutic management and following up on the course of the disease. By employing laboratory investigations and imaging procedures, clinicians can validate clinical impressions so that a greater understanding of the patient's status may be appreciated. Imaging, for instance, may illustrate classical pulmonary patterns of PCM or outline the distribution of disseminated disease. Also, ascitic fluid analysis in immunocompromised patients, who at times may present with atypical presentations such as chylous ascites, emphasizes the need for detailed differential diagnoses. Such evaluation not only aids in confirming PCM but also aids in treating co-existing conditions so that all possible complications are addressed in full. Through these multi-dimensional approaches of clinical evaluation and symptom assessment, clinicians are able to enhance diagnostic accuracy and treatment efficacy in the management of paracoccidioidomycosis (Figure 15.11).

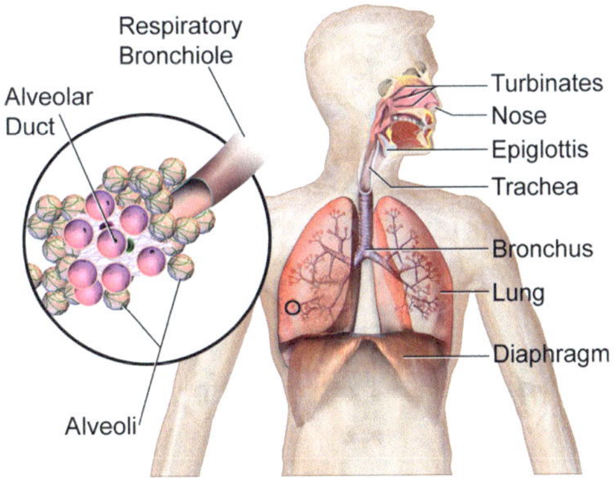

Figure 15.11. Sputum production.

Source: https://www.physio-pedia.com/images/thumb/a/af/Respiratory_System_basic.png/300px-Respiratory_System_basic.png.

15.3.2. Laboratory Tests and Imaging Techniques

For the diagnosis of Paracoccidioidomycosis, laboratory results and radiological studies play the key role in making the accurate diagnosis. As the conventional culture methods have limitations with decreased sensitivity, other techniques such as serologic tests, antigen detection, and molecular tests are gaining more prominence. These non-culture-based diagnostic techniques, though less researched, are rapid and confirm histopathological diagnosis. For instance, the identification of specific antibodies against *Paracoccidioides brasiliensis* can confirm exposure to the fungus and assist in clinical diagnosis, especially in immunocompromised patients. Notably, the validity of PCR-based assays can complement diagnostic correctness further by the direct identification of fungal DNA from clinical material, thereby accelerating the identification process crucial for patient management. It is thus paramount to employ a multimodal strategy incorporating a combination of various laboratory examinations to maximize diagnostic correctness for Paracoccidioidomycosis. Imaging techniques are also used in the diagnosis of Paracoccidioidomycosis, particularly in assessing the degree of lung involvement, which is common among patients with the disease. Chest X-rays in most instances are able to detect characteristic pulmonary lesions of this mycosis, such as reticulonodular infiltrates, nodules, or cavitary lesions. More sophisticated imaging techniques such as computed tomography (CT) scans are able to provide finer details and further assist in the differentiation of Paracoccidioidomycosis from other lung infections. This difference is especially useful in light of the increasing prevalence of opportunistic infections in immunocompromised patients, such as those with HIV/AIDS. For example, imaging findings can allow clinicians to distinguish Paracoccidioidomycosis from tuberculosis or other similar pulmonary infections, ultimately affecting appropriate management strategies. Imaging thus constitutes an essential adjunct to laboratory workups, further refining the diagnosis. The relationship between laboratory testing and imaging techniques is important for the correct management of Paracoccidioidomycosis, particularly for patients with complicated clinical manifestations. In patients who are also receiving antifungal therapy, routine culture techniques may yield false negatives due to the inhibition of fungal growth, as in breakthrough invasive fungal infections studies (Alastruey-Izquierdo et al., 2020).

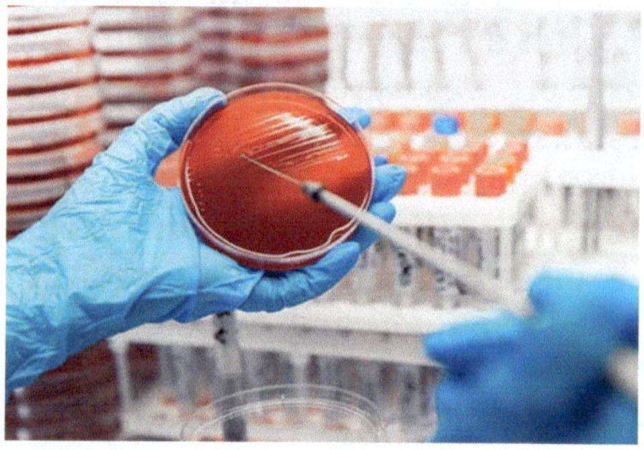

Figure 15.12. Given the challenges posed by traditional culture methods, which can exhibit reduced sensitivity, alternative diagnostic approaches such as serologic tests, antigen detection, and molecular methods are increasingly emphasized.

Source: https://myadlm.org/~/media/project/myadlm/myadlm/images/publications/cln/industry-i nsights/thermo-fisher/pg2723pjt9431col021281 shutterstock_ 2142832239_500.jpg.

This makes non-invasive diagnostic modalities like antigen tests and serologic assays essential in providing real-time information on the infections status. Secondly, as evidenced in recent medical literature, integration of clinical history with results of diagnosis is pivotal in managing co-infections that are common among some populations, especially among HIV-positive individuals (Antunes et al., 2003). Therefore, a multidisciplinary diagnosis based on both laboratory and imaging techniques is required in achieving an immediate and accurate diagnosis, which is essential for the successful management of Paracoccidioidomycosis (Figure 15.12).

15.3.3. Differential Diagnosis Considerations

Differential diagnosis is crucial in PCM clinical diagnosis due to the fact that symptoms are similar to other illnesses, particularly respiratory infections. Physicians must adequately screen diseases such as tuberculosis and histoplasmosis, which share similar respiratory manifestations. According to published literature, co-morbidity of tuberculosis has been observed among PCM patients and exhibited sensitivity to justify adequate investigation of a patient's history and onset symptoms. The geographical distribution and population of patients also complicate the diagnostic process, as PCM-endemic regions may at the same time have high frequencies of other fungal infections. Some clinical manifestations—such as lesions and immune response type—can distinguish PCM from these other diagnoses and direct corresponding and timely treatment interventions. Another critical element of differential diagnosis of PCM is the inclusion of autoimmune illnesses such as systemic lupus erythematosus and rheumatoid arthritis, which affect the lungs as well. The autoimmune diseases may have multifocal pulmonary manifestations that would mimic PCM, such as hemoptysis, cough, and pulmonary nodules.

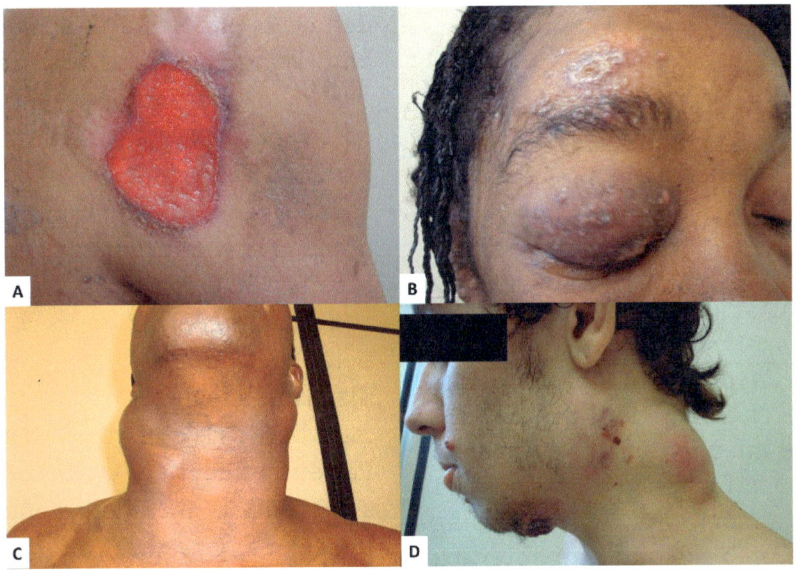

Figure 15.13. Differential diagnosis is a crucial aspect in the clinical evaluation of Paracoccidioidomycosis (PCM) due to the overlapping symptoms with various other diseases, particularly respiratory infections.

Source: https://www.mdpi.com/jof/jof-09-00946/article_deploy/html/images/jof-09-00946-g002.png.

These should be differentiated by thorough assessment of imaging studies and serological markers. The doctors must also be careful to see the formation of fungal balls or cavitary lesions that may be characteristic of certain illnesses but less common in PCM. Importantly, while PCM will have a chronic course, autoimmune illnesses are usually complicated by exacerbations whose multifaceted symptomatology renders it thus vital to re-evaluate the patients clinical history and clinical course to prior therapy with keen observation. Moreover, no underestimate must be made of the role played by co-infection in differential diagnosis of PCM. The interaction between PCM and HIV/AIDS has been noted in the literature that is relevant, particularly in regions where both diseases are endemic. Immunocompromise evoked by HIV has the potential to significantly alter the presentation of fungal infection, and often leads to atypical presentations, which complicate diagnosis as well as clinical management. In these instances, providers should be careful to watch for not only PCM, but also other opportunistic infections that can occur, including aspergillosis and cryptococcosis. The consistent mortality rate observed with PCM highlights the need for prompt and accurate diagnosis, as delays in the detection and treatment of co-infections can have a negative impact on patient outcomes and disease control overall (Figure 15.13).

15.4. Treatment

The management of paracoccidioidomycosis (PCM) is a multifaceted issue that depends on the severity of the infection and the patient's general condition. Antifungal medication is the mainstay of PCM treatment, with agents including sulfonamides, itraconazole, and amphotericin B. Antifungal medication choice depends on disease severity, comorbid conditions, and tolerance to drugs by the patient. A planned approach generally means initiating therapy with a more intense drug like amphotericin B in the case of severe infection and then a switch to oral azoles for long-term maintenance. An approach like this staggered treatment not only aims to eradicate the fungal pathogen but also to circumvent or minimize potential side effects, establishing a balance between efficacy and safety in treating patients, which is so critical for optimal outcomes in the long term. Patient monitoring during therapy is essential, as patients can frequently develop a variety of side effects from antifungal medications, thus requiring meticulous control. Regular review, both clinical and laboratory, helps to detect any emerging complications or side effects. In some cases, therapy needs to be adjusted on the basis of pharmacological response or drug resistance emergence. Furthermore, multidisciplinary management involving infectious diseases specialists, pulmonologists, and dentists plays a critical role in ensuring optimal therapeutic outcomes.

For instance, PCM oral manifestations may result in complications that require special attention; therefore, an early intervention by the dentist is important to achieve early detection and treatment of moriform lesions and other oral manifestations as highlighted in a recent case report wherein severe oral signs led to an accurate PCM diagnosis, and subsequently, to successful management (Baldo et al., 2022). After appropriate antifungal treatment, long-term care for PCM may involve prophylaxis against recrudescence. This is especially true in patients who have underlying immunocompromising diseases such as HIV/AIDS or diabetes and may be at risk of recurrence of the disease. Patient education on recurrence signs and symptoms is included, educating the patient to seek early medical intervention should they present. Follow-ups periodically and radiologic check-ups are an insurance mechanism for the early detection of recurrences or disease-related complications. Lastly, the efficient treatment of paracoccidioidomycosis relies on an extended program encompassing successful antifungal therapy, proper monitoring, and interdisciplinarity to ensure patients not only clinical cure but also better quality of life upon therapy (Colombo et al., 2008) (Figure 15.14).

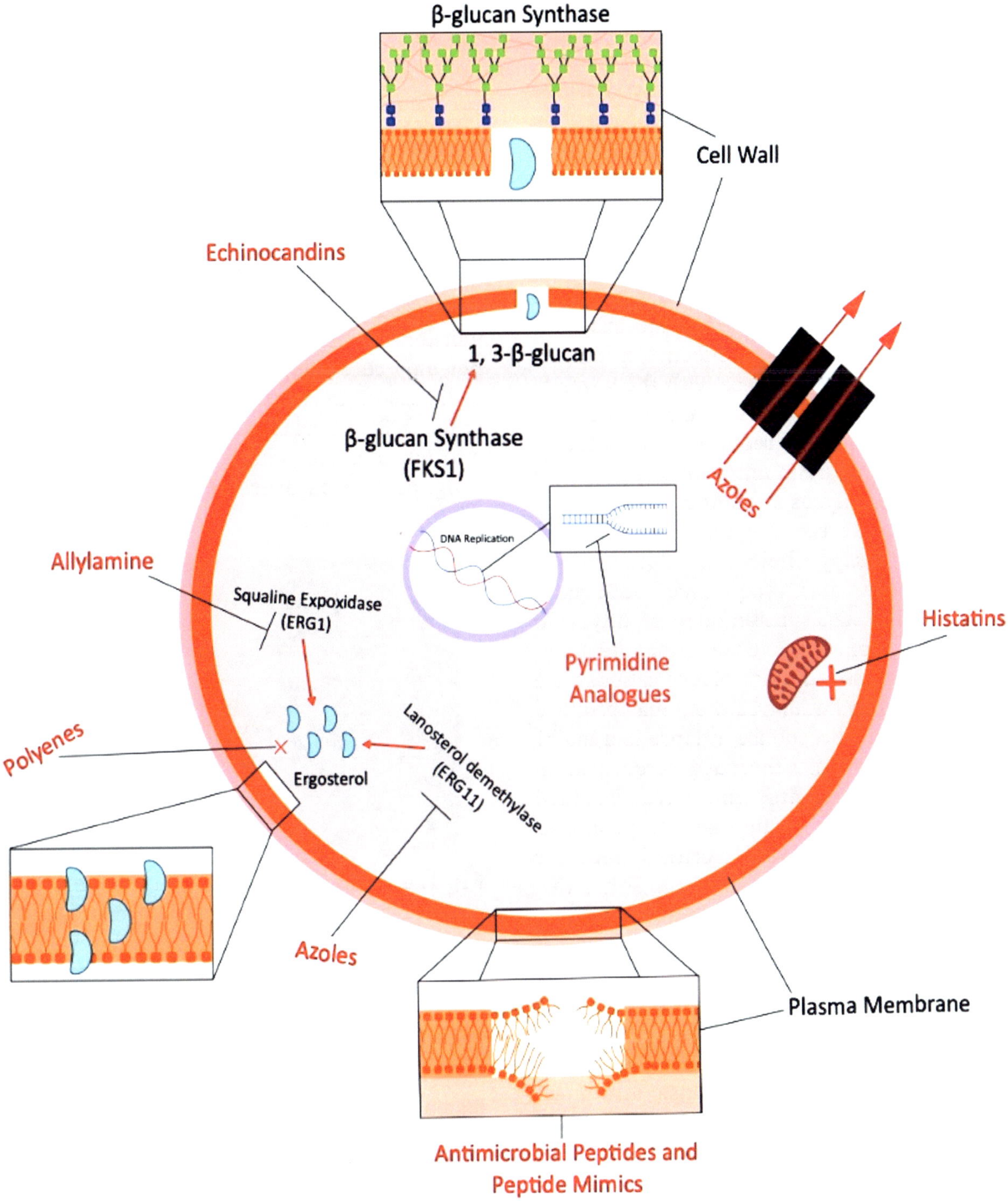

Figure 15.14. Antifungal therapy is the cornerstone of PCM management, primarily utilizing agents such as sulfonamides, itraconazole, and amphotericin B.

Source: https://www.mdpi.com/encyclopedia/encyclopedia-02-00118/article_deploy/html/images/encyclopedia-02-00118-g001.png.

15.4.1. Antifungal Medications and Their Effectiveness

Treatment of paracoccidioidomycosis, a subacute or chronic systemic fungal infection caused by the *Paracoccidioides brasiliensis* organism, is largely dependent on the efficacy of antifungal drugs. Triazoles, and specifically itraconazole and posaconazole, are among the first-line treatments and have proven to be effective in treating the disease. Itraconazole is frequently used because it has an excellent safety profile and excellent oral bioavailability. Although effective, treatment regimens vary in accordance with the severity and presentation of the disease, so that an individualized course is required. In individuals who have severe pulmonary or disseminated paracoccidioidomycosis, amphotericin B may be employed at the beginning of therapy. Antifungal therapy choice and duration are significant considerations, since inadequate treatment can cause substantial morbidity from paracoccidioidomycosis. Studies on the long-term effectiveness of antifungal medications have shown that while initial treatment may produce successful clinical response, relapse is a major issue. There are reports that suggest reactivation of disease in patients who have received azoles, particularly in immunocompromised individuals. This suggests a critical need for continued monitoring and potential adjunctive therapy to augment immune function alongside antifungal therapy. In addition, new data support the hypothesis that combination therapy may enhance the effectiveness of treatment, particularly in cases resistant to monotherapy. Effective paracoccidioidomycosis cure thus is not only a function of the intrinsic antifungal drug efficacy chosen but also of host condition control such as immune status and potential co-infection, which can complicate treatment. The impact of antifungal medication extends beyond efficacy at the single treatment level; it has also implications for public health policy in dealing with paracoccidioidomycosis in endemic regions. According to guidelines laid out in literature to this point, sensitization and early detection are important in treating the disease, particularly in high-risk groups. Furthermore, the ability of certain infections to cause comorbidities, such as adrenal insufficiency, underlines the importance of intensive treatment regimens. Adrenal gland infections can present with significant overlaps of clinical complications, creating a complex relationship that may influence the treatment options (Abraham et al., 2014). Knowledge of these relationships in-depth allows healthcare workers to enhance antifungal treatment to not only cure the infection effectively but also avoid associated health complications (Abraham et al., 2020). Overall, the dynamic character of antifungal medications is central in control and prognosis of paracoccidioidomycosis (Figure 15.15).

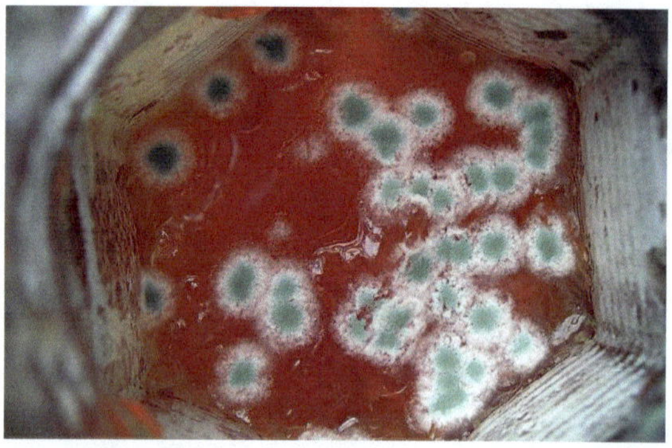

Figure 15.15. The treatment of paracoccidioidomycosis, a systemic fungal infection caused by the organism *Paracoccidioides brasiliensis*, heavily relies on the effectiveness of antifungal medications.

Source: https://di.myupchar.com/189/paracoccidioidomycosis-ke-karan-lakshan-ilaaj-bachav-upchar-in-hindi.jpg.

15.4.2. Duration and Management of Treatment

The management of paracoccidioidomycosis (PCM) demands an in-depth understanding of the diseases epidemiology, clinical manifestations, and effectiveness of the various regimens of treatment. Typically, antifungal therapy is the treatment of choice, and itraconazole and sulfamethoxazole-trimethoprim are typically employed. Duration of treatment could be largely dictated by the extent of infection and immunological status of patients. For mild cases, a minimum of six months of treatment is generally sufficient, while severe cases may be given long therapy lasting one to two years. Patient-specific variables such as co-morbidities and interactions with drugs also need to be considered by clinicians. Appropriate antifungal therapy should be started immediately since any delay in treatment will lead to complications and increased morbidity, thus emphasizing the importance of accurate diagnosis by various laboratory methods described in PCM diagnostic studies (Camargo et al., 2008). Follow-up monitoring of treatment efficacy is equally important as in the case of initial treatment. The use of antigen detection assays, as a means for quantifying gp43 and gp70, provides a valuable pathway along which to assess response to therapy and surveillance for risk of relapse. Antigen detection not only enhances diagnostic sensitivity but also provides a tool for monitoring for clearance of infection. Such methods provide physicians with responsible means of making decisions regarding continuation or adjustment of therapeutic regimens. Besides, an understanding of the nuances of PCM, especially in immunocompromised individuals, is essential to maximize management planning. With a significant number of cases occurring in returning travelers, being able to adapt in response to the evolving clinical scenario in a timely manner is essential to maximize patient outcomes (Committee et al., 2023). Overall, effective management of paracoccidioidomycosis is predicated on an intricate multifaceted system that synchronizes effective therapeutic interventions with vigilant monitoring of the course of disease. While antifungals represent the standard of therapy, treatment duration must be tailored to individual patient conditions by clinicians more on the basis of severity and co-existing health risks. The incorporation of newer diagnostic techniques, in addition to ongoing investigation of the microbiologic characteristics of the diseases, can further maximize the treatment modalities and minimize potential long-term complications. Ultimately, a thorough understanding of both the diseases lifecycle and its impact on various demographics will inform best practices in managing paracoccidioidomycosis and improving patient outcomes (Figure 15.16).

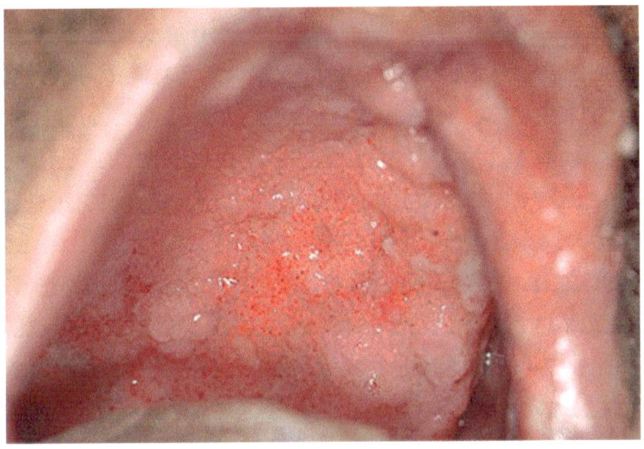

Figure 15.16. The management of paracoccidioidomycosis (PCM) necessitates a comprehensive understanding of the diseases epidemiology, clinical manifestations, and the effectiveness of various treatment regimens.

Source: https://www.researchgate.net/publication/45089090/figure/fig5/AS:267947977474051@1440895184095/Paracoccidioidomycosis-superficial-ulcers-on-palate-with-granular-aspect-and-hemorrhagic.png.

15.4.3. Challenges in Treatment Adherence and Resistance

Treat compliance in paracoccidioidomycosis is a serious issue, mainly because treatment lasts for a long period and antifungal agents can have some side effects. Gastrointestinal upset, fatigue, and other side effects are frequent, resulting in a failure to comply with treatment regimens. This is further compounded by the fact that the diseases are chronic, and this may lead to the understatement of illness severity by the patients, thus resulting in poor compliance with the treatment regimens. The health workers must, therefore, employ intervention strategies that address not only medical needs but also enhance patient education and psychosocial management. By encouraging increased disease and complete courses of treatment awareness, providers can increase levels of adherence and ultimately lead to better clinical outcomes. Resistant strains of fungus are another very important barrier to treating paracoccidioidomycosis effectively, complicating the disease to treat. Drug-resistant fungal infections have been caused by inadequate treatment adherence besides the abuse of antifungal drugs in both the clinical and agricultural spheres. This resistance makes the normal treatments less effective to the extent of leading to prolonged illness and increased mortality. Additionally, leukemia and AIDS patients who are immunocompromised are most vulnerable to these resistant strains, further indicating that new treatment approaches are needed. Improved understanding of the immune response in addition to the mechanisms of resistance of these fungal pathogens is needed so that novel strategies can be designed to induce patient responses while also improving cure rates, as emphasized in Alves et al., (2017). The global rise in paracoccidioidomycosis, particularly within regions of low healthcare resource availability, illustrates the necessity for multi-faceted public health initiatives that target both adherence to therapy and drug resistance. Poverty and poor access to healthcare contribute to these difficulties as underlying factors since patients cannot afford drugs or undergo routine treatment due to logistical barriers. Also, the co-infection dynamics of sicknesses such as tuberculosis, which also reflect growing patterns of resistance, render therapeutic solutions to populations under their grip increasingly challenging (Contini et al., 2017). Cure to treatment compliance and resistance is a multi-dimensional task that includes community engagement, better health infrastructure, and research on novel antifungal medications. It is only through concerted efforts that health systems can try to stem the risks of paracoccidioidomycosis and improve the quality of life for affected patients (Figure 15.17).

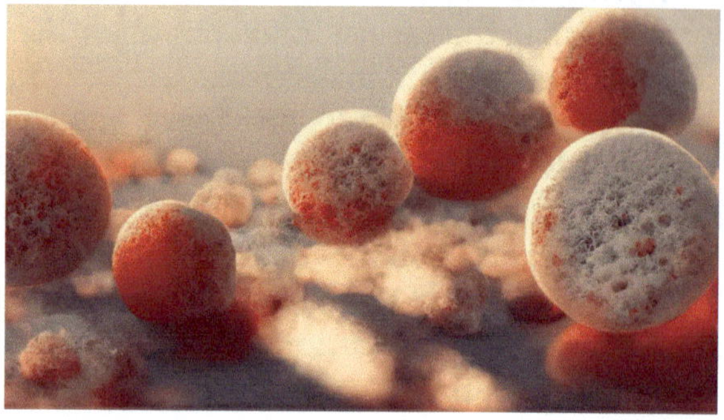

Figure 15.17. Resistant strains of fungi pose another formidable barrier to effective treatment of paracoccidioidomycosis, complicating the management of the disease.

Source: https://www.myco-academy.com/sites/infectiology/files/2024-06/Fungi%20are%20a%20diverse%20Desktop.webp.

SUMMARY

Paracoccidioidomycosis (PCM) is a systemic infection produced primarily by the pathogen *Paracoccidioides brasiliensis*, native to certain regions of Latin America. Focal points of immune response against PCM stress the predominance of cellular immunity, particularly macrophage function. Macrophages have been found to be involved centrally in regulating the infection through the induction of phagocytosis and cytokine production, specific and significant cytokines such as interferon-gamma (IFN-γ) and tumor necrosis factor (TNF). Such immune responses are critical in establishing a balance between protective immunity and inflammation, demonstrating how host factors may dictate the course and severity of the disease. Furthermore, the relative virulence of different *P. brasiliensis* strains necessitates a subtle understanding of the host immune interactions that determine outcomes in infected patients (Araujo et al., 2013). The suppressive effects of interleukin-10 (IL-10) take center stage in the debate regarding PCM. Evidence shows that while IL-10 in some scenarios can play a protective role, its upregulation during PCM can suppress immune responses, leading to heightened infection and host survival reduction. For instance, IL-10-deficient mice are more immune to *P. brasiliensis*, indicating that heightened levels of this anti-inflammatory cytokine can detrimentally affect the performance of macrophages. This process can suppress the production of critical antimicrobial mediators and delay the development of effective T cell immunity against the infection. Hence, the understanding of the regulatory activities of IL-10 is essential in developing therapeutic interventions to augment the hosts immunity in PCM (Araujo et al., 2013). Further, analysis of the macrophage activation dynamics gives valuable information on the pathogen's virulence. Experiments show that various strains of *P. brasiliensis* of varying virulence cause bone marrow macrophages to respond in a varied manner. Notably, co-stimulation of macrophages with IFN-γ and lipopolysaccharide (LPS) induces the high production of the antimicrobial effector molecule nitric oxide. This illustrates how the pathogen may hijack macrophage signaling for avoidance of host immunity during infection. These findings emphasize the need for additional exploration of the mechanisms by which macrophages interact with *P. brasiliensis* to further clarify PCM and identify potential therapeutic targets. The interface of virulence and immunity remains one of the primary areas in need of continued study as we seek means of reducing the impact of this severe fungal infection (Araujo et al., 2013).

A CLOSER LOOK

TUMOR NECROSIS FACTOR

Tumor necrosis factor (TNF) is a pro-inflammatory cytokine released by macrophages and T cells in most cases as a response to infection, injury, or immune stimulation. It plays a central role in regulating inflammation, immune responses, and apoptosis. While TNF is an important factor in fighting infection and controlling tumor development, overactive or dysregulated TNF has been associated with chronic inflammatory and autoimmune diseases such as rheumatoid arthritis, Crohn's disease, and psoriasis. TNF inhibitors are a class of biologic drugs used to inhibit its activity and manage these conditions.

REFERENCES

1. Abraham, G., Upadhyay, J., Trivedi, N., & Sudhindra, P. (2014). Tuberculosis of the adrenal gland: A case report and review of the literature of infections of the adrenal gland. https://core.ac.uk/download/193453332.pdf (accessed on 27th June 2025).
2. Abreu, L. G., Agostini, M., Andrade, B. A. B. de, et al. (2023). Oral Para coccidioidomycosis: A retrospective study of 95 cases from a single center and literature review. https://core.ac.uk/download/570980579.pdf (accessed on 27th June 2025).
3. Adebiyi, A. I., & Oluwayelu, D. O. (2019). Zoonotic fungal diseases and animal ownership in Nigeria. https://core.ac.uk/download/478436841.pdf (accessed on 27th June 2025).
4. Alastruey-Izquierdo, A., Gangneux, J. P., Hoenigl, M., et al. (2020). Diagnosis of breakthrough fungal infections in the clinical mycology laboratory: An ECMM consensus statement. https://core.ac.uk/download/388349973.pdf (accessed on 27th June 2025).
5. Almeida, J. N. de, Bagagli, E., Benard, G., et al. (2015). Matrix-assisted laser desorption ionization-time of flight mass spectrometry for differentiation of the dimorphic fungal species *Paracoccidioides brasiliensis* and *Paracoccidioides lutzii*. https://core.ac.uk/download/37742221.pdf (accessed on 27th June 2025).
6. Almeida, L. G. C. de, Araújo, M. A. C., Bezerra, J. V. de M., et al. (2023). Epidemiological aspects and oral implications of Para coccidioidomycosis infection: An integrative review. https://core.ac.uk/download/578691470.pdf (accessed on 27th June 2025).
7. Alvarado, P., Arechavala, A., Barker, B., et al. (2020). Genomic diversity of the human pathogen *Paracoccidioides* across the South American continent. https://core.ac.uk/download/343666396.pdf (accessed on 27th June 2025).
8. Alves, S. H., Loreto, É. S., Santurio, J. M., et al. (2017). Immunotherapy for fungal infections. https://core.ac.uk/download/322429348.pdf (accessed on 27th June 2025).
9. AMCLI Mycology Committee, Angheben, A., Conte, M., D'Aleo, F., et al. (2023). Endemic systemic mycoses in Italy: A systematic review of literature and a practical update. https://core.ac.uk/download/614217516.pdf (accessed on 27th June 2025).
10. Amorim, J. de, Magalhães, A., Munoz, J. E., et al. (2013). DNA vaccine encoding peptide P10 against experimental Para coccidioidomycosis induces long-term protection in presence of regulatory T cells. https://core.ac.uk/download/37739307.pdf (accessed on 27th June 2025).
11. Araujo, E. F. de, Bassi, Ê. J., Bazan, S. B., et al. (2013). In pulmonary Para coccidioidomycosis IL-10 deficiency leads to increased immunity and regressive infection without enhancing tissue pathology. https://core.ac.uk/download/pdf/37520231.pdf (accessed on 27th June 2025).
12. Bagagli, E., Barrozo, L., Bosco, S. M. G., et al. (2010). Road-killed wild animals: A preservation problem useful for eco-epidemiological studies of pathogens. https://core.ac.uk/download/pdf/37450114.pdf (accessed on 27th June 2025).
13. Baldo, M. E., da Silva Santos, P. S., Raffaele, R. M., et al. (2022). A diagnostic challenge in an individual with Para coccidioidomycosis during hospitalization in times of COVID-19. https://core.ac.uk/download/591028516.pdf (accessed on 27th June 2025).
14. Barbosa Neto, J. de P., Coelho, R. C., Damasceno, L. S., et al. (2021). Trends and patterns of mortality arising from fungal infections in Brazil in a period of 11 years. https://core.ac.uk/download/652318601.pdf (accessed on 27th June 2025).

15. Bartalesi, F., Bartoloni, A., & Zammarchi, L. (2014). Tuberculosis in tropical areas and immigrants. https://core.ac.uk/download/301568278.pdf (accessed on 27th June 2025).

16. Biolowons, G. K., Girotto, L. P. dos S., da Jaques, P. J. S., et al. (2021). Para coccidioidomycosis in the northern region of Rio Grande do Sul. https://core.ac.uk/download/386712718.pdf (accessed on 27th June 2025).

17. Bonan, P. R. F., Carvalho, E. J. de A., de Castro, J. F. L., et al. (2019). Oral Para coccidioidomycosis in a non-endemic region from Brazil: A short case series. https://core.ac.uk/download/250404496.pdf (accessed on 27th June 2025).

18. Calich, V. L. G., de Araújo, E. F., Loures, F. V., et al. (2020). Pulmonary Para coccidioidomycosis in AhR deficient hosts is severe and associated with defective Treg and Th22 responses. https://core.ac.uk/download/534004636.pdf (accessed on 27th June 2025).

19. Camargo, Z. P. de, Cotta Malaquias, L. C., Damaso, C. S., et al. (2014). Prevalence of Para coccidioidomycosis infection by intradermal reaction in rural areas in Alfenas, Minas Gerais, Brazil. https://core.ac.uk/download/37741220.pdf (accessed on 27th June 2025).

20. Camargo, Z. P., Faccini-Martinez, A. A., Falqueto, A., et al. (2018). A case of Para coccidioidomycosis due to *Paracoccidioides lutzii* presenting sarcoid-like form. https://core.ac.uk/download/328364104.pdf (accessed on 27th June 2025).

21. Cassone, A., Marques, A. F., Marques, A. F., Marques, A. F., Ribeiro, A. M., Pinto, A. R., de Bastos, A. S. R., et al. (2012). Therapeutic DNA vaccine encoding peptide P10 against experimental Para coccidioidomycosis. https://core.ac.uk/download/pdf/8688052.pdf (accessed on 27th June 2025).

22. Chies, J. A. B., & Ellwanger, J. H. (2021). Zoonotic spillover: Understanding basic aspects for better prevention. https://core.ac.uk/download/590924764.pdf (accessed on 27th June 2025).

23. Colombo, A. L. (2008). Para coccidioidomycosis: Advances and unmet needs 100 years after its initial description by Lutz. https://core.ac.uk/download/37707464.pdf (accessed on 27th June 2025).

24. Contini, C., di Nuzzo, M., Grilli, A., et al. (2017). The impact of tuberculosis among immigrants: Epidemiology and strategies of control in high-income countries—Current data and literature review. https://core.ac.uk/download/322429451.pdf (accessed on 27th June 2025).

25. de Camargo, Z. P. (2008). Serology of Para coccidioidomycosis. https://core.ac.uk/download/37733867.pdf (accessed on 27th June 2025).

26. Executive Committee of IJMS, IJMS. (2019). Abstracts of the XXVII Medical Academic Congress of Unicamp, CoMAU, 2018. https://core.ac.uk/download/270177732.pdf (accessed on 27th June 2025).

27. Fahal, A. H., Goodfellow, M., Maghoub, E. S., et al. (2014). The mycetoma knowledge gap: Identification of research priorities. https://core.ac.uk/download/43318713.pdf (accessed on 27th June 2025).

28. Feitosa, L. dos S., Guereschi, M. G., Konno, A. Y. de C., et al. (2012). *Paracoccidioides brasiliensis* GP43-derived peptides are potent modulators of local and systemic inflammatory response. https://core.ac.uk/download/37738222.pdf (accessed on 27th June 2025).

29. Fortes, R. M., Junqueira-Kipnis, A. P., & Kipnis, A. (2009). *Paracoccidioides brasiliensis* pancreatic destruction in *Calomys callosus* experimentally infected. https://core.ac.uk/download/pdf/8289035.pdf (accessed on 27th June 2025).

30. Ledeboer, A., de la Llave-Rincon, A. I., Oaklander, A. L., Jaggi, A. S., Marsh, B. J., Erridge, C., Fernandez-de-las-Penas, C., et al. (2013). Toll-like receptor signaling adapter proteins govern spread of neuropathic pain and recovery following nerve injury in male mice. https://core.ac.uk/download/323064514.pdf (accessed on 27th June 2025).

31. Lopera, D., Cano, L. E., Naranjo, T. W., González, Á., & Restrepo, Á. (2012). Pulmonary Para coccidioidomycosis: Clinical, immunological and histopathological aspects. https://core.ac.uk/download/322408707.pdf (accessed on 27th June 2025).

32. Pina, A., Restrepo, A., Restrepo, A., Restrepo-Moreno, A., Popi, A. F., Campanelli, A. P., Moreira, A. P., et al. (2011). Cell-free antigens from *Paracoccidioides brasiliensis* drive IL-4 production and increase the severity of Para coccidioidomycosis. https://core.ac.uk/download/pdf/8583707.pdf (accessed on 27th June 2025).

INDEX

C

D

E

F

G

H

I

N

O

P